fundamental and clinical bone physiology

Philadelphia · Toronto

J. B. LIPPINCOTT COMPANY

Edited by

MARSHALL R. URIST, M.D.

Professor of Surgery (Orthopedics)
Director of UCLA Bone Research Laboratory
UCLA Medical School
Los Angeles, California

12 contributors

fundamental

and clinical

bone

physiology

1 3 5 7 6 4 2

Library of Congress Cataloging in Publication Data

Main entry under title:
Fundamental and clinical bone physiology.

    Includes bibliographical references and index.
    1. Bone. 2. Bones—Diseases. I. Urist,
Marshall R. [DNLM: 1. Bone and bones—Physiology.
WE102 F981]
QP88.2.F86   612'.75   80-13436
ISBN 0-397-50470-5

The authors and publisher have exerted every effort to ensure that drug selection and dosage set forth in this text are in accord with current recommendations and practice at the time of publication. However, in view of ongoing research, changes in government regulations, and the constant flow of information relating to drug therapy and drug reactions, the reader is urged to check the package insert for each drug for any change in indications and dosage and for added warnings and precautions. This is particularly important when the recommended agent is a new or infrequently employed drug.

To our mentors

William F. Neuman
Fredrick K. Steggerda
Harold C. Hodge
Wayne O. Southwick
Carl W. Kuhlman, Jr.
Joseph D. Godfrey
Hector F. DeLuca
Fredrick C. Reynolds
Franklin C. McLean
Charles B. Huggins
F. Raymond Keating

contents

Herbert A. Fleisch, M.D., Department of Pathophysiology, University of Bern, Bern, Switzerland.

Harold M. Frost, M.D., Southern Colorado Clinic, Pueblo, Colorado.

Robert E. Kuhlman, M.D., Asst. Clinical Professor (Orthopedic Surgery), Washington University School of Medicine, St. Louis, Missouri.

Rajiv Kumar, M. D., Department of Endocrine Research, Mayo Clinic, Rochester, Minnesota.

James L. Matthews, M.D., Associate Dean, A. Webb Roberts Center for Continuing Education in the Health Sciences, Dallas, Texas.

William F. Neuman, M.D., Department of Radiation Biology and Biophysics, University of Rochester Medical Center, Rochester, New York.

Anthony W. Norman, M.D., Department of Biochemistry, University of California at Riverside, Riverside, California.

John A. Ogden, M.D., Professor of Surgery (Orthopedics) and Pediatrics, Yale University, School of Medicine, New Haven, Connecticut.

B. Lawrence Riggs, M. D., Endocrinology and Internal Medicine, Mayo Clinic, Rochester, Minnesota.

David J. Simmons, M.D., Department of Surgery, Washington University School of Medicine, Barnes Hospital, St. Louis, Missouri.

James T. Triffitt, Ph.D., MRC Bone Research Laboratory, Nuffield Department of Orthopaedic Surgery, University of Oxford, Nuffield Orthopaedic Centre, Oxford, England.

Marshall R. Urist, M.D., UCLA Bone Research Laboratory, Los Angeles, California.

contributors

Today's research on fundamental physiology of bone is tomorrow's new treatment of patients with disorders of bone. Nearly all important principles of biomedical research are applicable to skeletal system research. Nearly every significant advance in fundamental physiology of bone brings new understanding of unsolved orthopedic problems. Every important advance opens new fields for further investigation and exposes how much is not known about bone.

This multiauthored book is a compendium of knowledge of the physiology of bone for students and new research workers. The contributors, acknowledged leaders in the field, were invited to present the information in a style most suited to the subject matter. The coverage is intended not to be elementary but fundamental and to present knowledge for readers preparing for a career in either basic science or one of the applied clinical specialities. The manuscripts are published in the author's individual style. In the interest of publication before the material might become out-of-date, time was not invested in revising manuscripts solely for compliance with a standardized format.

In an effort to make the book interesting as well as informative, I have selected a broad scope of chapter titles with authorities representing a variety of disciplines. Several chapters deal with how the skeleton interacts with many other organ systems in normal and abnormal pathological physiology. How this interaction evolved is presented in Biogenesis of Bone, Handbook of Physiology, Vol. 7, published by the American Physiological Society, Washington D.C., 1976.

For present purposes, it is sufficient to note that in the evolution of vertebrate species from fish to man, bone became increasingly dependent upon other organ systems for its metabolic functions. When the study of bone was much less detailed, the emphasis was on calcium and phosphorus metabolism. Now cell differentiation, the central problem of all of biology and medicine, is the focus of attention of bone research. The subject goes far beyond the scope of mineral metabolism. A working knowledge of general physiology is a prerequisite for the study of bone. Molecular biochemistry is one field in which important discoveries about bone are

preface

being made. New biosynthetic products of bone cells are being isolated. New observations on enzymes and metabolites of bone are bringing new insight into diagnosis and treatment of bone disease. Normal and abnormal metabolic activities are observed not simply as localized in bone as a tissue but also as alterations in regional and systemic levels of function. On a regional level, biomechanics and bioelectric effects represent important subjects in bone physiology. For students pursuing careers in dentistry and orthopedic surgery, these subjects are reviewed in volumes 124 and 146 of CLINICAL ORTHOPEDICS AND RELATED RESEARCH.

The laboratory is now closer to the bedside than ever in the history of skeletal tissue research—so close that laboratory investigations are inseparable from everyday treatment of patients. From this association, there is every expectation that the etiology of nearly all diseases and disorders of bone will be discovered by the turn of this century. In anticipation of future discoveries, this book points out the direction in which bone research is headed.

I am grateful to the contributors for their diligence, skill, and prompt submission of manuscripts. An acknowledgement is owed to Mr. Stuart Freeman of J. B. Lippincott/Harper and Row Co. who persuaded me to organize this band of dedicated, hard-tissue scientists to the task of writing for novitiates.

Marshall R. Urist, M.D.

fundamental and clinical bone physiology

The highlights of bone physiology are the chapter headings of this book. The documentation is selected rather than complete. Each chapter is to be read and understood separately and wherever overlapping of subject matter occurs, the repetition is retained for emphasis. Teachers and veterans in the field will notice that progress has been evolutionary in some areas and almost revolutionary in others, but considering the paucity of knowledge of etiology of nearly every bone disease except rickets, the opportunities for discovery in bone physiology remain unlimited.

"An Introduction to the Physiology of Bone" (Bone, University of Chicago Press, 1955) by McLean and myself appeared in three editions, the last in 1968. The book was intended for recruitment of new workers in what in 1955 was a new field of biology. Since 1968, bone physiology has become an established field of endeavour in its own right. The subject is covered in detail in excellent reference books for advanced students by Vaughan (1970); Hancox (1969); Bronner and Comar (1960); Stein, Stein and Beller (1955); Sognnaes (1963); and Rasmussen and Bordier (1977). Exhaustive review articles can be found also in specialized periodicals like Calcified Tissue International (1980), 4 volumes on biochemistry and physiology of bone edited by Bourne (1978), a Simmons and Kunin (1979) book on laboratory methods of SKELETAL RESEARCH, the Basic science section of CLINICAL ORTHOPEDICS AND RELATED RESEARCH (1980), and a wide variety of other journals of clinical specialties. For citations of works, either omitted or unintentionally overlooked in this book, readers will want to consult the above reference books for advanced students.

In Chapter 2, James L. Matthews outlines current knowledge of the functional structure and ultra-structure of bone as a tissue, with landmarks on areas of uncertainty and controversy. In Chapter 3, James T. Triffitt summarizes the knowledge of the chemical composition of the organic matrix of bone including the important discovery of three newly defined components: gamma-carboxyglutamic acid-rich

MARSHALL R. URIST

1

introduction

protein; alpha-2HS glycoprotein; and bone morphogenetic protein. The three new components are presented against the background of modern knowledge of the molecular structure of other more or less well characterized matrix collagenous and non-collagenous proteins. In recent years, as the number of new non-collagenous constituents has increased, the weight of the bone matrix assigned to collagen has correspondingly decreased.

The chapter on bone mineral and the mechanism of calcification by William F. Neuman is one of the few important reviews, if not the only review, in which these two closely related subjects are considered simultaneously by a single authority. There are many very good articles on the problem of the composition of the bone mineral and many detailed articles on the enormous research effort to understand the mechanism of calcification, but Neuman's chapter is one place where in lively readable fashion the two related topics are integrated for the beginner to read and ponder.

In Chapter 5, John A. Ogden reviews the application of basic science techniques to the field of skeletal tissue development and bone growth that was once descriptive morphology and is now entirely multidisciplinary in approach. In Chapter 6, Robert E. Kuhlman presents a syllabus of up-to-date knowledge of the enzymes in developing, mature, and regenerating bone tissues. This chapter includes a summary of the author's personal experience with the enchanting subject of enchondral bone formation in deer antlerogenesis, in which serum alkaline phosphatase levels may rise almost as high as in Paget's disease and osteogenic sarcoma.

In Chapter 7, Harold Frost writes about internal remodelling of bone, a field he sowed in the 1960's and has cultivated ever since. Despite the fact that the concept of theoretical biology is not comparable to theoretical physics, in the strict sense of the word Harold Frost is the theoretician of bone biology. His concepts of osteons as functional units comparable to lymph nodes or kidney tubules or liver lobules have captured the imagination of clinicians and research workers striving to solve the unyielding problem of osteoporosis.

In Chapter 8, Anthony Norman, one of the earliest workers on the new Vitamin D metabolites, presents a succinct statement of the spectacular developments in the laboratory and in the clinical knowledge of Vitamin D and parathyroid and other hormonal interrelationships. In Chapter 9, Herbert Fleisch and associates present a unique summation of present knowledge of phosphate metabolism and, at the same time, dispel the long held idea that phosphate ion concentrations are unregulated in the fluids of the body.

In Chapter 10, David Simmons, a biologist now working in a clinical setting, presents the information about bone regeneration that is essential for an understanding of the healing of fractures. In Chapter 11, I have made a survey of laboratory and clinical concepts of bone graft physiology while in Chapter 12, I review the unsolved problem of heterotopic bone formation. Both chapters introduce the work on bone morphogenetic protein (BMP) by my colleagues and myself at the UCLA Bone Research Laboratory over the past quarter century. The presentation reflects our first hand knowledge, but not without consideration of alternative views of others working on osteoblast generating agents. In this connection, heterotopic bone formation is viewed not merely as an abnormality, but as a consistently reproducible experimental condition for investigation of cell differentiation, the central problem of bone biology. In Chapter 13, Rajiv Kumar and B. Lawrence Riggs, writing from direct experience with many patients, summarize knowledge of pathogenesis, diagnosis and treatment of osteoporosis, renal osteodystrophy, osteomalacia, and hyperparathyroidism—the 'big four' of the bone and stone clinics.

In recent years, striking advances in calcified tissue physiology have been made in research on bone resorption. The subject is presented in detail in a conference report on "Localized Bone Loss", edited by Horton, Tarpley, and Purvis in 1978, which includes the mode of action and interactions of parathyroid hormone, osteoclast activating factor, bone resorption factor, serum albumin, plasminogen activator, cyclic AMP, monocytes, macrophages, and osteoclasts in systems *in vitro*. How this knowledge of bone resorbing agents *in vitro* can be extended to conditions *in vivo*, to improve present understanding of rarifying diseases of bone, is a trenchant question. The coverage of bone resorption in this volume is almost exclusively derived from research on systems *in vivo* in laboratory animals and patients. Bone resorption is observed as a phase of bone remodelling, normally coupled by some unknown mechanism to bone formation, and is presented in terms of microanatomy by Matthews, histomorphometry by Frost, biochemistry by Norman, and pathologic physiology by Kumar and Riggs. The foremost challenge on the research frontier, from almost every point of view, is to characterize such bone resorption inhibitor and bone formation inducer molecules as can be found in the intact animal in health and disease.

Introduction

Bones vary in size and shape, ranging from the small ossicles to the heavy weight-bearing bones of the axial skeleton and the long bones of the appendicular skeleton. These mineralized, cellular structures are normally invested in a fibrous sheath, the periosteum, and are richly supplied with both blood vessels and nerves. Skeletal muscles gain attachment to these skeletal organs by collagenous fibrils of the muscle tendon being interwoven into and through the fibrillar and ground substance elements of the periosteum. Those portions of ligaments or tendons that are enmeshed in the periosteal matrix are called Sharpey's fibers. Forces mediated through these ligament and tendon Sharpey's fibers are distributed through the adjacent skeletal tissue, resulting in deformational stresses being directed through the bone. As a consequence, bone is modeled or remodeled to achieve a structure that is adapted to accomodate these conditioning forces intermittantly applied during normal locomotion, and also in response to the need to maintain functional posture in the continuous presence of gravitational force. Thus, bone is not a static deposit of mineralized matrix but is a dynamic structure in which the structural elements and the overall architectural plans are being continuously modified by bone cell activity. Obviously, genetic influence may dictate the general structural plan of a bone, but environmental influence and growth modify the structure significantly. Generally, the external configuration of each bone is genetically predictable, but the internal organization may vary widely, for example, change in the thickness of the compact layer, change in the overall diameter of the periosteum or marrow space, and the increase or decrease in number and the change in direction or quality of internal beams and struts. Early organ culture experiments of Fell showed that explants of rudiments of chick limb buds progressed to form typical young limb buds in the absence of any external force. Wolfe recognized the dynamic nature of bone and postulated the following law: bone forms and remodels in response to the forces applied to it.[24] This is dramatically illustrated in the thickened and

J. L. MATTHEWS

2

bone structure and ultrastructure

roughened points of muscle attachment in trained athletes and in the rarification of bones and loss of structural mass in persons with paralysis, or following long periods of bed rest, or the weightlessness experienced during space flights.

Flat bones and tubular bones

It is common practice to refer to flat bones and tubular (long) bones, although the casual observer readily recognizes that many complex shapes are found in certain bones. "Flat" bones are typically those of the cranial vault and "tubular" bones are characterized by the major bones of the appendicular skeleton. Tubular bones are classically divided into the following regions: epiphysis, metaphysis, diaphysis, and articulating surfaces. The articulation of bones of the appendicular skeleton is cushioned by a layer of hyalin cartilage at the articular surface of the opposed bones of a joint. Often, an additional island of cartilage is interposed between the two articulating surfaces of the bones. These weight-bearing surfaces are further assisted by a thin film of proteinaceous material, the synovial fluid, which is produced by the synovial membrane. The synovial membrane lies adjacent to the weight-bearing surfaces, lining a fibrous joint capsule that spans from the periosteum of one bone to the next.

Membrane bone and endochondral bone

In tracing the embryonal development of bones, two primary types of bone formation are described: (1) membrane bone or intramembranous ossification, and (2) ossification in cartilage—endochondral ossification.

The bones of the face, cranial vault, and clavicle are typically membrane bone, whereas the bones of the appendicular skeleton, vertebral column, and base of the skull are classified as endochondral. In some cases, bones may have ossification centers originating in both membrane and cartilage. The occipital bone is an ex-

ample, in which the flat portion ossifies in membrane and the basioccipitalis ossifies in cartilage.

This traditional classification is not sufficient to account for the subtle differences noted within different parts of bone, for example: bundle bone that is seen in fetal bones and in fracture callus, in which dense bundles of coarse collagen fibers are incorporated into the bone matrix; ossification in mesenchyme; ossification in aponeuroses, tendons, ligaments, sutures, and bone surface apposition, and so forth. All differ slightly in fiber size, content, distribution, cell number, and distribution. Nevertheless, certain general features may be attributed to these differences in membrane or cartilage origin.

Endochondral bone

Endochondral bone formation occurs as a consequence of the original formation of hyalin cartilage in the form and future location of bone. This cartilage model is subsequently replaced by bone. Remnants of the original cartilage model remain as articular cartilage and the growth plate of the epiphysis (Fig. 2-1). The first morphological change noted in the cartilage model prior to ossification (replacement with bone) is the hypertrophy of the chondrocytes in the midshaft (diaphysis) of the cartilage model. This region shows increased chondrocyte proliferation followed by hypertrophy, resulting in compression and thinning of the cartilage matrix surrounding the hypertrophic cells. Vascular buds from the perichondrial region invade the normally avascular cartilage. Within the matrix fibrils of this hypertrophic region, membrane-bound vessicles are found, around which the first hydroxyapatite crystals are forming. Subsequent coalescence of these crystal clusters result in mineralized cartilage matrix (Fig. 2-2). The hypertrophic cartilage cells in these mineral-bound lacunae die, presumably because of the reduction of free diffusion of essential nutrients and gases resulting from the mineralization. Cartilage is normally avascular, so its cells are dependent upon diffusion through the matrix for survival. Kuettner and colleagues have shown that a polypeptide of approximately 10,000 daltons can be extracted

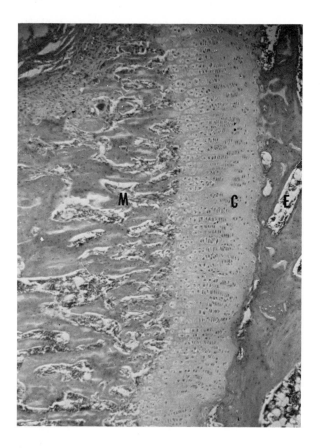

FIGURE 2-1 *Photomicrograph of endochondral bone showing epiphysis* **(E)**, *cartilage growth plate* **(C)**, *and primary spongiosa (trabeculae), of metaphysis,* **(M),** × 150.

from cartilage by guanidinium hydrochloride.[13] Extraction of this protein leads to vascular invasion, so it may act as an anticollagenase as well as an antiproliferation factor for endothelial cells. It has been suggested by some researches that hydroxyapatite can absorb this protein, so the events of matrix mineralization and vascular invasion may be coupled by changing concentrations of both inhibitor and inductor materials in these sites. The region of first mineralization is the primary ossification center.

Perichondrial changes accompany the central midshaft ossification. Cells in the perichondrium differentiate into osteoblasts and assume an osteogenic function, laying down a collar of "membrane" bone around the ossification center. This periosteal collar grows in length and thickness by appositional growth. The former perichondrium is now the periosteum. Osteoprogenitor cells accompany the invading vascular buds, and osteoblasts differentiate within the spaces formerly occupied by hypertrophic car-

tilage cells. Bone matrix (osteoid) is apposed by these newly activated osteoblasts upon the surfaces of mineralized cartilage. The new bone mineralizes, resulting in the formation of trabeculae of bone containing a mineralized cartilage core. Osteoclastic resorption of these primary trabeculae, accompanied by additional osteoblastic activity, ultimately replace this cartilage–mixed bone structure with bone.

The primary ossification center progressively moves toward the ends of the bone, with the sequence of hypertrophy, matrix mineralization, vascular invasion, and osteoblastic activity being repeated at the migrating ossification front. Some myeloid elements also migrate into the spaces between struts and within the boundaries of the extending periosteal collar, initiating the hematopoeitic activity in the marrow spaces.

In most tubular bones, secondary ossification centers are formed in the epiphyses, occurring at a later time but in the same manner as the primary center. Total removal of the cartilage model is not programmed. Rather, the articulating surface of the cartilage model is retained throughout the normal life of the bone, being eroded only in disease processes such as osteoarthritis. Usually, a zone of cartilage remains between the primary and secondary ossification centers, serving as a center for cartilage growth for several years, although it is ultimately replaced by bone. This cartilage growth plate is essential to the growth in length of the whole bone. Bone as a tissue grows only by apposition, that is, by forming on existing surfaces. Cartilage tissue, however, can grow both by apposition and interstitially. Cartilage matrix has sufficient plasticity to enable cartilage cells buried deep in lacunae to divide, secrete additional territorial and interterritorial matrix, and contribute to the overall mass and volume of cartilage matrix. If cartilage growth did not contribute to the growth in length of long bones, they would be extraordinarily thick and short.

Organization of the cartilage growth plate

The residual growth cartilage following endochondral ossification becomes a highly ordered structure, permitting the division of the cartilage into several functionally specialized zones characterized by unique zonal features of both cartilage cells and matrix. The cartilage zone on the epiphyseal surface of the growth cartilage is called the resting zone. The succession of zones progresses from epiphysis to metaphysis in the following order: resting zone, zone of proliferation, zone of matrix synthesis, zone of hypertrophy, zone of provisional calcification, and zone of ossification. Figure 2-3 illustrates the order of zones in the growth cartilage.

The zone of resting (reserve) cartilage is contiguous either with articulating cartilage or with bone tissue in those bones that have a secondary ossification center formed between the articular cartilage and the cartilage growth plate.

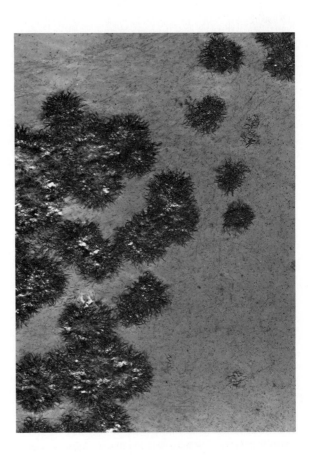

FIGURE 2-2 *Electron micrograph of mineralizing matrix, showing clusters of hydroxyapatite that begin as a few needles associated with vesicles and grow—ultimately coalescing into a solid mineral mass,* × *10,000.*

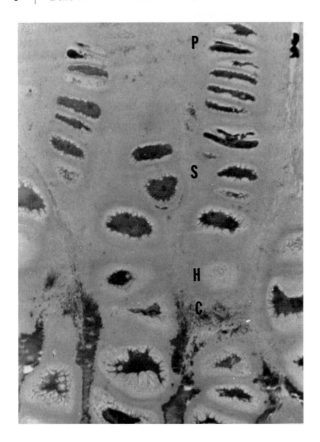

FIGURE 2-3 *Photomicrograph of cartilage growth plate, showing zone of proliferation* **(P)**, *zone of matrix synthesis* **(S)**, *zone of cell hypertrophy* **(H)**, *and zone of provisional calcification* **(C)**, × 600.

The chondrocytes of the resting zone are usually small and are randomly distributed.

The zone of proliferation shows the beginning of spatial orientation, with the chondrocytes arranged in columns that parallel the long axis of the bone. This columnar orientation of cells is maintained throughout the rest of the cartilage zones. Chondrocytes in this zone are active in mitosis, and are somewhat disc-shaped, resembling stacks of coins in each cell column. Each chondrocyte has numerous processes that radiate into the surrounding matrix. Because of the mitotic activity, more than one chondrocyte is often observed in one lacunae, with little or no matrix separating adjacent cells in a column. Intercolumnar matrix is thicker, allowing a clear definition of separate but parallel cell columns. Figure 2-4 shows the characteristic ultrastructure of chondrocytes of the zone of proliferation. Numerous mitochondria, rough endoplasmic reticulum, a small Golgi complex, and an elongated nucleus are typical of these cells.[17]

The zone of matrix synthesis is characterized by the evidence of this synthesis taking place in cells that were formerly of the zone of proliferation. Cells of this zone are larger, have a larger Golgi complex and many dilated cisternae in the endoplasmic reticulum. Each cell in the column is separated from the other cells by a layer of newly synthesized cartilagenous matrix, consisting of fine fibrils embedded in an amorphous ground substance. Cell processes extend marginally from these cells, sometimes extending midway into the longitudinally oriented matrix that separates cell columns. The extreme tips of these cell processes are often electron dense, and are rounded—resembling a small ball on the end of a process (Fig. 2-5). Recent work by Cecil and Anderson and Wuthier and colleagues with freeze-fracture techniques has clearly shown these processes with bulbous ends extending from the chondrocytes.[4,25] Examination of the fracture face of these end bulbs has shown them to be true extensions of plasma membrane.

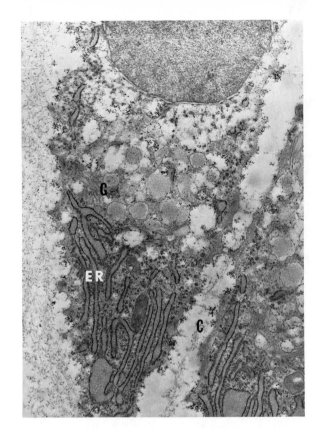

FIGURE 2-4 *Electron micrograph of chondrocytes from lower part of zone of proliferation. The cells are flat, spindle-shaped, and possess a developing Golgi complex* **(G)** *and extensive rough-surfaced endoplasmic reticulum* **(ER)** *and mitochondria (arrow). Newly formed collagen fibrils* **(C)** *lie between the recently divided cells,* × *12,000.*

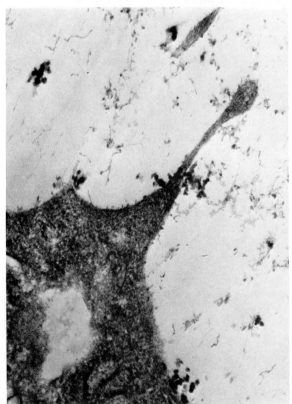

FIGURE 2-5 *Electron micrograph of chondrocyte process extending into surrounding matrix. The bulbous ends of these processes are believed to separate to form vesicles,* × *30,000.*

These extensions are presumed to be the source of matrix vesicles observed in the longitudinal septa. Freeze-fracture studies of matrix vesicles also indicate a typical trilaminar membrane envelope that is right side out. These vesicles are found at the center of mineral clusters in the zone of provisional calcification, and their presumed role in initiating mineralization is discussed fully in Chapter 4 in this book.

The zone of cell hypertrophy has larger lacunae, with the fibrils of longitudinal septa compressed together, enhancing recognition of collagen bundles. Some collagen fiber axial periodicity may be recognized here, although it is much more readily discerned in the mineralizing zone. The transverse septa that separate related column cells do not appear to be as compressed, they contain fine fibrils, and interestingly, they rarely mineralize. Two different morphological descriptions have been reported for these cells, the dissimilarities being due to differences in techniques used in tissue fixation. Hypertrophic cells viewed following routine aldehyde fixation

appear vacuolated and irregular in shape, often giving a prickle cell appearance. Conversely, cells of this zone obtained from tissues fixed in solutions containing polyanionic groups such as alcian blue appear as rounded cells that fully occupy the enlarged lacunae. Casual inspection of the cytoplasm of these cells suggests a paucity of organelles, with the Golgi complex scattered and with widely dispersed mitochondria and membranes of rough-surfaced endoplasmic reticulum. However, by using histomorphometric techniques, one finds the actual number of organelles per cell is equal to, if not greater than, that of the previous zone, suggesting that these cells are not dying as originally suggested by some workers, but are in fact cells capable of significant metabolic activity.

The zone of provisional calcification shows most cells with pyknotic nuclei and irregular margins, particularly those cells closest to the metaphyseal surface. This is true of the last two to three cells in the column even in tissues specially fixed to preserve cell integrity as already

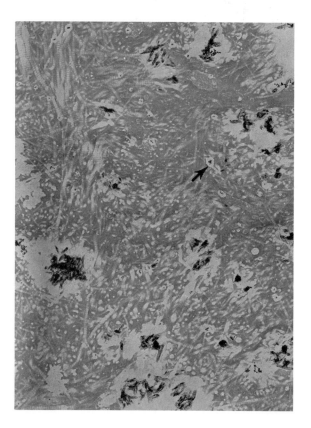

FIGURE 2-6 *Electron micrograph of microashed matrix, showing negative image of collagen and vesicles (arrow). Mineral within vesicles and in apatite clusters survives incineration and appear as dark structures,* × *10,000.*

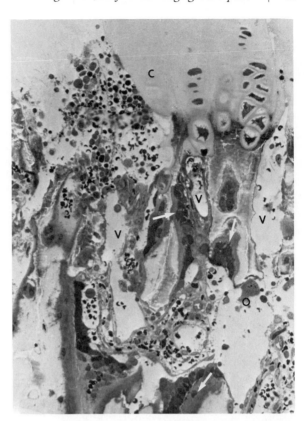

FIGURE 2-7 *Photomicrograph of metaphysis. Cartilage* **(C)** *is mineralized and blood vessels* **(V)** *penetrate the space formerly occupied by chondrocytes. Osteoblasts follow and appose new bone (arrows) upon the mineralized cartilage cores. These resultant primary trabeculae are later remodeled by osteoclasts* **(O)**, *×230.*

discussed. When fixed in special preparations such as those containing K-pyroantimonate, oxalate, and so forth, an interesting distribution of cation-rich precipitates (mostly calcium) are observed. This distribution of cations has been studied extensively by Brighton and Hunt, and Matthews and coworkers.[3,14] Cells in the intermediate zones of the cartilage growth plate have an abundance of calcium bound to the cristae of the mitochondria as well as to the plasma membrane. The last few cells in the column show a significant reduction in bound calcium. The significance of this distribution is unknown but may possibly be related to the events of matrix mineralization occurring in the longitudinal matrix septa. The beginning of matrix mineralization appears as small, isolated clusters of mineral crystals in the central area of the longitudinal septa. Chelation of sections of this zone has revealed membrane-limited vesicle remnants within the centrum of the resorbed crystals and microincineration also confirms their presence (Fig. 2-6). Clusters of crystals increase in size and

number, reaching an almost solid crystalline mass at the cartilage-metaphysis interface. A large part of this increase in crystalline mass is attributed simply to the physicochemical events associated with individual crystal growth. Extension of crystal formation within the septa invests the collagen fibrils within a mineral casing. Extensive modification of ground substance material and water loss occur in this mineralizing zone.

At the metaphysis interface, capillary buds and accompanying osteoprogenitor cells penetrate the transverse septa, gaining access to the large lacunae bounded laterally by mineralized septa. These mineralized cartilage walls serve as the surfaces on which bone matrix is deposited by the newly differentiated osteoblasts (Fig. 2-7). This orderly and spatially regulated formation of bone onto mineralized cartilage generates the parallel columns of bone trabeculae called the primary spongiosa, whose parallel array mimics the organization of cell columns in the cartilage. This region of ossification has been studied extensively by Schenk and colleagues.[21] Osteoclastic resorption of the primary spongiosa coupled with additional osteoblastic bone forming activity ultimately replaces the trabeculae-containing mineralized cartilage cores with a secondary spongiosa consisting of trabecular arrays without cartilage remnants.

The zonal organization of the cartilage growth plate imparts a longitudinal growth to the bone with the proliferative activity in equilibrium with the ossification activity, resulting in the maintenance of a relatively constant thickness of the growth plate for the duration of growth in length for that specific bone. Through genetic determinants, the growth plate of each bone ultimately ceases its proliferative and matrix synthesizing activity with the consequence that all of the growth cartilage ultimately becomes hypertrophic and ossifies. A ridge of bone, the terminal bar, marks the location of the growth plate that has been totally ossified when growth activity is arrested. The cartilage is subsequently totally replaced with bone and the growth plate or epiphysis is said to be "closed."

Histochemical procedures reveal several changes in the metabolism of the chondrocytes as they progress from one zone and state of activity to the next. Important changes that have been detailed occur in the activity of alkaline phosphatase, sulfatase, adenylate cyclase, phosphoproteins, phospholipids, and enzymes of oxidative phosphorylation and anaerobic glycolysis.

Examination of chondrocyte lacunae dyed with metachromatic stains such as toluidine blue reveals that the cartilage matrix is not homogeneous. Each chondrocyte is immediately surrounded with a zone that is periodic acid-Schiff (PAS)-positive and metachromatic. Kuettner and others have studied cartilage matrix extensively using various extraction procedures and fluorescent dyes and have enumerated the following regional features that are also shown in Figure 2-8.[12] A felt work of loosely woven fila-

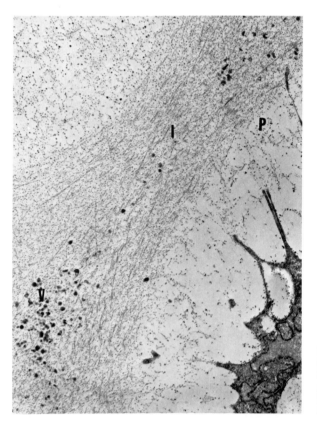

FIGURE 2-8 *Electron micrograph of cartilage, showing interterritorial matrix* **(I)** *between two lacunae. Matrix vesicles* **(V)** *are seen here. The perilacunar matrix* **(P)** *is metachromatic with some stains and appears here as a loose, filamentous mesh with ground substance particles,* × 13,965.

ments in immediate juxtaposition to the cell membrane is bounded by a wider territorial matrix consisting of definitive fibrils bound by a metachromatic amorphous cement, in which many of the fibrils follow a circumferential course, separated from other chondrocytes by interterritorial matrix. The interterritorial matrix contains larger, more parallel fibrils embedded in ground substance with less metachromatic capability. Additional loss of this territorial staining is noted around the cells of the zone of provisional calcification, indicating that removal and substitution of matrix constituents occur in association with mineralization events.

Intramembranous bone

Areas in which intramembranous bone formation will occur first appear as condensed layers of mesenchyme cells characterized by a polyhedral shape, with pale-staining cytoplasm, pale ovoid nuclei, and numerous slender processes, with processes of adjacent cells often in direct contact. Reticular fibers are irregularly dispersed between cells, and a proliferating vascular network is interspersed within the condensed mesenchyme field. Subsequent elaboration of additional collagenous matrix results in a bilayered collagenous envelop containing vascular elements, fibrocytes, mesenchyme cells, osteoprogenitor cells, and osteoblasts. Bone formation is initiated by the differentiated osteoblasts apposing new sheaths, as well as bundles of collagen fibers within the condensed region. Thus, no pre-existent model is made other than that afforded by the shape and limits of the fibrous mesenchyme condensates in sites where osteogenesis ultimately occurs.

Although the description presented represents the classic description of embryonal development, numerous sites of bone formation may be equated with intramembranous ossification, that is, a cartilage core is not required as a surface for new bone apposition. Examination of the periosteum of a developing bone, for example, reveals a fibrous (collagenous) layer containing both fibrocytes and undifferentiated cells as well as widespread vessels and nerves. Osteoblasts dif-

ferentiate within this layer, forming an "osteogenic layer." Successive lamellae of bone are deposited by these cells, without any prior evidence of resorptive activity. Bone formed in this manner could also be regarded as "membrane" bone.

Compact bone–vascular supply

As the volume of mineralized matrices enlarge, some special organization of cells and vascular elements are made, so that no cell is buried in the matrix more than 300 μ from a blood vessel. The fluid that bathes bone cells is unique, having ion concentrations and organic components that are different from those of general extracellular fluid. This suggests that either the endothelial cells of vessels within bone are different from those in other organs or that some other cellular layer serves to partition general extracellular fluid from bone fluid. It has been suggested that the osteoblasts serve as a functional membrane, separating these two fluid compartments. Experiments with tracer materials such as horseradish peroxidase (a protein with enzyme activity permitting one to identify its location through histochemical means) show that these proteins move from within blood vessels to the extracellular fluid by passing between endothelial cells. Tracer material is also observed between osteoblasts, within the subjacent interstices of the osteoid, within canaliculi, and surrounding all osteocytes. The rapidity with which tracer material reaches the deepest buried osteocytes (5–10 min) suggests that fluid movement through the canalicular network of bone is a continuous and rapid flow, facilitating either deposition into and/or release from bone mineral stores.

Periosteal vessels gain access to the marrow cavities by way of nutrient canals. The major number of intracortical vessels branch from penetrating vessels and run a course primarily parallel to the long axis of tubular bones and in a more irregular pattern in the compacta of irregularly shaped bones (Fig. 2-9).

Both arterioles and venules are found in these intracortical canals connected by capillaries of large luminal diameter (Fig. 2-10). Each vessel

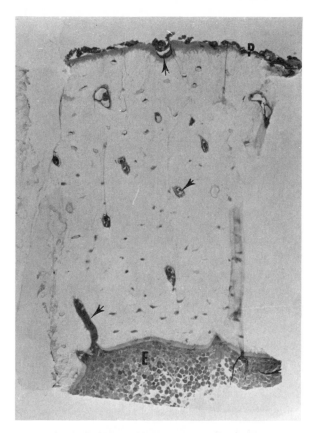

FIGURE 2-9 *Photomicrograph of compact bone, showing endosteal* **(E)** *and periosteal* **(P)** *surface. Blood vessels (arrows) penetrate the surface and course through the bone supplying the regional osteocytes. A Howship's lacuna with an osteoclast is seen on the periosteal surface (arrow), × 250.*

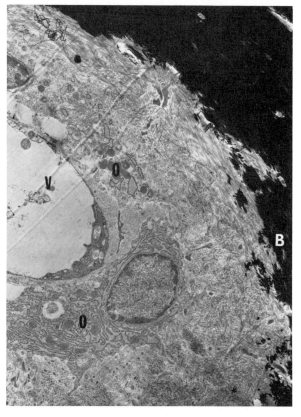

FIGURE 2-10 *Electron micrograph of blood vessel* **(V)** *in compact bone* **(B).** *Osteoblasts* **(O)** *are interposed between vessel and osteoid, × 9000.*

has surrounding lamellae and associated cells constituting a haversian system or **osteon.** Vessels that anastomose between haversian vessels are Volkman vessels in Volkman canals.

Haversian systems

Haversian systems have an average cross-sectional diameter of 300 μ and are approximately 3 to 5 mm long. Haversian systems or osteons are made on bone surfaces by successive periods of matrix apposition in the walls of trenches or grooves, ultimately encircling vessels that lie in the groove or by filling in spaces between trabeculae of spongy bone. Osteons formed by apposition onto periosteal or endosteal surface grooves or formed within the lattice of cancellous bone are called primary osteons. Osteons formed in tunnels made during the course of remodeling are called secondary osteons. The outer limits of secondary osteons or secondary haversian systems are readily identified because a cement line separates them from adjacent mineralized tissue. In remodeling, new haversian systems are generated in existing compact bone by a group of osteoclasts organized into a resorbing wedge or "cutting cone" moving progressively through older mineralized bone creating a new tunnel that parallels the adjacent haversian systems. The relative position of a new tunnel is not limited to the boundaries of a former haversian system, so parts of two or more haversian systems may be eroded away by the · osteoclasts in new tunnel formation. Thus partial haversian systems may be seen lying between other haversian systems. If one views a cutting cone in longitudinal view, the osteoclasts are readily observed at the resorbing end. Immediately distal to these cells, in the area in which excavation has already occurred, sprouts of vascular elements and a mixture of poorly differentiated cells and some cell fragments are observed. Distal to this small region, active osteoblasts are found depositing new bone lamellae upon the walls of the recently excavated tunnel. Successive periods of formation and rest create the multiple lamellae of the newly forming system. Cross-section views of compact bone show

the haversian systems to have relatively constant overall diameters but significant variation in internal diameters of the vascular canals lined by the osteoblasts (Fig. 2-11). Viewing the same specimen with x-ray micrographs or autoradiographs also clearly shows variance in the extent of mineral density in each lamellae and each haversian system in bones in which active remodeling is occurring.

The fate of the cells in a forming haversian system has been a controversial subject. Some researchers have theorized that the orderly succession of cells in a cone of compact bone could be explained by the leading population of cells—the osteoclasts—dissociating to single nucleated cells that become the successional osteoblasts. This theory has been refuted by the observations of dying osteoclasts and mitosis of other cells located between the osteoclasts and the osteoblast front.

The osteocytes are derived from the osteoblast population, representing those osteoblasts that are incorporated into the matrix components being secreted by the cells on all surfaces of the membrane as contrasted with the polarity of secretion to one side on those osteoblasts that do not become incorporated.

The cell-to-cell relationship in haversian systems, as well as in all bone, is essential to assuring adequacy of a fluid diffusion pathway to the buried osteocytes. The basilar aspect (bone surface) of osteoblasts is characterized by several short cell processes extending into the nonmineralized osteoid covering the mineralized surface. In addition to these short processes, one or more longer cell processes are seen in each section. These cell processes course through the osteoid and occupy canals (canaliculi) that radiate through the mineralized matrix. These long processes make specific cell-to-cell junctions with processes of the buried osteocytes (Fig. 2-12). These cell junctions are of the gap junction type. Other tissues that have gap junctions include cardiac and smooth muscle. In these muscle sites, the gap junctions serve as special low-impedance cell contacts through which certain ion fluxes are facilitated. These morphologically similar junctions in bone cells suggest a certain functional syncytial organization, as simple

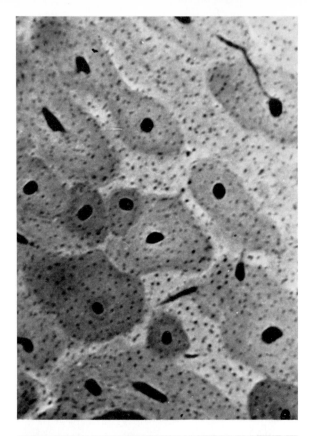

FIGURE 2-11 *A radiograph of osteons of compact bone. Osteocytes are regularly spaced in lamellae. Varying diameters and levels of mineral maturation are seen in neighboring osteons, × 200.*

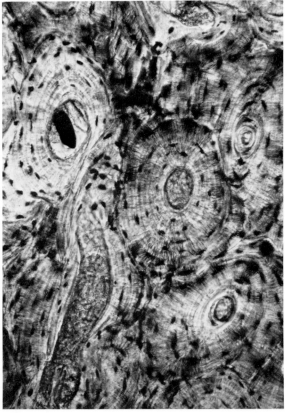

FIGURE 2-12 *Photomicrograph of haversian systems. Osteocytes in adjacent lamellae communicate through canaliculi, × 350.*

cell-to-cell junctions such as desmosomes observed between epithelial cells are not found joining bone cells. Gap junctions are found uniting processes of osteocytes to osteoblasts and also are found uniting processes of osteocytes to other osteocytes. The conjoined processes within the canaliculi are separated from the mineralized lacunae wall by a thin layer of loosely organized matrix. This thin pericellular region serves as the diffusion pathway for bone fluid, connecting the subosteoblastic region with lacunae housing the junction-coupled osteocytes (Fig. 2-13).

In addition to large lumen capillaries and other vessels in haversian canals, nonmyelinated nerve fibers also are found in many haversian canals. These nerves arise primarily as collaterals from nerves distributed in the periosteum. Their size suggests that they are either postganglionic sympathetic fibers or small nonmyelinated afferent pain fibers.

Cancellous (Spongy) bone

The organization of cancellous bone is characterized by beams and struts of mineralized bone covered primarily by osteoblasts, but osteoclastic resorption on one surface, especially a free apex of a strut, is not uncommon. Large beam-like pieces are termed trabeculae, whereas the term spicule is used to connote the smaller strut-like pieces. The axis of the trabeculae, is usually positioned at 90° to deformational forces from muscle tension and weight-bearing. Cancellous bone is also called trabecular bone or spongy bone.

Trabeculae may contain a core of mineralized cartilage if they were formed in sites of endochondral ossification, but remodeling activity produces trabeculae that consist wholly of bone. The trabecular surface is covered by a thin layer of nonmineralized osteoid produced by the sur-

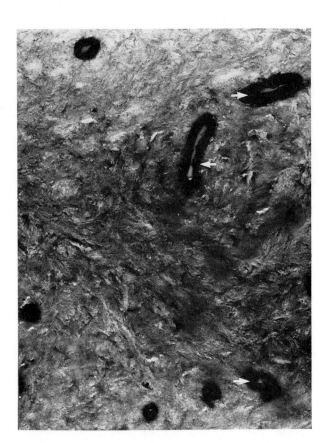

FIGURE 2-13. *Electron micrograph of canaliculi (arrows) in compact bone matrix. The dense periphery of the canalicular space is occupied by a heavy metal tracer injected into the veins 10 min before fixation, × 25,000.*

face osteoblasts. Because of the incremental synthesis of matrix, followed by increments of mineralization, discrete lamellae may be observed. Trabeculae may attain significant cross-sectional dimensions in regions of great functional stress, so osteocytes are also commonly observed in lacunae within the trabeculae. Adjacent osteocytes communicate with processes in canaliculi and with the covering osteoblasts by gap junction contact in a manner similar to that observed in compact bone. Figure 2-14 shows a region of the metaphysis in which trabeculae with and without mineralized cartilage cores are found. Osteoclasts occupy Howship's lacunae on some trabecular surfaces, whereas the greater surface is covered by active osteoblasts.

The number, size, and distribution of trabeculae are integrally related to the weight-bearing functions of bone as well as to the calcium storage their presence affords. In egg-laying birds, trabeculae disolution and reformation is a dynamic process, as the calcium

stored as hydroxyapatite in these mineralized structures supplies much of the calcium needed in rapidly forming the calcium carbonate egg shell. A cyclical activity results, in which periods of extensive osteoclastic resorption are followed by periods of new matrix formation and mineral deposition. Because of the transient need for large numbers of active osteoclasts, many of these cells appear to remain in the marrow spaces, even during periods of trabecular reformation. Active osteoclasts are characterized by a large, ruffled border consisting of motile microvilli separated from the surrounding environs. These cell margins appear as a clear zone because of the large number of contractile microfilaments that are concentrated in the cytoplasm at the brush border periphery. Inactive osteoclasts are more rounded, are not in direct contact with the bone surface, and have little or no brush border. Miller has described an interesting configuration for these inactive cells.[17] Complex invaginations of the cell membrane of the brush

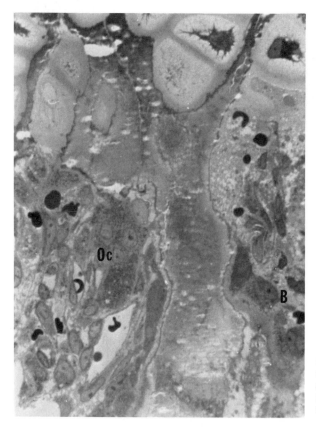

FIGURE 2-14 *Photomicrograph of primary trabeculae (adjacent to cartilage) containing cartilage cores. Osteoclastic resorption* **(Oc)** *and osteoblastic formation* **(B)** *will remodel these to form secondary trabeculae,* × 800.

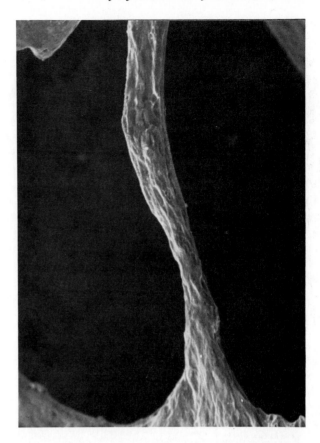

FIGURE 2-15 *Scanning electron micrograph of cell-denuded human bone trabeculum. Surface shows grooves caused by resorptive activity, × 100. (Provided by Arnold, J. S., Chicago)*

border flows to the opposite cell pole, becoming invaginated in the process. This action has been interpreted as a means whereby the cell preserves membrane that will be needed for the brush border when the cell re-enters the active state.

Trabecular thinning is also a common feature in diseased or older bone, likely representing the result of reduction in muscle activity and consequent loss of stimulus for sustained strong skeletal structure (Fig. 2-15).

Life cycle activities of bone cells

The cell that covers most of the surface of bone is the osteoblast. Other cells on the bone surface in special foci are osteoclasts. Although bare spots (surfaces of bone on which no definitive cell-bone relationship is noted) have been reported by some workers, more recent work using

serial sections of bone from young and aging individuals has shown bare spots to be minimal. One reason for the earlier reports of large bare spots may be related to the known difficulty of preserving cell integrity because of the shrinkage of soft organic elements from the mineralized surfaces during histologic preparation and the difficulty encountered in obtaining good penetration of embedding material into large segments of bone. Another likely reason for the disparity in descriptions lies in the fact that osteoblasts assume a variety of shapes that have been interpreted as being indicative of the functional state of the cell. Active osteoblasts, that is, those synthesizing and secreting matrix constituents during a phase of matrix formation, are large, polyhedral cells with a centrally positioned nucleus, extensive rough endoplasmic reticulum, and one or more large Golgi complexes. Inactive osteoblasts, especially those observed lining the channels of compact bone in persons over 65 yr of age may be squamous in shape, with thinned cytoplasm providing a meager membrane covering the bone. Some workers have suggested the term **lining cell** for osteoblasts, suggesting a fluid partitioning activity (bone fluid from general extracellular fluid) for these cells, regardless of their synthesizing activity or morphology.

Osteoblasts are usually organized into a single cell layer over the bone surface. Other adjacent cells may resemble osteoblasts morphologically, and may indeed represent differentiating osteoprogenitor cells. Osteoblasts lining endosteal surfaces of the inner circumferential lamellae or surrounding trabecular surfaces often are in direct contact with cells of the myeloid series of the hematopoietic system. Osteoblasts in periosteal regions are covered with collagen fibers of the periosteum, the osteoblasts composing the osteogenic layer, with the outer fibrous part consisting of ordered collagen bundles with typical fibrocytes extending their processes between and along the surfaces of the bundles.

The haversian system remodeling is a classic example of the scheme postulated by Frost: an activation of cells that occurs in sequential order with resorption preceding formation, that is, a period of osteoclastic resorption is followed by osteoblastic formation.[6] This remodeling scenario has been abbreviated to the ARF (activation-resorption-formation) phenomenon. The population of cells, osteoblasts, osteoclasts, osteocytes, progenitor cells, and related vascular cells that engage in the ARF sequence in a given site constitute a functionally related group of cells called the BMU (bone metabolic unit). Conceptually, a BMU may be likened to the functional unit of other organs such as the nephron, pneumon, or hepatic lobule. The life span of one BMU, starting with activation and proceeding through completion of formation, is designated by the symbol σ. The duration of σ is relatively constant for BMUs in common locations within bones, and varies with different vertebrate species.

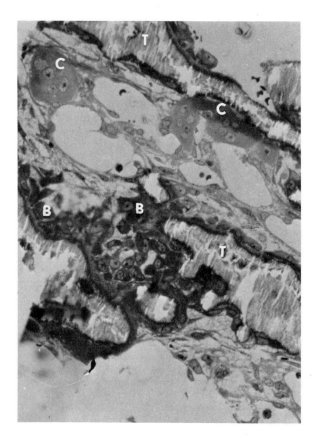

FIGURE 2-16 *Photomicrograph of trabeculae, showing both osteoblasts* **(B)** *and osteoclasts* **(C)** *on the trabeculae* **(T)** *surface. The dark-staining surface is the nonmineralized osteoid,* × 230.

Bone cells

Osteoblasts

Cells that lie directly on bone surface osteoid are osteoblasts. These cells vary in size and shape, depending upon species, age, metabolic activity, and hormonal influence. All organic components of bone matrix are synthesized and secreted by these cells. In addition to their activity of matrix synthesis, they are also believed to play a role in the initiation of mineralization and modulating electrolyte fluxes between the extracellular fluid and bone fluid.

Osteoblasts constitute a single layer of cells, separated from the mineralized matrix by a nonmineralized osteoid. Osteoblasts are said to be "active" when they are engaged in matrix production. Active osteoblasts are usually rounded, pyramidal, or cuboidal, having a characteristic basophilic cytoplasm. The basophilia is associated with the ribosomal fraction of the rough endoplasmic reticulum that occupies the greater part of the cytoplasm of these protein synthesizing cells (Fig. 2-16). A large juxtanuclear Golgi complex and scattered mitochondria are always present. Interestingly, no presecretory granules *per se* are present. The organization of cellular components is ordered, much like that of simple epithelia, with most of the nuclei and other cell components occupying a similar position in adjacent cells of an actively synthesizing osteoblast population. Cells may occasionally present an overlapping (shingle-like) appearance or may occasionally be columnar. Inactive cells lose height and often are more fibrocyte-like, becoming as thin as endothelial cells.

The outer surface of osteoblasts often contact other cells that have the overall shape of osteoblasts but lack the cytoplasmic basophilia of the osteoblasts. These cells are presumed to be osteoblast progenitor cells for three reasons: (1) their proximity to osteoblasts, (2) their state of organellar differentiation, and (3) the distribution of labeled nuclei following the incorporation of tritiated thymidine, as reported by several investigators. Major processes of the basilar surface of osteoblasts may be seen with light microscopy.

Some of these may be followed through the osteoid into the canalliculi of the mineralized bone.

The ultrastructure of osteoblasts reveals additional characteristic features that are not resolved with routine procedures. The cytoplasm of active osteoblasts is primarily occupied by rough endoplasmic reticulum, consisting of a series of membranous tubes studded with ribosomes (Fig. 2-17). Free ribosomes are also readily observed. The membranous endoplasmic reticulum labyrinth surrounds the cysternal protein, the product of ribosomal-directed synthesis. In highly active cells, the cysternae of the rough endoplasmic reticulum is often dilated. Membranes of rough endoplasmic reticulum may be traced from points of attachment to the plasma membrane and to the nuclear membrane. The rough endoplasmic reticulum normally surrounds the Golgi complex (Fig. 2-18).

Interspersed between the rough endoplasmic reticulum are mitochondria, which are usually rounded, although tubular shapes may occur. The cristae appear as parallel shelves completely spanning the membranes of the opposing walls. Mitochondria consist of a double membrane, with the inner membrane folded and evaginated to form the characteristic cristae. Some mitochondria contain small granular mineral deposits attached to the outer cristae surface. Microprobe analysis of these dense granules shows a high concentration of calcium and phosphate, with traces of magnesium. Some organic component is also present, as microincineration of sections at 500° C reduces the granule size, although a sizable deposit of mineral ash remains. A few mitochondrial granules are completely removed by ashing. These latter organic structures are presumed to be lipid because of their high electron density in osmium-fixed tissue. The role of mitochondria in the cells energy cycle is well known, being the site for oxidative phosphorylation and the consequent production of adenosine triphosphate (ATP). A second important function is now recognized. Mitochondria are able to remove calcium ions from cell cytoplasm. Mitochondrial calcium is removed by coprecipitation with phosphate, resulting in the formation of mitochondrial granules. This is an essential capability that enables the regulation

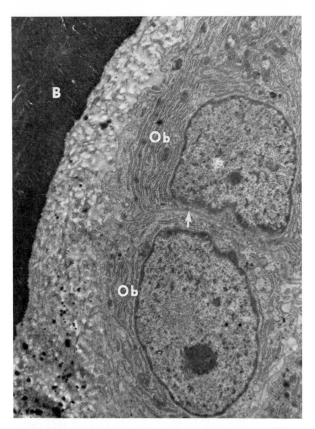

FIGURE 2-17 *Electron micrograph of two osteoblasts* **(Ob)** *separated from the mineralized bone* **(B)** *by osteoid in which a few scattered mineral nodules are dispersed. Only a narrow channel (arrow) separates these metabolically active cells evidenced by the extensive endoplasmic reticulum, × 700. (Matthews, J. L. and Martin, J. H., Atlas of Human Histology and Ultrastructure, Philadelphia, Lea & Febiger, 1971.)*

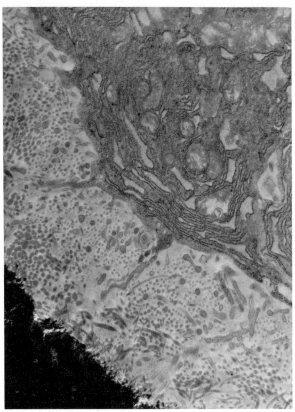

FIGURE 2-18 *Electron micrograph of basilar aspect of osteoblast, showing extension of processes into osteoid, × 12,800.*

of cytoplasmic calcium levels to normal ranges of 10^{-6} to 10^{-7} M. This inward gradient is ordinarily compensated for by the exchange of cell calcium for sodium at the cell membrane and some active extrusion of calcium by calcium-magnesium adenosine triphosphatase (ATPase). Transient rises above these normal intracellular levels are damped by the accretion of excess calcium in the mitochondria and in other cell structures with less calcium sequestrating capacity. Mitochondrial calcium is discharged back into the cytoplasm when cytosolic levels return toward normal levels. This latter process requires metabolic activity. Bone cells often show large numbers of mitochondrial granules, possibly because of the influence of bone effecting hormones upon cell membrane fluxes. Parathyroid hormone (PTH), for example, causes increased entry of calcium into cells, and is accompanied by an increase in the number of mitochondrial granules. Osteoblasts adjacent to newly mineralizing matrix often show increased mitochon-

drial granules, where osteoblasts in adjacent fully mineralized zones show less. This accumulation of calcium in cells in this stage has been interpreted by some to represent some level of cell involvement in the packaging of future matrix mineral. Severely damaged cells show accumulations of mitochondrial granules of sufficient number to initiate mineralization of the cell, particularly the mitochondria. X-radiation, for example, may cause some target cells to mineralize, a probable consequence of cell membrane leakage and consequent mitochondrial overloading. In some cells, calcium is deposited along the surface of cristae rather than in discrete granules. Fixation of tissues with K-pyroantimonate-osmium demonstrates this distribution pattern very well, and also enhances the density of mitochondrial granules in cells with that configuration. The K-pyroantimonate fixative reacts with cations, particularly calcium in low concentrations, producing a characteristic electron dense precipitate (Fig. 2-19).

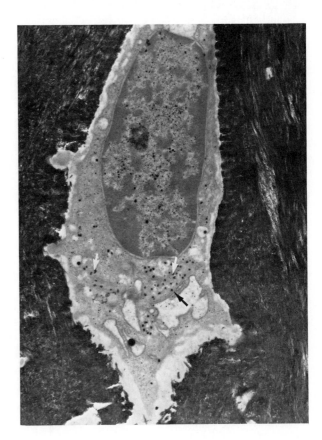

FIGURE 2-19 *Electron micrograph of osteocyte fixed with K-pyroantimonate to preserve calcium-phosphate granules in mitochondria (arrows), × 10,400.*

Cytoplasmic microtubules and microfilaments are also observed in osteoblasts, especially in those fixed in glutaraldehyde fixatives. Bundles of microfilaments course throughout the cytoplasm, occupying the interstitial spaces between rough endoplasmic reticulum, mitochondria, and Golgi complexes. A circumferential network of filaments surrounds the nucleus, with other filaments radiating to the plasma membrane. The latter also has filaments that course parallel to the membrane, occasionally terminating at the inner membrane surface. Studies by King and Holtrup and others, have confirmed that these microfilaments have properties similar to those of proteins of muscle cells.[10] Heavy meromyocin–staining of bone cells shows an "arrowhead" pattern on the microfilaments. The arrowhead pattern is produced by the alignment of the heads of the myosin molecule along the axis of the microfilaments. This technique, along with others that have used fluorescein conjugated antiactin immunoglobulins, has confirmed the actin-like nature of these proteins. Some myosin and troponin are also probable constituents of these filaments. The presence of contractile filaments makes sense for many reasons. Cell motility of bone cells has been observed by time-lapse cinematographic techniques, and remarkable changes in osteoblast shape have been observed when bone cells are exposed to microfilament effecting agents such as the fungal metabolite cytochalasen B. Bone cells exposed to this agent become spherocytes within 1 to 3 min and return to normal shape when the agent is washed off. These widely dispersed filaments undoubtedly provide a basis for motility but additionally give the cell an internal cytoskeleton that serves as a constraint to govern sol-gel cytoplasmic flow.

Microtubules, although present in the cytoplasm of the cell soma, are more abundant in the cell processes. These tubular structures are made by the association of several molecules of tubulin forming a microtubule with a cross-sectional diameter of approximately 7 nm. These structures function as the spindle apparatus of cells in the prophase-telophase stages of mitosis, but their function in the processes is not clearly established. One possible function may be to serve as flow conduits to facilitate transportation of electrolytes, water, or select organic substances. No experiments are reported on bone cells involving agents known to disperse microtubules into their tubulin subunits. Each bone cell has a cytocentrum consisting of two centrioles, satellite bodies, and microtubules. These structures are usually found in a concavity of the nucleus and are often adjacent to the Golgi complex. Visualization of these structures is dependant upon the plane of section, as they occupy a relatively small part of the cell volume. The paired, cylindrical centrioles are positioned in such a way that one centriole is oriented at a right angle to the axis of its paired member. The centrioles are 0.3 nm to 0.5 nm long with a diameter of 0.15 nm. Each centriole consists of nine sets of tubules with three tubules in each set. Triplets of tubules are coupled and positioned at the periphery of the centriole, giving an overall appearance of a gear with the triplets making the "teeth." Triplets are also coupled to adjacent triplets. Centrioles are self-replicating, and two centriole pairs are seen at each pole of a cell in mitosis (Fig. 2-20).

Structures resembling centrioles in their tubular organization are also found near the cell membrane. At least one of these centriole-like basal bodies is found in each bone and cartilage cell. Basal bodies serve as the attachment point (and source of origin) of additional filaments that form the core of cell membrane–covered cilia. Cilia found on osteoblasts are most often found on the cell surface facing the osteoid. The core of each cilium consists of nine pairs of tubules organized around two central tubules. The overall tubule arrangement resembles that of a centriole, differing in the number of tubules involved, and an organization into doublets rather than triplets. Basal rootlets extend from the basal body on the end opposite the cilium. These rootlets are crossbanded and are attached to microfilaments of the cytoskeleton. No special function has been attributed to cilia of bone cells, but their location in bone fluid poses the possibility that they may present a means of stirring the bone fluid to equilibrate ion concentrations.

Inclusions in osteoblasts are not abundant; occasional small vacuoles are observed that contain

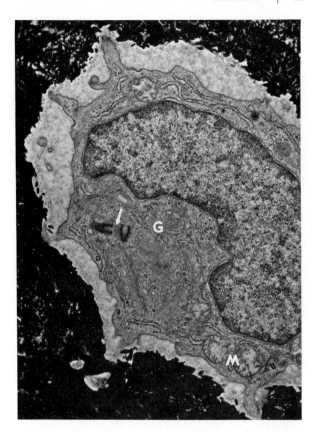

FIGURE 2-20 *Electron micrograph of osteocyte in lacunae. This cell posesses some rough endoplasmic reticulum, mitochondria* **(M),** *a Golgi complex* **(G),** *and a pair of centrioles* (arrow). *Microfilaments extend into processes,* × *10,400.*

homogeneous material of light density. No true secretory granules or storage granules are noted. Thus, in spite of the matrix synthesizing and secretion activity of these cells, the precollagen and ground substance synthesis appears to be coupled with a fast secretory release, rather than a cell storage phenomenon. Occasional lipid inclusions are found.

Some primary lysosomes occur in osteoblasts, but little evidence of secondary lysosomes or residual bodies is present. Osteoblasts that are in areas of injury resulting from x-radiation, incorporation of bone-seeking isotopes, or physical trauma may have an increased presence of these catabolic organelles, but more often areas of injury are invaded by macrophages and tissue histiocytes that phagocytize matrix and cellular debris. The osteoblast is thus regarded primarily as an anabolic specialist.

The nucleus of the osteoblast is limited by two membranes; the outer one often has attached ribosomes. Fusion of outer and inner nuclear membranes produce nuclear pores or annulae. These are seen as small single lines in profile, with the chromatin usually condensed adjacent to these structures. Nuclear pores observed en face, which occurs when the plane of section passes tangential to the nuclear surface, appear as round electron lucent spots. These pores represent the route of most materials that traverse this nuclear-cytoplasmic interface. The chromatin is widely dispersed, but the greater part of the heterochromatin is associated with the nuclear periphery in inactive cells, enhancing the outline of the structure in micrographs. Margination of chromatin is not as prevalent during synthesis. A small nucleolus may be seen, but it is not a prominent feature of osteoblasts. The chromatin is of two types, euchromatin and heterochromatin (clumped). When the DNA strands uncoil to participate in transcription, the resultant euchromatin threads are very small, making their microscopic resolution very difficult. Inactive, densely coiled chromatin is readily identified as large electron dense clumps called heterochromatin. The euchromatin : heterochromatin ratio is useful as one criterion of the state of cell synthesis. Active osteoblasts show a reduction in heterochromatin clumps.

The cell membrane of osteoblasts is a typical trilaminar structure, and the membrane has numerous projections—the microvilli. The membrane facing adjacent osteoblasts is often irregular in contour, often interdigitating with adjacent cells. Following hormonal stimulation, or in sites of newly differentiated cells, microvilli are also seen at these intercellular margins. The basilar (osteoid facing) surface has the greatest number of microvilli, and additionally has large processes that pass through the osteoid to contact processes of osteocytes, these contacts occurring within both the osteoid and the canaliculi. The cell contacts are of the special gap junction type, sometimes called a nexus (Fig. 2-21). These junctions are characteristic of muscle cells as well

as bone cell-to-cell contacts. In nexus (meaning "bond"), cells are separated by a very narrow space of 2 to 3 nm, which is seen by freeze-fracture techniques to be crossed by minute projections, each possessing a central pore allowing the rapid passage of ions and small molecules between adjacent cells. In muscle, this low-impedance-type junction is essential for rapid propagation of a muscle contractile impulse. The role of these structures between bone cells is unknown, but their presence suggests at least two possibilities: (1) calcium ions entering osteocytes may have a facilitated flow pathway through the bone cells, concentrating in the osteoblast for extrusion into the extrabone space postulated by Talmage[22]; (2) the presence of a high extracellular potassium and bone fluid level contrasted with general extracellular fluid reported by Neuman and Ramp[18] may be expected to produce a hyperpolarized membrane potential sensitive to physical deformation.[22] Responses of bone cell potential to local deformation would influence a local

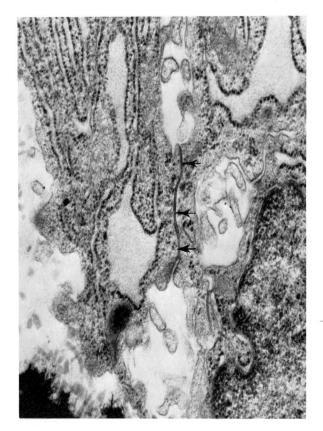

FIGURE 2-21 *Electron micrograph of gap junction (arrow) between adjacent osteoblasts,* ×43,890. *J. L. Matthews, J. H. Martin, J. W. Kennedy, & E. J. Collins: An ultrastructural study of calcium and phosphate deposition and exchange in tissue. In: Oggness, R. and Vaughan, J. (eds.): Hard Tissue Growth, Repair & Mineralization, p. 188, Amsterdam, Excerpta Medica, 1973.*

population of cells because of their syncytial-like gap junction coupling. Bone cell membrane physiology is a virgin field to date, resulting primarily from the difficulty of gaining access to bone cells for experimentation, as their mineralized matrix impedes manipulation. Cell cultures have not shown the necessary fluid partitioning to date, so this approach may not yield the kind of data needed.

Ordinarily, cells that line surfaces are united by either intermittant contact desmosomes (maculae) or a zonula ("little girdle") around the apical margins of cells, especially the margins of epithelial cells abutting lumina. Although osteoblasts form a continuous sheath of surface cells, they have no zonula. This is an important difference between bone cells and epithelial cells, as the zonula occlude intercellular passage of many molecules, requiring cell participation for translining transport. Zonula are not totally impervious however, and several substances pass through the zonula at the intercellular spaces. Bone cells do show some intercellular maculae of the simple trilaminar type. Epithelial cells often have a pentalaminar structure, with cell filaments (tonofibrils) attached to the inner junctional lamina in each abutted cell. Microfilaments of bone cells do not show a preferential concentration at the maculae sporadically binding adjacent bone cells. When epithelial cells rest upon a basal lamina (a fibrous connective tissue), special attachments of cell to matrix are made that resemble one half of a pentalaminar desmosome. These cell-matrix unions are called hemidesmosomes. No comparable structure is seen between bone cells and the adjacent fibrous matrix.

The absence of zonula between adjacent bone cells assures a more patent intercellular space. The patency between osteoblasts has been clearly demonstrated by using electron dense markers such as lanthanum nitrate, ferritin, horseradish peroxidase, and so forth. Injection of a marker substance into the vasculature followed serially by examination of body tissues reveals the time course and route of the marker into the tissue. Interestingly, markers move quickly into the innermost bone spaces within a matter of minutes, suggesting that fluid flow within bone, or diffusional activity within bone, is extraordinarily high. Markers injected into the femoral artery leave the distal capillaries by passing between endothelial cells and diffusing into the surrounding tissue fluid. Two to 5 min postinjection, marker is observed at the osteoblast surface, in the intercellular space between osteoblasts, and partially into the osteoid region. By 10 min, marker is also found in the canaliculi and in the lacunar fluid of deep osteocytes. Thus, ions of bone fluid and those in the general extracellular fluid are separated by narrow and tortuous, but nevertheless patent, pathways. Since these intercellular crevices are narrow, and are bounded by bone cell membranes, it is conceivable that some modification of electrolyte content can be achieved by cell metabolism. Obviously, change of cell shape or intercellular spacing induced by hormones and so forth would significantly alter the capacity for flow as well as the possibility for electrolyte modulation by cell activity. Changes in bone cell shape through membrane flow and cytoskeletal contraction seem an attractive mechanism for osteoblast influence upon exchange of electrolytes in bone. Some additional evidence for osteoblast modulation of bone fluid constituents is given by the observation of pinocytotic (endocytotic) vesicles on the bone fluid side of osteoblast membranes following stimulation of bone with PTH but not calcitonin. This selective cell response brings bone water and its associated organic and electrolyte constituents into the partitioning bone cells. Whether they are discharged on the opposite side or simply empty into the cytosol remains to be established.

Scanning electron micrographs of osteoblasts confirm the dynamic condition of these cells. Scanning electron microscopy (SEM) is advantageous in that it allows the investigator to observe whole fields of several hundred cells in one view. Unfortunately, the ultrathin sectioning required for transmission electron microscopy (TEM) requires that the tissue be embedded in plastic and trimmed to specimen dimensions of less than 1 mm². This limits the number of osteoblasts that can be seen in one field as does the size of the specimen support mesh and the limits of the viewing field with even the lowest magnification setting. Low-power scanning of the endosteal surface of diaphyseal bone is easily accomplished by washing away the marrow cells with buffer after a bone is fixed and split longitudinally. Hundreds of osteoblasts are viewed from their free surface aspect. Cells viewed from this perspective give a flagstone appearance as the cells move slightly apart during the drying process, exaggerating the intercellular width about 15% more than that observed in plastic-embedded sections observed with TEM. Small microvilli are seen projecting from the membrane. Osteoblasts from tissue culture show a ruffling of the surface membrane in addition to the microvilli, a modification in morphology attributed to some influence of culture conditions upon the cell structure (Fig. 2-22). Calcitonin has also been reported by Jones and Boyde to enhance membrane ruffling who compared PTH, calcitonin, and control bones in tissue culture. Matthews and colleagues, Krempien and colleagues, and Jones and Boyde and colleagues have all reported SEM observations on PTH-treated bones.[9,11,15] The osteoblasts show surface blebbing and elongate along the bone axis, closely orienting the cell axis parallel to subjacent collagen bundles. SEM has only recently been used to follow bone cell activity and promises to yield additional information that will help delineate cell responses to different stimuli and environmental conditions.

The osteocyte

ORIGIN

Osteocytes are osteoblasts that become totally entrapped in the matrix being synthesized. With subsequent mineralization of the newly formed matrix, the osteocyte is bounded by a mineralized wall, defining a lacunar space that is incompletely filled by the osteocyte. A thin, incomplete layer of nonmineralized pericellular "osteoid" separates the cell margin from the

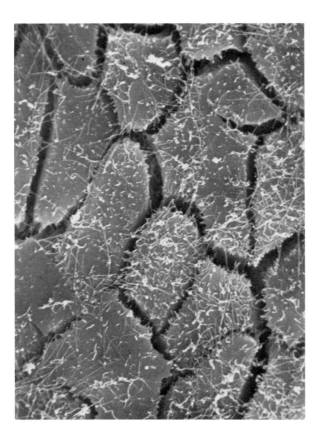

FIGURE 2-22. *Scanning electron micrograph of osteoblasts lining marrow cavity. Microvilli extend from free cell surface and lateral borders, × 2800.*

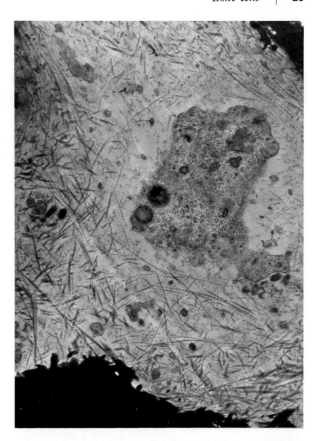

FIGURE 2-23 *Electron micrograph of tangential section of osteocyte lacunae, giving better view of fibrillar matrix that is interposed between the osteocyte (barely in the plane of section) and the mineralized wall × 16,000.*

mineralized lacunar wall (Fig. 2-23). The lacunar surface of the mineralized matrix is a hyperdense region of matrix and is referred to as the lamina densa. The lamina densa surface is usually smooth and is readily distinguished from the less dense interlacunar matrix. In some regions, the overall lacunar size is larger and more irregular in shape, with the lamina densa either missing or intermittant in distribution. The occurrence of these irregular and large lacunae have been intensively investigated by Baud.[1] Interest focused on these osteocytes and lacunae following the work of Belanger, who suggested that osteocytes have the capacity to release citrate, lactate, collagenase, and lysosomal enzymes that would cause erosion or "resorption" of bone around osteocytes.[2] He suggested the term osteocytic osteolysis for this phenomenon. The determination of large amounts of citrate and lactate in bone fluid confirms that some bone cells do release a significant amount of these acids. The irregularity of some lacunar margins and

the lack of lamina dura support this interpretation. However, additional studies are necessary to absolutely confirm this osteolytic concept. What is necessary is the ability to examine the same lacunae at differing stages in time, so that one can delineate between those lacunae that are so configured because they represent a stage of incomplete maturation from those that reached maturation with a smooth lamina densa and subsequently became eroded to larger, irregular lacunae.

Since the osteocyte results from entrappment of osteoblasts, young osteocytes have many of the features of active osteoblasts, that is, they contain an abundance of rough endoplasmic reticulum and they have a large Golgi complex, numerous mitochondria, large cell volume, and a nucleus that has significant amounts of chromatin in the euchromatin form. These young osteocytes are also easily recognized, as they are close to the osteoblast surface, and are often seen in stages in which they are bounded on three sides by fully mineralized matrix, but one side is invested in dense collagen, which shows only scattered deposits of newly forming crystals in the matrix (Fig. 2-24). A characteristic of these and all other osteocytes is the presence of several long, tapering cell processes that course primarily perpendicular to the osteoblast surface, although processes extend laterally as well. With continued maturation of the surrounding matrix with mineral, the processes occupy increasingly smaller canals, ultimately occupying most of the canaliculus, with only a thin layer of nonmineralized matrix separating the process from the mineralized canalicular wall. It is in this area that markers injected into the vasculature are found, confirming that fluid of adjacent lacunae have access for diffusion of essential nutrients and gases. The extension of processes governs the formation and retention of a canalicular network. Processes of adjacent osteocytes may unite end to end or may overlap, forming special nexus junctions at points of cell-to-cell contact. The

diffusional flow capacity through this canalicular system is likely the limiting factor on the thickness of bone produced between the deepest buried osteocyte and the tissue fluid bathing the osteoblast.

Osteocytes that are fully surrounded by mature bone are more sessile. Since little space is left for additional collagen to be deposited, the organellar machinery of the osteocyte is reduced. Rough endoplasmic reticulum is greatly reduced, with only occasional saccules present. Dilated cysternae are rare. The Golgi complex is reduced to a few lamellae, and few vesicles are seen on its secretory or formative face. The nucleus shows heavy margination of heterochromatin, and the nucleolus may be lacking. Mitochondria are larger than those of osteoblasts, and are less numerous. A centrosome is present, and a single cilium extends into the lacunar space (Fig. 2-25). Inclusions of small neutral lipid droplets, isolated vacuoles, and some electron dense microbodies are usually pres-

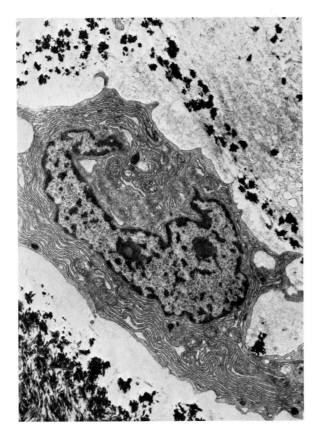

FIGURE 2-24 *Electron micrograph of incompletely walled osteocyte. This cell possesses many of the organelles typical of an active osteoblast or a cell in transition from an osteoblast to an osteocyte, × 14,000. (Matthews, and Martin, Atlas of Human Histology and Ultrastructure, Philadelphia, Lea & Febiger, 1971)*

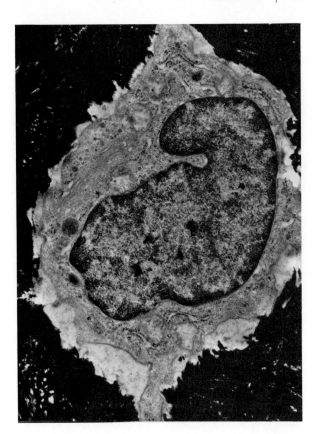

FIGURE 2-25 *Electron micrograph of osteocyte in completely mineralized lacunae. Cell contains several organelles, including a well-developed Golgi complex in the area of indented nucleus (centrosphere), × 10,000.*

ent (Fig. 2-26). From this appearance, the osteocyte has been relegated to a maintenance role, possibly producing some new matrix components to replace others that may be exchanged. Other possible functions that will require further work for elucidation are: (1) the regulation of the pericellular environment by exchange of electrolytes at the plasma membrane and the change of pH, which would certainly modify the crystal-fluid steady state for calcium and phosphate deposition or release, and (2) by alternately contracting and relaxing or by changes in cell hydration a pumping action of osteocytes may be imagined that would contribute to the direction and rate of fluid flow in and out of bone.

In bones of older animals, and in osteocytes of mature cortical bone, the sparse cytoplasm is even more devoid of organelles, and the nuclei are condensed, often spindle-shaped, electron dense, and occasionally pyknotic. Some empty lacunae may be seen. Two interpretations of this may be made, and both must be considered

whenever a histologic evaluation is being made. The features described could represent various stages of cell death or aging. Alternatively, consideration must be given to the fact that the diffusion path to these cells is long and tenuous, thus, they are the last to be fixed when specimens are immersed in fixatives in preparation for histologic study. By the time the fixative diffuses to these sites, significant time may have elapsed, allowing these cells to degenerate. Passage through the bone "sieve" may also modify the carefully prepared osmolality, pH, and concentration of the fixative, resulting in a chemical insult to the target cells. In order to make an appropriate interpretation, the investigator has to make certain that areas showing the features of cell deteriorization or "aging" were situated close to the fixative-exposed surface following excision of the specimen. Unfortunately, areas immediately adjacent to freshly cut surfaces must be ignored because of the physical trauma and deformation caused by passing a blade

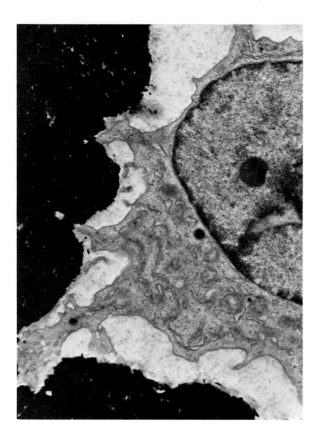

FIGURE 2-26 *Electron micrograph of mature osteocyte, showing some residual rough endoplasmic reticulum but no Golgi complex. Microfilaments continue into cell processes, × 12,000.*

through the resistant matrix. Possibly, many empty lacunae may be explained by the displacement with a dull blade of poorly impregnated cells from their hard-walled lacunae.

Osteocytes, like osteoblasts, show changes in electrolyte density following PTH and calcitonin, suggesting that these cells also must have receptors for these hormones. Histochemical or immunochemical studies are necessary to confirm their presence and distribution. Reaction with heavy meromyosin confirms that these cells, and particularly their processes, contain a large number of actin-like microfilaments. Other histochemical techniques show some lysosomes with acid phosphatase and a positive plasma membrane reaction for alkaline phosphatase, particularly those osteocytes situated in forming lacunae.

The osteoclast

The bone cell specialized for resorption is the osteoclast. In certain conditions involving local inflammation, macrophages may also participate in focal resorption.

The osteoclast is readily recognized by its large size, and multiple numbers of nuclei (see Fig. 2-16). Single nucleated osteoclasts are more difficult to recognize, but an additional identifying feature is the increased number of mitochondria. When osteoclasts are actively resorbing both mineral and organic parts of the matrix, a matrix surface irregularity is produced that becomes a concavity approximating the cell shape. These resorbed sites are termed Howship's lacunae (see Fig. 2-8). The presence of a cell in these concavities is not sufficient to call the cell an osteoclast, as Howship's lacunae are usually repaired and filled with new bone by osteoblasts that migrate into the field vacated by the osteoclast. A cement line demarcates the resorption surface that was filled in with new bone.

The origin of this cell has been extensively studied, and several postulates have been presented over the past few decades. One postulate has been that both the osteoblast and osteoclast differentiate from a common osteoprogenitor cell, forming either preosteoblasts or preosteoclasts. Upon appropriate activating signals, the preosteoclasts fuse to form the multinucleated osteoclast. This postulate is based upon studies involving autoradiography of bones from animals killed at varying times following injection of tritiated thymidine (Young and Owen).[19,26] Labeled nuclei of S-phase cells in the region adjacent to osteoblasts and osteoclasts are later observed in the nuclei of osteoblasts and osteoclasts. These observations clearly indicate that both dividing preosteoblasts and preosteoclasts are definitive cell populations but do not prove the commonality of a single stem cell. This was clearly recognized and discussed by these workers. The number of labeled nuclei in a given osteoclast varies depending upon the state of fusion at the time of administration of tritium-labeled thymidine. By following the ratio of labeled:nonlabeled nuclei sequentially for several days, it is evident that mature osteoclasts may fuse with additional cells, making even larger cells. It is also clear, however, that some nuclei may be extruded from osteoclasts, representing a turnover of nuclei within the cell. This latter finding, coupled with the observed distribution of cells in a cutting cone (resorbing front) in compact bone, led Rasmussen and Bordier to suggest that the advancing osteoclasts may dissociate into single nucleated osteoblasts.[20] This latter postulate has been strongly challenged by the observation of dying and fragmented osteoclasts in these sites and by the lack of any direct observation of cytokinesis in these cells. In the past few years, new evidence has been introduced that strongly supports the concept that the stem cells of osteoblasts and osteoclasts, and hence their intermediate stages, are from separate and unrelated cell populations. This evidence comes from two significant experimental studies. Inbred mutant strains of mice that are osteopetrotic, that is, having no functional osteoclasts, can be provided with an active osteoclast population by transplanting spleen cells from normal mice into these osteopetrotic mutants. A few human cases of osteopetrosis have been successfully treated by transplantation of thymic tissue following immunosuppression therapy. The studies of Walker, Milhaud and colleagues, and others clearly implicate the lymphoid organs as the location of osteoclast stem cells.[16,23] This origin would require that an osteoclast progenitor cell be blood-borne. The present leading candidate is a special monocyte that would be expected to undergo diapedesis from the vasculature into appropriate bone sites. The development of marker enzyme techniques, and chimera, make possible additional methods to trace the cell origins with confidence. Further research into these cells appears fruitful. Much additional work must be done to assess the mechanism of initiation of fusion, resorption activation, and so forth.

The ultrastructure of the osteoclast has been studied by several investigators. Recently, a grid system has been used to make precise histomorphometric analyses of cell size, volume, nucleus number, and most importantly, a determination of the total brush border area. The "brush border" is the "business end" of the osteoclasts, and actually consists of hundreds of microvilli directed at the resorbing surface (Fig. 2-27). The elegant movies of Hancox show these microvilli to be a highly motile portion of the osteoclast, sweeping back and forth across the resorbing face.[7] Morphometric techniques have established that inactive osteoclasts have little or no brush border, whereas those activated by PTH, vitamin D, prostaglandin, and so forth increase the number of microvilli, causing an overall increase in brush border area at the bone interface. Surface area changes are reported to occur within 30 min of activation. Additional numbers of osteoclasts develop several hours after activation. The work of Miller complements the morphometric data, as he has shown that membrane

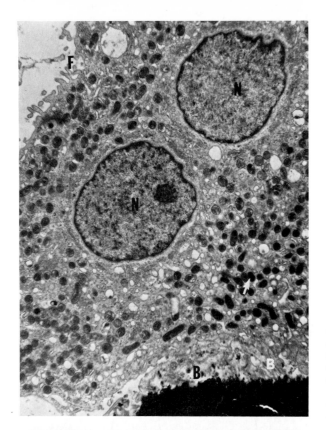

FIGURE 2-27 *Electron micrograph of multinucleate* **(N)** *osteoclast. This relatively inactive cell has a small brush border* **(B)**, *a few cytoplasmic vacuoles, and numerous mitochondria (arrows). Microfilaments and smooth endoplasmic reticulum circle the nuclei. Some microvilli are seen on the free cell surface* **(F)**, *× 9000. (Matthews, and Martin, J. H., Atlas of Human Histology and Ultrastructure, Philadelphia, Lea & Febiger, 1971)*

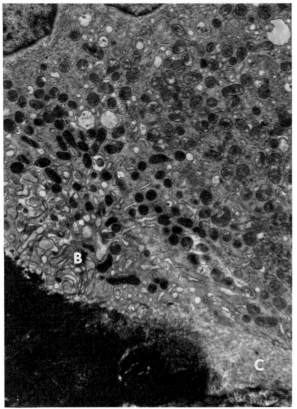

FIGURE 2-28 *Electron micrograph of brush border region* **(B)** *of osteoclast at resorption site. Extensive microvilli extend toward bone while invaginations of plasma membrane terminate in vesicles deeper within the cell. A clear zone* **(C)** *defines the lateral limits of the site of resorption, × 9000.*

flow occurs in osteoblasts, with the brush border membrane being stored as invaginations on the opposite surface of inactive cells.[17]

The membrane between microvilli of the brush border are invaginated in such a way that a series of vacuoles are formed that communicate with the resorption area by way of narrow necks (Fig. 2-28). Other vacuoles are abundant in adjacent areas and are found throughout the cell. Many of these vacuoles likely have their origin from pinched off invaginations, but some may be derived from the Golgi complex found between the nuclei. The matrix at the resorption front appears frayed because free ends of collagen fibers extend from the matrix into the spaces between microvilli with varying levels of electron density, indicating partial demineralization of the frayed matrix. Some apatite crystals and fragments of collagen fibrils may also be found in the space at the active border as well as within vacuoles (Fig. 2-29). It has been difficult to determine whether the mineral crystals observed here represent crystals that have been freed from matrix or whether they represent recrystalization of calcium and phosphate of acid solubilized matrix mineral. It is assumed that the modification of pH in this site is a major factor in demineralization, and it is clear that the osteoclast can produce a variety of organic acids. Whether this cell can produce free hydrogen ions is not determined. *In vitro* tests have indicated that it is necessary to demineralize collagen before collagenase can degrade the fibers. The presence of intact crystals within vacuoles in the osteoclast suggest that some organic material can be digested, freeing the crystals. Before this interpretation is accepted, studies must be made under strict controls that eliminate the conditions that would facilitate reprecipitation of dissolved salts in areas in which the ions are obviously concentrated.

The microenvironment at the resorption front is unique, primarily because the brush border area is sealed off from adjacent cells and tissue

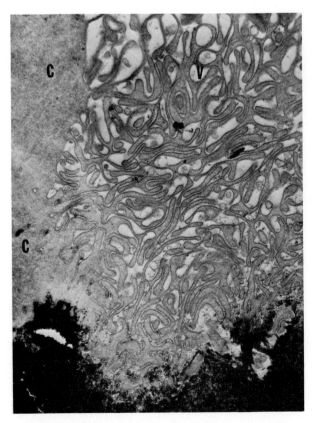

FIGURE 2-29 *Electron micrograph of osteoclast clear zone* **(C)** *and brush border region. Invaginations form vacuoles* **(V)**. *Demineralized collagen fibers extend between microvilli. Some free mineral is seen in invaginated membrane folds,* × 13,000.

fluids, much like a suction cup isolates its interior from the outside. The periphery of the brush border consists of cytoplasmic bulges, with the cell membrane closely abutting the mineralized surface; this arrangement walls off the microvillus area, creating the isolated microenvironment conducive to bone resorption. This boundary area of the osteoclast is called the clear zone, and is characterized by extensive numbers of microfilaments and an amorphous material that is essentially devoid of other organelles.

BONE MATRIX ULTRASTRUCTURE

The spatial organization of bone matrix components is a function of several factors, including age, rate of matrix formation, number and distribution of cells, and exogenous factors including vitamins, hormones, and physical stress. The basic tissue constituents consist of the cells and the intercellular matrix. The latter has varying amounts of connective tissue fibers, ground sub-stance, and interstitial fluid and free electrolytes. In bone and some areas of cartilage, a mineral phase is added in the form of crystals of hydroxyapatite and microcrystals of "amorphous" calcium phosphate. The latter is metastable in aqueous solution, has a lower calcium:phosphorus ratio, appears amorphous to x-ray diffraction techniques, and is readily extracted during routine histologic processing. The amorphous form is reported to be more abundant in bones of young animals. Ultrastructural demonstration of this mineral has been observed employing cryosectioning techniques that avoid aqueous phases during processing. Using this methodology, the amorphous mineral appears as a dispersed cloud of electron dense microparticles, often adherent to specific intrafibrillar zones of collagen fibers (Fig. 2-30). The apatite crystals *per se* are elongated and plate-shaped and have a mean size of 30 to 50 A in width and about 600 A in length.

The major bone matrix component is collagen,

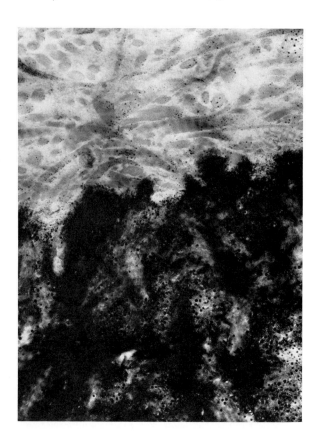

FIGURE 2-30 *Electron micrograph of matrix, showing amorphous mineral deposits within mature mineral and in association with collagen fibers in osteoid, × 51,300.*

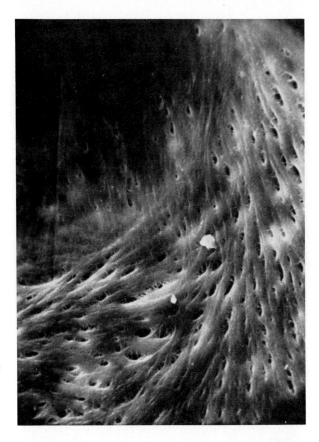

FIGURE 2-31 *Scanning electron micrograph of cell-denuded bone, showing matrix surface of mature mineralized bone (lower right) and bone surface covered by newly formed osteoid (upper left), × 2000. (Provided by Arnold, J. S., Chicago)*

making up 64% of the organic mass. Noncollagenous proteins contribute 14%. Bone collagen is classified as type I collagen, showing an axial periodicity of 640 A. Each collagen molecule is made of three polypeptide chains arranged in a helical array, with each chain containing a large amount of the amino acids glycine, proline, hydroxyproline, and hydroxylysine. The basic unit of extracellular collagen is tropocollagen (approximately 3000 × 16 A). Individual tropocollagen units are polymerized into long, slender microfibrils consisting of approximately five units of 44 A circumference, that is, they are formed into a hollow tube. These microfibrils are further polymerized into fibrils with cross-sectional diameters ranging up to 3000 A. Additional cross linking during maturation results in fibers with definitive spatial orientation, a feature most readily demonstrated by viewing sections with polarized light. Thus, lamellar bone with ordered collagen is readily distinguished from

bundle bone (seen in repairing tissue and embryonal tissue) by its birefringent orientation.

Collagen synthesis and secretion by osteoblasts is also accompanied by synthesis and secretion of noncollagenous matrix parts. Although extraction procedures have yielded much information about the presence of several classes of noncollagenous matrix components, that is, mucopolysaccharides, glycoproteins, phosphoproteins, phospholipids, and so forth, little is known at present about their precise distribution and function within the bone matrix. They have been assigned the role of mineralization nucleators and inhibitors, as well as serving as a glue that occupies the spaces between collagen fibrils. Undoubtedly, further histochemical studies of these substances will prove rewarding. Even less is known about the influence of bone affecting hormones on these noncollagenous parts.

The mineral relationship to the collagen fibrils is evident. By measuring the hole spaces in fi-

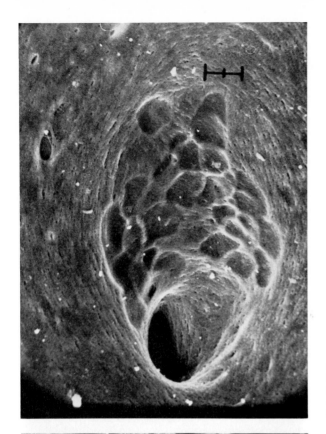

FIGURE 2-32 *Scanning electron micrograph of cell-denuded bone matrix of rabbit endosteal diaphysis, showing resorption cavities produced by osteoclasts on bone surface adjacent to a blood vessel foramen,* × 500. (*Provided by Arnold, J. S., Chicago*)

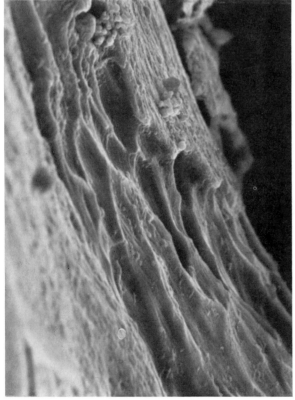

FIGURE 2-33 *Scanning electron micrograph of cell-denuded bone matrix, showing tangential view of resorption cavities produced by osteoclasts advancing along surface,* × 1000. (*Provided by Arnold, J. S., Chicago*)

brils produced by the quarter length lapping of microfibrils, one can account for approximately 50% of the mineral deposited. The remaining mineral is associated with the interfibrillar spaces and the intrafibrillar (intrafibril lumen) spaces. The fact that the mineral crystals have some continuity is adduced from the integrity of a fully ashed bone.

The osteoid that separates osteoblasts from mineralized bone represents a gradation of collagen maturation, ranging from the more coarse fibrous osteoid at the mineral surface to the more fibrillar collagen and yet-to-be polymerized tropocollagen at the osteoid-cell surface. No gradation of mineral density is noted in the osteoid using routine electron micrographic procedures (see Fig. 2-18). Rather, a definitive line demarcates the mineralized bone from the osteoid, albeit, islands of mineral clusters (bone nodules) are found dispersed in regions of osteoid. Interestingly, sites of osteoclast resorption rarely show resorptive activity on an osteoid sur-

face, but are usually found working on fully mineralized surfaces (Figs. 2-31–2-33). Some workers have thus assigned osteoid a function of resorption resistance. The width of the osteoid seam remains relatively constant in normal bone. The width may be increased significantly in osteomalacic bone. Experimentally, the osteoid seam may be greatly widened by partial nephrectomy, depletion of phosphate and vitamin D, and treatment with some diphosphonates. A classic failure of osteoid maturation is shown in Figure 2-34.

The interface between mature mineralized matrix and maturing osteoid is the site of additional accretion of new mineral. These sites are readily demonstrated by several markers, permitting the histomorphometrist to make meaningful measurements of the extent of new formation during time periods between exposure to two markers. One of the earliest markers used was alizarin Red, a dye that colored the newly mineralizing matrix red. Other materials such as

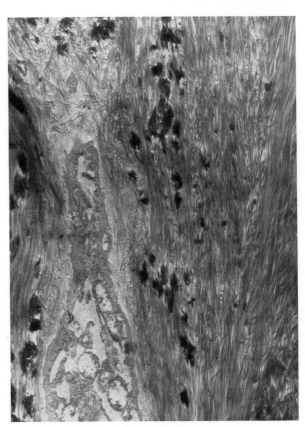

FIGURE 2-34 Electron micrograph of osteocyte and extensive osteoid from malacic bone of uremic patient. Extensive collagen matrix has only sparse nodules of mineral in recently formed matrix. The osteocyte shows some degeneration of organelles, × 11,000.

the tetracyclines are also concentrated in these sites. Their fluorescence emission in ultraviolet light provides a clear delineation of these active surfaces. Ultrastructural localization is also readily done with low doses of lead salts and autoradiographic techniques can be used to localize the site of accretion of bone seeking radionuclides. Ideally, the selective use of different markers at different time periods permits the most precise overall determination of bone growth and turnover.

Other chapters in this book will elaborate on histomorphometric techniques and upon the factors that modify the structure and ultrastructure of bone cells and the related matrix components.

References

1. Baud, C. A.: Submicroscopic structure and functional aspect of the osteocyte, Clin. Orthop. 56:227, 1968.
2. Belanger, L. F.: Osteocytic osteolysis, Calcif. Tissue Res. 4:1, 1969.
3. Brighton, C. T., and Hunt, R. M.: Histochemical localization of calcium in growth plate mitochondria and matrix vesicles, Fed. Proc. 35:143, 1976.
4. Cecil, R. N. A., and Anderson, H. C.: Freeze-fracture studies of matrix vesicle calcification in epiphyseal growth plate, Metab. Bone Dis. & Rel. Res. 1:89, 1978.
5. Fell, H. B., and Robison, R.: The growth, development and phosphatase activity of embryonic avian femora and limb-buds cultivated in vitro, Biochem. J. 23:767, 1929.
6. Frost, H. M.: Tetracycline-based histological analysis of bone remodeling, Calcif. Tissue Res. 3:211, 1969.
7. Hancox, N.: The Osteoclast. In: Bourne, G. H. (ed.): The Biochemistry and Physiology of Bone, p. 213, New York, Academic Press, 1956.
8. Holtrop, M. E., Raisz, L. G., Simmons, H. A.: The effects of parathyroid hormone, colchicine, and calcitonin on the ultrastructure and the activity of osteoclasts in organ culture, J. Cell Biol. 60:346, 1974.
9. Jones, S. J. and Boyde, A.: Scanning electron microscopy of some bone cells in culture. In: Copp, D. H. and Talmage, R. V. (eds.): Endo-crinology of Metabolism, p. 97, Amsterdam, Excerpta Medica, 1978.
10. King, G. J. and Holtrop, M. E.: Actin-like filaments in bone cells of cultured mouse calvaria as demonstrated by binding to heavy meromyosin, J. Cell Biol. 66:445, 1975.
11. Krempien, B., Ritz, E.: Effects of parathyroid hormone on osteocytes. Ultrastructural evidence for anisotropic osteolysis and involvement of the cytoskeleton, Metab. Bone Dis. Res. 1:55, 1978.
12. Kuettner, K., Sorgente, N., Croxen, L., Howell, D. S. and Pita, J. C.: Lysozyme in preosseous cartilage, Biochem. Biophys. Acta 372:335, 1974.
13. Kuettner, K. E., Harper, E. J., and Eisenstein, R.: Protease inhibitors in cartilage, Arthr. & Rheum. 20:(suppl.), 124, 1977.
14. Matthews, J. L., J. H. Martin and E. J. Collins: Metabolism of radioactive calcium by cartilage, Clin. Orthop. and Rel. Res., 58:213, 1968.
15. Matthews, J. L., Davis, W. L., Martin, J. H., and Talmage, R.: The endosteal cell response to exogenous stimuli, an electron microscope study. In: Slavkin, H. (ed.): Extracellular Matrix Influences on Gene Expression, p. 735, New York, Academic Press, 1975.
16. Milhaud, G., Labat, M. L., Graf, B., and Thillard, M. J.: Relation between the thymus and osteopetrosis. In: Cop, D. H., and Talmage, R. V. (eds.): Endocrinology of Calcium Metabolism, p. 143, Amsterdam, Excerpta Medica, 1978.
17. Miller, S. C.: Rapid activation of the medullary bone osteoclast cell surface by parathyroid hormone, J. Cell Biol. 76:615, 1978.
18. Neuman, W. F., Ramp, W. K.: The concept of a bone membrane: some implications. In Nichols, G. Jr., Wasserman, R. H., (eds.): Bone cells, calcification, and calcium homeostasis, p. 211, New York, Academic Press, 1971.
19. Owen, M.: Cell population kinetics of an osteogenic tissue, I. J. Cell Biol. 19:19, 1963.
20. Rasmussen, H., Bordier, P. J.: The Physiological and Cellular Basis of Metabolic Bone Disease. Baltimore, Williams & Wilkins, 1974.
21. Schenk, R. K., Wiener, J., and Spiro, D.: Fine structural aspect of vascular invastion of the tibial epiphyseal plate of growing rats, Acta Anat. 69:1, 1968.
22. Talmage, R. V.: Calcium homeostasis—calcium transport—parathyroid hormone and the movement of calcium between bone and fluid, Clin. Orthop. Res. 67:210, 1969.
23. Walker, D. G.: Spleen cells transmit osteopetrosis in mice, Science, 190:785, 1975.

24. Wolff, J.: Die Lehre von den functionellen Knochengestalt, Virchows Arch. 155:256, 1899.

25. Wuthier, R. E., Linder, R. E., Warner, G. P., Gore, S. T., and Borg, T. K.: Non-enzymatic isolation of matrix vesicles: characterization and initial studies on ^{45}Ca and ^{32}P-Orthophosphate metabolism, Metab. Bone Dis. & Res. 1:125, 1978.

26. Young, R. W.: Cell proliferation and specialization during endochondral osteogenesis in young rats, J. Cell Biol. 14:357, 1962.

Selected readings

Cartilage

Ali, S. Y.: Analysis of matrix vesicles and their role in the calcification of epiphyseal cartilage, Fed. Proc. 35:135, 1976.

Anderson, H. C., Cecil, R., and Sajdera, S. W.: Calcification of rachitic rat cartilage in vitro by extracellular matrix vesicles, Am. J. Pathol. 79:237, 1975.

Bonucci, E.: Fine structure of early cartilage calcification, J. Ultrastruct. Res. 20:33, 1967.

Borg, T. K., Runyan, R. B., and Wuthier, R. E.: Correlation of freeze-fracture and scanning electron microscopy of epiphyseal chondrocytes, Calcif. Tissue Res. 26:237, 1978.

Bozdech, A., and Horn, V.: The morphology of growth cartilage using the scanning electron microscope, Acta Orthop. Scand. 46:561, 1975.

Brighton, C. T., and Hunt, R. M.: Histochemical localization of calcium in growth plate mitochondria and matrix vesicles, Fed. Proc. 35:143, 1976.

Clarke, I. C.: Articular cartilage: A review and scanning electron microscope study. II. The territorial fibrillar architecture, J. Anat. 117:261, 1974.

Hirschman, A.: Staining of fresh epiphyseal cartilage with toluidine blue, Histochemie 10:369, 1967.

Hohling, H. J., Steffens, H., and Stamm, G.: Transmission microscopy of freeze dried unstained epiphyseal cartilage of the guinea pig, Cell Tissue Res. 167:243, 1976.

Holtrop, M. E.: The ultrastructure of the epiphyseal plate. I. The flattened chondrocyte, Calc. Tissue Res. 9:131, 1972.

Kashiwa, H., Lachtel, D. L., and Park, H. Z.: Chondroitin sulfate and electron lucent bodies in the pericellular rim about unshrunken hypertrophied chondrocytes of chick long bone, Anat. Rec. 183:359, 1975.

Matthews, J. L., Martin, J. H., Sampson, H. W., Kunin, A. S., and Roan, J. H.: Mitochondrial granules in the normal and rachitic rat epiphysis, Calcif. Tissue Res. 5:91, 1970.

Matthews, J. L., Martin, J. H. and Collins, E. J.: Metabolism of radioactive calcium by cartilage, Clin. Orthop. 58:213, 1968.

Matukas, V. J., Panner, B. J., and Orbison, J. L.: Studies on ultrastructural identification and distribution of protein-polysaccharide in cartilage matrix, J. Cell Biol. 32:365, 1967.

Schenk, R. K., Spiro, D., and Wiener, J.: Cartilage resorption in the tibial epiphyseal plate of growing rats, J. Cell Biol. 34:1, 275, 1967.

Schenk, R. K., Wiener, J., and Spiro, D.: Fine structural aspect of vascular invasion of the tibial epiphyseal plate of growing rats, Acta Anat. 69:1, 1968.

Scott, B. L., and Pease, D. C.: Electron microscopy of the epiphyseal apparatus, Anat. Rec. 126:465, 1956.

Zimny, M. L., and Redler, I: Scanning electron microscopy of chondrocytes, Acta Anat. (Basel) 83:398, 1972.

Cortical and trabecular bone

Carter, D. R., and Hayes, W. C.: Bone compressive strength: The influence of density and strain rate, Science 194:1174, 1976.

Frost, H. M.: Tetracycline-based histological analysis of bone remodeling, Calcif. Tissue Res. 3:211, 1969.

Merz, W. A., and Schenk, R. K.: Quantitive structural analysis of human cancellous bone, Acta Anat. (Basel) 75:54, 1970.

Parfitt, A. M.: Quantum concept of bone remodelling and turnover: implications for the pathogenesis of osteoporosis, Calcif. Tissue Int. 28:1, 1979.

Piekarski, K., and Munro, M.: Transport mechanism operating between blood supply and osteocytes in long bones, Nature 269:80, 1977.

Rasmussen, H., and Bordier, P. J.: The Physiological and Cellular Basis of Metabolic Bone Disease, Baltimore, Williams & Wilkins, 1974.

Schenk, R. K., Merz, W. A., and Muller, J.: A quantitative histological study on bone resorption in human cancellous bone, Acta Anat. (Basel) 74:44, 1969.

Sternstrom, A., Hansson, L. T., and Thorngren, K. G.: Cortical bone remodeling in normal rat, Calcif. Tissue Res. 23:161, 1977.

Osteoblasts and bone formation

Bernard, B. W., and Pease, D. C.: An electron microscope study of initial intramembranous osteogenesis, Am. J. Anat. 125:271, 1969.

Fell, H. B., and Robison, R.: The growth, development and phosphatase activity of embryonic avian femora and limb-buds cultivated in vitro, Biochem. J. 23;767, 1929.

Friend, D. S., and Gilula, N. B.: Variations in tight and gap junctions in mammalian tissues, J. Cell Biol. 53:758, 1972.

Hancox, H. M., and Boothroyd, B.: Electron microscopy of the early stages of osteogenesis, Clin. Orthop. 40A:153, 1965.

Harrel, A., Binderman, I., and Guez, M.: Tissue culture of bone cells: mineral transport, calcification and hormonal effects, Isr. J. Med. Sci., 12:27, 1976.

Jones, S. J.: Secretory territories and role of matrix production of osteoblasts, Calcif. Tissue Res. 14:309, 1974.

Jones, S. J., and Boyde, A.: Is there a relationship between osteoblasts and collagen orientation in bone? Isr. J. Med. Sci. 12:11, 1976.

Luk, S. C., Napajaroonsri, C., and Simon, G. T.: The ultrastructure of the endosteum, J. Ultrastruct. Res. 46:165, 1974.

Matthews, J. L., Davis, W. L., Martin, J. H., and Talmage, R.: *In* Slavkin, H. (ed.): Extracellular Matrix Influences on Gene Expression. The endosteal cell response to exogenous stimuli, an electron microscope study. p. 735, New York, Academic Press, 1975.

Matthews, J. L., Martin, J. H., Collins, E. J., Kennedy, J. W., and Powell, E. L., Jr.: *In* Talmage, R., and Munson, P. (eds.): Calcium, Parathyroid Hormone and the Calcitonins, Immediate changes in the ultrastructure of Bone Cells Following Thyrocalcitonin Administration. p. 376, Amsterdam, Excerpta Medica, 1971.

Owen, M.: Cell population kinetics of an osteogenic tissue, I. J. Cell Biol. 19:19, 1963.

Pritchard, J. J.: The osteoblast, *In* Bourne, G. H. (ed.): The Biochemistry and Physiology of bone, Vol. I., p. 19, New York, Academic Press, 1976.

Schenk, R. K., Olah, A. J., and Merz, W. A.: Bone Cell Counts, *In* Frame, B., Parfitt, A. M., and Duncan, H. (eds.): Clinical Aspects of Metabolic Bone Disease, p. 103, Amsterdam, Excerpta Medica, 1971.

Osteoclast and bone resorption

Belanger, L. F., and Migicovsky, B. B.: Histochemical evidence of proteolysis in bone: the influence of parathormone, J. Histochem. Cytochem. 11:734, 1963.

Bonucci, E.: The organic-inorganic relationships in bone matrix undergoing osteoclastic resorption, Calcif. Tissue Res. 16:13, 1974.

Gothlin, G., and Ericsson, L. E.: The osteoclast, Clin. Orthop. 120:201, 1976.

Hall, B. K.: The origin and fate of osteoclasts, Anat. Res. 183:1, 1975.

Hanaoka, H.: On the hypothesis of modulation of osteoclasts to osteoblasts on the endosteal bone surface, a critical review, J. Jap. Orthop. Ass. 51:613, 1977.

Hancox, N.: The osteoclast. *In* Bourne, G. H. (ed.): The Biochemistry and Physiology of Bone, p. 213, New York, Academic Press, 1956.

Holtrop, M. E., King, G. J., Cox, K. A., and Reig, B.: Time-related changes in the ultrastructure of osteoclasts after injection of parathyroid hormone in young rats, Calcif. Tissue Int. 27:129, 1979.

Holtrop, M. E., Raisz, L. G., and Simmons, H. A.: The effects of parathyroid hormone, colchicine, and calcitonin on the ultrastructure and the activity of osteoclasts in organ culture, J. Cell Biol. 60:346, 1974.

Jowsey, J.: Microradiography of bone resorption. *In* Sognnaes, R. F. (ed.): Mechanisms of Hard Tissue Destruction, p. 447. Washington, D. C., American Academy Advanced Sciences, 1963.

Kallio, D. M., Garant, P. R., and Minkin, C.: Evidence of coated membranes in the ruffled border of the osteoclast, J. Ultrastruct. Res. 37:169, 1971.

Kallio, D. M., Garant, P. R., and Minkin, C.: Ultrastructural effects of calcitonin in osteoclasts in tissue culture, J. Ultrastruct. Res. 39:205, 1972.

King, G. J., Holtrop, M. E., and Raisz, L. G.: The relation of ultrastructural changes in osteoclasts to resorption in bone cultures stimulated with parathyroid hormone, Metab. Bone Dis. Res. 1:67, 1978.

Lucht, U.: Acid phosphatase of osteoclasts demonstrated by electron microscopic histochemistry, Histochemie 28:103, 1971.

Lucht, U.: Osteoclasts and their relationship to bone as studied by electronmicroscopy, Z. Zelliforsch. 135:211, 1972.

Matthews, J. L., Martin, J. H., Race, G. J., and Collins, E. J.: Giant cell centrioles, Science 155:1423, 1967.

Miller, S. C.: Rapid activation of the medullary bone osteoclast cell surface by parathyroid hormone, J. Cell Biol. 76:615, 1978.

Schenk, R. K., Spiro, D., and Wiener, J.: Cartilage resorption in the tibial epiphyseal plate of growing rats. J. Cell Biol. 34:275, 1967.

Weisbrode, S. E., Capen, C. C., and Nagode, L. A.: Influence of parathyroid hormone on ultrastructural and enzymatic changes induced by vitamin D in bone of thyroparathyroidectomized rats, Lab. Invest. 30:786, 1974.

Young, R. W.: Cell proliferation and specialization during endochondral osteogenesis in young rats, J. Cell Biol. 14:357, 1962.

Osteocyte

Aaron, J. E.: Osteocyte types in the developing mouse calvarium, Calcif. Tissue Res. 12:259, 1973.

Baud, C. A.: Submicroscopic structure and functional aspect of the osteocyte. Clin. Orthop. 56:227, 1968.

Belanger, L. F.: Osteocytic osteolysis, Calcif. Tissue Res. 4:1, 1969.

Cameron, D. A.: The ultrastructure of bone. In Bourne, G. H. (ed.): The Biochemistry and Physiology of Bone, Vol. I, p. 191–201, New York, Academic Press, 1972.

Cameron, D. A., Paschall, H. A., and Robinson, R. A.: Changes in the fine structure of bone cells after the administration of parathyroid extract, J. Cell Biol. 33:1, 1967.

Jande, S. S., and Belanger, L. F. Electron microscopy of osteocytes and the pericellular matrix in rat trabecular bone, Calcif. Tissue Res. 6:280, 1971.

King, G. J., and Holtrop, M. E.: Actin-like filaments in bone cells of cultured mouse calvaria as demonstrated by binding to heavy meromyosin, J. Cell Biol. 66:445, 1975.

Krempien, B., Maregold, C., Ritz, E., and Bommer, J.: The influence of immobilization on osteocyte morphology, Virchows Arch (Pathol. Anat.) 370:55, 1976.

Krempien, B., and Ritz, E.: Effects of parathyroid hormone on osteocytes. Ultrastructural evidence for anisotropic osteolysis and involvement of the cytoskeleton, Metab. Bone Dis. Res. 1:55, 1978.

Lok, E., and Jaworski, ZFG.: Changes in the periosteocytic lacunae size observed under experimental conditions in adult dog. In Jaworski, Z. F. G. (ed.). Proceedings of First Workshop on Bone Morphometry. p. 297, Ottawa, University of Ottawa Press, 1976.

Marotti, G.: Osteocyte orientation in human lamellar bone and its relevance to the morphometry of periosteocytic lacunae. Metab. Bone Dis. and Rel. Res. 1:325, 1979.

Martin, J. H., and Matthews, J. L.: Mitochondrial granules in chondrocytes, osteoblasts and osteocytes, Clin. Orthop. 68:273, 1970.

Tonna, E. A.: Electron microscopic evidence of alternating osteocytic-osteoclastic and osteoplastic activity in the perilacunar walls of aging mice, Connect. Tissue Res. 1:221, 1972.

Wasserman, R., and Yaeger, J. A.: Fine structure of the osteocyte capsule and of the wall of the lacunae in bone, Z. Zellforsch. Mikrosk. Anat. 67:636, 1965.

Bone and cartilage matrix components

Anderson, C., and Danylchuk, K. D.: Scanning electron microscopic observations on bone, Arch. Pathol. Lab Med. 101:19, 1977.

Boyde, A., and Hobdell, M. H.: Scanning electron microscopy of bone, Calcif. Tissue Res. 2:(Suppl.), 4, 1968.

Boyde, A., and Hobdell, M. H.: Scanning electron microscopy of lamellar bone, Z. Zellforsch Mikrosk Anat. 93:213, 1968.

Carneiro, J., and Leblond, C. P.: Role of osteoblasts and odontoblasts in secreting the collagen of bone and dentin, as shown by radioautography in mice given tritium labeled glycine, Exp. Cell Res. 18:291, 1959.

Frank, R. M., and Frank, P.: Autoradiographie quantitative de l'osteogenese en microscopie electronique a l'aide de la proline tritiee, Z. Zellforsch. 99:121, 1969.

Frasca, P., Harper, R. A., and Katz, J. L.: Collagen fibre orientations in human secondary osteons, Acta Anat. (Basel) 98:1, 1977.

Jackson, S. F.: The fine structure of developing bone in the embryonic fowl, Proc. R. Soc. Lond. 146B:270, 1957.

Knese, K. H., and Knoop, A. M.: Uber den Ort der Bildung des Muckopolysaccharide-Protein-Komplexes im Knorpelgewebe-Electronenmikroskopische und histochemische Untersuchen, Z. Zell-forsch 53:210, 1961.

Kuettner, K., Sorgente, N., Croxen, L., Howell, D. S., and Pita, J. C.: Lysozyme in preosseous cartilage. Biochem Biophys. Acta 372:335, 1974.

Revel, J. P., and Hay, E.: An autoradiographic and electron microscopic study of collagen synthesis in differentiating cartilage, Z. Zellforsch. Mikrosk. Anat., 61:110, 1963.

Robinson, R. A., and Cameron, D. A.: Electron microscopy of cartilage and bone matrix at the distal epiphyseal line of the femur in the newborn infant, J. Biophys. Biochem. Cytol. (Supl.) (4) 2:253, 1956.

Salomon, C. D.: A fine structural study on the extracellular activity of alkaline phosphatase and its role in calcification, Calc. Tissue Res. 15:201, 1974.

Scherft, J. P.: The ultrastructure of the organic matrix of calcified cartilage and bone in embryonic mouse radii, J. Ultrastruct. Res. 23:333, 1968.

Weinstock, M.: Radioautographic visualization of ^{3}H-fucose incorporation into glycoprotein by osteoblasts and its deposition into bone matrix, Calcif. Tissue Int. 27:177, 1979.

Whitehouse, W. J., Dyson, E. D., and Jackson, C. R.: The scanning electron microscope in studies of trabecular bone from a human vertebral body, J. Anat. 108:481, 1971.

Mineralization

Anderson, H. C.: Introduction to the second conference on matrix vesicle calcification, Metab. Bone Dis. Res. 2:1, 1978.

Ascenzi, A., and Bonucci, E.: The osteon calcification as revealed by the electron microscope. *In* Fleisch, H., Blackwood, H. J., and Owen, M. (eds.): Calcified Tissues, p. 104, Berlin, Springer-Verlag, 1966.

Bonucci, E.: The locus of initial calcification in cartilage and bone. Clin. Orthop. 78:108, 1971.

Eisemann, D. R., and Glick, P. L.: Ultrastructure of initial crystal formation in dentin. J. Ultrastruct. Res. 41:18, 1972.

Glimcher, M. J.: Specificity of the molecular structure of organic matrices in mineralization, p. 421–487, *In* Sognnaes, R. F. (ed.) Calcification in Biological Systems, Washington, D. C., American Association for the Advancement of Science, 1960.

Molnar, Z.: Development of the parietal bone of young mice: I. Crystals of bone mineral in frozen-dried preparations, J. Ultrastruct. Res. 3:39, 1959.

Salomon, C. D.: A fine structural study on the extracellular activity of alkaline phosphatase and its role in calcification, Calcif. Tissue Res. 15:201, 1974.

Schraer, H., and Gay, C. V. : Matrix vesicles in newly synthesizing bone observed after ultracryotomy and ultramicroincinesation, Calcif. Tissue Res. 23:185, 1977.

Thyberg, J.: Electron microscopic studies on the initial phases of calcification in guinea pig epiphyseal cartilage, J. Ultrastruct. Res. 46:206, 1973.

Wuthier, R. E.: The role of phospholipids in biological calcification. Distribution of phospholipase activity in calcifying epiphyseal cartilage, Clin. Orthop. 90:191, 1973.

When considered as an organ any bone consists of a variety of tissues (Fig. 3-1). The articulating surfaces are covered with a layer of cartilage beneath that is subchondral spongy (cancellous) bone tissue. Cartilage is present in the growth plates of growing animals; the metaphysis contains cancellous bone tissue; and the marrow contains hematopoietic elements and stromal cells. A fibrous and cellular envelope, the periosteum externally and the endosteum internally, covers the bone tissue surfaces and tendons, ligaments and muscle attachments are in serted into the bone wall. Blood vessels and nerves permeate and penetrate these various regions; therefore in any biochemical analysis of bone tissue it is important to minimize contamination from these adjacent tissue elements.

Most investigators have appreciated this difficulty in working with bone tissue and have selected the compact bone of the shafts of long bones for their starting materials. This is the least heterogenous sample of bone tissue that can be obtained in quantity. In certain studies, particularly when development and growth of bone is a major feature of the experiments, it is almost impossible to obtain a pure sample of bone tissue for study, and these observations are limited by the presence of other tissues. Therefore, only those organic materials that have been isolated from compact bone tissue will be discussed here.

In biological terms the organic matrix of any tissue is most simply described as the organic material between the cells. The complete biochemistry of the organic matrix of bone tissue deals with the nature of the extracellular organic constituents of bone, their functions, and the chemical changes they undergo in the course of the activity of living bone—ultimately in the hope of describing precise chemical structure-function relationships in an integrated manner. In this chapter the nature of the organic materials that have been isolated from bone tissue will be described and some aspects of their formation, origins, and possible functions will be discussed.

Bone has two major functions that are very different from each other in nature. First, and most obvious, bone serves a mechanical function by providing a rigid internal skeleton whose

J. T. TRIFFITT

3

the organic matrix of bone tissue

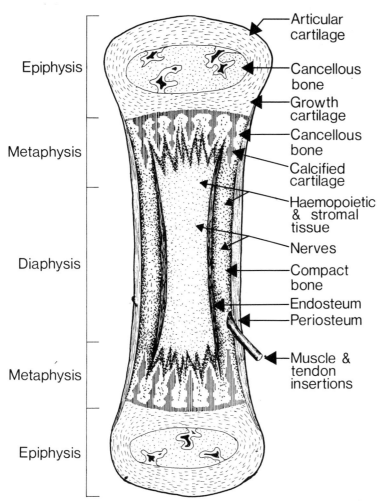

Epiphysis

Metaphysis

Diaphysis

Metaphysis

Epiphysis

Articular
cartilage

Cancellous
bone

Growth
cartilage

Cancellous
bone

Calcified
cartilage

Haemopoietic
& stromal
tissue

Nerves

Compact
bone

Endosteum

Periosteum

Muscle &
tendon
insertions

FIGURE 3-1 *Diagrammatic representation of bone as an organ to show the tissues associated with bone tissue.*

separate pieces are moved by the leverage action of attached muscles and by the provision of joints or articulations. The chief function of some parts of the skeleton appears to be the protection of delicate organs; the brain, for example, is almost completely surrounded by the skull. Second, the vertebrate skeleton serves as a reservoir of mineral ions and plays a part in calcium and phosphate homeostasis. With respect to the organic matrix of bone, however, its general contribution to the structural integrity of the tissue is the most obvious. It is perhaps less obvious that the organic matrix plays a role in mineral homeostasis but this too is dependent upon the relationship between the mineral and the matrix,

and this association affects the availability of the constituent calcium and phosphate ions to the circulatory fluids. Particular organic molecules could influence the release of these ions by binding to mineral surfaces and, by the inherent nature of their affinity for calcium, also function as a readily accessible store for this biologically important cation.

The question of the precise mechanism of bone mineralization has fired the enthusiasm of all involved in bone research, and the idea that bone organic matrix contains specific factors essential to this process is a fervent belief of many investigators in this field. As will be discussed later, this may be true in certain respects, but it would appear more probable that such unique materials would be located at the actual site of mineralization. This latter view can be appreciated if certain aspects of the formation of bone tissue are considered. Formation of new bone tissue must occur by the laying down of new tissue on the pre-existing surfaces, as the hardness and rigidity of calcified bone precludes deposition within the mineralized regions. If this occurs on a scaffolding of cartilage as, for example, in the epiphyseal ends of the shafts of long bones, the process is termed endochondral ossification. When bone is formed at a site at which bone is not preceeded by cartilage as, for example, in the periosteal region of the shafts of long bones or on the walls of the tunnels (haversian canals) carrying blood vessels through the bone substance, the process is called membranous ossification. In both types of bone formation, bone-forming cells (osteoblasts) synthesize an organic matrix (osteoid) as a narrow zone of extracellular material between themselves and the underlying calcified bone. Although there is a time lag between osteoid synthesis and its mineralization, this preosseus tissue very rapidly undergoes calcification. The calcium phosphate mineral deposited initially is amorphous to x-ray diffraction techniques and is thought to consist of a particular mineral phase that subsequently transforms to a more crystalline, highly substituted hydroxyapatite phase.[59] The interface between the osteoid tissue and the calcified bone is the site of active mineralization (calcification front). The specific reactions resulting in the formation of calcified bone occur at this location, and the biochemical entities actively engaged in this process are present at this site. Therefore it is likely that such constituents would represent only a small proportion of the organic matrix of compact bone tissue and that the majority of the matrix has a purely structural function in the integration of the organic and mineral phases into a functional unit.

The extracellular matrix of bone tissue is obviously different from most other connective tissue matrices by its content of calcium phosphate minerals. Up to the present time it has not proved possible to assign conclusively all the chemical moieties that have been isolated—even

from the relatively more homogenous samples of compact bone tissue—to the extracellular location, as all bone tissue used for analysis contains cells. This is illustrated in Fig. 3-2, which demonstrates the location of numerous bone cells (osteocytes) in lacunae surrounded by intercellular material. The latter material is permeated by tiny canals (canaliculi) containing cell processes, many of which interconnect in a syncytial network. It has been estimated that there are approximately 26,000 osteocytes/mm^3 of bone tissue.[7] Also present are blood vessels with associated cellular and extracellular elements—nerves and cells actively involved in bone formation (osteoblasts) and bone remodeling (osteoclasts).

The ratio of extracellular to cellular volume in compact bone tissue is relatively high—the cells making up only 5 to 8% of the volume of the calcified matrix of the tissue.[63] Therefore those materials that are present in abundant quantities in the sample of bone tissue used for analysis are presumably extracellular. Similarly located are the bulk of those organic constituents (e.g., collagen, proteoglycans) that have been found to be located mainly in the extracellular space in other connective tissues and that are detectable by staining and microscopy. However, as more of the minor constituents of bone tissue are discovered and investigated, precise localization studies become increasingly important.

The matrix of bone, as that of other connective tissues, contains many diverse materials that are dependent on the bone type and on the species, age, and development of the animal. So proteins, glycoproteins, proteoglycans, glycosaminoglycans, peptides, carbohydrates, lipids, and others are present. However, it was recognized many years ago that the bulk (about 90% w/w) of the organic material was made up of a single protein, collagen. Evidence is accumulating that the majority of the remainder of the bone matrix, the noncollagenous material, is made up mainly of noncollagenous proteins. So, if a sample of carefully prepared mammalian compact bone is considered, an estimate can be made of the approximate relative weights of the major organic constituents in the extracellular and cellular compartments of bone (Fig. 3-3).

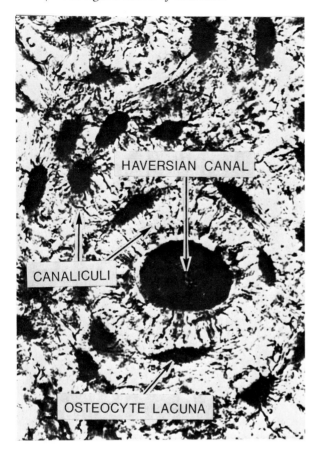

HAVERSIAN CANAL

CANALICULI

OSTEOCYTE LACUNA

FIGURE 3-2 *Transverse section of rabbit cortical bone stained to demonstrate osteocyte lacunae and canaliculi.*

These values are calculated from the results and assumptions of various authors for compact bone tissue of various species. The basic premises are:

1. Cells and their processes in bone may make up a maximum of 7% of the total bone volume.[63]
2. Fresh compact bone is composed of water (9% w/w), organic material (22% w/w), and inorganic material (69% w/w).[28]
3. Cell density = 1 g/ml.
4. Protein content cells = 10% w/w.[16]
5. Collagen makes up 90% w/w of the organic material.

This suggests that cell protein may make up a maximum of about 16% of the weight of noncollagenous protein. In the event that a single cell protein makes up 10% w/w of the total cell protein we may expect this protein to contribute 1.6% to the weight of the total bone noncollagenous protein. Thus, it reasonably may be assumed that if an isolated bone protein constit-

uent makes up greater than 2% of the total non-collagenous matrix it most probably resides in the extracellular matrix site. This is a rule of thumb that depends of course upon the preparation and nature of the bone sample used for analysis. Cancellous bone and bone from embryonic tissues with higher cell contents, and more difficult removal of adhering tissues may be expected to have greater proportions of their organic contents associated with cells.

Before defining the materials isolated from bone tissue more specifically there is one further concept that must be borne in mind. The matrix of bone is impregnated with calcium phosphate mineral, which itself has a particular affinity for organic materials, and certain constituents may be found in bone because of this affinity. Bone tissue has been proved to act as a sink for many materials artificially introduced into the organism, some of which are of continuing concern to toxicologists and radiobiologists, and certain

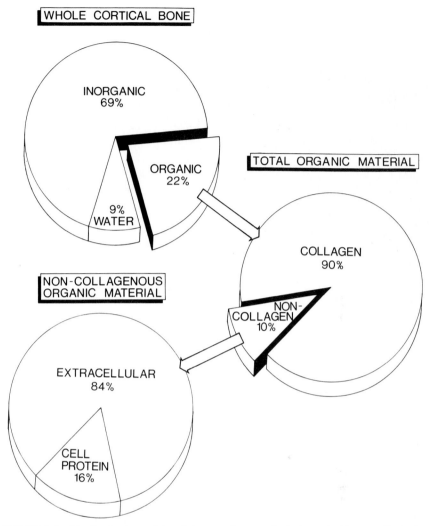

FIGURE 3-3   *Distribution by weight of the constituents of whole cortical bone to illustrate the proportion of cell protein in the organic material.*

naturally occurring substances may be accumulated in a similar manner. This will be discussed more fully in a later section.

General procedures for the isolation of constituents of bone organic matrix

The presence of hard insoluble mineral and the nature of the organic material in bone has made the application of standard biochemical techniques for the isolation of undenatured constituents very difficult. Initially, dilute acids (e.g., N

HCl, 0.05 N acetic acid) were used to decalcify the bone, but acid hydrolysis of labile constituents may occur. Progress has been made in defining general extraction schedules for the hydrophilic noncollagenous components, but these will be adapted for isolation of specific constituents in the future.[30]

To increase the efficiency of extraction of bone materials the mineral phase must be removed initially. This procedure is most satisfactorily performed by powdering the bone at liquid nitrogen temperature and subsequently using the calcium-chelating agent ethylenediaminetetraacetic acid (EDTA) in solutions at 4° C and buffered at physiologic pH over extended periods of the order of 1 wk. During this time—to inhibit bacterial growth and minimize endogenous enzyme action—inhibitors of these processes are added to the extraction solution.

The solution so obtained contains appreciable quantities of the noncollagenous components (about 68% of original) with only small amounts of collagen (1–2%) and can be subjected to further study, but a large proportion of the organic matrix remains insoluble. This is mainly collagen associated with the remaining 32% of the noncollagenous materials, and most of the latter can be released for study by employing highly purified collagenase enzyme to degrade the collagen. Unless converted into gelatin by boiling or by treatment with denaturing solvents (e.g., guanidinium chloride, urea, potassium thiocyanate), investigations on the mainly insoluble bone collagen requires special and direct reaction with chemicals (e.g., cyanogen bromide, sodium borohydride, periodate) or enzymes (e.g., trypsin, pepsin) to produce specific fragments that may be analyzed further. By using organic solvents, hydrophobic constituents (lipids) have been extracted from whole powdered bone tissue or from the residue obtained after EDTA extraction.

Bone collagen

General properties

Collagen is the major structural protein of the animal kingdom, and a tremendous research effort by many investigators over the past 25 yr has resulted in a detailed picture of its structure and biochemistry. Bone organic matrix consists almost entirely of this molecule, and its relative abundance in bone has resulted in it being investigated much more extensively than any other organic constituent present in this tissue. Only the salient features of this unique material that are related to an understanding of the nature of bone matrix will be described, and reference should be made to the following basic reviews of the biosynthesis, structure, and function of col-

lagen for a fuller discussion of the particular points mentioned.[4,22,48,49]

Collagen gives strength to, and makes up the structure of, various tissues and organs. A measure of this strength is described by the fact that a weight of 10 to 40 kg is necessary to break a collagen fiber of 1-mm diameter, and this high tensile strength combined with the resistance to compression of hydroxyapatite governs the unique load-bearing properties of the skeleton—an integrated structure that probably contributed to the evolutionary success of the vertebrates.[13] Bone contains generally parallel fibrils of collagen of even diameter, whose orientation changes through the thickness of the tissue, which is presumably related to the orientation of the secretory cell. Scanning electron microscopy of bone surfaces shows that adjacent collagen fibrils branch and interconnect in an intricate woven pattern (Fig. 3-4). Bone collagen fibril diameters vary widely in different species, but there is a general trend to being more closely packed and to having increased diameters with increasing age. The structure and arrangements of fibers, however, is similar to that seen in other tissue sites, and from x-ray diffraction data bone collagen does not differ markedly from other sources, nor are there any marked differences using the electron microscope.[18] With the electron microscope the collagen in bone and other tissues is seen to be made up of parallel microfibrils that have, when the tissue is stained, a characteristic pattern of cross-striations, or bands, with the most prominent bands being about 68 nm apart.

A major difficulty in the study of bone collagen, apart from the presence of mineral, is its almost complete insolubility regardless of the age of the animal from which the sample was derived. Its insolubility contrasts with the situation in soft tissues, in which collagen can be extracted by neutral salt solutions and dilute acids, and indicates that in bone collagen strong bonds cross-link and stabilize the constituent molecules to form an insoluble network. Earlier studies have dealt with the small proportion that can be solubilized and isolated in purified form, rather than the bulk of the insoluble material. More recently, however, attention has been di-

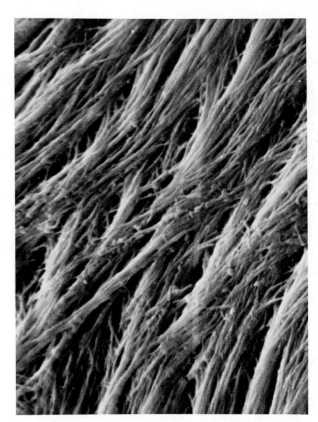

FIGURE 3-4 *Scanning electron micrograph of the surface of an adult rabbit bone matrix, showing how the collagen fibrils branch and interconnect in an intricate, woven pattern × 4800. (Provided by Dr. A. Boyde)*

rected toward the organization of the latter, quantitatively more important fraction.

Molecular and fibrillar structure

Analyses of soluble collagens isolated from numerous tissues have indicated that there is a basic molecular unit upon which the collagen fibers are built. This molecule has been named tropocollagen and it is a rod-like asymmetric molecule that in solution is approximately 300 nm in length and 1.5 nm in diameter. This protein molecule is built up of three individual polypeptide chains that have been called α-chains. In bone, two of the α-chains—denoted as α_1-chains—are identical, whereas the third, denoted as an α_2-chain, has a slightly different amino acid composition. Each α-chain contains about 1000 amino acid residues and has a molecular weight of about 95,000. For the majority (95%) of its length each α-chain is coiled in an extended helical conformation with no intra-

chain hydrogen bonding between the constituent amino acids. Still mainly in helical conformation, in the case of bone and certain other soft tissue collagens such as tendon and skin, two α_1-chains and one α_2-chain are coiled together in a super helix to form a triple helical collagen molecule of rope-like structure (Fig. 3-5**A**). Interchain hydrogen bonding between certain constituent amino acids of the α-chains are partially responsible for stabilizing the structure of the tropocollagen molecule. These bonds can be broken by denaturing agents or under suitable conditions of temperature change, and in newly synthesized collagen these bonds predominate. When the triple α-chain molecules aggregate to form fibers, there is a rapid introduction of more stable covalent bonds, which contributes to increased stability. These intermolecular bonds are formed between the terminal portions of the α-chains, which are not in the helical conformation already described, and the helical region of an adjacent molecule. The nonhelical regions of the tropocollagen molecule of some 15 to 30

a)

TRIPLE HELIX

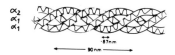

b)

PRIMARY STRUCTURE-TYPICAL AMINO-ACID SEQUENCE

GLY - PRO - Y - GLY - X - Y - GLY - X - HYP - GLY -

c)

PACKING OF TROPOCOLLAGEN MOLECULES IN THE COLLAGEN FIBRIL

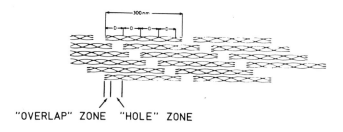

"OVERLAP" ZONE   "HOLE" ZONE

d)

APPEARANCE OF COLLAGEN FIBRIL IN ELECTRON MICROSCOPE

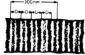

FIGURE 3-5 *Diagrammatic representation of* **(a)** *three constituent α-chains of tropocollagen wound into the superhelix;* **(b)** *typical amino acid sequence of the major portion of the tropocollagen molecule;* **(c)** *tropocollagen molecules approximately quarter-staggered with respect to each other in adjacent rows and showing overlapping of the ends of the molecules;* **(d)** *electron micrograph of negatively stained collagen fibril, showing the image resulting from relatively high amounts of electron-dense stain in the "hole zone" compared with the "overlap zone." (Bailey, A. J., and Robins, S. P.: Sci. Prog. (Lond.) 63:419–444, 1976)*

amino acid residues are called the telopeptides and are referred to as N- or C-terminal telopeptides depending upon their location. These regions are of great importance in linking the molecules in the final fiber and in fibrillogenesis. They are also the major antigenic regions of the collagen molecule and may be regarded as the remains of much longer nonhelical sequences that exist at each end of the molecule at an earlier intracellular stage.

This unique helical structure of the majority of the collagen molecule is a result of a peculiar amino acid sequence with a repeating structure, in which a glycine residue occupies every third amino acid residue position. This is an absolute requirement for the triple helical, coiled-coil structure of the molecule and does not exist in the telopeptide extension. The repeating tripeptide gly-X-Y frequently has a proline residue at X, and hydroxyproline residues are almost exclusively confined to position Y (Fig. 3-5**B**), these two imino-acid residues being in roughly equal proportions and together making up 21% of the total amino acids. The small glycine residues are located on the inside of the helical molecules and form hydrogen bonds with the amide group of the peptide bond of the adjacent chain. Hydroxyproline appears to stabilize the molecule by its hydrogen-bonding capacity, and another unusual amino acid, hydroxylysine, is present to the extent of 6 residues/1000 total amino acid residues. This amino acid carries the carbohydrate groups that are present in the molecule and is involved in the extremely important process of linking the molecules together in the intact fibers.

The pattern of bands seen with the electron microscope results from the tropocollagen molecules being arranged in the microfibril in a precise manner. Adjacent, parallel molecules are approximately quarter-staggered with respect to each other with a gap or "hole" of about 41 nm between the ends (Fig. 3-5**C**). This produces areas through the fibril in which the molecules overlap completely ("overlap zones") or in which they do not ("hole zones"). In negatively stained collagen fibrils the latter zones are filled with electron dense stain to give the axial periodicity of about 68 nm (Fig. 3-5**D**). There are also five charged regions on the tropocollagen molecule that are approximately 68 nm apart and that can be stained with electron dense stains. Because of the stagger of the molecules these polar regions are in the same plane through the fibril and a similar periodicity of about 68 nm is seen.

The way in which the collagen molecules are arranged and are packed three-dimensionally in the microfibril has been studied by using electron microscopic and x-ray diffraction techniques, and various models have been postulated, none of which are thought to define exactly the native situation. The most well-accepted concept that five tropocollagen molecules, in quarter-staggered array, are rolled into a cylinder yields a visualization (Fig. 3-6) of the five-stranded rope model of Smith.[67]

It was thought initially that all collagens, whatever the tissue of origin, had the basic structure of two α_1-chains and one α_2-chain, as already described. This was shown not to be the case, however, by the demonstration that cartilage contained three identical α-chains, having similar but not identical composition and chromatographic properties to the α_1-chains from bone, skin, or tendon collagens.[50] The latter, most prevalent collagen type was named, therefore, type I collagen and the constituent α_1-chains were designated α_1-type I or α_1 (I), to given a tropocollagen chain composition of $(\alpha_1 (I))_2\alpha_2$. The cartilage collagen was designated type II collagen with a chain composition $(\alpha_1 (II))_3$ or $(\alpha II)_3$. Other collagen types have been discovered in other tissue sites and the nomenclature extended to describe these additional molecules as shown in Table 3-1. This is an active area of investigation and it is likely that additional collagen types will be described in the near future.

With the detailed analysis of the individual α-chains it is apparent that marked chemical differences exist between the collagen types and that they are genetically distinct and have been called "isocollagens."[48] Bone tissue, however, consists almost entirely of type I collagen.[19]

Biosynthesis

To understand the make-up of bone organic matrix it is necessary to discuss certain aspects of the biosynthesis, carbohydrate content, and linking of the molecules in the type I collagen fiber.

The osteoblast synthesizes most of the constituents of the intercellular matrix in bone and collagen is no exception. It has been found that the insoluble extracellular protein is derived from a soluble cellular precursor molecule, and there is a complex sequence of reactions leading from the soluble monomeric collagen molecules within the cell to the assembly of the fibers in the extracellular space. The basic sequence of these steps is as illustrated in Fig. 3-7 but the exact order of the various intracellular and extracellular steps of collagen biosynthesis remains uncertain.

Collagen is synthesized on membrane-bound ribosomes and it appears that the three constituent α-chains are synthesized simultaneously,

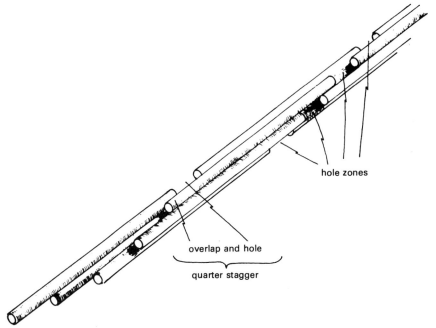

FIGURE 3-6 *Diagram illustrating the proposed three-dimensional organization of tropocollagen molecules in an approximately quarter-staggered, pentafibril arrangement.* (*Provided by Dr. A. J. Bailey*)

and the unmodified translated protein has been named "protocollagen."[22]

HYDROXYLATION

After translation, the primary structure of the α-chain is modified by hydroxylation of certain proline and lysine residues by specific enzymes to form the amino acids characteristically present in collagen—hydroxyproline and hydroxylysine. These hydroxylase enzymes require α-ketoglutarate, molecular oxygen, ferrous ion,

and ascorbic acid as cofactors, and if the supply of these cofactors is restricted by using, for example, the iron chelating agent $\alpha\alpha^1$ dipyridyl or by anaerobosis, inhibition of hydroxylation occurs and collagen secretion from the cell is inhibited. In scurvy the lack of ascorbic acid leads to decreased hydroxylation and gives rise to particular skeletal lesions with the bone cortex becoming thin and fragile and osteoid formation being reduced.[76] Once the helical structure of the molecule is formed, no further hydroxylation occurs and an almost complete helical structure is required before secretion from the cell.

TABLE 3-1 TYPES OF COLLAGEN

TYPE	MOLECULAR FORMULA	TISSUE	HYDROXYLYSINE RESIDUES/10^3 AMINO ACID RESIDUES	CARBOHYDRATE (% HYDROXYLYSINE GLYCOSYLATED)
I	$[\alpha 1(I)]_2\alpha 2$	Bone, dentine, skin, tendon, blood vessel wall, gastrointestinal tract	6–8	<20
II	$[\alpha II]_3$	Cartilages	20–25	50
III	$[\alpha III]_3$	Skin, blood vessel wall, synovial membrane, gastrointestinal tract, dentine	6–8	15–20
IV	$[\alpha IV]_3$?	Basement membranes	60–70	80
V	$[\alpha B]_2\alpha A$?	Basement membranes	6–8	20

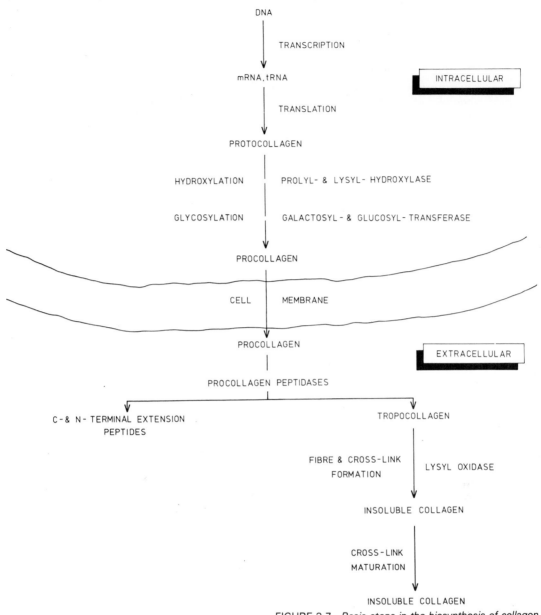

FIGURE 3-7 *Basic steps in the biosynthesis of collagen.*

GLYCOSYLATION

At certain positions in the molecule, specific hydroxylysine residues are further modified by attachment of a monosaccharide (galactosyl) residue or a disaccharide (glucosylgalactosyl) residue, so that by its content of carbohydrate residues collagen can be classified as a glycoprotein. Although tissue variation exists in the glycosylation of the different collagens and in the proportion of monosaccharide or disaccharide substitutions, no particular function can as yet be definitely allotted to these moieties.

PROCOLLAGEN

The various biosynthetic reactions result in a collagen molecule in the cell that, when compared with the basic building block of the fiber—tropocollagen—has extension peptides on

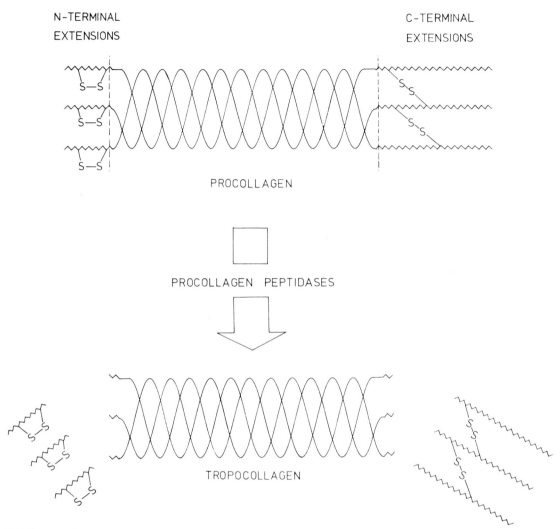

FIGURE 3-8 *Conversion of procollagen to tropocollagen in the extracellular space with the release of the C-terminal and N-terminal extension peptides.*

each α-chain having a molecular weight of about 15,000 at the N-terminus and of about 35,000 at the C-terminus. This molecule has been named procollagen. The C-terminal peptide has interchain disulfide bonds and may be involved in registering the molecule in an array suitable for triple helix formation. These extension peptides may also aid transport from the cell through the cell membrane and extracellular space. Extracellularly the extension peptides are cleaved intact from the soluble procollagen by specific endopeptidase enzymes—the procollagen peptidases (Fig. 3-8). A hereditary defect in cattle, dermatosparaxis, results in a deficit in the procol-

lagen peptidase responsible for cleavage of the N-terminal extension peptides. This apparently interferes with the deposition of the molecules, so that the fibers are abnormally formed and cross-linked. The C-terminal peptide is thought to be cleaved by another enzyme. In dermatosparaxis the collagen framework is less abundant than in normal bone, but the chemical differences compared with normal bone are relatively small. This reduction in collagen content is accompanied by an increased mineral content indicating that although abnormal collagen is formed, calcification does occur.[53]

The subsequent fate of the peptides released

from the procollagen molecule in bone tissue has not been established. It is possible that they may be retained in the matrix by an affinity for the bone mineral or by specific interaction with the organic constituents, and it has been suggested that they may exert feedback control on collagen synthesis.

CROSS-LINK FORMATION

The resultant, mainly helical tropocollagen molecules are virtually insoluble in physiologic fluids and are built up into stable microfibrils by intermolecular cross-linking. The cross-links are formed by oxidative deamination of specific lysine or OH-lysine residues in the nonhelical N- and C-telopeptides by a copper-dependent amino-oxidase enzyme, lysyl oxidase. The

C-terminal telopeptides are thus restricted to intermolecular cross-linking, whereas the N-terminal telopeptides may also participate in intramolecular cross-link formation but to a much lesser extent. Intramolecular cross-links, between the constituent α-chains of the tropocollagen molecule, are probably insignificant in bone tissue and most if not all cross-links are intermolecular between the tropocollagen molecules. The aldehydes produced are then believed to condense with mainly ε-NH_2 groups of OH-lysine in the helical region of adjacent molecues to form a bonding network of intermolecular cross-links. The major cross-links in bone collagen are derived from two residues of hydroxylysine or to a lesser extent from one residue of hydroxylysine and one residue of lysine (Fig. 3-9). The relative amounts are governed by the

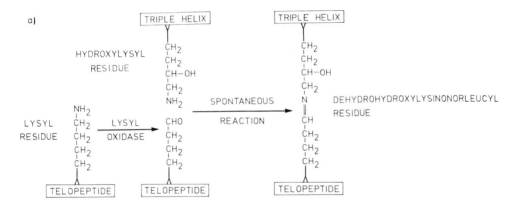

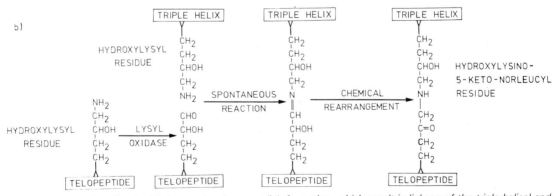

FIGURE 3-9 *Reactions involved in intermolecular cross-link formation, which result in linkage of the triple helical and telopeptide portions of adjacent tropocollagen molecules. The chemical cross-link formed by reaction* **(a)** *(aldamine type) is chemically less stable than that formed by reaction* **(b),** *in which a chemical bond (keto-imine type) is derived from two hydroxylsyl residues. The type of cross-link formed by reaction* **(b)** *is predominant in bone tissue.*

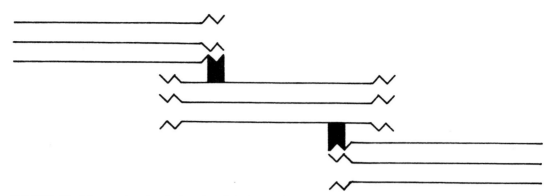

FIGURE 3-10 *Diagram showing the location of the intermolecular cross-links in the collagen fibril and involving the N- and C-terminal telopeptides. (After Bailey, A. J., and Robins, S. P.: Sci. Prog. 63:419–444, 1976)*

extent of hydroxylation of the lysine residues in the telopeptide regions, and in bone the hydroxylation process at this site is almost complete. This pattern of cross-linking may contribute significantly to the distinctive solubility properties of bone collagen, but interactions of the collagen microfibrils with other matrix components are almost certainly involved. Thus the intermolecular links are between the N- or C-terminal telopeptide and the triple helical portions of the tropocollagen molecules, and furthermore, it is the overlap regions near the ends of the helical regions that are involved (Fig. 3-10). These cross-links predominate in young tissue, but with age and maturity of the tissue other more complex interfibrillar cross-links form. These are most probably derived in some way from the reducible cross-links already described. The nature of these mature cross-links, however, remains to be elucidated. It has been suggested that cross-links also form between the tropocollagen helices but this is considered unlikely and no direct evidence is available for their existence.[44]

STRUCTURE-FUNCTION RELATIONSHIPS

Since the amino acid compositions and sequences of the corresponding α-chains of type I collagens from different tissues of the same species are remarkably similar, the post-translational changes and chemical interactions between other matrix components are of major importance in determining the properties characteristic of the tissues of origin.[45]

In bone collagen the molecules appear to be spaced further apart than in the soft tissues and this could be of importance in providing space for the deposition of mineral in the definite pattern that is observed.[36] A great deal of effort has been directed toward determining whether bone collagen has specific chemical properties that would explain why this tissue mineralizes, whereas the soft tissues containing the same collagen type do not mineralize. Hydroxylysine content and glycosylation vary widely between and within collagen types (see Table 3-1), and there is no obvious relationship between the amount of hydroxylation or glycosylation and calcification. In the future much more work will be designed to assess the post-translational modifications at different sites that confer the specific tissue properties. As mentioned earlier, the pattern of cross-linking is different in bone compared with soft tissue collagen and appears attributable to the relatively large amount of hydroxylysine in the bone telopeptide, even though bone collagen generally tends to have a relatively low content of hydroxylysine.[6] However, cross-linking does not affect calcification, since in lathyritic bone, in which administration of the sweet-pea extract β-amino propionitrile (BAPN) inhibits lysyl oxidase and subsequent cross-link formation, calcification does occur. The use of BAPN to form lathyritic bone has proved extremely useful in studies on bone collagen, as the lack of cross-linking results in soluble collagen that can be characterized chemically.

The suggestion that bone collagen is involved in the organization of the initial crystal nuclei[20] has been challenged by observations that although earlier collagen preparations initiated *in vitro* precipitation of calcium phosphates from metastable solutions, highly purified reconstituted collagen fibrils function poorly in this respect.[3] Also, *in vivo* initial calcification is seen to occur in association with the interfibrillar ground substance rather than with the collagen fibers.[9,70] However, Cohen-Solal and colleagues[12] have shown that highly purified chicken bone collagen contains 20% of the total protein-bound organic phosphorus in the bone, and that it is present principally in the α_2-chains. This phosphorus is not present as a phosphorylated hydroxy amino acid, as a phosphoamidated amino acid, or a phosphorylated sugar, and there are four to five atoms of organic phosphorus molecule of collagen. It is suggested that at least part of the bone collagen organic phosphorus is present as phosphorylated glutamic acid, and this organically bound phosphorus could be of importance in the interactions with mineral ions during calcification.

In any event, it is obvious that the proper structure of bone tissue depends on the normal biosynthesis of its major constituents and on the normal remodeling processes. The majority of the collagen that is synthesized by the cell and deposited in the matrix in bone remains after calcification until specific extracellular and intracellular enzymic reactions are initiated by the osteoclasts and osteocytes or, abnormally, by invasive cancerous cells. The degradation of collagen fibers during remodeling processes is therefore under cellular control, and an account of these processes is presented elsewhere in this book. Any defects occurring in the genetic machinery of the osteoblast and in subsequent transcription, translation, and post-translation processes may be expected to impart varying degrees of defect in the structural integrity and functioning of bone. Various diseases of the muscular-skeletal system, which have been described in humans and are under current investigation, have been attributed to collagen abnormalities. A form of Ehlers-Danlos syndrome (type VI hydroxylysine deficiency disease) results from a specific enzyme defect of lysyl hydroxylase with alteration in cross-linking.[57]

Ehlers-Danlos syndrome type VII is analogous to dermatosparaxis in the calf with a defect in the enzymic conversion of procollagen to collagen.[43] Some forms of osteogenesis imperfecta may result from a reduction in the amount of type I collagen in bone tissue, which in some unknown way leads to the brittle bones present in this condition.[51,56] As more knowledge is gained of the biosynthesis and structure of collagen the molecular basis of the defects occurring in certain bone diseases will become more fully understood.

Noncollagenous constituents of compact bone tissue

The noncollagenous constituents of bone tissue are defined as the constituents of the organic material of compact bone that are not accounted for by the collagen content. The collagen content is calculated from hydroxyproline analysis or from the susceptibility to the specific bacterial collagenase enzyme. Whether or not they contain remnants of the procollagen molecule, for example, has not been determined.

These constituents make up approximately 10% of the weight of the organic matrix and are chiefly noncollagenous proteins with smaller proportions of proteoglycans and lipids. Quantitatively they are minor constituents of bone tissue, but the noncollagenous proteins especially are receiving increasing attention with respect to their possible involvement in the structural integrity and in the physiologic properties and function of bone tissue. These proteins are mainly glycoproteins that are macromolecules containing protein and carbohydrate linked together by covalent bonds. They are defined by Gottschalk[21] and are characterized by their carbohydrate prosthetic groups that have a relatively low number of sugar residues that show no repeating pattern along the chains. The increase in attention given to the noncollagenous components is not only because of the application of new methods of extraction, separation, and analysis but also because of the continuing quest to define the biochemical changes resulting in mineralization of the matrix. Also, until the constituents of normally mineralized tissue are more completely defined biochemically, it is impossible to investigate how they may influence the process of mineralization and difficult to assess the relevance of any changes that may occur in the bone matrix in certain bone diseases.

As mentioned earlier, it must be remembered that samples of bone tissue, even compact bone, contain cellular elements. An unknown but probably small proportion of these elements are derived from the many blood vessels present throughout the tissue and from connective tissues in the haversian canals and on the periosteal and endosteal surfaces. The presence of blood plasma, which contains 7% protein (w/w), in the bone blood vessels also contributes to the nonhomogeneity of the starting material for biochemical study. These factors, together with the presence of newly synthesized noncalcified matrix at microscopic sites, emphasizes the need for cautious interpretation of the origins and location of certain of the materials discovered to be present in any bone sample. This will become apparent as the noncollagenous constituents that have been isolated from bone tissue are described in more detail.

Noncollagenous proteins

In the section on procedures for isolating bone matrix constituents it was noted that mild extraction of the organic constituents of powdered bone requires the removal of mineral with solutions of EDTA at about a neutral pH. The resultant solution contains up to about two thirds of the noncollagenous proteins. This does not necessarily mean that these substances are directly associated with the mineral phase in the tissue. Mineral removal could merely allow their release from diffusion-locked sites—this being dependent, of course, upon their solubility in the EDTA solution used and on their lack of interaction with the remaining insoluble matter under the extraction conditions. Because of the relative ease of its preparation, many studies have concentrated on these materials extracted by EDTA solutions. The one third of the noncollagenous proteins that remain insoluble and are associated with the mainly collagenous residue after this

treatment have been studied in more detail recently and have been credited with having some very interesting properties that will be mentioned later. Certain of these constituents can be released for study by using commercially available purified bacterial collagenases that have little detectable protease activity. Although some of these constituents are related to those extracted by EDTA solutions, others appear specifically released by this digestion procedure. Little work has been done on the small amounts of material that remain after collagenase digestion, but it has been suggested this may be involved in the structure of bone and is similar perhaps to the structural glycoproteins seen in other connective tissues.[62]

It is not intended here to survey the whole spectrum of the many noncollagenous proteins in bone tissue. Only those proteins that have been isolated in a form pure enough for meaningful chemical analysis or whose identities have been established by other means will be described.

SIALOPROTEINS

Studies by Vaughan[75] on the peculiar location of the transuranic elements in bone tissue showed that there was a particular association of plutonium with the bone surfaces and that these stained strongly positive with the periodic acid-Schiff (PAS) technique. This led to comprehensive studies culminating in a detailed description of the purification of a protein, from EDTA extracts of bovine bone, which contained high levels of sialic acid (15.9% w/w) and was named sialoprotein.[31] During the next decade the chemical and physiochemical properties and ion-binding characteristics were investigated[27] and until relatively recently bone sialoprotein could be described as "the best characterised connective tissue glycoprotein in terms of both structure and properties."[1]

The amount of sialoprotein in bovine bone has been calculated from the average sialic acid content of bovine sialoprotein, and the proportion of the total bone sialic acid that is present in sialoprotein separated chromatographically on Diethylaminoethyl (DEAE)-cellulose. It is found to make up about 8% (w/w) of the noncollagenous matrix of bone tissue. Other studies indicated heterogeneity in the sialic acid content of different preparations. This possibly results from the greater ease of extraction of sialoprotein with high sialic acid content. Thus more efficient extractions, with higher yields, result in preparations of lower sialic acid content (about 14% w/w). Most of the sialic acid is present as N-acetylneuraminic acid with about one tenth of the total sialic acid as the N-glycolyl derivative. Carbohydrate residues make up about 40% by weight of the molecule, and sialic acid can account for up to half of this value. Mild acid and alkali hydrolysis and periodate oxidation studies suggest that the carbohydrate is contained in a single, highly branched group of unusually high molecular weight (9220). Sialic acid and fucose residues occupy terminal residue positions, and the probable sequence of the other carbohydrate residues is as shown in Figure 3-11, which is a diagrammatic representation of the tentative structure of bovine sialoprotein.

The amino acid composition of bovine bone sialoprotein (Table 3-2) shows that acidic residues—aspartate and glutamate—together make up 40% of the total amino acid residues,

and 80% of these are present in the acid form rather than as the amide derivatives. Also present are 2 to 4 mol of phosphate/mole of protein, most probably as serine esters, which further increases the acidic nature of the polypeptide chain. Neither the amino acid sequence nor the N-terminal amino acids are known, and no free N-terminal amino group can be detected. Proteolytic digestion by using the enzyme pronase has been used to produce small peptides containing carbohydrate (glycopeptides). Analysis of these glycopeptides showed that those containing 20 to 25 amino acid residues contained only 7 to 9% acidic amino acid residues. Thus, it is suggested that the carbohydrate is linked to regions in the protein that are relatively devoid of acidic residues. This must mean, therefore, that the rest of the polypeptide chain has over half its total amino acids as aspartate or glutamate.

Molecular weight measurements obtained by using the ultracentrifuge show that the molecular weight of sialoprotein is about 25,000 when isolated from EDTA extracts or 21,800 when isolated from phosphate-extracted, acid-demineralized bone. An increased polydispersity of the molecule extracted by the latter method was suggestive of greater degradation, which possibly explains the observed decrease in molecular weight. It was also found that the molecule extracted by the former method sedimented slower in the ultracentrifuge than would a spherical molecule of the same molecular weight and density. This could result from a nonspherical, elongated structure or from a spherical structure having an expanded and open network.

As described earlier, the original object of the studies on sialoprotein was radiobiologic in nature, and the binding of "bone-seeking radionuclides" to this glycoprotein and to other fractions isolated during the course of these studies has been well documented.[26] It has been found that the high binding of plutonium by sialoprotein could partially account for its distinctive location in bone. But other glycoprotein and chondroitin sulfate fractions were found to bind plutonium strongly also, although binding to collagen was low.

Possibly of more significance to the normal physiology of bone are studies on calcium bind-

STRUCTURE OF BSP

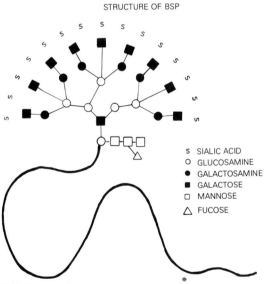

S SIALIC ACID
O GLUCOSAMINE
● GALACTOSAMINE
■ GALACTOSE
□ MANNOSE
△ FUCOSE

FIGURE 3-11 *Possible structure of bovine bone sialoprotein. (Herring, G. M.: In Bourne, G. H. (ed.): The Biochemistry and Physiology of Bone, 2nd edition, Vol. 1, New York, Academic press, 1972)*

TABLE 3-2 AMINO ACID COMPOSITIONS OF SIALOPROTEINS ISOLATED FROM VARIOUS SPECIES (EXPRESSED AS AMINO ACID RESIDUES/1000 RESIDUES)

AMINO ACID	BOVINE[27]	HUMAN[65]	RABBIT[46]	RABBIT[11]
Asp	174	166	128	120
Thr	111	125	105	49
Ser	80	76	199	52
Glu	229	233	210	193
Pro	49	41	42	78
Gly	122	102	136	70
Ala	40	47	84	99
Cys	13			9
Val	31	28	24	69
Met	0	0	0	0
Ile	25	26	9	28
Leu	29	26	10	68
Tyr	22	41	0	18
Phe	11	29	17	26
Lys	29	33	24	57
His	12	13	15	47
Arg	12	15		17
Trp	11			

ing that demonstrate a binding of calcium to sialoprotein that, although relatively low, is significantly higher than that for chondroitin sulfate. The fact that calcium is bound by sialoprotein is not surprising in view of its overall acidic nature, but removal of sialic acid by mild acid hydrolysis seems to have little effect on this binding. This is an interesting observation as at physiologic pH, sialic acid is said generally to be strongly and preferentially complexed with calcium ions,[35] but it appears that the free carboxyl groups in the peptide chain of sialoprotein contribute almost entirely to its calcium-binding activity.

When added to buffered solutions of calcium and phosphate ions, sialoprotein reduces the amount of calcium phosphate precipitate deposited initially. With time, a second precipitate appears that is more difficult to separate by centrifugation and is thought to be of different crystalline nature. As the concentration of sialoprotein is raised, more protein is found associated with the second precipitate, and this has been interpreted to mean that the physicochemical nature of the calcium phosphate produced is altered. This may have some relevance to the nature of the bone mineral produced *in vivo*, and these preliminary experiments should be reinvestigated.

So far, no glycoprotein of similar characteristics has been isolated from other connective tissues, and it is possible that this material is specific to bone tissue. It occurs in the free state in bovine bone, but in complexed form it may be involved in the structural make-up of bone, as will be described when bone proteoglycans are discussed. Its identity and homogeneity as a single molecular species has been based on the criteria of having a single peak in the ultracentrifuge and a single band on cellulose acetate electrophoresis. With the advent of more critical criteria for protein homogeneity since this work was performed, it is important that these techniques be applied to bovine sialoprotein preparations. Although possibly a difficult substance to raise antibodies against, because of its low molecular weight and highly acidic character, immunochemical criteria would help to resolve the specific localization of sialoprotein in bone tissue.

Nevertheless, there is no doubt that bone tissue from various species (ox, human, rabbit, rat, fish, sheep) contains sialic acid-rich protein molecules (sialoglycoproteins) that are readily detected by their strong binding to anion exchangers. None of those analyzed so far contain the very high levels of sialic acid seen in bovine bone, and human bone sialoprotein is the only one that has been isolated, albeit in low yield (13 mg from 100 g bone), with closely similar composition (see Table 3-2). Sheep bone lacks free sialoprotein but does have sialic-acid complexes associated with proteoglycan similar to the bovine situation. Rabbit bone has been noted to contain a quite different sialoglycoprotein fraction[11] (see Table 3-2) and here the situation is complex. Some of the sialic acid is associated with a keratan sulfate-like substance linked to a sialoglycoprotein core[46] (see Table 3-2), and our recent studies indicate that there are a number of other sialoglycoproteins present. New methods of separation of these constituents from rabbit bone need to be developed before their characteristics can be determined. Studies on the function and metabolism of these macromolecules in bone awaits clarification of the chemical nature of the individual sialoglycoproteins in a more convenient experimental animal than the ox.

The plasma membranes of cells may contain up to 3% sialic acid by weight of protein,[77] with individual proteins having a higher content, and it is probable that at least some of the sialoglycoproteins present in bone extracts are located in cells. Estimates of the amount of bovine sialoprotein in bone seem too large to be accounted for as a cellular constituent and on this basis this component is present in the extracellular matrix.

PHOSPHOPROTEINS

Proteins containing 0.15 to 0.3% of phosphate have been isolated as single components from bovine femur cortex and jaw bone and from chicken metacarpal bone by a series of chromatographic procedures.[68] In these molecular species the phosphate is bound to the hydroxyl group of serine residues to give a primary phosphate ester group, producing phosphoserine (Fig. 3-12). Almost any phosphate-containing compound has a strong attraction for calcium, and the presence of this moiety in bone tissue is of interest, as it has been proposed that matrix-bound organic phosphorus plays an essential role in the initiation of calcification.[20] However, the phosphate content is relatively low compared with other phosphate-containing compounds isolated from tooth dentin (4% phosphorus w/w),

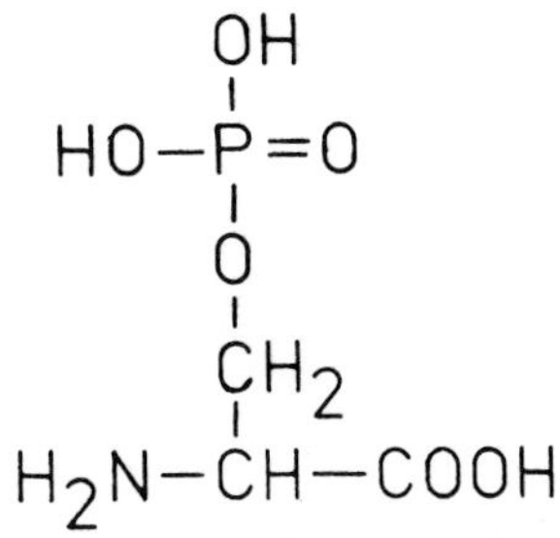

FIGURE 3-12 *Chemical structure of phosphoserine.*

and there is no similarity in general composition between these substances isolated from the two different calcified tissues. The bone phosphoproteins have high levels of glutamic and aspartic acids and relatively low levels of serine, whereas the dentine phosphoproteins ("phosphophoryns"[15]) are very rich in aspartic acid and serine. The "phosphophoryns" are found as EDTA-soluble and insoluble forms; the latter are thought to be intimately associated with dentin collagen and covalently bound by way of the disaccharide groups on the glycosylated collagen molecule. This does not seem to be the case in bone, for although periodate cleavage[66] or collagenase digestion[39,40] of bone collagen releases components containing low amounts of phosphate, their compositions are very different from those soluble in EDTA. Recently Cohen-Solal and colleagues[12] have concluded that none of the phosphoproteins in chicken bone are covalently bound to collagen. A small proportion (5–10%) of the total phosphoproteins seem more intimately bound to the collagen than those extractable by EDTA solutions, but these can be dissociated from the collagen by denaturant solutions.

γ-CARBOXYGLUTAMIC ACID-CONTAINING PROTEINS

γ-Carboxyglutamic acid is a newly discovered amino acid, whose structure has been established by mass spectrometry and is indicated in Figure 3-13**A**. As can be seen from this structure, γ-carboxyglutamic acid (Gla) can be derived from glutamic acid (Fig. 3-13**B**) by substitution of a carboxyl group on the γ-carbon atom. It has been found that this modification occurs *in vivo*

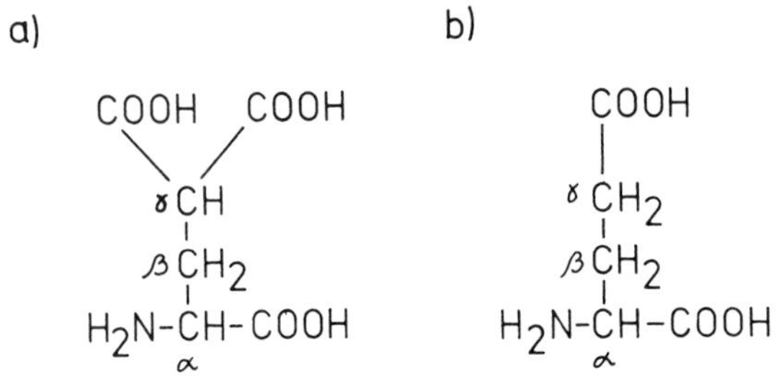

a)

COOH COOH
  \   /
   δCH
   |
   βCH$_2$
   |
H$_2$N-CH-COOH
       α

b)

COOH
 |
δCH$_2$
 |
βCH$_2$
 |
H$_2$N-CH-COOH
       α

FIGURE 3-13 *Chemical structures of* **(a)** *γ-carboxy-glutamic acid and* **(b)** *glutamic acid.*

when the glutamic acid is in peptide linkage by an enzymic reaction that requires vitamin K and bicarbonate ion.

This amino acid was first found in prothrombin, and specific glutamic acid residues at selected sites on the polypeptide chain are converted to Gla in post-translational events. Subsequently, other blood clotting factors (factors VI, IX, and X) and other blood proteins were found to contain Gla, and this discovery provided a molecular basis for elegant studies on the requirement of vitamin K in the blood coagulation process.[69] Gla residues in these proteins act as calcium-binding sites that are essential for calcium- and phospholipid-dependent activation of hemostasis. Thus, during vitamin K deficiency, or when vitamin K metabolism is antagonized with dicoumarin or warfarin, the conversion of glutamic acid to Gla is inhibited, and the synthesized proteins lack these residues. In these cases only weak interaction with calcium ions occurs, probably caused by nonspecific binding mainly to sites rich in carboxyl groups. This association of calcium binding by proteins with Gla content has led to the suggestion that any protein exhibiting calcium binding should be assessed for its Gla content.

In the blood coagulation system protein-phospholipid interactions occur that result in controlled proteolytic activation of the various factors. These complex processes are mediated through calcium binding to Gla residues present in the protein coagulation factors. The features of this system led two American groups working in Boston and La Jolla to search for the presence of Gla-containing proteins in bone tissue. Independent confirmation of components that contained this amino acid and were isolated from chicken and bovine bone resulted, and were named osteocalcin by the Harvard group and Gla-protein by the California group. This nomenclature will be retained here to distinguish the results of the studies performed by these two groups, which are referred to in recent publications by Nishimoto and Price[52a] and by Lian and colleagues.[42] These proteins are species equivalents and Gla-containing proteins are indeed present in dentine and bone tissue from a wide selection of vertebrates ranging from swordfish to humans. Some of the Gla-containing proteins have been purified and this amino acid has been shown to be present also in the proteins associated with the mineral deposits in renal calcium-stone disease and in atherosclerotic plaque. Calcified cartilage from elasmobranchs or from calf epiphyses, and tooth enamel were reported initially to contain only insignificant amounts of this amino acid[59a]. Recently these calcified cartilages have been shown to contain significant amounts of Gla[20a]. The most calcified bovine cartilage fractions contained as much Gla as did bone tissue. However, the whole calcified cartilage tissue contained only 2 residues of this amino acid per 10^5 total amino acid residues, compared with 45 residues of Gla per 10^5 total amino acid residues found in whole cortical bone. Uncalcified epiphyseal bovine cartilage contains insignificant, and bovine enamel undetectable, amounts of this amino acid.

There are important differences in the amino acid composition of the chicken and bovine Gla-containing proteins (Table 3-3). Thus although neither protein contains threonine or methionine, the chicken protein also contains no hydroxyproline, cysteine, histidine, lysine, or trytophan, unlike the bovine protein. The lack of hydroxyproline in the initial description of bovine Gla-protein was reported to be in error, and similarly the number of total amino acid residues in the molecule has been reduced from 59 to 49.

Since almost all the Gla in bone is contained in a single protein, the amount of this protein can be calculated from the total Gla content of bone. Such a calculation shows that this protein makes up 0.5 to 1% of the total amount of all proteins in bone—or about 5 to 10% of the noncollagen-

TABLE 3-3 AMINO ACID COMPOSITIONS (AMINO-ACID RESIDUES PER MOLE) OF GLA-CONTAINING BONE PROTEINS

	BOVINE[58]	CHICKEN[24]
Gla	3	4
Hyp	1	0
Asp	6	6
Thr	0	0
Ser	0	3
Glu	3	7
Pro	6	7
Gly	3	6
Ala	4	6
Cys ½	2	0
Val	2	3
Met	0	0
Ile	1	1
Leu	5	4
Tyr	4	3
Phe	2	3
His	2	0
Lys	1	0
Trp	1	0
Arg	3	4
Total residues	49	57

elimination of the γ-carboxyl group as carbon dioxide under acidic conditions. Nevertheless, the interest in these materials is directly related to their content of this peculiar amino acid that confers specific properties to these molecules. Analyses of Gla in proteins is now relatively easily performed by the use of alkaline hydrolysis procedures before amino acid analysis, since under these conditions the amino acid is stable.[23]

The sequence of amino acids in the polypeptide chain has been established for the 49-residue Gla-protein (Fig. 3-14). There is no homology in the amino acid sequence of this protein when compared with the blood proteins that contain Gla, and the molecular weights and amino acid compositions are very different. The presence of Gla in bone, therefore, cannot be accounted for by the accumulation of these factors in bone tissue. The three Gla residues in the molecule occur at positions 17, 21, and 24, and a disulfide bond links positions 23 and 29. Swordfish Gla-protein is reported to have a very similar sequence with three Gla residues and a disulfide bond in identical positions to those found in the bovine protein.

The synthesis of Gla-containing proteins has been shown to be vitamin K–dependent in the case of chick and bovine bone. Thus chicks fed a diet that is vitamin K–deficient or that contains dicoumarin show a reduced bone Gla content as do chick embryos treated with warfarin. The bone osteocalcin from chicks fed with vitamin K antagonists contains 50 to 80% less Gla than do controls, and the purified osteocalcin shows sev-

ous organic material—and is a true constituent of the extracellular matrix. So the Gla-containing proteins are some of the most abundant of the noncollagenous proteins in bone and were probably detected in bone fractions studied by earlier workers, and certainly materials with similar general properties have been described.[2,68] Gla was not discovered earlier, however, since the free amino acid released during routine acid hydrolysis for amino acid analysis of these materials is rapidly converted to glutamic acid by

Tyr-Leu-Asp-His-Trp-Leu-Gly-Ala-Hyp-Ala-Pro-Tyr-Pro-Asp-Pro-

        17   21   24
Leu-Gla -Pro -Lys-Arg-Gla -Val -Cys-Gla -Leu-Asn-Pro-Asp-Cys - Asp-

Glu-Leu-Ala -Asp-His-Ile -Gly -Phe-Gln -Glu-Ala -Tyr- Arg - Arg -Phe-

Tyr-Gly - Pro -Val

FIGURE 3-14 *The sequence of amino acid residues in the bovine Gla protein, showing the presence of Gla at positions 17, 21, and 24 and the presence of a disulfide bond between positions 23 and 29. (After Price, P. A., Poser, J. W., and Raman, N.: Proc. Natl. Acad. Sci. (USA) 73:3374–3375, 1976)*

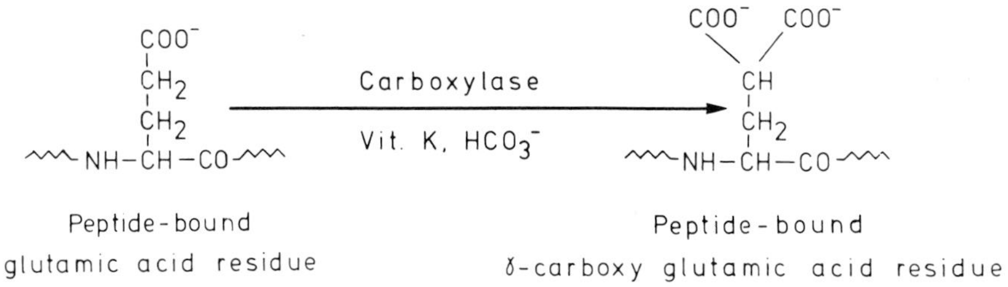

FIGURE 3-15 *Synthesis of peptide-bound γ-carboxyglutamic acid by a vitamin K–dependent, post-translational, enzymic reaction.*

eral under-carboxylated species containing two and three Gla residues/molecule rather than the four residues as seen in control birds. Bone defects have been noted in fetuses and children of women who have received anticoagulant therapy during pregnancy. In *in vitro* culture, embryonic chick bone from the limb, mandible, or calvarium, or trabecular or cortical bone from the metacarpals of calves have all been shown to synthesize the particular Gla-containing proteins. Incorporation of radioactivity from ^{14}C-labeled bicarbonate into chick bone osteocalcin or from ^{3}H-proline into bovine bone Gla-protein showed this synthesis. The appearance of osteocalcin in the chick embryo has been shown to coincide with the onset of mineralization, but what effect the protein has on this process is not known.

The microsomal carboxylase enzyme system that synthesizes Gla and that is present in liver, kidney, and placenta has also been demonstrated in microsomes prepared from embryonic bone. The carboxylation process is diagrammatically represented in Fig. 3-15.

It has been conclusively demonstrated, therefore, that the cells present in the bone specimens used by these two groups are responsible for the synthesis of the Gla-containing proteins. Whether this ability is related to particular cells cannot be decided on the evidence available. With the production of specific antibody now achieved in California,[52a] this and other important questions concerning the origins and metabolism of these proteins doubtless will soon be resolved.

Binding of calcium by chick osteocalcin was first shown by the reduction in electrophoretic mobility of the molecule in agarose gels in the presence of calcium ions compared with the situation in which calcium ion concentrations was reduced by chelation with EDTA. More precise and extensive quantitative measurements of the calcium-binding affinity by equilibrium dialysis methods show both high- and low-affinity calcium binding sites for chick osteocalcin, but only low affinity sites for bovine Gla-protein.

Gla-protein has been shown to bind to hydroxyapatite selectively *in vitro* with little affinity for amorphous calcium phosphate. This suggests a particular orientation of the binding sites on the protein molecule that is responsible for the interaction with the crystal surface, as both types of mineral phase contain ionized calcium and phosphate groups. This could also explain the observed inhibition of precipitation of hydroxyapatite from supersaturated solutions that is caused by this protein by the inhibition of growth of crystal nuclei by specific protein binding. Osteocalcin also inhibits the phase transformation that occurs before hydroxyapatite is formed *in vitro*. Whether the Gla-containing proteins exert an influence on these processes of mineral formation or on the subsequent stability and solubility of the mineral once it is formed *in vivo* is unknown, and the fact remains that no definite function *in vivo* has been found.

The presence of Gla-containing proteins in bone may be adventitious because of their affinity for crystals—albeit possibly a remnant of an unknown biochemical event occurring locally in the tissue. The accumulation noted in extraskeletal sites in artherosclerotic plaque and in renal calcium stone disease could also be purely by accumulation from the surrounding tissue fluids.

A large amount of speculation has resulted from the inference that Gla-containing proteins

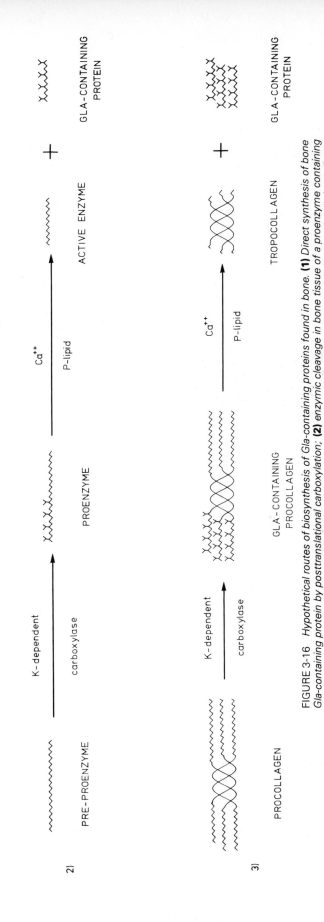

FIGURE 3-16 Hypothetical routes of biosynthesis of Gla-containing proteins found in bone. (1) Direct synthesis of bone Gla-containing protein by posttranslational carboxylation; (2) enzymic cleavage in bone tissue of a proenzyme containing Gla residues and release of the Gla-containing protein as a fragment; (3) release of Gla-containing proteins during collagen fibril synthesis. The ratio of tropocollagen to osteocalcin found in bone tissue is 1:1 or 2:1 but because of its small molecular size, it is possible that a proportion of the Gla-containing protein is lost from the calcified matrix. (After Lian, J. B., Hauschka, P. V., and Gallop, P. M.: Fed. Proc. 37:2615–2620, 1978)

in bone tissue may have similar biochemical transformations to the Gla-containing factors operative in blood coagulation. The presence of phospholipids at the mineralizing front adds further credence to this concept. Some of the possibilities published recently are described in Fig. 3-16 and doubtless these will be tested in future research.

PLASMA PROTEINS

A sample of compact bone tissue contains small but variable amounts of blood vessels, and it is not surprising to find that blood plasma proteins are found in the solutions used to extract these samples. Plasma albumin, γ-globulins, and α-glycoproteins have been detected in extracts by electrophoretic and immunochemical means and were originally considered to reflect the contents of the bone vascular spaces. In most other tissues of the body, however, the proteins found in plasma are also found in extravascular sites because of the variable leakiness of the blood capillaries. The possibility exists that a similar situation occurs in bone.

In order to describe recent findings in our laboratory it is necessary to consider the major extravascular compartments in compact bone. These compartments are shown diagrammatically in Figure 3-17**B** with the actual appearance of a cross-section of rabbit femur cortex presented in Figure 3-17**A**. It should not be assumed that at a particular horizontal plane in bone there is a direct connection—by way of the canalicular-lacunar network—of one side of the bone with the other, and the diagram serves merely to show the major bone compartments.

The "space" outside the blood vessels and outside the cells in bone is potentially available for molecules originating from the blood plasma, if these molecules can penetrate the bone blood vessel walls and the continuous cellular membrane of the bone cells. This extravascular-extracellular space can be subdivided further into:

1. The space between the cells and their processes and the calcified matrix (designated "bone fluid"; **BF** in Fig. 3-17**B**).
2. The calcified matrix itself (designed **CM** in Fig. 3-17**B**).

Because of its low water content and high surface charge, the calcified matrix presents a formidable barrier to the diffusion within it of any molecular species.[52] The "bone-fluid" space, however, is more aqueous and probably has characteristics similar to the gel-like extracellular matrices of soft tissues.[38]

Plasma albumin

In fact, it has been found that plasma proteins are present in extravascular sites in bone.[55] Measurements of the quantity of plasma albumin in rabbit compact bone show that it is present in much higher amounts than can be accounted for by the measured plasma volumes of these specimens. After injection of radioactively labeled ^{125}I-albumin, autoradiographic studies show that albumin is present throughout the bone-fluid space already referred to, and this labeled albumin can be removed by simply washing in isotonic salt solutions (Fig. 3-18). It is also present in the calcified matrix at the sites corresponding to the position at which mineralization was occurring at the time of injection of the radioactive label, when the levels of radioactively labeled albumin in the blood were relatively high. The albumin in the calcified matrix cannot be removed by simple washing in isotonic saline but requires demineralization for its release (Fig. 3-19).

The transient nature of the labeled albumin in the bone fluid compartment and the direction of its general movement from endosteal to periosteal surfaces indicates that there is a continual circulation of albumin, and presumably of other plasma proteins, through this interstitial fluid matrix. This is of obvious importance for the carriage of essential factors to and from the bone cells, as plasma proteins generally act as transporters of hormones, metals, ions and other metabolites and maintain the osmotic pressure of body fluids. The amount of plasma albumin incorporated into calcified matrix of bone is calculated to be a small amount (0.5%) of the total albumin that passes through the tissue fluid of bone, even in rabbits that are actively growing. In these animals there is 1 to 3 mg albumin/g of fresh bone, but only 16% of the total albumin is found in the vascular compartment, with about 27% in the bone fluid and the majority in the calcified matrix. It is considered most likely that the albumin in the calcified matrix is adsorbed to the mineral phase during the formation of the calcified tissue and that it remains there until the bone is resorbed. A relatively uncharged radioactively labeled polymer, polyvinylpyrrolidone, does not show this accumulation in the calcified matrix, as it has little affinity for apatite. This indicates that simple entrapment of molecules in the calcified matrix does not occur, but a definite chemical affinity for the insoluble organic or inorganic components is necessary. Albumin

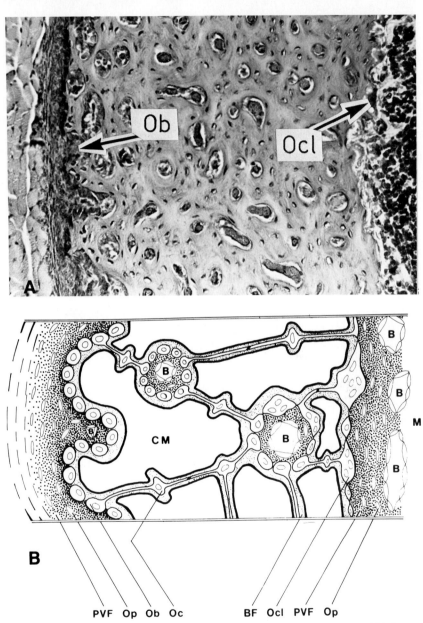

FIGURE 3-17 **(A)** *Cross-section of bone wall from the midshaft of young rabbit femur: marrow cavity is on the right; muscle is on the left. Ocl = osteoclast, Ob = osteoblast.* **(B)** *Diagram of the compartments in the bone wall. M = marrow, B = blood vessel, Ocl = osteoclast, Ob = osteoblast, Op = osteoprogenitor cell, Oc = osteocyte, CM = calcified matrix, PVF = perivascular "fluid," BF = bone "fluid." (Owen, M., Howlett, C. R., and Triffitt, J. T.: Calcif. Tissue Res. 23:37–45, 1977)*

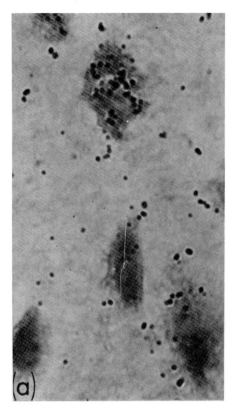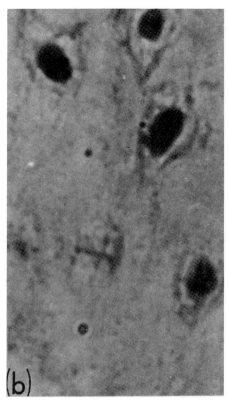

FIGURE 3-18 **(a)** *Autoradiograph showing radioactively labeled albumin associated with osteocyte lacunae a short time (15 min) after intravenous injection.* **(b)** *Autoradiograph of bone tissue from the same animal as in* **(a)** *but taken after washing the tissue block in sodium chloride solution, showing that this process removes the label from the tissue. (Owen, M. E., Triffitt, J. T., and Melick, R. A.: In Hard Tissue Growth, Repair and Remineralisation, Amsterdam, Associated Scientific Pubs., 1973)*

makes up about 3% (w/w) of the noncollagenous matrix of bovine bone, but its influence on the nature of the matrix is unknown.

Plasma α_2HS-glycoprotein

In studies conducted in our laboratory we have been concerned with the composition of the organic matrix of bovine bone and the composition and the metabolism of the organic matrix of rabbit bone. Our investigations have lead to the discovery that a particular plasma glycoprotein may be of some importance in the metabolism of bone tissue, and it constitutes a normal constituent of bone matrix.[2,71,72]

From neutral EDTA extracts of either bovine or rabbit bone, a fraction was prepared that contained a large proportion of the total noncollagenous proteins. One of the major glycoproteins present in this fraction has been purified

and found to have a molecular weight of about 50,000. Antibodies prepared against the purified proteins show that these components are also present in the blood plasma. The proteins in the particular species occur at a level of 20 mg/dl in

TABLE 3-4 THE CONCENTRATION OF PLASMA α_2HS-GLYCOPROTEIN IN CALCIFIED TISSUES

SAMPLE	CONCENTRATION FACTOR*
Ox bone	100–250
Rabbit bone	40–60
Human bone	30–60
Human dentine	100

* The concentration factor is a measure of the concentration of plasma α_2HS-glycoprotein relative to plasma albumin in bone compared with blood plasma.

i.e., Concentration factor

$$= \frac{\alpha_2\text{HS in bone/albumin in bone}}{\alpha_2\text{HS in plasma/albumin in plasma}}$$

bovine plasma and between 100 and 300 mg/dl in rabbit plasma depending on the age of the animal. When measured in relation to the content of albumin and other plasma proteins in bone extracts, there is a concentration of this particular glycoprotein in bone over the same ratio in plasma. This concentration factor varies from 40 times in young rabbits and 60 times in old rabbits up to 250 times in adult bovine bone, and

it is also concentrated in human dentine and bone tissue (Table 3-4). The selective concentration of plasma α_2HS-glycoprotein in calcified tissues can be mimicked by *in vitro* precipitation of calcium phosphate by the addition of calcium and phosphate ions to blood plasma or serum. Depending upon how much precipitate is formed, the relative concentration in the mineral phase ranged from factors of 20 to more than 300

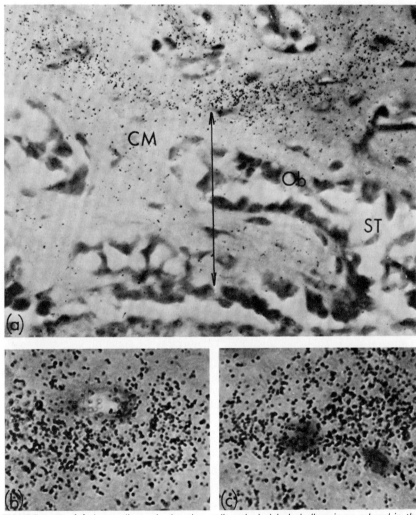

FIGURE 3-19 **(a)** *Autoradiograph showing radioactively labeled albumin as a band in the calcified matrix of bone tissue, 3 d after intravenous injection. The arrows indicate the growth of bone since the injection.* **CM** = *calcified matrix,* **Ob** = *osteoblast,* **ST** = *soft tissues.* **(b)** *and* **(c)** *Autoradiograph of similarly labeled band as in* **(a)** *before* **(b)** *and after* **(c)** *extraction of the tissue block with sodium chloride solutions, showing that this process does not remove albumin once it has been incorporated into the calcified matrix. (Owen, M. E., Triffitt, J. T., and Melick, R. A.: In Hard Tissue Growth, Repair and Remineralisation, Amsterdam, Associated Scientific Pubs., 1973)*

and so could account for the values observed *in vivo*.

This concentration effect is not seen in the soft tissues such as skin, kidney, intestine, muscle, and aorta, and it appears to be specifically accumulated in calcified tissues. The blood vessel content of rabbit bone is such that only 0.5% of the total amount of this protein that is present in bone tissue can be accounted for in the blood plasma in bone tissue, and the vast majority of the protein is located in the intercellular matrix.

It has been shown that this glycoprotein cannot be synthesized by bone tissue in *in vitro* culture conditions. However, perfused liver incorporates a radioactively labeled glycoprotein precursor, ^{14}C-glucosamine, readily and secretes the labeled protein into the perfusion fluid. *In vivo*, therefore, it appears that this glycoprotein is synthesized by the liver, released into the blood plasma, and subsequently accumulated in bone tissue.

A survey of the plasma proteins present in human cortical bone, and their immunochemical quantitation by using commercially available antisera, demonstrates that only one plasma protein, named plasma α_2HS-glycoprotein, shows a concentration effect similar to the rabbit and bovine proteins. These glycoproteins from the three species also have similar molecular weights, electrophoretic mobilities, carbohydrate compositions, and amino acid contents, and it has been concluded that these proteins are analogous to each other and are the species-specific equivalent proteins. By the use of fluorescently labeled antibody to α_2HS-glycoprotein it has been shown that it is localized in mineralized regions in 12-week-old human fetal bone matrix.[14]

The reason for the somewhat selective adsorption to the mineral phase is unknown, but the α_2HS-glycoprotein has been found to have an affinity for calcium ions 40 times greater than albumin. One report suggests that the α_2HS-glycoprotein has opsonic properties and renders certain bacteria susceptible to phagocytic attack *in vitro*.[74] If such a "recognition factor" role is operative *in vivo*, it may be speculated that the presence of α_2HS-glycoprotein in bone matrix may aid resorption of bone by activation of specific bone-resorbing cells. It must be em-

phasized, however, that no known physiologic function has been found for this protein.

The α_2HS-glycoprotein accounts for about 40% of the glycoprotein components in bone matrix synthesized from radioactively labeled glucosamine during bone formation in young rabbits. This, together with the fact that it is enriched in permanent tooth dentine in which remodeling does not occur, suggests that the glycoprotein interacts with the mineral phase during its formation, although a possible function at sites of bone resorption cannot be ruled out. Transformation of an amorphous calcium phosphate phase to hydroxyapatite is known to be delayed by certain serum fractions.[8] The influence of this particular plasma glycoprotein on the transformation rate and on the nature of the mineral phase may give some clue as to the effect of its accumulation in bone tissue.

Collagenase-released matrix components

Herring[28] pioneered the use of bacterial collagenase enzyme to release and solubilize components that are not soluble when bone powder is extracted with neutral EDTA solutions, and which are thought to have a particular association with collagen in the bone matrix. These "collagenase-released components" are found to make up about 3% (w/w) of the bone organic matrix with about 1% (w/w) of the total matrix remaining insoluble.

Using this technique, Leaver and colleagues[39] found that enzymic digestion of the EDTA-insoluble residue of bovine bone released two main components that were separated by chromatographic methods. They were partially characterized and were found to contain low levels of phosphate. One component was found to be a glycoprotein, and the other component consisted of over 90% protein. This more proteinaceous material was similar to the phosphoproteins described earlier.[66]

It is not known how firmly these materials are attached to the insoluble residue remaining after the EDTA extraction procedure. This residue is made up mainly of collagen, and enzymic digestion could release components that are either electrostatically or covalently bound to this molecule. There is interest in materials that are firmly associated with collagen not only because of their possible relevance to the structural organization of bone but also because of the peculiar property of insoluble bone matrix to induce certain cells in extraskeletal tissue sites to form bone tissue when this matrix is implanted into the animal. This fascinating property of bone organic matrix is described in detail in Chapter 13 by Urist, who is a leader in this field of research. It has been suggested that the moiety that could be responsible for the alteration in cell phenotype is a noncollagenous protein, which has been named "bone morphogenetic protein." A soluble noncollagenous constituent with bone morphogenetic properties has been separated from bone matrix by digestion with purified bacterial collagenase and separated by affinity chromatography procedures that recognize specific carbohydrate groups on molecules. This solubilized material could therefore be a glycoprotein molecule or could possibly be made up of molecular aggregates, and it appears to contain

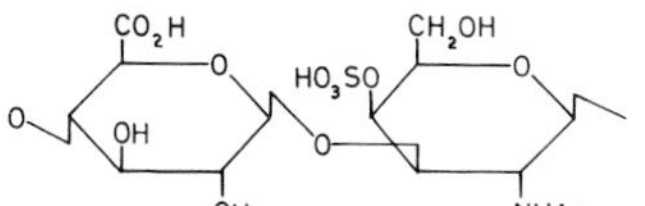

CHONDROITIN 4-SULPHATE

HYALURONIC ACID

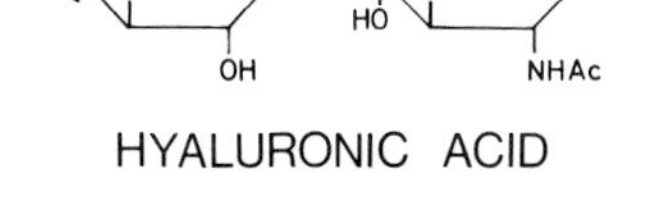

KERATAN SULPHATE

FIGURE 3-20 *The repeating units of the glycosaminoglycans found in bone tissue.*

disulfide bonds.[73] Now that a soluble active preparation has been achieved, the isolation and complete characterization of this material that appears to reside in bone organic matrix is a matter of obvious importance.

Proteoglycans and glycosaminoglycans

Proteoglycans are conjugated proteins that have carbohydrate prosthetic groups and are high-molecular-weight polymeric substances. The prosthetic groups are named glycosaminoglycans and contain linear repeating units consisting of two sugars. One of these sugars is a hexosamine residue (D-glucosamine or D-galactosamine) that can carry a sulphate group at various positions, and the other sugar is usually a uronic acid residue, but it can be a galactose residue. The linear repeating units that occur in the glycosaminoglycans found in compact bone tissue are shown in Figure 3-20. This description of the constituent glycosaminoglycans belies the complexity of their chemical structure, and any impression that simple chemical formulae can be applied to these complex substances should be regarded as an idealized situation. So components of a particular glycosaminoglycan chain may exhibit similarities to each of these structures.

The glycosaminoglycans normally exist in connective tissues covalently bound to proteins as proteoglycans, and these substances provide support to the tissues by forming a highly hydrated, compression-resistant network between the collagen fibrils. Because of their highly polyanionic character they exhibit characteristic physicochemical properties that influence the distribution and transport of ionized materials through the tissues.[38]

Very few studies have been performed on the proteoglycans of cortical bone. Usually the experimental methods involve digestion of the demineralized bone with proteolytic enzymes that degrade the protein moiety and release the glycosaminoglycans for further fractionation and study. Thus Meyer and his coworkers in 1956[47] used the enzymes pepsin and trypsin to digest acid-demineralized bovine compact bone, and by fractional precipitation with ethanol found only chondroitin sulfate at a level of 0.25% of the organic matrix. Methods were subsequently devised to separate the glycosaminoglycans in a clearer manner by using fractional precipitation or column chromatography of the complexes formed by these materials and the cationic detergent cetylpyridinium chloride. This led Hjertquist and Vejlens[32] to investigate dog cortical bone, in which chondroitin 4-sulfate was found to be the major glycosaminoglycan component and was identified by its infrared spectrum. It was found to constitute about 0.35% of the organic matrix, and the presence of hyaluronic acid at a level of 3% of the total glycosaminoglycans was reported, but no keratan sulfate could be detected. The size of the chondroitin sulfate chains was estimated to correspond to a molecular weight of about 50,000 from their chromatographic elution positions and from sedimentation data. Herring[25] demonstrated that at least some of the glycosaminoglycans in bovine bone exist as proteoglycans. EDTA extraction of the compact bone was followed by ion exchange chromatography to obtain the chondroitin sulfate fraction, which was repeatedly precipitated with cetylpyridinium chloride and finally with 9-aminoacridine. The resultant fraction still had a protein content of 11% and was resolved into three components by DEAE-cellulose column chromatography. Two of these fractions contained appreciable amounts of protein, and the third fraction resembled relatively pure chondroitin sulphate both in general composition and in electrophoretic mobility on cellulose acetate. The amino acid analyses of the two major protein-containing fractions were similar and were said to have close resemblance to the bovine sialoprotein that in the pure state is entirely free of sulphate and uronic acid. Furthermore, alkaline hydrolysis of the first of these fractions released two components; one had an electrophoretic mobility on cellulose acetate similar to but slightly faster than bovine sialoprotein and one had an mobility identical to pure chondroitin sulphate. It was concluded that the two fractions, containing both protein and chondroitin sulphate, represented proteoglycans with a sialoglycoprotein core very similar to sialoprotein, which differed in the number and length of attached chondroitin sulphate chains. The presence of free chondroitin sulphate chains may

have resulted from enzymic digestion of the proteoglycans during the extraction procedures or during bone formation or from the synthesis of free glycosaminoglycan by the bone cells.

The presence of proteoglycans consisting of chondroitin sulphate chains attached to sialoglycoproteins have also been reported in both sheep and human compact bone. Engfeldt and Hjerpe[17] used the method of discontinuous gradient centrifugation to separate and isolate microparticles from powdered human compact bone samples. The particles of different density are said to represent areas in bone of different degrees of mineralization. This technique has been used by many investigators in the past to study the nature of the changes that occur with increasing mineralization of the tissues. The glycosaminoglycans were investigated by the cetylpyridinium method after papain digestion and were shown to be mainly chondroitin 4-sulphate with perhaps a very small amount of hyaluronic acid. The proteoglycans were studied by methods previously developed extensively for the characterization of cartilage proteoglycans. The bone density fractions were extracted with EDTA solutions containing 4 M guanidinium chloride and subsequently separated by gel column chromatography. By this means it was shown that the bone proteoglycans are of much smaller molecular size than those present in cartilage, and each proteoglycan molecule in bone is considered to carry only a few glycosaminoglycan chains, as was suggested by earlier workers. With increasing degrees of mineralization the molecular size of the glycosaminoglycans decreased somewhat, and there was a change in molecular size of the proteoglycans.

So in most species studied, chondroitin 4-sulphate with minimal quantities of hyaluronic acid are the constituent glycosaminoglycans of the proteoglycans found in bone tissue. However, there is evidence from a number of laboratories, the author's included, that in rabbit compact bone a proteoglycan is present that resembles keratan sulphate or a sulphated glycoprotein in characteristics and composition. This material makes up an appreciable proportion of the proteoglycan fraction, but the significance of this species difference is unknown.

It has been suggested that proteoglycans play a role in biologic calcification and as much more is known of the structure of cartilage proteoglycans, most investigations have dealt with their possible role in endochondral bone formation. There is a decrease in proteoglycan size and concentration from the zone of resting to the zone of mineralized cartilage, presumably as a result of enzymic digestion of the proteoglycans. These molecules have been credited with having initiating and inhibitory roles in the calcification process, but current evidence suggests that they function mainly to inhibit calcification.[33] The proteoglycans isolated from bone tissue are very different in size and structure from their cartilage counterparts. They do, nevertheless, inhibit mineral deposition *in vitro* at concentrations similar to those used to demonstrate inhibition by bovine bone sialoprotein. Furthermore, removal of the protein moiety by protease digestion showed that the free glycosaminoglycan chains had lost this inhibitory action.[29] Thus, this may be relevant to the *in vivo* situation, as proteoglycans are known to be removed from the osteoid at the onset of mineralization in rat tibial cortex.[7a]

Other Constituents

PEPTIDES

The presence of dialyzable peptides in bone was reported as early as 1960, and these substances were subsequently studied by Leaver and his associates in Liverpool.[40] The low-molecular-weight materials released by acid and EDTA dimineralization of bone were fractionated by gel filtration, ion exchange chromatography, and high-voltage electrophoresis into a large number of fractions. Similar fractions were also detected when EDTA was used to decalcify the bone, and therefore they do not seem to be produced by the acid extraction conditions. Autolytic processes may lead to such materials, but it is thought that they represent actual constituents of the bone matrix. The characteristics and amino acid compositions of these fractions have been reviewed recently, and they are said to make up about 8% (w/w) of the noncollagenous bone matrix.

LIPIDS

Lipids are a very heterogenous group of substances defined by their ready solubility in low-polarity organic solvents (e.g., ether, chloroform, benzene) and their relative insolubility in water. There are numerous classes of lipids, and the lipids present in bone and other calcified tissues have been investigated extensively by Irving, Wuthier, and Shapiro.[64] Particular interest in bone lipids was generated by the observation of Irving that at the site of mineralization in cartilage and bone tissue there is material present that stains with Sudan black B dye under appropriate conditions (Fig. 3-21). This histochemical reaction is thought to change the nature of the lipids at the mineralization sites to render them sudanophilic.

Earlier observations suggested that the total lipid content of bone was very low and made up about 0.07 to 0.09% by weight of dry bovine bone. The constituent lipids were found to be mainly triglycerides, with smaller amounts of cholesterol and its esters, and trace amounts of phospholipids. It is difficult to obtain a reliable estimate for the lipid content of bone tissue, as the marrow contains fatty elements. So values of over 1% lipid have been reported, but these are made up mainly of triglycerides and are probably due to contamination by this adjacent tissue.

A major effort to identify the lipid materials associated with mineralizing sites was originated in the early 1960s by Irving and his coworkers. It was found that although most of the neutral lipids could be removed by a simple extraction with chloroform-methanol solvents, the complete extraction of acidic phospholipids required demineralization of the bone with EDTA followed by the use of acid solvents. It was considered that these latter phospholipids represented the material responsible for the Sudan black staining at the calcifying sites. Phospholipids were found to make up about 0.02% by weight of mature compact bovine bone and are therefore a small proportion of the total lipid content. The components extracted from powdered calcified bone by simple extraction with chloroform-ethanol made up 69% of the total phospholipids and consisted mainly of sphingomyelin, lecithin, and phos-

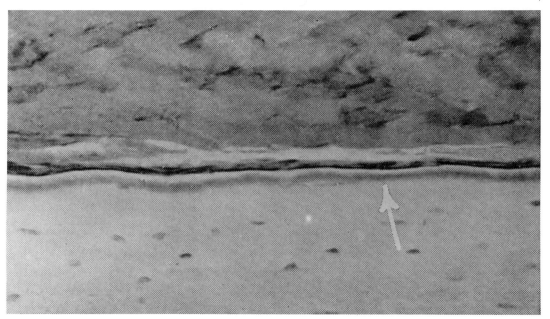

FIGURE 3-21 *Horizontal process of palatine bone stained with Sudan black after hot pyridine treatment. Note the sudanophil line (arrow) at the junction of the preosseus matrix and calcified bone, × 220. (Irving, J. T.: Clin. Orthop. 17:92–101, 1960)*

phatidylethanolamine. Demineralization yielded a further 28% of the total phospholipids of similar composition as the first fraction but phosphatidylserine, phosphatidylinositol, and phosphatidic acid were also present. The acidified solvent released the remaining 3% of the total phospholipids and lecithin; phosphatidylserine and phosphatidylinositol were the major components, and because of their possible association with mineralization were considered the most interesting. To explain the difficulty of extraction, these workers suggested that the various components were bound to the inorganic and organic phases of bone in stable complexes. However, recent experiments by Boskey and Posner[10] show that when powdered, calcified bone is exhaustively extracted with chloroform methanol alone with the aid of ultrasonic waves, more than 96% of the lipid content of bone can be extracted. These authors have isolated a calcium-phosphate-acidic phospholipid complex from rabbit and bovine compact bone, and the complex is more prevalent in young bone samples than in old. The phospholipids in the complex were mainly phosphatidylserine and phosphatidylinositol (Fig. 3-22), and they were associated with calcium and inorganic phosphate

to give a molar ratio of calcium to total phosphate of unity. These are the same phospholipids that Irving's group suggested might be involved in mineralization. It is thought that the calcium is bound to the polar phosphate groups and carboxyl groups in the phosphatidylserine complex and to the phosphate and hydroxyl groups in the phosphatidyl inositol complex.

The calcium-phosphate-acidic phospholipid complex has been shown to induce hydroxyapatite formation from metastable solutions of calcium and phosphate *in vitro* more efficiently than the uncomplexed phospholipids, but less so than when crystals of hydroxyapatite are used to seed the precipitation. Precipitation occurs even when uncomplexed phospholipids are used, but there is a delay in this case that may be due to the formation of the complex before nucleation takes place, with subsequent growth of the crystals.

The isolated complex is not considered to be an artifact, but the functions or locations of these materials in bone are unknown. Acidic phospholipids are common constituents of cell membranes and are also found in the vesicles that are present in the matrices of tissues, such as cartilage, dentin, and embryonic bone, in which mineralization is being initiated. The presence of matrix vesicles in compact bone is uncertain, however. Even if these structures are present, the cellular content of bone could account for the majority of the phospholipid content, and whether or not they are present in significant amounts in the extracellular matrix is unknown. Obviously, the relationship of phospholipids to the function of the vitamin K–dependent Gla-containing bone proteins will stimulate renewed interest in their functions in bone tissue.

Concluding remarks

Thus, the constituents of organic matrix of bone are varied and numerous, which may be expected because of the complexity of the structure of the tissue. The approximate amounts of the major molecular species in compact bone tissue that have been investigated up to the present time are indicated in Table 3-5. The fact that any bone sample taken for study is heterogenous in the biologic structures it contains suggests that gross analysis of the chemical composition may give only a limited insight into the various functions of the tissue, and this has proved to be the case.

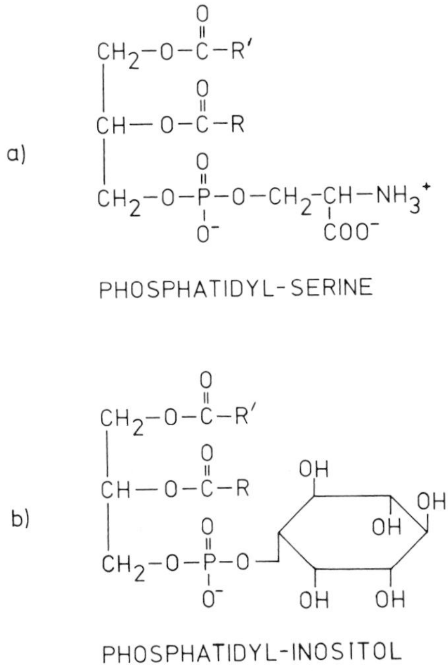

a)

PHOSPHATIDYL-SERINE

b)

PHOSPHATIDYL-INOSITOL

FIGURE 3-22 *The major acidic phospholipids thought to be associated with mineralizing sites.* **R** *and* **R**′ = *long-chain fatty acid groups.*

TABLE 3-5 APPROXIMATE AMOUNTS OF THE NONCOLLAGENOUS CONSTITUENTS OF THE ORGANIC MATRIX OF COMPACT BONE TISSUE

CONSTITUENT	% W/W*
Sialoprotein	8–12
Chondroitin sulphate	8
Gla-containing proteins	5–10
Albumin	3
α_2HS-glycoprotein	4
Lipids	4
Peptides	8
"Structural glycoproteins"	8.5

* As % of non-collagenous material

The bulk of the bone volume is designed for its structural role in body support, and normally only a fraction of this volume is involved in active mineralization. The important structural role of collagen in bone and all connective tissues has been emphasized earlier, and defects in bone structure are apparent when collagen biosynthetic patterns are impaired or altered, although mineralization in most cases seems little affected. The glycoprotein and proteoglycan components of connective tissue matrices are also important structurally in interactions leading to collagen fibril formation, orientation, and stability.[1,45] Few studies have dealt with the interaction between the tissue-specific constituents isolated from bone matrix, and studies on the physicochemical inter-relationships of these materials should lead to a better understanding of bone structure.

Many of the constituents of bone matrix have been implicated in mineralization, as indicated in the descriptions of the individual matrix components, but the precise nature of the mechanism of this process remains obscure. It is highly improbable that a single constituent isolated from bone tissue acts to initiate mineralization, and such a concept could lead to inaccurate conclusions in model systems. It is possible that interactions between organic constituents at the mineralization site results in organization into complex active structures that catalyze mineral deposition in a controlled fashion. In some way the osteoblast programs this event to occur at a precise location. The concept of small packets of

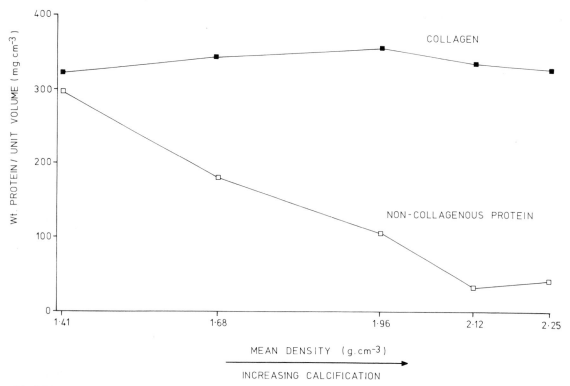

FIGURE 3-23 *Graph showing the collagenous and noncollagenous protein contents of bone fractions separated by density, showing that as calcification increases the amount of noncollagenous protein decreases, whereas the collagen content per unit volume remains relatively constant. (After Lapiere, C. M., and Nusgens, B. V.: In Balasz, E. A. (ed.): Chemistry and Molecular Biology of the Intercellular Matrix, Vol. 1, New York, Academic Press, 1970)*

membranous structures originating from bone-forming cells, the so-called "matrix vesicles," and seen with the electron microscope in tissues undergoing calcification, may take this initial organization away from the organic matrix components. However, once it is started, mineralization proceeds rapidly, and many components of the matrix could serve to influence the deposition in an orientated manner.

Exactly how the substances detected in the calcified matrix are involved in these processes is unknown and is complicated by the remarkable affinity of bone mineral for ionically charged molecular species. So it is possible that the presence of mineral in bone matrix determines the nature of at least some of the noncollagenous materials that have been found there. This binding, which could be considered to be adventitious, may, even so, influence the nature of the mineral phase and subsequent physical, chemical, and biochemical properties of the bone tissue.

Since only a small proportion of the bone tissue is actively engaged in the laying down of mineral, the bulk of noncollagenous components isolated may bear little relationship to the constituents at the active sites. They may merely represent the "fossilized" molecules or remains of molecules, which may or may not have been involved in calcification or have been accumulated from tissue fluids. On this basis a molecular species of crucial importance in the mineralization process could be lacking from bone matrix if there is no interaction with the insoluble elements of bone. The localization of specific organic entities in bone and their topochemistry would answer the uncertainties about the distribution of many of these materials. So it appears obvious that studies on the importance of the organic matrix in bone mineralization requires specific investigations on the changes occurring exactly at the sites at which this extracellular event is happening.

Mineralization is initiated in a matrix that contains 30 to 50% noncollagenous materials—the osteoid layer, and these materials decrease markedly in amount as the operation goes to completion. The fact that the amount of collagen in a given volume of bone remains constant and that water is lost as the tissue calcifies has been known for many years.[52] Recent evidence indicates that the decrease in water content is accompanied by decreasing amounts of noncollagenous constituents (glycoproteins and proteoglycans) as the degree of mineralization increases. This has been shown by Pugiarello and colleagues,[61] who dissected out osteoid and individual osteones of different degrees of calcification, and by Lapiere and Nusgens,[37] who separated bone fractions according to density (Fig. 3-23). Whether this decrease occurs simply to provide space for mineralization as it occurs is unknown, but histologic and electron microscopic evidence also shows that this removal of noncollagenous constituents does occur. It has been suggested that this removal is a necessary part of the mineralization process, as in cartilage in which the presence of proteoglycans especially are thought to have an inhibitory role and require removal for mineralization to begin.[33] There is, therefore, circumstantial evidence for supposing that noncollagenous constituents play an important role in the mineralization process.

The bulk of the matrix components are synthesized by the osteoblasts,[41] and using suitably radioactively labeled precursor, all the glycoprotein and proteoglycan fractions are labeled.[71] Still, this is a complex area to investigate in *in vivo* studies, as bone tissue does accumulate plasma proteins and possibly other substances from the interstitial fluids. This complicates interpretation of *in vivo* studies, and bone has to compete with other more metabolically active tissues when many of the radioactively labeled precursors of bone matrix constituents are used. *In vitro*, cultures of embryonic bone or incubations of bone fragments do not mineralize normally, and tissues are known to change qualitatively and quantitatively their synthetic patterns under culture conditions. The development of an *in vitro* system of pure bone tissue that undergoes "physiologic" mineralization would be of tremendous value in this sphere of research and, indeed, in all studies related to the mineralization process. The particular changes that occur as the matrix changes from an unmineralized, soft tissue state to a mineralized, relatively dehydrated state are poorly understood, and it is anticipated that efforts to achieve this ideal model will be actively pursued in the future. In any event, the ever-increasing interest in the biochemistry of bone tissue and in the structure-function relationships of its multitude of organic components will continue to provide fascinating problems for research scientists.

References

1. Anderson, J. C.: Glycoproteins of the connective tissue matrix, Int. Rev. Connect. Tissue Res. 7:251–322, 1976.
2. Ashton, B. A., Triffitt, J. T., and Herring, G. M.: Isolation and partial characterisation of a glycoprotein from bovine cortical bone, Eur. J. Biochem. 45:525–533, 1974.
3. Bachra, B. N.: Nucleation in biological systems. *In* Zipkin, I. (ed.): Biological Mineralization, pp. 845–881, New York, John Wiley & Sons, 1973.
4. Bailey, A. J., and Robins, S. P.: Current topics in the biosynthesis, structure and function of collagen, Sci. Prog. 63:419–444, 1976.
5. Bailey, A. J., Robins, S. P., and Balian, G.: Biological significance of the intermolecular crosslinks of collagen, Nature 251:105–109, 1974.
6. Barnes, M. J., and Lawson, D. E. M.: Biochemistry of bone in relation to the function of vitamin D. *In* Lawson, D. E. M. (ed.): Vitamin D, pp. 267–302, New York, Academic Press, 1978.
7. Baud, C. A.: The fine structure of normal and parathormone-treated bone cells. Excerpta Medica International Congress Ser. No. 120, pp. 4–6, Fourth European Symposium on Calcified Tissues, 1966.
7a. Baylink, D., Wergedal, J., and Thompson, E.: Loss of protein-polysaccharides at sites where bone mineralisation is initiated, J. Histochem. Cytochem. 20:279–292, 1972.
8. Blumenthal, N. C., Betts, F., and Posner, A. S.: Effect of carbonate and biological macromolecules on the formation and properties of hydroxyapatite, Calcif. Tissue Res. 18:81–90, 1975.

9. Bonucci, E.: The locus of initial calcification in cartilage and bone, Clin. Orthop. 78:108–139, 1971.

10. Boskey, A. L., and Posner, A. S.: Extraction of a calcium-phospholipid-phosphate complex from bone. Calcif. Tissue Res. 19:273–283, 1976.

11. Burckard, J., Havey, R., and Dautrevaux, M.: Etudes des proteines et glycoproteines de l'os compact du lapin, Bull. Soc. Chim. Biol. 48:851–863, 1966.

12. Cohen-Solal, L., Lian, J. B., Kossiva, D., and Glimcher, M. J.: Identification of organic phosphorus covalently bound to collagen and non-collagenous proteins of chicken bone matrix, Biochem. J. 177:81–98, 1979.

13. Curry, J. D.: Strength of bone, Nature 195:513–514, 1962.

14. Dickson, I. R., Poole, A. R., and Veis, A.: Localisation of plasma α_2HS-glycoprotein in mineralising human bone, Nature 256:430–432, 1975.

15. Dimuzio, M. T., and Veis, A.: Phospho-phoryns—major noncollagenous proteins of rat incisor dentin, Calcif. Tissue Res. 25:169–178, 1978.

16. Dowben, R. M.: General Physiology: A Molecular Approach, New York, Harper & Row, 1969.

17. Engfeldt, B., and Hjerpe, A.: Glycosaminoglycans and proteoglycans of human bone tissue at different stages of mineralisation, Acta. Pathol. Microbiol. Scand. 84A:95–106, 1976.

18. Engstrom, A.: Aspects of the molecular structure of bone. *In* Bourne, G. H. (ed.): The Biochemistry and Physiology of Bone, 2nd edition, Vol. 1, pp. 237–257, New York, Academic Press, 1972.

19. Epstein, E. H., and Munderloh, N. H.: Isolation and characterisation of CNBr peptides of human $[\alpha1(111)]_3$ collagen and tissue distribution of $[\alpha1(I)]_2\alpha2$ and $[\alpha1(111)]_3$ collagens, J. Biol. Chem. 250:9304–9312, 1975.

20. Glimcher, M. J.: Composition, structure, and organization of bone and other mineralized tissues and the mechanism of calcification. *In* Greep, R. O., and Astwood, E. B. (eds.): Handbook of Physiology, pp. 25–116, American Physiol. Soc., 1976.

20A. Glimcher, M. J., Kossiva, D., & Roufosse, A.: Identification of phosphopeptides and γ-carboxyglutamic acid-containing peptides in epiphyseal growth plate cartilage. Cal. Tiss. Int. 27:187–191, 1979.

21. Gottschalk, A.: Definition of glycoproteins and their delineation from other carbohydrate-protein complexes. *In* Gottschalk, A. (ed.): Glycoproteins, BBA Library, Vol. 5, pp. 20–28, Amsterdam, Elsevier Pub. Co., 1966.

22. Grant, M. E., and Prockop, D. J.: The biosynthesis of collagen, New Eng. J. Med. 286:194–199, 242–249, 291–300, 1972.

23. Hauschka, P. V.: Quantitative determination of γ-carboxyglutamic acid in proteins, Anal. Biochem. 80:212–223, 1977.

24. Hauschka, P. V., and Gallop, P. M.: Purification and calcium-binding properties of osteocalcin, the γ-carboxy glutamate-containing protein of bone. *In* Wasserman, R. H., Corradino, R. A., Carafoli, E. et al (eds.): Calcium-Binding Proteins and Calcium Function, pp. 338–347, New York, North Holland, 1977.

25. Herring, G. M.: Studies on the protein-bound chondroitin sulphate of bovine cortical bone, Biochem. J. 107:41–49, 1968.

26. Herring, G. M.: Mucosubstances and ion-binding in bone, Bibliotheca Nutritio et Dieta. Nr. 13, pp. 147–154, 1969.

27. Herring, G. M.: The organic matrix of bone. *In* Bourne, G. H. (ed.): The Biochemistry and Physiology of Bone, 2nd edition, Vol. 1, pp. 127–189, New York, Academic Press, 1972.

28. Herring, G. M.: Methods for the study of the glycoproteins and proteoglycans of bone using bacterial collagenase. Determination of bone sialoprotein and chondroitin sulphate, Calcif. Tissue Res. 24:29–36, 1977.

29. Herring, G. M., Andrews, A. T. de B., and Chipperfield, A. R.: Chemical structure of bone sialoprotein and a preliminary study of its calcium-binding properties. *In* Nichols, G., and Wasserman, R. H., (eds.): Cellular Mechanisms for Calcium Transfer and Homeostasis, pp. 63–73, Academic Press, New York, 1971.

30. Herring, G. M., Ashton, B. A., and Chipperfield, A. R.: The isolation of soluble proteins, glycoproteins and proteoglycans from bone, Prep. Biochem. 4:179–200, 1974.

31. Herring, G. M., and Kent, P. W.: Some studies on the mucosubstances of bovine cortical bone, Biochem. J. 89:405–414, 1963.

32. Hjertquist, S.-O., and Vejlens, L.: The glycosaminoglycans of dog compact bone and epiphyseal cartilage in the normal state and in experimental hyperparathyroidism, Calcif. Tissue Res. 2:314–333, 1968.

33. Howells, D. S., and Pita, J. C.: Calcification of growth plate cartilage with special reference to

studies on micropuncture fluids, Clin. Orthop. 118:208–229, 1976.

34. Irving, J. T.: Histochemical changes in the early stages of calcification, Clin. Orthop. 17:92–101, 1960.

35. Jacques, L. W., Brown, E. B., Barrett, J. M., Wallace, S. B., and Weltner, W.: Sialic acid: a calcium-binding carbohydrate, J. Biol. Chem. 252:4533–4538, 1977.

36. Katz, E. P., and Li, S-T.: Structure and function of bone collagen fibrils, J. Mol. Biol. 80:1–15, 1973.

37. Lapiere, C. M., and Nusgens, B. V.: Maturation related changes of the protein matrix of bone. *In* Balazs, E. A., (ed.): Chemistry and molecular biology of the intercellular matrix, Vol. 1, pp. 55–79, New York, Academic Press, 1970.

38. Laurent, T. C.: The ultrastructure and physicochemical properties of interstitial connective tissue, Pflügers Archiv. Eur. J. Physiol. (Suppl.) 336:S21–S42, 1972.

39. Leaver, A. G., Holbrook, I. B., Jones, I. L., Thomas, M., and Sheil, L.: Components of the organic matrices of bone and dentine isolated only after digestion with collagenase, Arch. Oral Biol. 20:211–216, 1975.

40. Leaver, A. G., Triffitt, J. T., and Holbrook, I. B.: Newer knowledge of the non-collagenous proteins in dentine and cortical bone matrix, Clin. Orthop. 110:269–292, 1975.

41. Leblond, C. P., and Weinstock, M.: Radioautographic studies of bone formation. *In* Bourne, G. H., (ed.): The Biochemistry and Physiology of Bone, 2nd edition, Vol. III, Development and Growth, pp. 181–200, New York, Academic Press, 1971.

42. Lian, J. B., Hauschka, P. V., and Gallop, P. M.: Properties and biosynthesis of a vitamin K–dependent calcium binding protein in bone, Fed. Proc. 37:2615–2620, 1978.

43. Lichtenstein, J. R., Martin, G. R., Kohn, L. D., Byers, P. H., and McKusick, V. A.: Defect in conversion of procollagen to collagen in a form of Ehlers-Danlos syndrome, Science 182:298–300, 1973.

44. Light, N. D., and Bailey, A. J.: Changes in crosslinking during aging in bovine tendon collagen, Febs. Letters 97:183–188, 1979.

45. Lindahl, U., and Höök, M.: Glycosaminoglycans and their binding to biological macromolecules, Ann. Rev. Biochem. 47:385, 1978.

46. Masubuchi, M., Miura, S., and Yosizawa, A.: Glycosaminoglycans and glycoproteins isolated from rabbit femur, J. Biochem. (Tokyo) 77:617–626, 1975.

47. Meyer, K., Davidson, E., Linker, A., and Hoffman, P.: The acid mucopolysaccharides of connective tissue, Biochim. Biophys. Acta 21:506–518, 1956.

48. Miller, E. J.: Biochemical characteristics and biological significance of the genetically distinct collagens, Mol. Cell. Biochem. 13:165–192, 1976.

49. Miller, E. J.: Collagens of extracellular matrices. *In* Last, J. W., and Burger, M. M. (eds.): Cell and Tissue Interactions, Gen. Physiologists Ser. 32, pp. 71–86, New York, Raven Press, 1977.

50. Miller, E. J., and Matukas, V. J.: Chick cartilage collagen: A new type of $\alpha 1$ chain not present in bone or skin of the species, Proc. Nat. Acad. Sci. (U.S.A.) 64:1264–1268, 1969.

51. Muller, P. K., Lemmen, C., Gay, S., and Meigel, W. N.: Disturbance in the regulation of the type of collagen synthesized in a form of osteogenesis imperfecta, Eur. J. Biochem. 59:97–104, 1975.

52. Neuman, W. F., and Neuman, M. W.: The Chemical Dynamics of Bone Mineral, Chicago, The University of Chicago Press, 1958.

52a. Nishimoto, S. K., and Price, P. A.: Proof that the γ-carboxyglutamic acid-containing bone protein is synthesized in calf bone, J. Biol. Chem. 254:437–441, 1979.

53. Nusgens, B., and Lapière, Ch. M.: Bone in dermatosparaxis. II. Chemical analysis, Calcif. Tissue Res. 21:37–45, 1976.

54. Owen, M., Howlett, C. R., and Triffitt, J. T.: Movement of ^{125}I-albumin and ^{125}I-polyvinylpyrrolidone through bone tissue fluid, Calcif. Tissue Res. 23:103–112, 1977.

55. Owen, M. E., Triffitt, J. T., and Melick, R. A.: Albumin in bone. *In* Ciba Foundation Symposium 11, Hard Tissue Growth, Repair and Remineralisation, pp. 263–293, Amsterdam, Associated Scientific Pubs., 1973.

56. Penttinen, R. P., Lichtenstein, J. R., Martin, G. R., and McKusick, V. A.: Abnormal collagen metabolism in cultured cells in osteogenesis imperfecta, Proc. Natl. Acad. Sci. (U.S.A.) 72:586–589, 1975.

57. Pinnell, S. R., Fox, R., and Krane, S. M.: Human collagens: differences in glycosylated hydroxylysines in skin and bone. Biochim. Biophys. Acta 229:119–122, 1971.

58. Poser, J. W., and Price, P. A.: A method for decarboxylation of γ-carboxyglutamic acid in proteins, J. Biol. Chem. 254:431–436, 1979.

59. Posner, A. S.: Crystal chemistry of bone mineral, Physiol. Rev. 49:760–792, 1969.
59A. Price, P. A., Otsuka, A. S., Poser, J. W., Kristaponis, J., Raman, N.: Characterization of a γ-carboxyglutamic acid-containing protein from bone. Proc. Nat. Acad. Sci. USA. 73:1447–1451, 1976.
60. Price, P. A., Poser, J. W., and Raman, N.: Primary structure of the γ-carboxyglutamic acid–containing protein from bovine bone, Proc. Natl. Acad. Sci. (U.S.A.) 73:3374–3375, 1976.
61. Pugliarello, M. C., Vittur, F., and de Bernard, B.: Chemical modifications in osteones during calcification. Calcif. Tissue Res. 5:108–114, 1970.
62. Robert, A. M., Robert, B., and Robert, L.: Chemical and physical properties of structural glycoproteins. *In* Balazs, E. A. (ed.): Chemistry and Molecular Biology of the Intercellular Matrix, Vol. 1, pp. 237–242, New York, Academic Press, 1970.
63. Robinson, R. A.: Chemical analysis and electron microscopy of bone. *In* Rodahl, K., Nicholson, J. T., and Brown, E. M., (eds.): Bone as a Tissue, pp. 186–250, New York, McGraw Hill Book Co., 1960.
64. Shapiro, I.: The lipids of skeletal and dental tissues: their role in mineralisation. *In* Zipkin, I. (ed.): Biological Mineralisation, pp. 117–138, New York, John Wiley & Sons, 1973.
65. Shetlar, M. R., Hern, D., and Chien, S. F.: Isolation and characterisation of human bone sialoprotein, Texas Reports Biol. Med. 30:339–345, 1972.
66. Shuttleworth, A., and Veis, A.: The isolation of anionic phosphoproteins from bovine cortical bone via the periodate solubilization of bone collagen, Biochem. Biophys. Acta. 257:414–420, 1972.
67. Smith, J. W.: Molecular pattern in native collagen, Nature 219:157–158, 1968.
68. Spector, A. R., and Glimcher, M. J.: The extraction and characterisation of soluble anionic phosphoproteins from bone, Biochim. Biophys. Acta 263:593–603, 1972.
69. Stenflo, J., and Suttie, J. W.: Vitamin K–dependent formation of γ-carboxy glutamic acid, Ann. Rev. Biochem. 46:157–172, 1977.
70. Thyberg, J.: Electron microscopic studies on the initial phases of calcification in guinea pig epiphyseal cartilage, J. Ultrastruct. Res. 46:206–218, 1974.
71. Triffitt, J. T., and Owen, M.: Studies on bone matrix glycoproteins. Incorporation of [1-¹⁴C]-glucosamine and plasma [¹⁴C] glycoprotein into rabbit cortical bone, Biochem. J. 136:125–134, 1973.
72. Triffitt, J. T., Owen, M. E., Ashton, B. A., and Wilson, J. M.: Plasma disappearance of rabbit α₂HS-glycoprotein and its uptake by bone tissue, Calcif. Tissue Res. 26:155–161, 1978.
73. Urist, M. R., Mikulski, A., and Lietze, A.: Solubilized and insolubilized bone morphogenetic protein, Proc. Natl. Acad. Sci. (U.S.A.) 76:1828–1832, 1979.
74. Van Oss, C. J., Gillman, C. F., Bronson, P. M., and Border, J. R.: Opsonic properties of human serum α₂HS-glycoprotein, Immunol. Commun. 3:329–335, 1974.
75. Vaughan, J.: The effects of radiation on bone. *In* Bourne, G. H. (ed.): The Biochemistry and Physiology of Bone, pp. 729–765, New York, Academic Press, 1956.
76. Vaughan, J. M.: The Physiology of Bone. Oxford, Clarendon, 1975.
77. Warren, L.: The distribution of sialic acids within the eukaryotic cell. *In* Rosenberg, A. and Schengrund, C-L. (eds.): Biological Roles of Sialic Acid, pp. 103–121, New York, Plenum Press, 1976.

Physicians and researchers, even those with a minimal training in chemistry, are exposed to elementary theory concerning the solubility properties of sparingly soluble salts. At least in the textbook examples the subject is simple to grasp conceptually and simple to work with in practical applications. Compendia are available of the solubilities of thousands of compounds, each expressed to several significant figures as a "thermodynamic solubility product."

Thus, it is surprising, if not alarming, to the beginning student of bone physiology to learn that the circulation of mammals is in rapid equilibration exchange with the skeleton, in which resides a relatively huge mass of sparingly soluble calcium phosphate salt. Yet the ion product of the constituent ions in the circulation can be shown to vary markedly in both health and disease.

Obviously, this is not an example of the suspension of physicochemical principles by the intervention of mysterious "vital forces." It is, however, another instance in which evolutionary processes have selected nonequilibrium boundary conditions in order that the system retain flexibility and a susceptibility to regulation by cellular activity.

Imagine the problems that would ensue if the mineral phase of bone did in fact exhibit a fixed solubility and was in a solubility equilibrium with serum. Calcium, phosphate, and hydroxyl ion concentrations would be locked into a fixed relationship and, depending upon the vagaries of dietary intake, the hapless individual would alternate between tetany (from hypocalcemia) and renal failure (from hypercalcemia). His skeletal mass would wax (drinking milk) and wane (drinking beer).

Conceptually then, it is easy to appreciate *why* evolutionary processes selected a regulated steady state disequilibrium upon which to impose hormonal homeostatic controls. However, the complexities of this steady state disequilibrium have so frustrated investigators and has proved to be so refractory to investigation, in

WILLIAM F. NEUMAN

4

bone material and calcification mechanisms*

* Supported in part by NIH Grant No. AM-17074 and in part by a contract with the U.S. Department of Energy and assigned number UR-3490-1683.

fact, that the problem was not clearly perceived until the 1950s. Now, after 25 years of investigation, it remains unsettled in many details. Nonetheless, although there is still room for debate over details, the general features of the system are clearly delineated. In this chapter, these features will be presented with the realization that with continuing investigation, changes in emphasis and modifications in substance will ensue.

The biologic requirements to be met by the system can be briefly stated as follows:

1. The metabolic requirements of cells and organ systems mandate that the variations in ionic levels of serum $[OH^-]$ and $[P_i]$ be kept within definite limits and those of $[Ca^{++}]$ within very narrow limits.

2. The skeletal mineral phase must provide a buffering depot for these ions in order to complement the homeostatic activities of the gut and kidney. For example when no calcium is ingested, neither the gut nor the kidney can prevent calcium losses, and the skeleton must provide the necessary reserves.

3. For growth and remodeling, skeletal processes must cause mineralization to occur in new areas and to disappear in old areas while continuously providing a strong mechanical framework.

Our first task, then, is to define the first requirement: the normal limits of variation of the levels of the constituent ions in the various fluid compartments.

The state of calcium and phosphate in body fluids

The concentrations of Ca^{++} and P_i in serum

Because ionic calcium has been selected to serve as a control or signaling mechanism in a bewildering variety of biologic functions (muscle contraction, nerve conduction, synaptic transmission, hormonal response, secretory processes) the level of Ca^{++} in serum is controlled with better efficiency than is that of perhaps any other substance. It has been referred to as "Nature's Constant."

With few exceptions, the total calcium concentration in the sera of a wide variety of species is 2.5 mM or 10 mg/dl. Not only is this value relatively species-invariant, but it also does not vary significantly with age or food intake.

Long before the advent of ion-specific electrodes, McLean and Hastings established that roughly one third of the total calcium was inactive biologically (as detected by the frog heart), apparently associated with the serum proteins. This association does not represent specific ion binding, although the literature frequently refers to the fraction as "protein-bound calcium." Rather, the highly anionic serum proteins (especially albumin, which has 18 negative charges per molecule) acquire halos of loosely immobilized cations (gegen ions) in order to achieve electroneutrality. These immobilized gegen ions are not bound in the strict physicochemical sense. That is, they are not chelated to group-specific sites. However, they are effectively removed from the solution by this immobilization in charge neutralization. The principal cation of serum, Na^+, is the main participant in this charge neutralization, but the hydrated Ca^{++} ion with its higher charge density and polarizability is relatively more attractive. Thus, the ratio of Na^+ to Ca^{++} free ions is greater than 100:1, whereas the ratio of protein-associated ions is only about 10:1 (15 to 1.5/mole of albumin, respectively).

In any event, the protein and sodium contents of serum are themselves relatively constant. It is unusual, then, for the proportion of protein-associated calcium to vary from its customary 35 to 40% of the total calcium present. Nonetheless, in renal dysfunction, in starvation, in hyper- or hypoproteinemia, and so forth, this distribution of calcium can deviate markedly, and the clinician is well advised to employ the commercially available electrode method for estimation of free calcium ion activity, a Ca^{++} that normally is about 1.25 mM.

The difference between free (1.25 mM) and total ultrafilterable calcium (1.5 mM) is small (~0.25 mM) and can be calculated to be complexed with citrate, bicarbonate, inorganic phosphate, pyrophosphate, and other minor constituents. In sum, the normal concentration in serum of free, ionic, biologically active Ca^{++} is almost always 1.25 mM, irrespective of species, time of day, diet, sex, or persuasion.

Conversely, the levels of inorganic phosphate in serum are much more variable. There are species variations (the normal fasting rat, 3 mM), age variations (the normal newborn human, 2 mM), diurnal variations, postprandial variations, and so forth. The normal fasting adult human value, however, is conveniently close to an easily remembered value, 1 mM. This figure represents the *total* concentration, and we must consider which proportion is free, which is ionic, and of the ionic proportion which of three possible forms is present: $H_2PO_4^-$, $HPO_4^=$, or $PO_4^{\equiv}$. As it turns out, the question is of little consequence.

Although the literature generally refers to a small amount of protein binding, there is no real evidence that anionic phosphate interacts with anionic protein. The confusion arises from the erroneous application of a Donnan factor to ultrafiltration data. Moreover, since the pH, temperature, and ionic strength are all essentially constant under physiologic conditions, the distribution of phosphate in serum among its various ionized forms is also a constant: roughly 80% $HPO_4^=$, 20% $H_2PO_4^-$, and less than 0.01% $PO_4^{\equiv}$.

One can, therefore, legitimately employ a physiochemical shortcut by expressing the relative degree of saturation of body fluids as a simple ion product $(Ca^{++}) \cdot (P_i)$ (1.3 mM $\times$ 1 mM or 1.3 mM^2). It must be remembered at all times, however, that this expression contains inherent assumptions concerning the Ca:P ratio, pH, temperature, and ionic strength. When comparisons of experimental data under divergent conditions are to be made, all solution values must be converted to thermodynamic ion activities.

The concentrations of Ca^{++} and P_i in extracellular fluid

Within the limits of present information concerning the constituent ions discussed here, there appear to be no significant gradients between the serum and the general extracellular fluids. The extracellular fluids may contain variable amounts of extravascular protein, and as a consequence the *total* calcium may vary accordingly, but except for specialized fluid compartments having strong barriers to diffusion, the transcapillary rates of ionic diffusion are so great that the general extracellular fluid is regarded as equivalent to serum in electrolyte composition (free ions).

The concentrations of Ca^{++} and P_i in cartilage fluid

It cannot be assumed that the fluids of connective tissue are isoionic with serum in electrolyte composition. These tissues are, in general, relatively avascular, dynamic in a cellular sense, and possess an extracellular matrix dominated by the local cell population in compositional and metabolic terms. Thus, it is reasonable to assume that compositional differences might exist in, say, the cartilage fluid compartment. The question of what these differences were, however, remained moot until Howell[2] and his associates developed techniques for the direct sampling and analysis of microvolumes of fluid withdrawn from living cartilage *in vivo*. The sampling area was in the region of the hypertrophic chondrocytic septa of the hind limb of the rat. In the normal animal, the major findings were as follows:

1. Protein content was surprisingly high, 41% that of serum.
2. This protein, unlike serum protein, did not render much Ca^{++} nonultrafilterable.
3. The ultrafilterable Ca^{++} was 93% that of serum, an insignificant difference.
4. P_i like Cl^- was slightly lower than that of serum (possibly because of the high fixed anionic charge of cartilage matrix).
5. The nucleotide content, though higher than serum ($2\times$) was very low in absolute amounts.
6. The pH was surprisingly high, 7.6 compared with serum 7.4 at comparable CO_2 tensions.

Thus, although differences were measurable, the composition of cartilage extracellular fluid is essentially comparable to that of serum, except for a slightly more alkaline pH.

The concentrations of Ca^{++} and P_i in the extracellular fluid of bone

The problem of evaluating the composition of the extracellular fluids of bone has proved intractable to direct investigation. Attempts to penetrate bone by micropipette or microelectrodes have proved unsuccessful. Nor can fluid be recovered from bone (powdered while frozen) even when subjected to high separation forces in an ultracentrifuge.

Lacking a direct approach, an indirect method was applied. Frozen bone has been powdered and then equilibrated at 37° C with synthetic buffers. The buffer was analyzed, and a fresh specimen of powdered bone was equilibrated with new synthetic buffer having its electrolyte composition adjusted to match that of the previous equilibration. This process was repeated until no measurable changes occurred during the equilibration. The composition of this final buffer differed in major respects from that of the extracellular fluids. The Ca^{++} level was lower, by 50%; the K^+ level was higher, by fivefold. All other components, notably Cl^-, HCO_3, and P_i and Mg^{++}, were essentially normal.

We now realize that these results were obtained with nonviable bone and that solid phase changes occur in dead bone. We are forced then to *deduce* the composition of bone fluid by even more indirect methods.

The experimental problems are immense, and the results are fraught with uncertainty. Our best information has been collected from studies of live calvaria clamped in specially designed chambers *in vitro*. From isotope uptake and release it has been found that the influx of ions and substrates is a passive, concentration-dependent process. The effluxes, too, are largely passive, only slightly affected by the acute application of metabolic inhibitors or hormones. The fluxes themselves are very large and appear to be *inter*cellular. Thus, the cellular membranes and intercellular syncitium appear to offer only a minor barrier to the free diffusion of ions, and it follows that concentration gradients in electrolytes, if they exist at all, must be small in magnitude or large only in a small number of sites of limited volumes.

The question of a bone membrane

For those familiar with recent history in this field, this last conclusion is somewhat discouraging. Our thinking has undergone a complete cycle. Twenty years ago, lacking information to the contrary, it was *assumed* that bone extracellular fluid and the extracellular fluid in general were quite comparable. Then there appeared a variety of reports that seemed to refute this idea. It appeared that the potassium concentration of the noncellular fluids of bone is inexplicably high, severalfold higher than in serum. Merely cutting embryonic bones in two (rupturing membrane integrity) caused the bones to mineralize *in vitro* and to alter metabolic pathways in the cells (lactate production). In contrast to bones with intact membrane structure, stripped or dead bones were unable to support physiologic levels of Ca^{++} and P_i in equilibration buffers.

Initial attempts to explain these findings postulated a membrane having a "pump-leak" system, that is, that Ca^{++} and P_i passively diffused across a membrane barrier into the bone fluids down a concentration gradient, and calcium ions, at least, were actively pumped back to the circulation. Secondarily, it was postulated that the metabolism of bone cells influenced local conditions. Bone cells are unusual in their handling of carbohydrate. They evince aerobic glycolysis (an "impaired" Pasteur mechanism) and produce huge quantities of lactic acid even when well oxygenated. Thus it seemed reasonable to suppose that all this acid production within the confines of a "tight" membrane enclosure could produce a localized lowering of pH.

We now realize that with respect to H^+, Ca^{++}, and P_i at least, the membranes are simply too "leaky" to support a leak-pump mechanism. Energetically, the system would be totally impractical. Moreover, by the rapid exchange of K^+, HCO_3^-, and P_i, even a lactate-produced proton gradient would be rapidly modulated to very small magnitudes as far as pH is concerned.

Is there, then, no bone "membrane"? Unfortunately, the facts upon which the concept was founded remain:

1. The K^+ content of bone is inexplicably high.

TABLE 4-1 CALCIUM AND PHOSPHATE COMPOUNDS

FORMULA	NAME	MOLAR Ca/P	ABBREVIATION
$Ca(HPO_4) \cdot 2\ H_2O$	Dicalcium phosphate dihydrate	1.0	DCPD
$Ca_4H(PO_4)_3$	Octacalcium phosphate	1.33	OCP
$Ca_9(PO_4)_6$ (var.)	Amorphous calcium phosphate	1.3–1.5	ACP
$Ca_3(PO_4)_2$	Tricalcium phosphate	1.50	TCP
$Ca_5(PO_4)_3OH$	Hydroxyapatite	1.66	HAP

2. Intact living bone supports higher levels of Ca^{++} and P_i than does denuded or killed bone.

3. Rupturing of membranes alters the metabolic activity of the cells themselves.

4. Morphologically, every element of bone extracellular matrix is surrounded by cells or cell membranes.

This is an unsettled area that only future research can resolve. However, we believe that the most likely resolution of this problem involves the following postulate: although the cells and membranes that surround all elements of bone are relatively permeable to substrates, electrolytes, and protons, they do markedly impede the flow and free diffusion of *macromolecules*.

Thus, proteins, polypeptides, proteoglycans, proteolipids, and even microstructures such as vesicles are locally produced by cells within an effective "container." It is the combination of these materials that affect the cells themselves and the controlled maturation of extracellular elements, both organic and mineral. This idea will be developed more fully in a later section.

Briefly stated, we have no direct evidence concerning the composition of the extracellular fluid of bone. It appears unlikely that there are any major differences between Ca^{++} and P_i in bone and Ca^{++} and P_i in serum. Distribution studies of the pH indicator, the weak acid 5,5-dimethyl-2,4-oxazolidenedione (DMO), suggest that the pH in mature bone is at serum pH or slightly less (pH 7.3 to 7.5) and in rapidly mineralizing tissue at serum pH or slightly more (pH 7.4 to 7.5) as in mineralizing cartilage. With respect to protein content, however, there is no comparison. As described in the previous chapter, collagen fibers and fibrils, sialoproteins, proteoglycans, osteocalcin and a variety of as yet uncharacterized macromolecules are either unique to bone or unique in their concentrations and ratios.

The mineral phase of hard tissues

The aqueous calcium-phosphate system

A variety of specific compounds of calcium and phosphate exist. These all can be prepared, isolated, and studied by analytical and structural techniques: x-ray or electron diffraction, infrared spectroscopy, nuclear magnetic resonance or electron spin resonance technology, and transmission and scanning electron microscopy (EM). Some of these characterized substances are listed in Table 4-1 (in order of decreasing acidity, decreasing solubility, and increasing thermodynamic stability:

The first compound is relatively stable at acidic pH only. Above pH 7.0, all the compounds except hydroxyapatite (HAP) are more or less unstable and, given an aqueous environment, will recrystallize or undergo solid state conversions to form the thermodynamically stable HAP.

A remarkable feature of this system of compounds is that structurally, the architecture is dominated by the phosphate groupings and as a consequence the structure of each substance, though unique to itself, has features in common with the structures of others in the series. Thus a structural plane of dicalcium phosphate dihydrate (DCPD) or otacalcium phosphate (OCP) can be shown to be essentially identical to a comparable plane of HAP. This opens the theoretical possibility of "sandwich" mixtures or "surface compounds," that is, a layer of DCPD or OCP on a base crystal of HAP, for example. A sample of this structural overlap is illustrated in Figure 4-1.

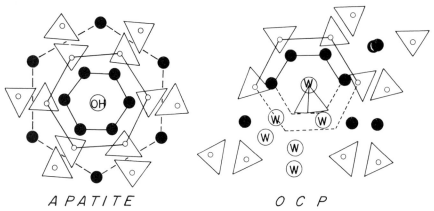

FIGURE 4-1 *This modification of a projection of the structure of OCP given by Brown is compared with a projection of a hexagonal column of the apatite HAP. It shows that the two structures have a similar form, namely, a hexagon of phosphates enclosing a hexagon of calcium ions. However, in OCP the hexagons are incompletely filled and contain water molecules.* (Simpson, D. R., Clin. Orthop. 86:260–286, 1972)

Another remarkable feature is that the thermodynamically stable end product, HAP, is microcrystalline, that is, under physiologic circumstances it never forms crystals of dimensions greater than a few hundred angstroms in length, breadth, or thickness. As a consequence, HAP always presents an enormous specific surface, 50 to 250 m^2/g. Thus, the possibility of sandwich or surface compounds becomes of practical significance. This means that a preparation of HAP, depending upon its mode of preparation or the medium to which it has been exposed, can exhibit chemical and solubility properties of members preceding it in the calcium phosphate series. Given these properties, it is understandable that controversies and arguments abound in the cumulative literature on "solubilities" and the nature of the calcium phosphates derived from biologic structures.

Another remarkable feature of the system relates to the formation of a solid phase from solution. The thermodynamic end product, HAP, cannot be formed *de novo* from its constituent ions in solution. Its smallest unit of crystallographic structure, the unit cell, contains 18 ions ($Ca_{10}[PO_4]_6[OH]_2$). There is no conceivable means by which a nidus of such complexity can form by collision processes directly. Thus it appears that as the concentrations of Ca^{++} and P_i are increased, the first solid to separate is the simplest—DCPD. *This* can be formed by a bimolecular or stepwise single ion collision process. If the pH is less than 6.0, DCPD is sufficiently stable to separate as a crystallographically identifiable solid phase. If the pH is greater than 7.0 or the temperature is elevated, DCPD is transient (so transient it may be unobserved), and the first solid isolated is frequently OCP or ACP. Thus, by adjusting conditions, any member (or mixture of members) from DCPD to HAP can be "precipitated" from solution. It is not at all certain that all sequential members are obligatory steps in the conversion of the initial DCPD to the final HAP crystals. At low supersaturation levels, HAP can catalyze its own formation directly from solution, for example. Nor is it certain to what degree solid state transitions and recrystallization processes (dissolution and redeposition) may be involved in these interconversions. What is commonly observed is that early precipitates exhibit a low calcium:phosphorus ratio from 1 to 1.5, whereas aged precipitates show a calcium:phosphorus ratio that is considerably higher, from 1.4 to 2 or even greater. Usually, the first transient phase isolated analyses near 1.3, suggesting the presence of OCP. Later, preparations with a ratio of 1.5 can be shown to contain HAP (ratio 1.66). It is clear that the solid phase cannot be inferred from the calcium:phosphorus ratio alone.

However, in practical terms, *when solid phase and nucleating catalysts, are lacking, it is the K_{sp} of DCPD that controls the stability of calcium-phosphate solutions under physiologic conditions of pH, ionic strength, and temperature.* From laboratory experience, a $(Ca^{++}) \cdot (P_i)$ ion product of less than 6 mM² can be prepared, and the resultant solution is stable indefinitely at pH 7.4. At concentrations above this critical product, spontaneous precipitation occurs. Once precipitation begins, the solid phase undergoes its spontaneous, autocatalytic conversion toward the thermodynamically stable end product, HAP. Depending upon time of standing and other conditions the "final" $(Ca^{++}) \cdot (P_i)$ is quite variable, reflecting the mixture of solid phase surface compounds, and "sandwiches" of phases present at the time of observation. In general terms, this ion product becomes quite low, only a fraction of the concentration product found in serum or in the extracellular fluid.

A point to be emphasized is the fact that *once formed, HAP crystals will autocatalytically promote further crystal formation at $(Ca^{++}) \cdot (P_i)$ products at or even below adult human serum levels.* This presents us with the "Lot's Wife Problem." Left to their own devices, the five or more pounds of HAP crystals found in our skeletons should grow and grow and grow—as long as they are provided with a normal extracellular fluid environment. Indeed, what is it that prevents us all from turning into pillars of salt? We shall return to this question subsequently. In general, the normal ion products in the body fluids of higher mammals (from 1.3 mM² [adult human] to 2.6 mM² [perinatal infant] to 4 mM² [adult rat]) all fall in the region of *metastability* of the aqueous calcium-phosphate system. They are well below the point of spontaneous precipitation, but well above the effective solubility of any solid phase or mixture of solid phases likely to be stable under physiologic conditions.

The solid phases of calcium phosphate in bone

From the preceding discussion, it should be easily understood that the solid phases of bone and cartilage have been most difficult to characterize

definitively. Controversy and disagreement have been common and persistent.

Historically, there has been general agreement only that *some* HAP is present. From compositional analyses, various investigators have suggested the presence of admixed $CaCO_3$ and other compounds. These suggestions have not survived. A little over a decade ago, the presence of large amounts of amorphous calcium phosphate (ACP) was claimed. Its presence was inferred mainly from the lack of ordered structure to be expected in the x-ray diffraction pattern of HAP. Understandably, though, it is difficult to quantitate that which cannot be seen by x-rays, and the estimates of the amounts of ACP present in bone have been repeatedly revised downward. Some years ago, our laboratory presented chemical evidence for the presence of $CaHPO_4 \cdot 2\text{-}H_2O$ in rat bone, and most recently high resolution NMR has confirmed, if not its presence, at least considerable quantities of P_i, having an electronic environment comparable to that of DCPD. In low density fractions of *very* recently deposited bone mineral, the presence of DCPD has been unequivocally demonstrated by diffraction techniques. In other words, at the present time it would seem that the bone mineral represents a complete array of the intermediates seen in the transition of solution Ca^{++} and P_i to solid phase HAP. The younger or more recent calcified structures contain solid, which predominates in DCPD and ACP. The more mature structures are predominantly HAP. Although OCP has never been directly demonstrated, it seems reasonable to presume that it, too, may be present in the intermediate stages of maturation, if not in a form sufficiently ordered to diffract x-rays, in layered surfaces or sandwich layers.

The striking feature is that this modern view of bone mineral is suggestive of two correlates: (1) that the same or at least a comparable sequence of phase transitions that occur physicochemically *in vitro* are also occurring *in vivo*, and (2) that the conversion process is frozen in bone. Conversions that *in vitro* require only minutes and hours, require days, months, and even years in living bone. We shall return to this feature later.

Impurities in the mineral phase

Although it is clear that the mineral of the calcified tissues mirrors the events observed in purified, synthetic physicochemical systems, it must be recognized that the extracellular fluids are enormously complex. Bone mineral forms in a medium containing many more ions and substances than simply Ca^{++}, P_i, or OH^-. When it is recalled that the HAP system is microcrystalline with surface areas of up to 200 m^2/g, the opportunities for adsorption, surface exchange, and so forth are seen to be enormous. It is no accident that HAP is commonly used as an adsorbant and in column chromatography.

It has been found that a variety of ions can substitute for certain constituent ions within the lattice of the crystal structure itself. Among the prominent examples are Sr^{++} or Pb^{++} for Ca^{++}, F^- for OH^-; and $CO_3^=$ for $PO_4^=$. An even wider range of possibilities exists at the particle surfaces at which spatial and charge requirements are less restrictive. Examples of this type of heteroionic exchange are Mg^{++}, Sr^{++}, Ra^{++}, Pb^{++}, and Na^+ for Ca^{++} and $Co_3^=$, citrate, phosphate esters, diphosphonates, pyrophosphate, and amino acids for phosphate.

Thus the overall composition of the mineral phase is a variable composite. It contains considerable quantities of $CO_3^=$, citrate, Mg^{++}, Na^+, and F^-, plus traces of many other substances. The composition reflects dietary history, and overall it exhibits the composition of a calcium-deficient apatite, that is, a residual calcium : phosphorus ratio of less than the theoretical 1.66 for HAP. This is no doubt a reflection of the presence of transition phases, all of which have a ratio of 1.5 or less.

The location of the apatitic crystals in cartilage and bone

These microcrystals of impure HAP and its solution antecedents are not found floating around as a loose suspension in the body fluids. Rather, the crystalline habit is influenced by the matrix, and conversely, the properties of the matrix are greatly influenced by the presence of the crystals.

Location in bone and dentine

Mature lamellar bone represents the best example and the clearest evidence of the interaction between crystals and matrix at the molecular level. Admittedly, the technical problems are immense in establishing the inter-relations on such a scale. The possibilities of artifacts arising in the preparation of specimens for study (swelling, contraction, translocation, dissolution, recrystallization, and so forth) are almost always present and are difficult to control and evaluate. Nonetheless, so much agreement has accumulated in this field that we can be confident that in the overall outline, current concepts must be substantially correct. It is difficult to believe that so many different laboratories employing such a variety of techniques could all produce the same artifacts.

From the earliest x-ray observations that showed preferential crystalline orientation in long bones to the present, most sophisticated ultrastructural delineations, there has been an ever-growing recognition that in mature lamellar bone, the crystals of HAP are located *within* the collagen fibrils. Perhaps not all, but 80 to 90% are so situated. The crystallographic c-axes of the crystals are parallel to the long axes of the fibers, and the earliest seeds appear at prescribed sites that correspond to the same periodicity as found in collagen fibrils themselves, that is, 700 A. An example of this close inter-relationship is given in Figure 4-2.

The exact architecture of the three-dimensional packing of the polymerized collagen rods themselves has not been settled. It may vary from tissue to tissue. However, the current proposals vary in detail, not in kind, and are an outgrowth and modification of the original two-dimensional model of Hodge and Petruska (see ref. No. 4.)

Because of these uncertainties, it is not possible at present to be dogmatic about the precise location of the crystals within the fibrils and fibers. Two relatively current models are presented in Figures 4-3 and 4-4. The general concensus is that mineralization begins as a "haze" of increased density primarily in the "hole" regions and that with maturation this density increases

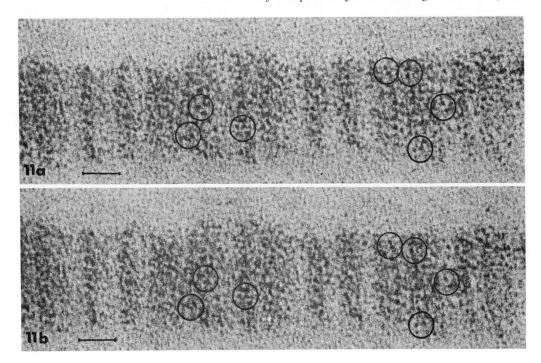

FIGURE 4-2 *Consecutive exposures at the same electron micrographic focus setting of bone collagen block-stained with alcoholic uranyl acetate. Regions represented by circles indicate the same particles in the two exposures — other matching regions may be found. The particles indicated are 0.8 to 1.2 nm in diameter. The point-to-point resolution is of the same order of magnitude. Detail can be accepted as real because it is found in consecutively exposed negatives. Formaldehyde-fixed, cacodylate buffer was used. Bars = 10 nm. (Booth-royd, B.: Clin. Orthop. 106:290–309, 1975)*

to form small plate-like structures. At full maturation, geometric considerations suggest that almost all of the "holes" and "pores" must be mineralized (in order to accommodate the mineral present). Since it is estimated that the collagen fibrils occupy roughly 85% of the extracellular space, there is very little room for extrafibrillar mineral to accumulate. And because the "hole" and "pore" volumes within a fibril are interconnected and continuous, full mineralization presents us with the possibility that both the organic and the inorganic phases are more or less *continuous.* This may explain a very old and often observed phenomenon, namely, that a bone retains its form and some structural strength whether one removes the organic (by ashing) or the inorganic (by acid or ethylenediaminetetraacetic acid [EDTA]) phases. This phenomenon is illustrated in Figure 4-5.

In mature dentine, like lamellar bone, this same intimate structural inter-relationship between mineral and collagen has been repeatedly described.

Location in woven bone and cartilage

From the point of view of function, woven bone, endochondral cartilage, and healing fracture callus cartilage are all intended as temporary structures. As the old saying goes: "it takes time to make good wine." Apparently it also takes time to produce the precise cocrystalline three-dimensional architecture of mineralized collagen seen in mature lamellar bone. In any event, the relationship between collagen and mineral in these temporary structures is much less striking. The collagen fibrils themselves are smaller, less-well developed, more random in array, and fill up much less of the total extracellular space. Beginning mineralization does not appear to be directly associated with the fibrils themselves. Rather, it appears to be associated with extracel-

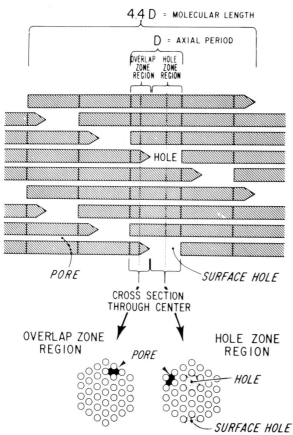

FIGURE 4-3 *Diagrammatic representation of the organization of the collagen macromolecules in a collagen fibril according to the general model proposed by Hodge and Petruska. The presence of both "holes" and "pores" in the hole-zone region and of "pores" only in the overlap region is depicted according to the model of the collagen fibril suggested by Glimcher, M.: Handbook of Physiology-Endocrinology VII, Baltimore, Williams & Wilkins Co., 1976)*

lular membrane-bound structures, matrix vesicles, and appears as "sunbursts"—extrafibrillar collections of crystals that give the appearance of having grown by autocatalytic nucleation from a central seed or nidus. An illustration is given in Figure 4-6—a section of embryonic woven bone. In these temporary structures, the general impression is that of a loose fibrillar network whose interstices are impregnated with randomly oriented tiny crystals. This is in sharp contrast to lamellar bone, which is a close-packed, ordered network of mineralized fibers.

All this makes sense from a functional point of view. The temporary "scaffolding" of cartilage and woven bone is much more available for disassembly than is the cement-like structure of lamellar bone. In cartilage, both the organic matrix and the mineral are easily available to attack by cellular secretory products—acids, chelators, and enzymes. In bone, by contrast, each phase protects the other. Enzymes simply cannot contact the fibrils, and the interstitial mineral is protected by severely restricted diffusional pathways.

Mechanisms of calcification

General considerations

We have discussed the state of the extracellular fluids and the general processes by which solid phases of calcium phosphate separate from solution. We have seen that with respect to calcium and phosphate the body fluids are *metastable*— below the saturation needed for spontaneous precipitation and yet well above the saturation needed to support crystal growth and maturation once a nidus or seed has been formed. There are then two possible types of mechanisms by which the mineralization process may be initiated:

1. A "booster mechanism" by which the concentration of either Ca^{++} or P_i is caused to be elevated above the critical ion product, 6 mM^2, in some isolated fluid volume, or

2. a "catalytic nucleation mechanism" that causes a beginning nidus or seed to form from the otherwise stable extracellular fluid.

There is no difficulty in finding one such example. Rather, examples of both phenomena abound and our first problem is in identifying which, if any, such mechanisms are operative, and where and when. Our second difficulty arises from the aforementioned "Lot's wife problem." It is one thing to initiate crystallization, it is quite another matter to keep the process from going too fast and too far. If the maturation of early transition states of the crystallization process were not slowed and arrested, all of the crystals would very soon be converted to HAP, the solubility of which is too low to be compati-

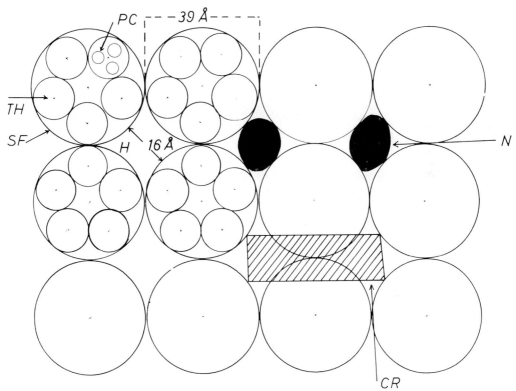

FIGURE 4-4 *Diagrammatic cross-section through the model of a tetragonal arrangement of subfibrils in the collagen fiber, according to Miller and Parry. On the left are shown the elements of the collagen structure; on the right are shown calcium-phosphate nuclei* **(N)** *and crystals* **(CR)**, *which may develop in the fiber.* **SF** = *subfibrils,* **TH** = *triple helix,* **PC** = *protein chain,* **H** = *hole region between the subfibrils. (Höhling, H. J., Ashton, B. A., and Koster, H. D.: Cell Tissue Res. 148:11–26, 1974)*

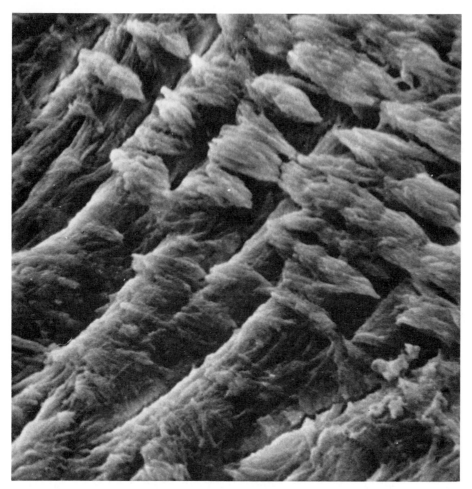

FIGURE 4-5 *A scanning electron micrographic visualization of the mineralizing front in an adult human lamellar bone. Mineralization is largely confined to the collagen fiber bundles. The collagen and matrix have actually been removed by a hot 1,2 ethylenediamine extraction, yet the fiber is easily visualized as a more or less continuous mineralized structure. (Jones, S. T., and Boyde, A.: Isr. J. Med. Sci. 12:98–107, 1976)*

ble with the homeostatic controls needed for maintenance of the proper electrolyte composition of the extracellular fluid. In the rapidly growing animal, uninhibited crystal growth and formation at the many bone formation sites would literally drain the extracellular fluid of its calcium and P_i content at rates much faster than the gut could restore or the kidney conserve. As a counterpart, then, to the two types of mechanisms for initiating crystals, two general mechanisms are needed to slow and regulate the mineralization process:

1. *Nucleation inhibition*, by which formation of nuclei of early transition forms of calcium phosphate is prevented in areas in which mineralization is *not* desirable.
2. *Crystal growth inhibition*, by which already formed nuclei are prevented from growth and autocatalytic seeding at uncontrolled rates.

Booster mechanisms

THE ROBISON HYPOTHESIS AND ALKALINE PHOSPHATASE

Historically, the first suggestion of a booster mechanism was that of Robison (see reference No. 1) who observed the formation of phosphate

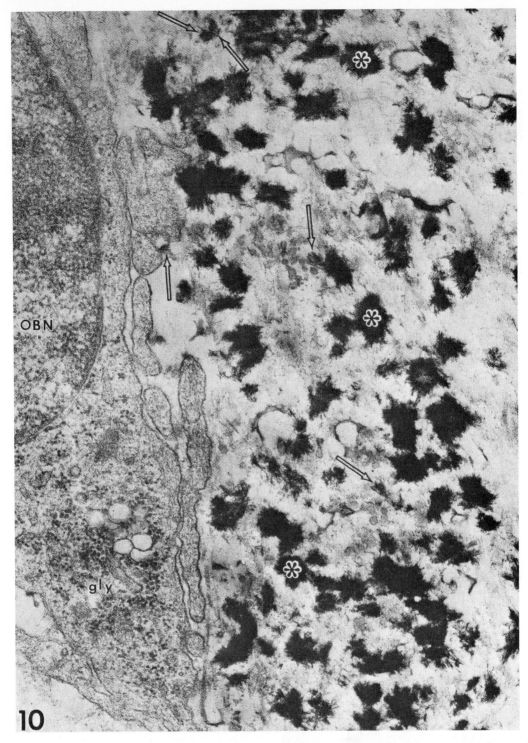

FIGURE 4-6 *In this section of early temporary woven bone it is seen that the fine, immature collagen fibers are relatively unrelated to beginning mineralization. There are portions of an osteoblast with nucleus* **(OBN)** *and glycogengranules* **(gly)** *appearing in the cytoplasm. There are numerous membrane-bound vesicles with HAP crystals within and around them (arrows) within the extracellular matrix. Spheroidal nodules of bone mineral (asterisks) appear among the fine fibrillar collagen and the ground substance,* × 48,000. (Marvaso, V., and Bernard, G. W.: Am. J. Anat. 149:453–467, 1977)

precipitates during early attempts to isolate the enzyme alkaline phosphatase. He reasoned that the enzyme could produce localized concentrations of P_i if it were provided with a suitable substrate of some ester phosphate. Further investigation revealed that the enzyme seemed to be closely associated and invariably present at sites of calcification. However, a suitable substrate in appropriate amounts extracellularly was never identified. Moreover, the enzyme (or one very much like it—it is fairly nonspecific) could be found in areas that did not calcify. This concept flourished for decades, fell into disuse, was revived, failed again, but has never been officially buried. We can be sure only that it will continue to survive until some function or functions for the enzyme in the processes of overall calcification have been fully agreed upon. One current opinion is that the enzyme is functioning

not so much as a "booster" of P_i as a necessary means of removing esterified phosphate inhibitors of the initiation and crystal growth processes (nucleotide phosphates, substrate phosphates, pyrophosphates, and so forth). This aspect is discussed more fully later.

INTRACELLULAR BOOSTER MECHANISMS

A variety of intracellular organelles have been shown to be capable of concentrating calcium to a remarkable degree. First and foremost is the mitochondrion. This organelle, by virtue of its oxidatively supported proton ejection mechanism, normally maintains a membrane potential estimated to be of the order of 180 mV, negative inside. From the Nernst equation, it can be calculated that this potential alone would lead to a millionfold concentration of calcium inside, rela-

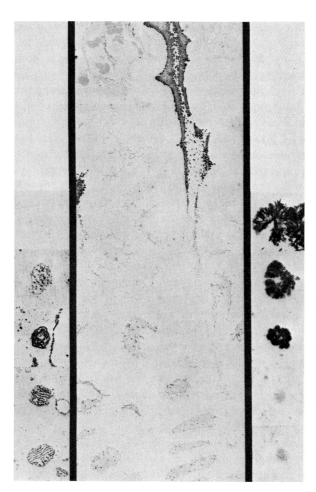

FIGURE 4-7   *A montage of electron micrographs of the zone of the hypertrophic cells of a control animal, which were stained with potassium pyroantimonate.*

The micrographs on the extreme right show the mitochondria of cells at different levels in the zone, × 21,000. The levels of these cells are indicated by the centrally placed micrographs, which show cells at different stages of maturation, × 750. Note that progressing down the zone of cells, the amount of black antimony–calcium complex in the mitochondria decreases.

The micrographs on the extreme left show matrix vesicles located at the same levels in the zone as those of the cells containing the mitochondria shown on the right, × 68,000. Note the gradually increasing accumulation of calcium in the vesicles located farther and farther down in the zone, as well as the crystal formation in the lowest vesicle. (Brighton, C. T., and Hunt, R. M.: J. Bone Joint Surg. 60A:630–639, 1978)

tive to the external cytosolic concentration outside. The calcium ion activity in the cytosol is generally very low, ca 10^{-7} M, which could lead to an internal $[Ca^{++}]$ of 0.1 M! Obviously, in the normally functioning cell this does not occur. The external membrane is quite impermeable to Ca^{++}, and an adenosine triphosphate (ATP)-activated pump, directed outward, keeps the mitochondrion from being inundated. However, if isolated mitochondria are provided with an energy source (substrate or ATP), Ca^{++}, and a permeable anion, they will literally stuff themselves to death. If P_i is present, the mitochondrion will become filled with a precipitate identified as ACP or even, occasionally, with some apatitic crystals.

On the basis of these observations, Lehninger and others have suggested that mitochondria may function normally as a means of initiating crystal formation in bone and cartilage. This seems rather unlikely given the many other less costly means of initiating crystal formation to be discussed. The mitochondrion, after all, is a very complicated structure that represents an enormous investment in terms of energy and biosynthetic activity. To deploy such an organelle (and its parent cell) for simple crystal initiation seems a poor choice from an evolutionary standpoint. Nonetheless, it must be admitted that any pathologic condition that renders the cell membrane permeable (thus flooding the cell cytoplasm with calcium) will invariably lead to mineralization of the mitochondria (CCl_4 acting on hepatocytes for example). Other pathologic states or even normal states of cell disruption (the hypertrophic chondrocytes for example) would follow a similar course. It is likely that such released mineralized mitochondria *could* catalyze further crystal initiation and growth in the extracellular environment into which they are released. Such a correlation between cell disintegration, mitochondrial uptake of calcium, and extracellular mineralization has been described as seen in Figure 4-7.

In the chorioallantoic membrane of the chicken egg and in the epithelia of intestinal mucosa, another calcium-concentrating organelle, the membrane vesicle, has been described. As is well known, the plasma membrane of all mammalian cells possesses an energized Ca^{++} pump, cal-

cium-ATPase (adenosine triphosphatase), which ejects calcium ions and keeps the cellular cytosol at micromolar concentrations or less. In these two tissues, a simple infolding of the membrane occurs. In the vesicle thus formed, the calcium pump is naturally directed *inward* and is fully energized (by cytosolic ATP). Thus, these vesicles concentrate Ca^{++} to a remarkable degree; the *total* Ca^{++} content has been estimated as 15M. These vesicles are apparently engaged in the transmural transport of calcium. The calcium-laden vesicle moves through the cell to the inside of the external tight junction and fuses again with the plasma membrane releasing its calcium content to the intercellular or capillary space. This is a unique means of transferring Ca^{++} across a barrier and up an electrochemical gradient, without disturbing the cell's control of its low cytosolic Ca^{++} content. These vesicles have not been described or studied in calcifying tissues. They remain, then, an untested possible mechanism for producing localized, transient high concentrations of Ca^{++} ions.

Other intracellular structures have been shown to concentrate calcium ions. The sarcoplasmic reticulum in particular is highly specialized in this regard. It is reported that the membrane protein of this organelle is almost made up entirely of the unique calcium-ATPase involved in Ca^{++} translocation.

This smooth endoplasmic reticulum stands as a highly specialized structure involved in the control of muscle contraction and relaxation. It has not been suggested to be a participant in normal mineralization processes. However, smooth endoplasmic reticulum is seen in other tissues, including osteoclasts. Other membrane-bound vesicles are commonly seen in cells in general and in bone cells in particular. With respect to calcification processes they have not been adequately studied.

EXTRACELLULAR ORGANELLES

There are, however, vesicles that have been extensively observed and analyzed. These are the extracellular matrix vesicles, of cartilage in particular. First described as discrete membrane-enclosed particles containing electron dense material they have since been shown to contain

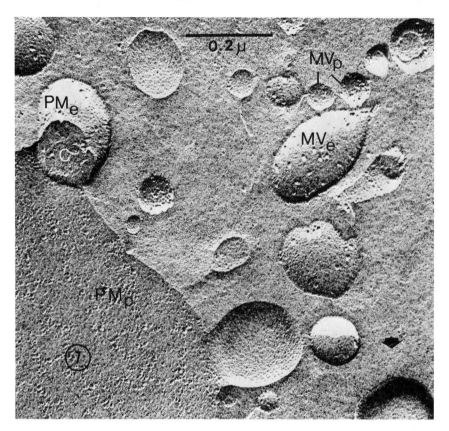

FIGURE 4-8 *A high-powered view of a freeze-fractured specimen, showing matrix vesicles have already formed and are in the process of budding from the edge of a chondrocyte (epiphyseal growth plate). (Cecil, R. N. A., and Anderson, H. C.: Metab. Bone Dis. Res. 1:89–95 1978)*

ACP or even more mature HAP crystals. Methods for isolation of these vesicles have been devised and even some success at dissolution and reconstitution has been achieved. They are thought to arise from a simple outfolding of cellular processes as illustrated in Figure 4-8. However, their membrane composition is not representative of the chondrocytic plasma membrane from which they are presumed to arise. They are, rather, enriched in alkaline phosphatase and in acidic (serine-containing) and inositol phospholipids. This observation of selectivity in composition is one of the best pieces of evidence that the isolated vesicles are not artifacts mechanically produced by the maceration and enzymic treatments employed in the isolation and purification procedures. It is frequently reported or postulated that these vesicles can ac-

tively accumulate Ca^{++}. This seems most unlikely, and there is no real evidence that they can. In the first place, in their formation by outfolding, the calcium pumps of the selected membrane surface would be *outwardly* directed, hardly a means for concentrating Ca^{++}. If the electromicrographic evidence is wrong, and the vesicles form by infolding and subsequent extrusion, this would not help matters. In such a case, the Ca^{++} pumps would be oriented in the right direction, inward, but they would have no energy source (ATP) by which to operate. The nucleotide content of cartilaginous extracellular fluid has been shown by direct measurement to be very low.

This is not to say that extracellular matrix vesicles are inoperative in cartilaginous mineralization. As will be discussed shortly, they may well function as nucleation centers. However, as participants in a booster mechanism the extracellular matrix vesicles seem unlikely prospects at the present time. As an alternative, a number of intracellular mechanisms for producing high localized concentrations of Ca^{++} exist, but these are *intra*cellular structures and have not as yet been implicated in normal calcification processes.

Nucleation Systems

COLLAGEN

It would seem that evolutionary selection has picked nucleation mechanisms over booster mechanisms as a means of getting calcium phosphate crystals to form when and where needed. Experimentally, the first and best studied example of such heterogenous nucleation is that of collagen. As early as 1958 two research groups demonstrated independently that purified collagen preparations will initiate HAP formation from metastable solutions well below the critical ion product, $Ca^{++} \times P_i$, of 6 mM^2 needed for spontaneous precipitation.

Since then it has been shown that only the normally occurring 700 A repeating crystallographic form of collagen is effective. Really active preparations will seed at concentration products, $Ca^{++} \times P_i$, as low as 1.3 mM^2, the levels seen in adult human serum. Occasionally in fact, collagen is more effective than even HAP crystals themselves. An unfortunate aspect, which has retarded the general acceptance of collagenous nucleation in bone, is the fact that a wide variety of collagens can be demonstrated to exhibit nucleation properties in the laboratory. These include collagen from sources that do not mineralize normally (rat tail tendon and skin) as well as those that may (turkey tendon and bone). Because of this phenomenon it has been suggested that a specialized activation process may account for specificity *in vivo:* (1) the presence of a special molecular adjunct (polysaccharide, polypeptide, phosphoprotein) that cocrystallizes with the collagen molecules as they form fibrils; or (2) the phosphorylation of very specific sites at selected areas on the collagen fibril.

With respect to (1), it is difficult to refute this possibility. However, it has been general experience that the purer the collagen, the more effective it is as a nucleator. Purified collagens have been recrystallized as many as ten times and show improved, not deteriorated, nucleation ability. Thus it cannot be excluded that a "helper" molecule may participate, but it certainly does not appear to be a requirement.

With respect to (2), it is clear that collagen can serve as a substrate phosphate acceptor in phosphorylating systems. Moreover, collagen forms a covalent linkage (serine phosphorylation) with inorganic P_i in incubation *in vitro*. Since this is without an energy source, some entropy contribution by a configurational change must be involved. The number of sites in both cases is very small. In addition, although the phosphorylated collagens are somewhat better nucleators, there is no direct evidence that phosphorylation is a necessary, or even normal, activation step.

The force of this idea was greatly weakened by the finding that exposure of a non-nucleating tendon to a high P_i-containing solution activated its nucleation properties not by phosphorylation but rather by the extraction of a high molecular weight nucleation inhibitor.

Structurally, the mineralization of collagen fibers *in vitro* follows the same course of events temporally observed *in vivo*, although the time course may be much accelerated. The initial seeding is between the major striations, predominantly in the "hole" regions, and is largely amorphous, and of low calcium : phosphorus ratio. Moreover, as expected, a partially mineralized collagen preparation is even more effective as a nucleator, fostering crystal initiation and growth at very low calcium $\times P_i$ products.

Thus, the case for collagen as a nucleator of and by itself seems almost unassailable. There remains, however, the question: "Why do not all collagens, in all places, undergo spontaneous nucleation?"

The answer to this question seems, at present to be threefold. First of all, collagens are *not* identical. Even the type I collagen of bone appears to be structurally unique. The pore size of bone collagen is large, ~6 A, large enough to accommodate the low diffusion of the large phosphate anion, ~ 4 A. By contrast, most collagens evince a pore size of only ~ 3 A. Second, the presence of specific inhibitor molecules (mentioned earlier) and other inhibiting substances (to be described) can easily render an otherwise effective collagen incapable of catalytic nucleation. Finally, any collagen that is not impregnated early in its life will by maturation and increasing cross-linking become more and more impermeable to the inner diffusion of ions and therefore ineffective in catalytic activity.

OTHER NUCLEATING AGENTS

As might be expected, any nonspecific matrix that contains preformed crystallites of Ca^{++} and P_i will, by their presence, be capable of catalyzing further crystal initiation and growth. This has plagued unwary investigators and no doubt will continue to do so. For example, the matrix vesicles described earlier were said to be effective nucleators. Careful study, however, showed that much of this ability was due to the presence of preformed ACP in the matrix vesicles as isolated. Fortunately, for all concerned, it was subsequently found that matrix vesicles whose calcium and P_i content was removed by exposure to acidic buffers retained a residual, albeit reduced, ability to nucleate when replaced in buffers at 7.6, the native pH of cartilage fluid.

A wide variety of other preparations have been claimed to possess nucleating ability. In general, these have not been studied as carefully (lack of preformed mineral) or as extensively (varying calcium:phosphate ratios and products) as one might desire. The list, however, is interesting and impressive. It includes tendon, phospholipids, proteolipids, phospholipid-calcium-P_i complexes, lysozyme, phosphoryn, noncollagenous proteins, and elastin, to mention only the most prominent candidates.

Thus the case for collagen as a nucleator in bone seems well founded. There is still some uncertainty whether other collagen-associated molecules assist in nucleation. In addition, cell organelles, membranous debris, blood vessel wall, and so forth all possess the propensity for initiating mineralization under special circumstances.

Inhibiting systems

With such an array of mineralization nucleators, it is appropriate to return to the "Lot's Wife Problem." How do cellular processes prevent us from turning into pillars of HAP?

IONIC INHIBITORS

In the extracellular fluid there exists a variety of low molecular weight substances that are inhibitory to initiation and/or growth of calcium phosphate crystals. For the most part these are effective in both spontaneous precipitation and catalyzed nucleation. Among the naturally occurring substances, the most important are Mg^{++}, citrate, and pyrophosphate. All three render solutions more stable and stabilize the early transient forms of calcium phosphate, ACP in particular. Although these three substances contribute on approximately equal terms, their concentrations are of course not all comparable: Mg^{++}, 10^{-3} M; citrate$^{\equiv}$, 10^{-4} M, and pyrophosphate$^{\equiv}$, 10^{-6} M. Thus pyrophosphate is by far the most powerful. Other polyphosphates, the nucleotides (guanosine triphosphate [GTP], adenosine triphosphate [ADP], and so forth,) are also relatively powerful inhibitors. In the cell cytosol, with its high Mg^{++}, citrate concentrations, low pH, nucleotide phosphates and low Ca^{++} levels, precipitation of calcium phosphates by spontaneous or nucleation mechanisms (membrane lipids) is virtually an impossibility. In mitochondria the high and continuously maintained levels of ATP ensures that a calcium-P_i phase, if formed, would be stabilized in a rather soluble and dynamic form of ACP.

A series of nonphysiologic substances that are inhibitory also exists. Among these are Sr^{++}, tetracycline, phosphonoacetate, and the synthetic diphosphonates.

These substances show differential actions on various steps of the overall process and have permitted Wadkins[6] to dissect out a multistep series: (1) Ca^{++} binding; (2) formation of $Ca(P_i)_1$; (3) formation of $Ca(P_i)_2$; (4) hydrolysis or phase conversion to HAP. His diagrammatic representation of the stepwise catalytic nucleation process and its inhibition is given in Figure 4-9.

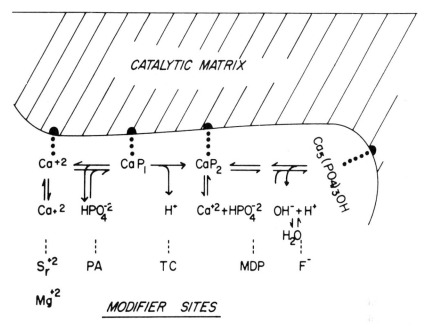

FIGURE 4-9 *This diagrammatic representation illustrates the multiple-step pathway in the nucleation by collagen of HAP from ions in solution. The first step, binding of Ca^{++} ions, is inhibited by competing cations Sr^{++} or Mg^{++}. The second step, the addition of a phosphate ion to form a surface compound analogous to DCPD is inhibited by phosphonoacetate. This product is stabilized and its ionization H^+ is inhibited by tetracycline. The further hydrolysis and addition of phosphates is inhibited by methylene diphosphonate. Finally, at critical concentrations, F^- may inhibit the final conversion to HAP. (Wadkins, C. L., Luben, R., Thomas, M., and Humphreys, R.: Clin. Orthop. 99:246–260, 1974)*

MACROMOLECULAR INHIBITORS

Very early in the history of the study of the mechanisms of calcification it was suggested that the control of mineralization might involve the state or content of macromolecules in the matrix. From histochemical staining at the level of the light microscope, it appeared that disappearance or at least depolymerization of mucopolysaccharides in the "ground substance" seemed to precede immediately the onset of deposition of Van Kossa staining material, calcium phosphate, in the cartilaginous growth plate.

Since then, there has accumulated a bewildering variety of substances that have been shown in one way or another to inhibit the nucleation or at least the growth and autocatalytic conversion of early mineral deposits to HAP. These include highly polymerized proteoglycans, phosphoproteins, phosphoryn, lysozyme, osteocalcin (the carboxyglutamic–containing polypeptide) and three other protein and polypeptide fractions of the EDTA-soluble, noncollagenous proteins extracted from powdered bone preparations. In general terms, these substances seem to be strongly attracted to HAP and/or preapatitic forms and they produce surface compounds and effectively remove these forming minerals from contact with the bathing solutions. Thus, they are capable of preventing the initiation or of arresting the maturation of forming HAP crystals. They are generally very powerful and by extrapolation from laboratory conditions, their concentration in bone is sufficiently high to more than cause a complete arrest of the mineralization process.

The mineralization processes in cartilage and bone

General considerations

It seems likely that quite different sets of mineralization processes exist in cartilage and bone. The contrasts between the tissues are enormous.

In cartilage, the matrix is loose, the collagen fibrils are small, immature, and disordered, the crystals seem unrelated to the collagen—located in bursts of unordered aggregates, and there exists an abundance of matrix vesicles. Most important, as the progenitor chondrocytes divide, they retreat from the advancing calcification front leaving behind the maturing chondrocytes, which, having synthesized a calcifiable matrix filled with vesicles, become hypertrophic, use up their stored energy supplies, and literally give up their ghosts and die. It is left for invading capillaries and cells to remove the calcified bridge left behind. In contrast, in bone the progenitor osteoblasts do not retreat from the calcifying front, but the product cells they leave behind make for themselves a more or less permanent home in the mineralized matrix that they cause to be produced. These cells, having become osteocytes, are forced to accomplish two things in order to survive. To maintain communication with the outside world, in terms of substrates and waste products, they must elaborate a complex network of interconnecting cell processes, the canaliculae, and, most important, they must elaborate agents that prevent the mineralized matrix from squeezing them to death. That matrix carries with it the potential to seed autocatalytically the further mineralization of any space available. If the osteocytes did not prevent it, their lacunae would fill up with mineral (and frequently do on the death of the osteocyte). Not only do the osteocytes prevent mineralization of their lacunae but they also can and do (under the stimulus of a bolus of parathyroid hormone (PTH), for example) act like osteoclasts by enlarging their living space through the removal of both mineral and matrix. This has been termed osteocytic osteolysis.

Finally, there is the matter of homeostatic regulation. The overall electrolyte economy of the young, growing animal can afford to have a limited fraction of the total skeleton accreting mineral in a more less controlled way. After all, dietary intake is high and a highly positive calcium balance is being maintained. In the cartilage, then, a calcium "sink" can be tolerated. This cannot be true of the skeleton as a whole. If the entire skeleton were to behave as a calcium "sink" it would be impossible to maintain blood levels of Ca^{++} and P_i within the prescribed homeostatic limits. In bone, then, the requirements for control of mineral accretion rates are much more stringent. In fact, it is necessary that the extracellular not have access to free hydroxy apatite surfaces with their incompatibly low solubilities. Understandably, associated with this high degree of control is a very slow appositional rate of growth. In a variety of species, including humans, the rate of advance of the calcification front in lamellar bone has been estimated at 1 μ/d (by successive tetracycline labelings). Imagine what such a limitation would mean in the metaphyseal cartilage. The long bones of our teenagers would lengthen only 2 mm every 3 yr. If cartilage were as limited in its growth rate there would be very few basketball players.

Mineralization in cartilage

With the emphasis on rapid growth and mineralization, with little regard for permanence in strength or viability, evolutionary processes could select the simplest of all possible mineralizing mechanisms for cartilage: the cells could simply create a relatively incompressible volume and then seed it. It could be left to the extracellular fluid and circulation, with their high content of Ca^{++} and P_i, to finish the job.

There were only two problems in the development of this simple mechanism: (1) selection of the seeding mechanism to be employed, and (2) the development of some inhibitor system to prevent the calcification front from advancing too fast. It is conceivable that the front could engulf the dividing prechondrocytes.

Since the chondrocytes are doomed to die anyway, the simplest mechanism for seeding would seem to be that of sloughing off small bits and pieces of selected membrane surfaces, the matrix vesicles. Their interior membrane surfaces contain proteolipids capable of seeding, and their membranes effectively prevent the entry of any macromolecular inhibitors. The high membrane content of phosphatases ensures the lack of penetration of pyrophosphate or nucleotides polyphosphates, and that is it. There is no need for pumps, membrane potentials, energy input, specialized substrates, or cofactors. Indeed, "dead" nonenergized, mineral-free, isolated matrix vesicles have been shown to seed *in vitro* in simple solutions having the composition of cartilage fluid. Once a nidus has started only the slight deterrent caused by Mg^{++} and citrate can slow the formation of HAP. Once HAP has formed the internal $[Ca^{++}]$ must fall, creating an electrochemical gradient, causing Ca^{++} and P_i to flow into the matrix vesicle interior until the vesicle must literally burst. Such crystal-stuffed matrix vesicles with rupturing membranes have been described in ultrastructure studies.

There seems to be a reluctance on the part of those investigating matrix vesicles intensively to accept such a simple passive role for these fascinating particles. Indeed, despite the attractiveness of Occam's razor in these matters, there is a hint that there may be somewhat more complexity to the system than that just described. There is a suggestion that ATP as a source of P_i may be somewhat more effective than P_i alone. The alkaline phosphatase of the matrix vesicles seems to contain a distinctive nonenzymatic subunit (a modifier?). The nucleotide concentration of cartilage fluid, though very low (compared with cytosol), is somewhat higher than that in the general extracellular fluids. Thus the possibility remains that alkaline phosphatase may function as a phosphorylating enzyme in addition to its role in destroying inhibitors. It may be that the phosphorylation of a specific site on the membrane interior, possibly inositol, provides a nucleation site. These are refinements that will require future research for delineation. In broad outline, the just-described system seems reasonably established and makes good sense.

Concerning the inhibition of mineralization in the region of dividing prechondrocytes and their subsequent maturation, our knowledge is sparse and imperfect. The noncollagenous proteins of epiphyseal cartilage have not been systematically studied, particularly with respect to their ability to inhibit nucleation and/or growth of HAP. Only one such inhibitor has been described (perhaps only one is needed). In their analysis of nanogram quantities of cartilage fluid withdrawn

directly by micropipette, Howell and his associates have described a high molecular weight proteoglycan that is strongly inhibitory to the nucleation and maturation of HAP.[2] Upon depolymerization this inhibitory action is lost.

It would seem that the early maturing chondrocytes would be well adapted to secrete the proteoglycan (and other inhibitors) simultaneously with the collagen and other ground substance constituents. The enzymes for depolymerization and destruction of inhibitory activity could be secreted at the same time, provided that their action was slow. Better, the secretion of such enzymes would accompany a later stage of chondrocytic maturation as does the appearance of lysozyme (and alkaline phosphatase). Perhaps the rupturing of the hypertrophied chondrocytes is sufficient to affect the release of the required enzymatic activities. Both in cartilage and in bone, this aspect of the mineralization processes—the formation and destruction of inhibitor molecules—has been neglected.

Mineralization in bone

As we have seen, the homeostatic electrolyte requirements of the animal as a whole places stringent requirements upon the control of mineralization in the skeleton. In fact, the end product of the process, HAP, can be considered a *threat* to the life of the animal itself. If there is space around an HAP crystal and an inadequate supply of inhibitors it will literally scavenge Ca^{++} and P_i ions from the extracellular fluid. In fully mineralized bone this presents no real problem. The space is practically filled with mineralized fibers, and the diffusion paths are so restricted that even though apposition probably continues throughout life, the diffusion rates are many orders of magnitude slower than free diffusion in solution. These rates have actually been calculated by Marshall in his study of the "diffuse" exchange of ^{45}Ca and other bone-seeking isotopes in established bone. His calculated rates fall roughly midway between diffusion in solution and diffusion in a solid (10^{12} times slower). At the edges of lacunae and at all the growing and exposed surfaces of bone, however, the extracellular fluid must be prevented from "seeing" bare HAP crystals.

There seems to be at least two means by which this can be accomplished. The first is to have the crystals initiate and grow *within* the collagen fiber itself. Again, the diffusion paths are highly restrictive (~6 A compared with ~4 A for the phosphate group) and the rates of growth and maturation therefore comfortably slow. Besides, such a process is limited to the rate of synthesis of new collagen by the cells.

Another means of shielding HAP crystals is to

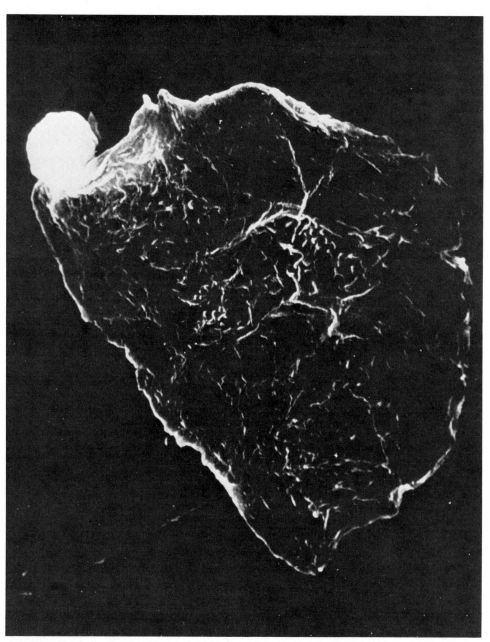

FIGURE 4-10   *A scanning electron micrograph of an "osteoblast" isolated from embryonic rat calvarium. Note the relatively enormous membrane surface in relation to the small size of the cell. (Provided by Dr. W. Peck)*

provide polypeptides and other macromolecules that strongly interact with the transient forms of calcium-P_i solids, slowing their maturation to HAP. An extension of this principle is inhibitor molecules that interact strongly with an HAP crystal surface. In such an instance, the extracellular fluid interacts essentially with a protein surface, and the HAP crystal is thus effectively removed from solution.

This argument is admittedly speculative. However, it is true that the kinetics of the disappearance of administered $^{45}Ca^{++}$ clearly demonstrate that only a very small fraction of the total mineral surfaces in the bony skeleton is readily accessible to the extracellular fluid. In amount, this is estimated as about 5 g of Ca^{++} in the adult human. If all the crystals' surfaces were available, it can be calculated from the crystal size that 200 g would be readily available for rapid exchange. Thus, we find that nearly 98% of the HAP surfaces are, in fact, "hidden."

Moreover, there is in the noncollagenous protein fractions of bone a surfeit of macromolecules that strongly inhibit the nucleation and maturation of crystal formation by HAP seeds. This problem is only beginning to come under investigative attack, but it is already apparent that the strength of this inhibition and the concentration of these substances is so high that it is difficult to see how the collagen molecules manage to mineralize at all. Perhaps these macromolecules cannot penetrate the collagen fibrils and thus prevent only *interstitial* seeding, limiting mineralization to the fibers themselves. Such a system would remove the threat of engulfment for the resting osteocyte.

This construct also explains otherwise puzzling observations concerning the importance of bone membranes. The histologists find that all bony elements are not "bare" but are covered by cell bodies or cell membranes. If one kills bone or macerates its membrane structure, the preparation will not support physiologic levels of calcium and P_i in its surrounding fluid medium. Rather it catalyzes the formation of new mineral crystals at the expense of the solution. In contrast, intact living bone preparations will support physiologic levels in their equilibration buffers.

It would seem that the cell membranes of intact bone act as a container, preventing the loss and/or enzymatic destruction of the inhibitor molecules. Their rupture, then, leads to a loss of this inhibition-control, with the resultant massive mineralization *in vitro*.

In any event, it is clear that a vesicle-initiated seeding mechanism in lamellar bone would be a real nuisance. The formation of interstitial clusters of HAP crystals could only interfere with the ordered mineralization of the collagen fibrils. Such crystals could not physically translocate from outside to inside the fibers. The fibers themselves are not phagocytic. The presence of such crystals would not elevate local concentrations, if anything they would lower them and induce interstitial mineralization.

Finally, such interstitial crystals would not go away. They cannot dissolve in the extracellular fluid of bone and could only be removed by invading cells, either phagocytic or osteoclastic in properties. Yet there are strong proponents of vesicular participation who would challenge these arguments. Fortunately for this presentation, the case for matrix vesicles in lamellar bone is weak. Moreover, the possibilities for artifacts are great. This is a great problem for would be vesicle proponents. The bone cell pictured in Figure 4-10 is a highly membranous structure, and it is common experience that it is difficult to avoid the spontaneous formation of vesicles in membrane preparations. They are routinely prepared from soft tissues for transport studies (e.g., kidney and liver). To underline this difficulty, recent studies have shown that simple mechanical pressure to a histologic tissue slice will produce a "shower" of vesicles not otherwise present. Thus, the presence of a few vesicles in electromicrographic sections of lamellar bone must be interpreted with caution.

Similarly, the participation of intracellular activities in the mineralization of lamellar bone seems unlikely. Given the low intracellular concentration of Ca^{++}, 10^3 lower than the extracellular fluids, it would seem unnecessary and pointless work to "packet" calcium phosphate particles for cellular export. This is particularly true when the desired result is the slow, controlled mineralization of the collagen fibers, *not* the seeding of a random interstitial collection of crystals. Yet it must be admitted that there are several claims that bone cells *in situ* contain unusually high histochemically demonstrated concentrations of Ca^{++}. Many of these claims can be discounted. The translocation of small amounts of Ca^{++} from the surrounding calcified matrix during the processing cannot be easily dismissed. Even with isolated cell preparations, the contamination with small amounts of calcified matrix can explain much of the literature. Still, the idea that bone cells may be unusually high in calcium content cannot be totally discounted. Whether this is a result of their calcified environment or a cause of it cannot be decided with finality.

To summarize, the current preferred view is that osteoblasts of lamellar bone secrete collagen molecules that spontaneously form expanded fibrillar structures. Special sites are capable in and of themselves of catalyzing nucleation and maturation of mineral crystals within their own molecular domains—the "holes" and "pores." These same bone cells secrete several inhibitors, both small and large molecules that slow the formation, maturation, and growth of calcium-P_i aggregates in the interstitial and nonmatrix areas.

Other mineralized structures

WOVEN BONE

Mostly embryonic and temporary, woven bone seems to be best described as having processes analogous to the mineralization described for cartilage. The collagen fibrils are irregular and immature. The mineralization is more interstitial and disordered, and numerous matrix vesicles are present.

DENTINE

Mature dentine appears to match the structure of lamellar bones, that is, a highly ordered structure of collagen fibers and a high degree of structural correlation between the crystals and the collagen. Conversely, in early odontogenesis, there is a poor relationship between mineral and

fibers, and there is evidence of the participation of matrix vesicles at the early dentinoenamel junction. Whether this is merely a transitory stage remains to be established.

ENAMEL

Enamel represents a very special case. It is perhaps the best example of the importance of the organic *milieu* in specifying and directing the course of calcium-P_i mineralization. The crystals appear to form within the extended cell processes of the receding ameloblasts. The crystals themselves mature into long, heavy, ribbon-like strips that are thousands of angstroms in length (along the c-axes). Such large crystals cannot be formed *in vitro* under any conditions. Somewhat larger, longer crystals, a bit more like enamel crystals, can be formed *in vitro* at acid pH.

To what extent intracellular pH and/or the specialized enamel proteins (collagen is absent) are responsible for these remarkable crystalline developments is not known. Pure enamel is difficult to obtain, and its total protein content is so low that careful seeding studies by purified enamel constituents are practically nonexistent.

ECTOPIC CALCIFICATION

From the discussion thus far, it should be clear that ectopic calcification is merely a specialized version of the persistent "Lot's Wife Problem." In the normal state we are presented with highly supersaturated extracellular fluids. Any pertubation of the normal complex system of controls is apt to initiate unwanted mineralization. These disturbances include (1) any trauma or inflammatory response that causes a localized concentration of alkaline phosphatase and collagen fibrogenesis; (2) local conditions that cause membrane lysis or functional loss, that is, an influx of Ca^{++} that may result in mitochondrial loading; (3) localized deposition of acidic phospholipids, particularly in association with fibrin, and (4) hypervitaminosis D (which in combination with various traumatic manipulations has been exploited under the term calciphylaxis.)

In fact, given the ease with which metastable solutions of Ca^{++} and P_i are destabilized, and given the large variety of substrates and molecules that can catalyze this destabilization, it is indeed a wonder that instances of ectopic calcification are not more common.

So it is that in the more than five decades since Robison, investigators have valiantly struggled to elucidate the mechanisms of calcification. We can confidently predict that the pendulum has finally swung back past center, and the next decades will see major efforts to elucidate the mechanisms by which mineralization is prevented. In fact we will predict that future editions of books on bone, such as this one, will require a separate chapter on "The Mechanisms of Nonmineralization."

References

Historical development

1. Neuman, W. F., and Neuman, M. W.: The Chemical Dynamics of Bone Mineral, University of Chicago Press, Chicago, 1958.

Cartilage fluids

2. Howell, D. S., and Pita, J. C.: Calcification of growth plate cartilage with special reference to studies of micropuncture fluids, Clin. Orthop. 118:208–229, 1976.

Matrix vesicles

3. Anderson, H. C., and Howell, D. S. (eds.): Second conference on matrix vesicle calcification, Metab. Bone Dis. 1 83–242, 1978.

Collagen nucleation

4. Glimcher, M. J.: Composition, structure and organization of bone and other mineralized tissues and the mechanism of calcification. *In* Handbook of Physiology-Endocrinology VII, pp. 25–116, Baltimore, Williams & Wilkins Co., 1976.

Other nucleation systems and general biochemistry

5. Urist, M. R.: Biochemistry of calcification. pp. 1–57, *In* Bourne, G. H. (ed.) The Biochemistry and Physiology of Bone, Vol. IV, 2nd edition, New York, Academic Press, 1976.

Physical chemistry of calcium-P_i solids

6. Wadkins, C. L., Luben, R., Thomas, M., and Humphreys, R.: Physical biochemistry of calcification, Clin. Orthop. 99:246–266, 1974.

Pre- and postnatal chondro-osseous development

An adequate comprehension of the morphological and histologic changes characterizing prenatal and postnatal chondro-osseous development is important from a number of standpoints.

First, the developing human skeleton is subject to a multitude of inherited and acquired diseases affecting the ability to form the normal, genetically determined skeletal morphology.[20,52] In particular, skeletal dysplasias, infections such as metaphyseal osteomyelitis and septic arthritis, and progressive joint displacements such as congenital hip disease may have profound effects on the growth capacity of major chondro-osseous regions, leading to deformed skeletal components at full maturity.

Second, a better understanding of postnatal development can only lead to a better approach to treatment of those particular diseases that progressively change with time. For example, understanding the complexity and changing susceptibility to occlusion of the cartilage canal vascular system of the developing proximal femur has led to changes in the treatment of congenital hip disease in an effort to minimize, if not totally avoid, the major complication of ischemic necrosis early in the child's development.[67,69]

Third, to understand the differences in mechanisms of chondro-osseous growth in the various animal species, we must develop better concepts of how species-specific skeletal morphological changes might respond to environmental and internal demands and contribute to species evolution.[42,45,94] In particular, there is significant variation in types of bone as well as in types of cartilage. The mouse and rat are relatively small mammals that may have open physes ("lapsed union") throughout life.[16,17] They have no preexistent vascular supply in the epiphyseal cartilage, they calcify the epiphysis very promptly over a short period,[5] and then they ossify the entire epiphysis by invasion from a peripheral blood vessel (Fig. 5-1**A**), not unlike the initial development of the primary ossification center of the cartilaginous skeletal model (anlage) by the irruption artery. In contrast, larger mammals have increasingly complex vascular systems

JOHN A. OGDEN

5

chondro-osseous development and growth

within the epiphyseal cartilage that play a major role in patterns of calcification and ossification that occur within the epiphysis and proceed outward in a centrifugal fashion (Fig. 5-1**B**). Similar differences may be found in certain large reptiles (e.g., varanids, leatherback turtle), which exhibit a well-developed epiphyseal vascular system (Fig. 5-1**C**), in sharp contrast to most reptiles. In large mammals such as the elephant or the whale (Fig. 5-2) blood vessels cross the growth plate in regular patterns, whereas in the skeletally immature human these vessels are present infrequently, tend to be toward the physeal periphery, and may play a role in the spread of infection from one side of the growth plate to another.

Fourth, the macro- and microscopic types of bone differ significantly. The presence of osteon or mature haversian bone (lamellar) is minimal in small mammals, but yet gains in amount and complexity in increasingly larger mammals. Furthermore, even in the human, such bone is present to only a minor degree in the diaphysis of the femur, and nowhere else, within the well-formed cortices of the neonatal skeleton. It must be appreciated that important changes beyond mere growth and enlargement continue throughout the postnatal maturation of the musculoskeletal system, whether we are dealing with the human or any other type of mammal.

Fifth, the chondro-osseous skeleton, unlike most other organ systems within the body, undergoes considerable modulation among three primary tissue modes—fibrous, cartilaginous, and osseous—in both the prenatal and postnatal phases. Subtle gradations from one tissue type to another are very evident.

Patterns of growth

Development proceeds concomitantly with growth—which may be defined as an increased mass—of previously differentiated cellular components over a given period of time.[83] Development may be accomplished by several means: (1) differentiation or modulation of connective tissue cells into a skeletogenic mode (the pluripotential mesenchymal or osteoprogenitor cell), (2) mitosis of already differentiated cartilaginous and osse-

ous components (e.g., chondroblast, osteoblast), (3) increased synthesis of extracellular structural proteins (e.g., chondroid, osteoid), (4) increased intracellular water uptake, with accompanying shifts of water content between the intracellular and extracellular spaces, and (5) elaboration of increasing amounts of extracellular matrix must be formed in both the cartilaginous and osseous phases.[89,92] A sixth pattern of growth, cellular necrosis, is not completely established as a mechanism, but there is substantial evidence to suggest that certain cell groups do die to be replaced by other cell types (e.g., at the physeal-metaphyseal junction to create primary spongiosa).[82]

Organization and function of the skeletal system

CLASSIFICATION OF SKELETAL TISSUES

Skeletal tissues may be classified broadly into four types: (1) bone—intramembranous and endochondral, cellular and acellular, cancellous (trabecular), and lamellar; (2) cartilage—hyaline, elastic, acellular; (3) dentine, and (4) enamel.

Bone certainly is the most common skeletal tissue. As a tissue, it fulfills another major role—mineral homeostasis—by serving as a reservoir of calcium, phosphate, and citrate ions, among others. As an organ, bone serves as a location within which hematopoiesis may occur.

Although each chondro-osseous tissue may appear grossly similar, components of the skeleton evolve into individual organs that react selectively and temporally to external and internal demands. This response leads to the formation of different concentrations and patterns of tissue elements within each bone. The relative amounts of cartilage, fibrocartilage, trabecular bone, periosteal-derived cortical (laminar) bone, and osteon (haversian, lamellar) bone will each vary considerably within a given bone and from bone to bone. Each bone, as an individual organ composed of varying tissue and cellular types and concentrations, will respond in different ways to biologic stresses, both physiologic and pathologic.

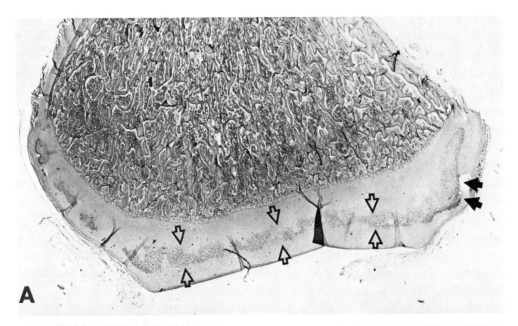

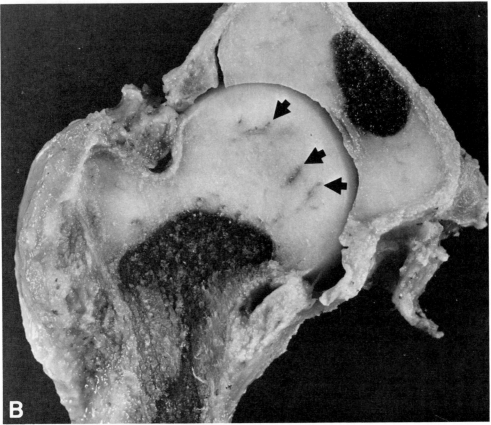

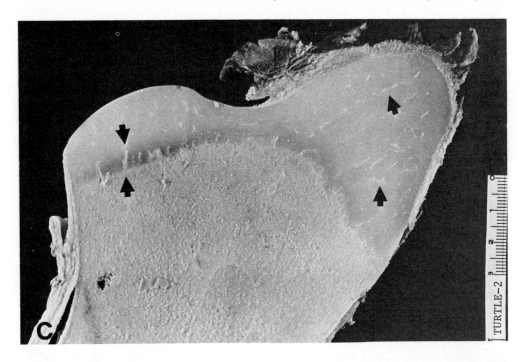

FIGURE 5-1   **(A)** *Distal femur from a monotreme (platypus). This animal appears to hypertrophy and calcify a considerable portion of the epiphyseal cartilage prior to any ossification (open arrows). There is no pre-existent intraepiphyseal blood supply. Vascular invasion (solid arrows) occurs from the margin and rapidly ossifies this prepared tissue.* **(B)** *Pre-existent cartilage canals (arrows) penetrate the proximal femoral epiphyseal cartilage in a newborn human. The ossification center will not appear until 4 to 6 mo of age in this particular epiphysis.* **(C)** *Proximal humerus from the leatherback turtle, apparently the only extant marine reptile to evolve vascularized chondroepiphyses as well as endochondral- and membranous bone formation comparable to marine mammals. A well-developed vasculature is present in both the capital humerus and the greater tuberosity (arrows). Interestingly, this species retains unossified chondroepiphyses, with the bones being capable of continued growth throughout life.*

THE BIOMECHANICS OF BONE

The organization of the skeletal system is best understood by considering the various functions both as a group of tissues and as a set of organs. The *primary role* of all skeletal systems, whether cartilaginous, fibrous, or osseous, is biomechanical: to provide protection, support, and motion. The size, shape, and position of the skeletal organs, as well as their internal and external structural arrangements and modes of articulation, accurately reflect this primary functional requirement. Biomechanical demands are further reflected in the histologic composition of the various skeletal organs. Vertebrate skeletal tissue, which includes all possible variations of fibrous, cartilaginous, and osseous tissue types, forms a continuous spectrum of connective tissues that

individually respond to specific functional demands.

The composition and structural arrangement of skeletal tissues accurately reflect the external biomechanical forces usually imposed upon them. Bone provides a relatively high degree of structural rigidity as well as mechanical protection, whereas cartilage is more useful in situations requiring elasticity or growth. In all of these skeletal tissue types, further refinements of histologic composition are functionally related. For example, hyaline cartilage is well suited to withstand compressive forces, and thus is found on the articular surfaces of most long bones. When shearing forces are applied, however, fibrocartilage is encountered, since this tissue type best withstands such forces (e.g., tibial tuberosity).[68] The preferential arrangement of both col-

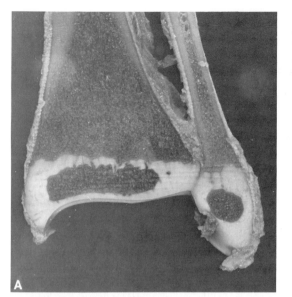
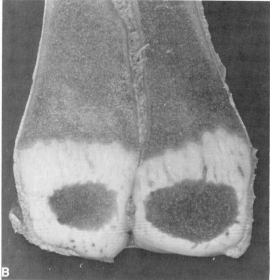
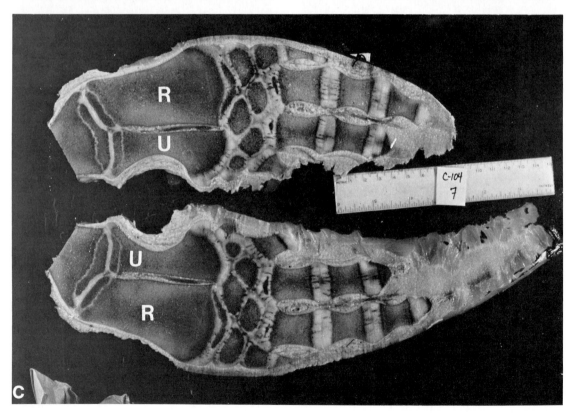

FIGURE 5-2 *Sagittal sections of the distal tibia and fibula* **(A)** *and distal radius and ulna* **(B)** *from a 3- to 4-month old Indian elephant, showing vasculature crossing the growth plate in numerous areas.* **(C)** *Sagittal sections of flipper of young whale (Globicephala macrorhyncha), showing extensive intra- and intercartilaginous vessels from the distal radius* **(R)** *and ulna* **(U)** *through the carpals into the phalanges. Many of these vessels cross the growth plates, and in certain instances cross the vestigial joints.*

lagen fiber bundles and interspersed cells in all skeletal tissue types is an excellent indication of areas upon or through which external forces are applied. Conversely, random arrangements of these same structural elements are a good general indication of areas that are subjected to minimal external loadings.

Bone is vital, dynamic tissue, not in any way to be regarded as "dead" or fixed in either its structure or composition. In a real sense, bone is in a constant state of flux, in terms of both its composition and structure. The histologic differences among reticular or woven bone, trabecular or cancellous bone, and compact bone indicate specific osseous responses to differing functional demands. The usually transitory masses of woven bone are laid down rather rapidly, and have a less-directed biomechanical function, whereas compact bone, whether laminar, lamellar or osteonal, is formed more slowly. The thin trabeculae, serving as internal trajectories, are easily reconstructed if the nature of the imposed loads varies. The ease of resorption and redeposition of trabecular bone also makes it admirably suited to serve as a mineral reservoir.

CELL DIFFERENTIATION IN SKELETAL TISSUE

Basic cell types produce each of the various skeletal tissues. The presumed undifferentiated base cell has several names, including scleroblast and osteoprogenitor cell, which implies that the tissues represent a family of tissues with close affinities to each other. Such initial cells may be mesodermal, ectodermal, or ectomesenchymal (from the neural crest) in derivation.[39,40,44] The first basic modulation of the cell type is into individual cells such as the osteoblast, which produces bone, the chondroblast, which produces cartilage, the odontoblast, which produces dentine, and the ameloblast, which produces enamel. The dynamics of representative cells and tissues within each osseous organ must be considered.

The aforementioned diversification of chondro-osseus (skeletal) cell types in a multicellular organism is presumably due to differential functioning of specific genetic loci in the various cells. It seems unlikely that cellular activity is independent in each of these definitive specialized cells. The more likely possibility is that many cells composing a given specialized type are mitotically derived from a smaller number of precursor cells in which the tissue-specific loci first became active, with subsequent retention of that activity (or at least the potential capacity for the activity) in the mitotic progeny of each of the precursor cells. Each of these mitotic lineages from a genetically determined precursor cell type can be considered a clone, and all skeletal differentiation occurs clonally from one or more progenitor cells (clonal initiator cell). Each clone represents a cellular lineage of perpetuated special genetic function that becomes a critical developmental unit.[92]

The first sign that skeletogenesis is imminent is condensation of mesodermal (or ectomesenchymal) cells to form the anlage or primordium of the bone. The position of the condensation within the embryo defines the subsequent position of the bone within the adult. The shape of the condensation defines the future basic shape of the bone. However, since skeletal tissues are extremely susceptible to modulations from environmental factors, both extrinsic and intrinsic to the embryo (prenatal) and developing animal (postnatal), the basic shape can be changed significantly. The condensing cells either arise locally in the position the bone will occupy subsequently, as in the formation of the vertebrae, or they migrate from elsewhere in the body to the site at which skeletogenesis is to occur, as in the migration of ectomesenchymal cells into the lower jaw. The factors responsible for condensation are largely unknown, although cell adhesion and migration may play a significant role.

The position of the condensed mesoderm or ectomesenchyme, and the shape, size, and rate of growth of the condensed cells are determined by interaction with adjacent ectoderm, (epithelial-mesenchymal interactions). These interactions may involve the two-way interchange between a stationary layer of ectoderm and local mesoderm, as in the formation of the limb, or the establishment of an association between mobile (migrating) mesoderm and/or ectoderm.[8]

Mesodermal cells adjacent to the specialized

ectodermal ridges, but outside the mesodermal condensation, can also form skeletal tissues, but only the tissues within the mesodermal condensation normally do form skeletal tissues. A good example is the formation of the cartilaginous primordia of the long bones of the limb in the embryonic chick. Any mesodermal cell in the limb bud is capable of producing either cartilage or muscle up to Hamilton-Hamburger state 24 (about 4½ days).[90] Thereafter, only the cells in the central condensed mesoderm form cartilage, and these are the cells most closely associated with the specialized ridge of ectoderm (apical ectodermal ridge). During development, local environmental factors probably stabilize the genome of cells in specific sites for skeletogenesis and further influence what type of skeletal tissue will form.

After mesenchymal cells condense, skeletogenesis begins. Depending on the site within the body and local epigenetic factors, the scleroblast may differentiate into different types of tissue. Each is characterized by a particular extracellular product and by a particular macro- and microscopic structure. Once the cells begin to differentiate, a three-dimensional structure develops. At first, the individual cells within the condensing mesoderm are randomly arranged, but as these cells begin to synthesize extracellar matrix and differentiate further, they orient relative to the long axis of the condensation and initiate a pattern and direction to the growth and shape of the anlage. From then on factors other than the direct genetic constitution of the component cells may come into play. A study of the determination of the morphology of particular bones within the skeleton sheds considerable light on the relative contributions of genetic and "epigenetic" factors. Bone does mold and adapt—the concept being based on the trajectory theory of Wolff that the form of a bone is, in large measure, molded by the external forces acting upon it.[56] However, it turns out that inherent genetic control is more important than was previously thought. Most theories have been based on the bone alone, rather than on the more pliable pre-existent cartilage. It is important to realize that many of the transformations, particularly in human disease, initially affect car-

tilaginous development, and the bone forms only secondarily in the already deformed cartilaginous epiphysis or early anlage.

The attainment of the fundamental form (the initial three-dimensional morphology) and considerable linear growth of a chondro-osseous element are *independent* of functional demands, and most likely are under direct genetic control.[25] This genetic control involves the expression of the inherent rates of cell division, cell hypertrophy, and amounts and types of intercellular matrix produced per cell. Once this fundamental form is established, the development of minor architectural features of the bone, such as ridges for attachment of muscle and ligaments, is much more responsive to functional demand and certainly can be modified by extraneous factors. The appearance of these minor architectural features establishes the final form of the bone, and the continued action of mechanical factors during postnatal development is necessary to maintain that form.

Stages of skeletal development

Skeletal development can be divided into two major stages—the morphogenetic phase and the cytodifferentiation phase.[77] The former is characterized by cellular movements and cellular interactions that determine the basic skeletal shape, whereas the latter is concerned with cellular differentiation and modulation and is featured by the elaboration of and changes in the extracellular matrix, which is composed principally of hyaluronic acid, chondroitin sulfate–protein complexes, and collagen. Essential to mesenchyme-cartilage-bone modulations are two important changes on the molecular level—the appearance of the enzyme hyaluronidase and the quantitative increase in chondroitin sulfate. Quantitatively, there appears to be an inverse relationship between hyaluronic acid and chondroitin sulfate in the prenatal intercellular matrix. The earliest phases of the morphogenetic (mesenchymal) stage are characterized by hyaluronic acid production, but as cellular differentiation continues, chondroitin sulfate becomes the primary intercellular molecule of the cartilaginous stage, and hyaluronic acid is removed by increased hyaluronidase production. Hyaluronic acid appears to be necessary for cellular aggregation and may be essential to the accumulation of a sufficient number of precartilage cells to initiate the transition from the morphogenetic phase to the differentiation phase. Quantitative deficiencies may prolong cellular transition and lead to skeletal reduction deformities. The effects of hyaluronic acid can be antagonized by some growth-promoting hormones, especially thyroxine, but the effects at early stages of development are poorly understood.[44]

Collagen appears to go through similar molecule transitions. The characteristic collagen of adult skin and bone has two α-1 and one α-2 units and is designated $(\alpha$-1$)_2\alpha$-2. In contrast, collagen of hyaline cartilage has three α-1 chains and is designated $(\alpha$-1$)_3$. Furthermore, the α-1 chains of both types of collagen appear to have slightly different amino acid sequences. Additionally, there are translational changes that occur in the molecules through the mechanisms of cross-linkage, hydroxylation of proline and lysine, and the glycosylation of hydroxylysine. Collagen of the precartilage (mesodermal) stage appears similar to adult bone, namely $(\alpha$-1$)_2\alpha$-2 molecule. More recently a third type of collagen has been demonstrated in the hypertrophic cartilage of the physis, $(\alpha$-3$)_3$.[100]

Thus, at the biochemical level there exists a timing element—the sequential, inter-related appearances of specific collagen types in the anlage, and a spatial element—the separation of at least two different collagen types within the mesenchymal tissues that eventually will become cartilage, bone, fibrous tissue, and muscle. This differentiation of collagen components also appears during later stages of development; the collagen of osteoid appears to have a higher degree of hydroxylation of lysine than the collagen in mature (lamellar) bone matrix. It is important to realize that each of these changes in collagen types parallel changes in structure and/or function.

The third intercellular molecular component is chondroitin sulfate (types A and B), which complexes with proteins to form glycosaminoglycans (mucopolysaccharides). These various glycosaminoglycan moieties interact with colla-

gen. This interaction seems important to morphogenesis and the overall properties of the cartilage matrix, particularly in areas such as the growth plate, in which cell column formation requires a certain degree of structural integrity.

The individual constituents of the skeleton begin as mesenchymal condensations during the embryonic period.[23,29,31,32,66] These mesenchymal cells are derived from the primary germ layers, usually under the mechanical or chemotactic influence of other tissue structures (e.g., notochord, neural tube, apical ectodermal ridge). Some of these cellular condensations ossify directly to form the membrane-derived or intramembranous bones (cranial and facial skeleton, clavicle). However, most of the postcranial skeleton is derived from the transformation of the mesenchymal model into a cartilage model and subsequently into an ossified structure by two discrete processes: (1) the formation of a primary osseous collar and subsequent vascular invasion to form the primary ossification center, which will become the diaphysis and metaphyses, and (2) a later (usually postnatal) vascular-mediated ossification in the epiphysis to form the secondary ossification center. Selected areas of cartilage, termed growth plates (physes) and capable of rapid growth longitudinally and latitudinally, develop between the primary and secondary ossification processes. This gradual replacement of a pre-existent cartilage model by osseous tissue is termed endochondral ossification. These two types of bone formation (intramembranous and endochondral) refer only to the primary pattern of development. Subsequent growth after this initial differentiation may involve juxtaposed areas of both patterns. Endochondrally derived bones have intramembranous ossification with appositional growth from the periosteum. Similarly, membrane-derived bones may undergo subsequent growth by a modified endochondral process (e.g., proximal clavicle).

Congenital defects may result from aberrations in the developmental stage or the growth stage, or both stages.[4,26,34,71,91,102] For example, hemimelia may be due to the primary failure to form the fibrous or cartilaginous anlage (developmental error) or the primary failure to synthesize appropriate quantities at the appropriate time of collagen or mucopolysaccharide (glycosaminoglycan moieties) that will allow further cellular changes (growth error). Once a developmental error has been introduced into the sequential developmental pattern of the skeleton, numerous associated abnormalities may sequentially ensue because of the extremely interrelated patterns of development of each of the skeletal components. Defects having origin in the embryonic phase have a greater likelihood of concomitant multisystem abnormalities, whereas those occurring in the fetal period tend to be more localized abnormalities.

Membranous bone formation

Primary membranous bone formation forms the cranial vault, facial bones, and, in part, the clavicle and mandible, whereas the axial and appendicular bones become involved in membranous bone formation only secondarily. The membrane-derived bones are formed from proliferative (ecto) mesenchymal tissue condensations that are structural analogues of the presumptive bone, similar to the cartilaginous precursors in endochondral ossification. At the site of the presumptive primary ossification, small groups of cells differentiate, undergo mitotic proliferation, and aggregate in short, irregular strands running in random directions.[30] Concomitantly, these cells form a fibrous, intercellular matrix, which is quickly followed by calcification and ossification to form the primary trabeculae. Some of the osteoblasts become encased in the mineralizing osteoid tissue and modulate into osteocytes, whereas most cells remain on the periphery as osteoblasts. Intramembranous ossification then spreads out from these primary ossification centers in such a way that relatively large areas of the fetal skull and facial bones are covered rapidly by a dense, protective tissue layer that is undoubtedly essential to effective, rapid development of the intracranial contents and characteristic facial features (Fig. 5-3).

The major bones of the cranium are characterized by primary trabeculae radiating parallel to the surface of the presumptive skull. These primary trabeculae increase in length by accretion at their free ends (the area of major osteoblastic activity). Smaller secondary trabeculae form at right angles to add further thickness to the central region. This process creates spaces that fill with vascular connective tissue. The overall result is a dense mass of bone that composes the primary ossification center. This center expands by two mechanisms: (1) further formation or extension of peripherally located trabeculae, and (2) coalescence with small islands of bone arising in the more peripheral regions of the expanding fibrocellular anlage. This pattern is referred to as open reticular-bordered plate bone. As the ossification centra expand toward each other, the peripheral trabeculae become more organized and interconnected, and centrifugal expansion rates decrease, although the growth of the peripheral areas continues slowly by additional bone along the sutural margins. Concomitant with the decreased rate of centrifugal expansion, a new osteogenic process commences with the formation of a distinct periosteum over the outer surface of the cranial vault. This tissue has a thick outer fibrous layer, a layer of mitotic cells, a fibrovascular layer, and an inner layer of mature osteoblasts. Periosteal osteogenesis now becomes the major growth

TRANSFORMATION

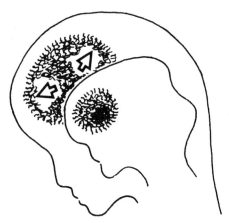

FIGURE 5-3 *Membranous ossification in the fetal skull. This process of modulation of mesenchymal tissue into woven bone is termed* **transformative growth**.

TRANSLATION

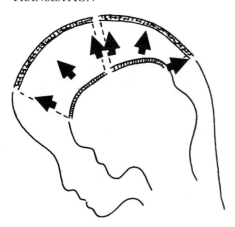

FIGURE 5-4 *The cranial plates arising by transformative membranous ossification are progressively shifted outward and away from each other. This translative growth is characteristic of the cranial membranous bones, whereas facial membranous and secondary membranous (long bone) formation progressively build on the "nonmoving" antecedent bone and necessitates extensive remodeling with continued growth.*

process. The bones of the cranial vault accommodate the growth of the brain by changing contours through outer surface bone deposition and inner surface bone resorption. There is a small amount of osteogenesis at the inner layer. Furthermore, like expansion of the acetabulum through the mechanism of the triradiate cartilage, the cranial sutures allow displacement of the cranial plates away from each other as a response to the enlarging cranial contents (translative growth). This allows the plates to be moved integrally with brain growth, without any need for the inner table to be replaced completely (Fig. 5-4).

The cranial membranous bones arise, grow, and are maintained while embedded in what can be conceived as a neurocranial capsule capable of expanding and protecting the enclosed neural mass. As the capsule expands, the embedded calvarial bones are passively carried outward (translative growth). Transformative osteogenetic processes, along with bone deposition and resorption, occur within these bones. However, such transformative growth is not the primary event causing the bones to grow outward, but rather is the secondary and compensatory remodeling process by which the translated bones

respond to the need to cover increasingly larger neurocranial vault areas and also to compensate for changes in vault curvature. Thus, there are two primary types of membranous bone tissue growth: transformative and translative. The former is an active process that alters size, shape, and structure of the bone tissue, whereas the latter is a passive process by means of which this bone tissue is relocated in space, even while it is being transformed simultaneously.

At birth the bones composing the cranial vault consist of a single plate of reasonably compact bone with small intertrabecular spaces. The trabeculae are primarily composed of coarse-fibered (woven) bone. Postnatally, significant changes occur. The outer surface (outer table) becomes a dense, recognizable structure through rapid subperiosteal new bone formation, whereas the inner surface, which is undergoing both resorption and deposition, forms a less prominent inner table. The middle zone is cancellous and is referred to as the diploe. This becomes an area of intense hematopoietic activity in infancy and childhood. The developing postnatal bone is increasingly compact, fine-fibered lamellar bone.

In other membrane bones (e.g., facial bones) ossification proceeds in a similar fashion, except that the central plate (primary ossification center) develops more rapidly and has smoother, relatively nontrabeculated margins and infrequent bone islands. This is termed smooth-bordered plate bone. Because of functional demands, multiple muscle attachments, and considerable angularity compared with the plate bones of the cranial vault, the trabecular patterns tend to be more complex than the radiating pattern of the vault bones.

The clavicle is the first fetal bone to ossify (membranous ossification), followed rapidly by the mandible, with both bones ossifying by the eighth week.[28] According to some studies, the clavicle initially forms two ossification centers that soon coalesce to form a single primary ossification center.

Some membrane bones, particularly the clavicle and the mandible, form hyaline epiphyseal cartilage, but only after primary ossification is well under way. This cartilage, sometimes re-

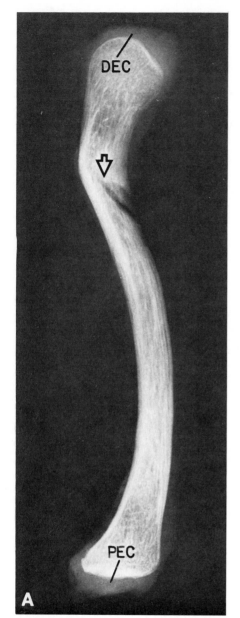

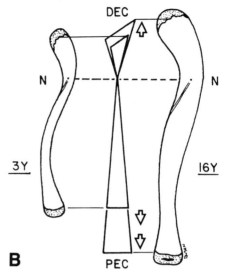

FIGURE 5-5 **(A)** *Radiograph of a clavicle from a skeletally immature child, showing nutrient artery foramen (arrow) and cartilaginous areas at both the acromial **(DEC)** and sternal **(PEC)** ends. **(B)** Schematic showing how each epiphyseal cartilage contributes to the overall growth of the clavicle relative to the nutrient artery **(N)**. Most growth occurs from the proximal (sternal) physis, which eventually develops a secondary ossification center in late adolescence and is one of the last physes to close (midtwenties).*

ferred to as *secondary* cartilage, is characterized by cells that tend to be larger and that have less intercellular matrix than the hyaline cartilage of the endochondral bones. The fate of such cartilage is quite variable.[39] Nonetheless, this cartilage may form a modified growth apparatus (physis), and it modulates the further growth of these bones (Fig. 5-5). Histologically, these cartilaginous areas either resemble the nonepiphyseal ends of the small longitudinal bones (distal end of the clavicle and mandible) or form a rudimentary epiphysis (proximal clavicle). These regions are unique in that blood vessels in synovial or fibrous tissue reflections may run along portions of the joint surface, since the sternoclavicular and acromioclavicular joints have minimal motion. This vascular arrangement also exists in the temporomandibular joint, but disappears as the joint becomes functional and generates high joint-reaction forces.

Some of the axial and appendicular skeletal elements also are involved in subsequent intramembranous ossification. The metaphyseal and diaphyseal cortices of developing tubular bone are derived from specialized mesenchyme (periosteum) investing the cartilage model.[22] This process is quite dramatic in childhood osteomyelitis, in which the original diaphysis may become a sequestrum, and the elevated periosteum forms a totally enveloping shell of new bone (involucrum) that is completely intramembranous in origin (Fig. 5-6).

Endochondral ossification

Endochondral bone formation is the primary developmental process of axial and appendicular skeletal components and may recur even in adult life in the normal process of fracture repair (formation and maturation of callus). Basically, it is the synchronous replacement of a cartilaginous precursor by osseous tissue.[24] This overall process is a continuum that can be divided arbitrarily into a number of steps (Fig. 5-7):

1. Formation of a highly cellular mesenchymal condensation (anlage).
2. Increased cellular activity to form precartilage.
3. Extensive ground substance elaboration to form the hyaline cartilage model.
4. Further interstitial enlargement of the entire anlage and selective hypertrophy of the central chondrocytes.
5. Formation of a primary bone collar by conversion of perichondrium to periosteum.
6. Increased enzymatic activity (especially alkaline phosphatase) in the hypertrophic cells and subsequent calcification within this central region.
7. Penetration of the primary bone collar by the fibrovascular irruption tissue, part of which will develop into the nutrient artery.
8. Cartilage replacement by bone centrally, with subsequent extension of the periosteum and bone collar process and accom-

panying extension of the periosteum and bone collar longitudinally toward the ends of the anlage (this forms the primary ossification center, which becomes the diaphysis and metaphyses).

9. Establishment of an orderly arrangement to the ossification-growth mechanism (the physis or epiphyseal growth plate) and an actively remodeling metaphysis.
10. Vascularization of the chondroepiphysis by the cartilage canal system.
11. Appearance of secondary ossification centers in the chondroepiphyses (this is primarily a postnatal process, although a few centers, especially the distal femoral ossification center, may form just before birth).

These steps will be covered in more detail in the ensuing sections specifically concerning limb bud, vertebral, and epiphyseal development.

This method of initial bone formation leads to two apposed structures termed endochondral cones (Fig. 5-8). The apices of these cones juxtapose at the site of the primary ossification center and nutrient artery. The bases of the cones, which are a composite of epiphysis and physis, grow away from the apex at variable rates.[88] For example, the proximal humeral cone grows four times as fast as the distal humeral cone. Concomitantly, the physis and epiphysis grow diametrically, increasing the size of the base. The surrounding bone collar concomitantly enlarges by membranous ossification to fill in the shaft and create the diaphyseal cortical bone.

Chondro-osseous cells

No matter what the pattern of initial or secondary chondro-osseous formation, certain basic cell types characterize skeletal tissue:

Undifferentiated mesenchymal cells

The data indicate that the majority of bone cells initially arise from the undifferentiated mesenchymal cells forming within the embryonic tissue planes (prenatally) and cartilage and bone

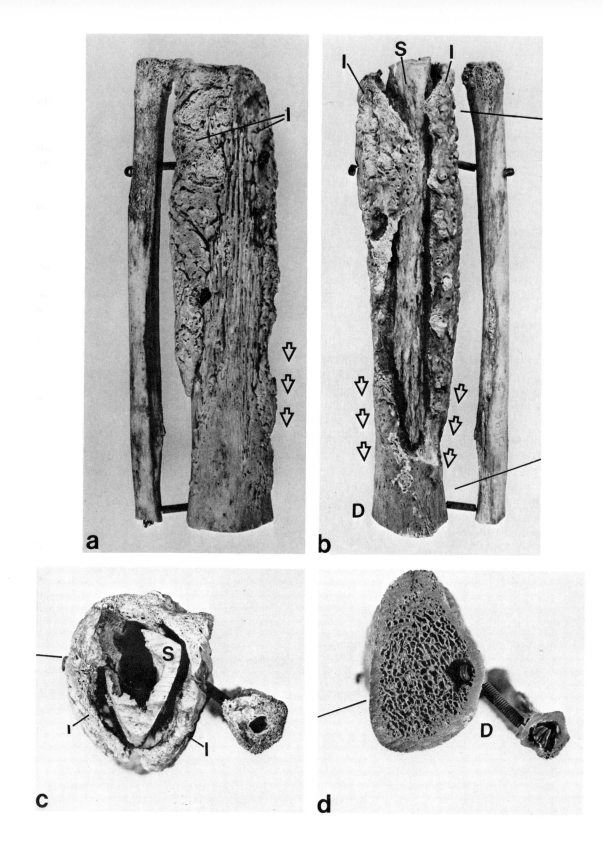

(postnatally). Tritiated thymidine initially will remain in the nuclei of undifferentiated mesenchymal cells (osteoprogenitor cells) adjacent to blood vessels, rather than being applied directly to the surface of newly forming osteoid or bone. If sequential studies are then done, the next cells to be filled will be the osteoblasts and osteoclasts, and finally the osteocytes will be filled. Similarly, with cartilage the chondroblasts become labeled before chondrocytes. This occurs particularly in the zone of Ranvier.

The primary function seems to be one of replication, with the daughter cells being the ones that eventually will migrate to become the functioning chondro-osseous cells.

Chondroblast

These cells are present primarily in three regions: (1) in association with the epiphyseal perichondrium, (2) in association with the zone of Ranvier, and (3) in the pericanalicular tissues of the cartilage canals. In all regions they give rise to the primary functioning cells of the epiphysis and physis—the chondrocyte. A separate cell population may be in the subarticular region to give origin to the articular chondrocytes. These cells are germinal, but they also elaborate significant amounts of intercellular chondroid. Once the cell has divided and produced a pocket (lacuna) surrounded by matrix, metabolic function becomes less, and the cell becomes a chondrocyte. On rare occasions mitotic division may be seen in these chondrocytes, implying that under certain conditions a chondrocyte may modulate back to a chondroblast.

Chondrocytes

Throughout most of the epiphysis, these cells lie in lacunae surrounded by extensive amounts of extracellular matrix (chondroid). The prime function is maintenance of the matrix during growth and prior to ossification. However, con-

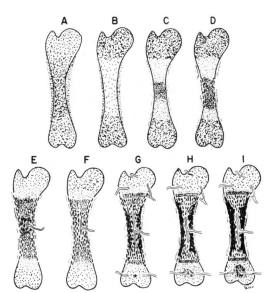

FIGURE 5-7 *Schematic of the progressive stages of endochondral ossification in the human femur. (A) Mesenchymal model. (B) Central chondrification. (C) Central hypertrophic cartilage. (D) Formation of the bone collar. (E) Vascular irruption. (F) Rapid formation of the primary ossification center. (G) Formation of cartilage canals in the chondroepiphyses. (H) Formation of an epiphyseal preossification center by cartilage hypertrophy. (I) Formation of a secondary center of ossification in epiphysis. (See text for details.)*

trary to popular belief, they are within reasonable distances from blood supply or an articular surface, from which they can derive nutrition. Human epiphyseal cartilage is profusely filled by canal systems.

The cell surface is irregular and has numerous short cell processes extending out of the matrix, although these do not extend long distances through canaliculi. Modifications in chondrocyte morphology are seen in the growth plate, in which the various metabolic and physiologic demands on the cell necessitate differences in the amounts of intracytoplasmic organelles and the morphology of the cell. These cells apparently participate significantly in the production of matrix collagen and protein polysaccharides. Pro-

◄ FIGURE 5-6 *Specimen of tibial segment, showing extensive subperiosteal new bone formation consequent to osteomyelitis. This new bone, the involucrum (I), eventually blends into the uninvolved diaphysis (open arrows) through the periosteal continuity. The original diaphyseal segment becomes isolated and is termed a **sequestrum (S)**. Distally (D) the bone is unaffected.*

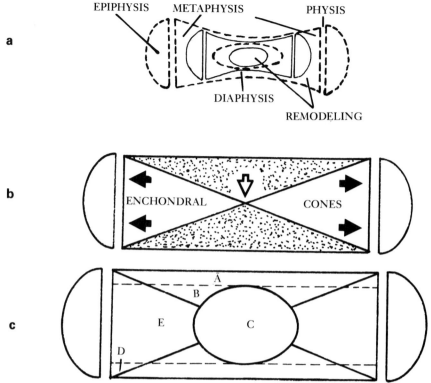

FIGURE 5-8 **(a)** *Regions of a growing bone and major sites of remodeling.* **(b)** *Schematically, the physes grow away from each other (solid arrows) and from a central reference point (the original site of entry of the irruption artery—open arrow, which becomes the nutrient artery). The space between these two diverging cones is filled in with bone formed by the periosteum (stippled areas). This bone is membranous.* **(c)** *In a terrestrial mammal, major changes occur commensurate with growth.* **A** = *the formation of lamellar (osteon) bone;* **B** = *endosteal new bone;* **C** = *tubulation to form a marrow cavity;* **D** = *peripheral metaphyseal remodeling; and* **E** = *central metaphyseal remodeling (primary spongiosa replaced by secondary spongiosa).*

tein is produced in the rough endoplasmic reticulum, moves to the Golgi zone, in which sugars and sulfates are added, and is then excreted into the extracellular matrix. As one traces chondrocytes from the germinal region to the hypertrophic degenerating regions of the growth plate, there is a progressive disappearance of organelles in a fairly predictable pattern, whereas the nuclear fragments and plasma membranes remain intact the longest.[9] At the end of the growth plate in the degenerating region, there is still some speculation about whether these cells die or whether they are capable of modulation into osteoblasts.[15,48,50] This is an area of significant ongoing research and still has not been completely solved.

The articular chondrocytes, although histologically the same as other epiphyseal chondrocytes, apparently become a histochemically defined population early in development. Because they become "fixed," modulation to more primitive states is less likely, and repair of cartilage defects and injuries is not common. Similarly, other cartilage cells appear incapable of modulating to this histochemical pattern to replace damaged articular chondrocytes.

Osteoblast

The osteoblast is the primary bone cell concerned with making protein (osteoid). These cells are characteristically found wherever new bone matrix is being formed. They generally lie alongside trabeculae, whether in woven or cortical bone. They frequently polarize to the extent that the nucleus lies at the end of the cell opposite the bone surface. These cells contain an abundance of endoplasmic reticulum, a characteristic of cells that manufacture protein. Protein production is a rapid phenomenon, integrated with the synthesis of protein polysaccharides, which are also formed by the osteoblasts.

Osteoblasts contain numerous cytoplasmic processes, especially on the side next to the bone matrix. These processes extend through the matrix, and some of them branch and enter bone by numerous canaliculi. It is incompletely determined whether these cells also play a role in the transport of calcium from the extracellular fluid to the bone matrix or in the mineralization of osteoid.

Typically, the cells are tightly packed in a single layer covering active, forming surfaces such as trabeculae and the subperiosteal region of developing bones. Fine cytoplasmic processes extend from the cells and form continuous networks between adjacent cells and preosteoblasts. The osteoblast apparently is not capable of cell division.

Osteocytes

Osteocytes represent the mature cells that lie in lacunae within the various types of bone. Whether an osteocyte of trabecular bone (primary spongiosa or secondary spongiosa) or cortical bone (laminar and lamellar) of the metaphysis or diaphysis, they all appear to be the same basic cell. Whether they represent different cell populations with genetically determined biochemical mechanisms specific for the various macroscopically and microscopically different regions of bone is still unknown. These cells do lie in lacunae and are uniformly oriented with respect to the longitudinal and radial axes of the bone lamellae. They have a sufficient component of cytoplasmic organelles, which indicates that they are actively functioning cells. Osteocytes are separated from the mineralized osteoid by a pericellular space containing protein, lipids, collagen fibrils, and protein polysaccharide. It has

been suggested that under certain circumstances, particularly in the remodeling metaphysis, they also may be stimulated to resorb bone (osteocytic osteolysis),[6,55,103] although this theory has recently come under question. Numerous processes (canaliculi) extend from these cells to contact comparable processes from other osteocytes. This is probably the mechanism whereby chemicals can be transported from cells that are closer to the central neurovascular process of the osteon to the cells that are more centrifugally located. The overall surface area of the cells within the lacunae, as well as the cytoplasmic extensions through the canaliculi, is very large and must have a significant role in bone physiology, particularly calcium homeostasis. This is of critical importance, since the serum calcium ion concentration is one of the most closely monitored concentrations in the human body because of its vital role in maintenance of cell functions, which include cell membrane transport, muscle contraction, and nerve irritability.

Osteocytes probably represent osteoblasts that have been engulfed by matrix (osteoid) that they subsequently mineralize. They thus represent the mature sequence of a cell that begins as undifferentiated mesenchyme. These cells continue to metabolize, but at a much lower rate than the osteoblasts. Osteocytes maintain the viability of mature bone tissue and are quite sensitive to the presence of an adequate and functioning vascular system.

Osteoclasts

Osteoclasts are multinucleated, probably syncytial cells. However, they represent a discrete mode of cellular differentiation, and do not represent an amalgam of osteocytes. They contain very little endoplasmic reticulum, but do contain a moderate number of ribosomes, polyribosomes, and smooth vesicles. They also have a very distinct brush border, which lies alongside the areas of bone that are being remodeled (resorbed). This infolding of the plasma membrane greatly increases the functional surface area. The brush border, which is seen only along disrupted bone surfaces, contains numerous channels ending in vesicles, within which lie numerous mineral crystals and collagen fibril fragments, presumably from the breakdown of the bone being resorbed. These cells contain high levels of enzymes—particularly acid phosphatase, collagenase, and other hydrolytic enzymes—that break down osseous tissue. The specific chemical and physical mechanisms of osteoclastic osteolysis remain unknown.

Whether these cells actually initiate the process of bone resorption or move into areas in which the process has been started by other cells has not yet been determined, but they certainly do play a major role in removal of mineral and matrix and are evident anywhere that bone is being resorbed.[19] The osteoclast gouges out a piece of bone tissue surface, probably by a combination of acid dissolution and pycnocytosis, forming a Howship's lacuna. The elaboration of proteolytic enzymes necessary to the digestion of matrix is accompanied by similar enzymatic cytolysis of the osteocytes. Apparently the osteocyte nuclei requires further degradation, which may occur within the osteoclast.[95]

Bone patterns

The aforementioned basic cell types may be arranged into several different micro- and macroscopic patterns of bone. These patterns differ with respect to amounts of matrix, orientation of matrix and cells, and types of associated vascularity.

Woven bone (fibrous, nonlamellar)

Bone tissue with an irregular unorganized pattern of collagen orientation and of lacunar distribution has been termed woven bone. Normally, it is found in areas of endochondral ossification (primary and secondary spongiosa) and at sites of tendinous or ligamentous attachments. It is usually reabsorbed and is eventually replaced by lamellar bone. It is also characteristic of the initial bone formation within fracture callus or adjacent to local inflammatory processes, and may also be found as tumor-induced new bone. It also appears as the initial bone formed by the periosteum, particularly if the periosteum is

pathologically stressed to undergo more rapid than normal bone formation.

This bone shows a marked variation in mineral density, particularly when comparing endochondral woven bone with periosteal woven bone. Woven bone should be considered to have a limited degree of organization, since short bundles of oriented collagen are present. These tend to be aligned at right angles to each other, giving a "warp and woof" appearance.

Woven fibrous bone responds biomechanically in a different fashion than does mature osteon bone. The physical properties of woven bone show no directional preferences, resulting from the lack of structural orientation, less organization, and relatively low density and high water content, all of which combine to give it greater flexibility and a lower modulus of elasticity, and certainly less strength in that it is unable to resist the same forces as lamellar bone without deforming significantly. These properties make it well suited for the embryo and the early developing skeleton, particularly in the metaphyseal ends of bone, which must be a lot more pliant than the more rigid components of the diaphyseal shaft. These properties of woven bone allow a certain resistance to encountered biologic forces, while concomitantly allowing for rapid growth. The lack of orientation permits it to be laid down rapidly and probably facilitates later remodeling features, which also enhance its usefulness in repair at all ages, since irritative processes such as osteomyelitis must be walled off during healing.

Trabecular bone

Trabecular bone is a three-dimensional lattice work of woven osseous plates and columns that may be found throughout the skeleton, and is a particular feature of the vertebral centra, the secondary ossification centers, and the metaphyses of developing bone. The entire metaphysis is generally filled with this osseous pattern. In the short and round bones, it is the predominant mode. In the metaphyseal region, it is subjected to constant remodeling. It becomes less prominent along the diaphyseal region, although in the metaphysis and diaphysis trabecular bone is continuous with the inner surface of the cortex

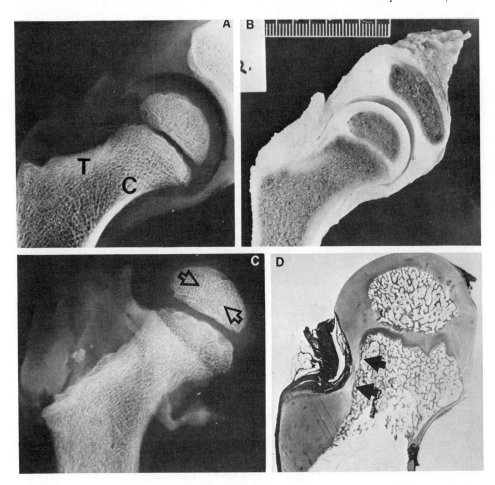

FIGURE 5-9 *Changes occur in trabecular bone of the metaphysis, especially when it is subjected to structural modifications. (A) Slab section of proximal femur, showing early development of compression (C) and tension (T) trabeculae in metaphysis. (B) Morphologic appearance of section shown in A. One can see the extent of cartilage in both femur and acetabulum. (C) Roentgenogram of intact specimen, showing extension of compression trabeculae through the central portion of secondary center of ossification (arrows). (D) Histologic section, showing continuity of epiphyseal cartilage along femoral neck (arrows). This area contributes to an increase in the width of the neck.*

(endosteal bone). In the major long bones there is minimal trabecular bone in the diaphyseal regions (primarily endosteal).

Trabecular bone changes patterns with time, and particularly seems to provide support for transmitting applied loads. The most obvious portion is the progressive development of the trabeculae in the capital femoral ossification center and femoral neck transmitting the load from the hip joint to the calcar (Fig. 5-9). As a general observation, trabecular bone is oriented to provide maximum strength while utilizing minimum osseous material.

The basic architecture for cancellous bone comprises oriented plates of compact bone interconnected by rod-shaped supports running perpendicular to the plates. The plates do not form layers in all locations, and they vary in width. Any description must consider trabecular bone from a three-dimensional standpoint, rather than the usual two-dimensional pattern obvious on normal histologic slides. There appear to be at least three patterns of trabecular plates. One pattern occurs in the proximal humerus, in which equally spaced plates of the same caliber exist. A second type occurs in the vertebra, in which slightly curved plates extend between the cortical end plates. The third pattern occurs in the femur, in which a mixture of smaller, evenly spaced plates, as in the humerus, and coarser, more widely spaced plates form a trajectorial system.

Much of the descriptive work on adult trabecular bone does not totally apply to developing trabeculae because these latter patterns are constantly changing. In particular, the development of the cortical end plates is a phenomenon occurring only toward the end of skeletal maturation. Prior to that there is a resilient layer of cartilage that amounts to an epiphysis at each end of the vertebral body. However, the basic pattern remains the same. The vertebral trabecular bone, which begins as a spherical ossification center, gradually begins to orient the trabecular bone in slightly curvilinear patterns that correspond to a sector of the surface of the sphere and tend to be laid down parallel to each other and also parallel to the contour of the end plate above or below. There is a great deal of concentricity to the lamellar pattern.

Lamellar bone

Lamellar bone is mature and biomechanically responsive. It has a lamellated structure, with the collagen fibrils in each of the multiple lamellae running in different directions, similar to plywood. In cancellous bone the lamellae usually run parallel to the trabeculae, whereas in cortical bone several patterns occur. This is especially evident in the osteons, in which concentric orientation of multiple layers occurs around vascular canals.

The functional basis for this lamellated appearance is controversial. The most commonly accepted theory assumes that each lamella contains two layers of collagen, with fibers in each layer running parallel to each other, whereas the separate layers cross at 90° angles. Others have questioned the concept that all bands contain equal amounts of collagen and have presented evidence to support an alternate theory suggesting fiber-rich and fiber-poor layers. The predominant theory favors the view that the lamellar organization of bones is determined by the orientation of collagen fibers.

The lamellae appear biphasic when viewed under polarized light. One layer is isotropic and the other is anisotropic (birefringence). When examined under polarized light, three types of osteons have been identified according to the direction of collagen bundles and successive lamellae. In the first type, the prevalent direction of fiber runs along the longitudinal axis of the osteon. The inner and outer perimeters of the osteon, however, often contain a few concentric lamellae running transversely around the osteon axis. In the second type of osteon, the majority of bundles run concentrically around the osteon axis. The third type of osteon shows alternating light and dark lamellae under polarized light. The mechanical properties of individual osteons vary according to the basic lamellar pattern, with longitudinally oriented osteons having greater tensile strength, and transversely oriented osteons having greater compressive strength. In the developing skeleton, these structures will have variable importance and appearance, depending on the type of stress that the child applies to the bone. Furthermore, as the bone grows and mechanical axes change, there will be shifts in the pattern of the osteons that necessitate continual remodeling in response to the normal physiologic stresses.

Each lamella should be considered to contain individual, highly oriented collagen bundles that do not branch. Overall, collagen has a basically parallel orientation, but the fibers form a continuum (syncytium) with frequent inner connections from one bundle to another, not only within the lamella. Many fibers probably traverse the interlamellar zone as they pass from one lamella to another. Such an arrangement would undoubtedly increase the resistance of bone to mechanical stress. Collagen fibrils, however, do not cross cement (reversal) lines, which probably explains why cement lines are biomechanically weaker than interlamellar planes. Again, in the developing skeleton, these patterns are constantly changing and undoubtedly remodeling and strengthening to respond to biologic stress.

Cortical bone

In comparison to trabecular bone, cortical bone has a dense texture, although on close inspection there are areas that are relatively porous, particularly in the metaphysis of the developing skeleton (Fig. 5-10). Although no well-defined mineral distinction exists between the two major types of bone, they can be arbitrarily differentiated by the apparent density. Trabecular bone (especially the subperiosteal type) is converted into cortical bone by compaction and modeling, as occurs in certain parts of the metaphysis during growth and as results when the woven (laminar) bone formed by the periosteum gradually is incorporated into the lamellar cortical pattern. Lamellar cortical bone usually replaces laminar cortical bone as the skeleton becomes increasingly mature. The relative quantity of cortical versus trabecular bone varies from bone to bone and even between different parts of the same bone. The cortical shell may be very thin, as in vertebra, or thick, as in most long bones. However, in either case, it is usually composed of lamellar bone. The organization of lamellae, however, varies markedly from place to place within the bone, as well as with time.

Cortical bone contains an elaborate system of anastomosing canals through which blood vessels permeate every region of the bone. Basically, the canals are incorporated as new bone is deposited during periods of endosteal or periosteal growth. The term primary canals refers to those canals incorporated initially, whereas secondary canals result from remodeling activity beginning with resorption along a primary canal and followed later by bone deposition. All canals, whether primary or secondary, usually follow a

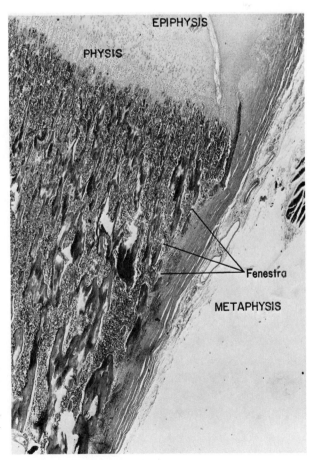

FIGURE 5-10 *The metaphysis is the site of extremely active bone change. Central primary spongiosa forms around a cartilage core (remnant of the longitudinal septae of a physis). Peripherally, the periosteum is forming a discontinuous cortex with multiple metaphyseal fenestrations. This area may be penetrated by infection and is structurally weaker at certain ages, allowing certain fracture patterns characteristic of childhood.*

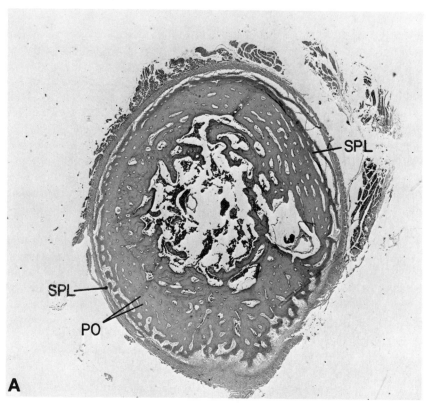

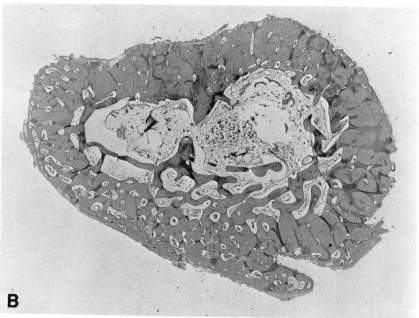

FIGURE 5-11 **(A)** *Transverse section of a neonatal femur.* **(B)** *Transverse section of tibia of 5-mo-old child. Both mid-diaphyseal sections show reasonably solid-appearing cortices. No haversian systems are evident in the tibia. The femur is beginning to develop primary osteons* **(PO)**. *Note the regional differences of subperiosteal laminar* **(SPL)** *new bone.*

predominantly longitudinal course in periosteal-derived cortical bone. Those canals in the bone of endosteal origin may be arranged more irregularly. Some vascular channels may be oriented in a radial direction perpendicular to the long axis of the shaft. These canals are called Volkmann's canals, in contrast to Haversian canals, which represent the longitudinal system.

Many early canals, particularly the ones that characterize cortical bone of a newborn infant, lack a surrounding ring of concentric lamellae (Fig. 5-11). A primary canal surrounded by a variably developed, elongated cylinder of concentric lamellae is known as a primary osteon. These primary osteons usually contain only a few layers of lamellae, so overall they rarely approach the size of the more mature, better-defined secondary osteons. Primary osteons are more common in young bone, particularly embryonic and fetal bone, and the incidence decreases with increasing age.

The best known canals in bone are the central canals of secondary osteons or Haversian systems. The secondary osteon resembles the primary osteon, but it results from remodeling activity along a pre-existing primary canal. Any type of primary canal can be reconstructed into a secondary osteon, so the general distribution of secondary osteons is largely determined by that of the primary canals. The conversion of a primary osteon to a secondary osteon begins with resorption and ends with new bone deposition. All stages of this process can be seen in cortical bone. This remodeling mechanism gives bone greater adaptability in its response to physical and probably metabolic stimuli, since it allows alteration of internal structure without significantly changing overall size or shape. With increasing age, therefore, higher concentrations of secondary osteons characteristically develop at definite locations within each bone. These areas correspond to sites of greater stress. Many small mammals such as the mouse and rat do not remodel cortical bone extensively; consequently, secondary osteons are not as characteristic, which limits their usefulness as model systems for the study of human skeletal physiology and disease.

Haversian systems, which represent the distinguishing feature of compact bone in the maturing human skeleton as well as the adult cortex, are irregular cylindrical structure composed of concentric lamellae of bone and osteocytes surrounding a central canal containing blood vessels as well as other structures, particularly unmyelinated nerves. Haversian systems are present only in selected areas of the mid-femur in the human at birth, but progressively develop in all the long bones. These Haversian systems (osteons) usually run longitudinally, although they branch frequently and anastomose extensively with one another.[13] The direction and orientation of the osteons, which may spiral around the bone axis as well as follow the longitudinal axis, usually follow pre-existing vascular channels, so the basic overall pattern of Haversian systems is undoubtedly established when the vessels are initially incorporated into bone during appositional, periosteal, and endosteal bone growth. Minor changes in the anastomotic network undoubtedly occur during remodeling, by revision of established anastomoses, by the addition of new communications, or by the obliteration of old ones. The fact that an occasional osteon ends blindly suggests that individual vessels may be able to grow in a new direction by burrowing out resorption spaces in previously formed bone. Throughout the central portion of the cortex, concentric lamellae are invariably present along a Haversian system, but the internal structure of the canal may vary strikingly, particularly at the ends at which point only partly formed osteon structures are present, alternating with the resorption spaces. The ends of these osteons are the more active portions and would be expected to be growing further in response to the biomechanical demands of maturation. These growth patterns will be discussed in detail subsequently.

Axial skeletal development

The early morphological development of the neural, muscular, and axial skeletal elements is intimately related to both the notochord and a more generalized biologic process—metamerism.[101,104,105] Metamerism is the linear repetition of anatomically similar segments, a process that originally evolved in high invertebrates and which forms the basic pattern of early vertebrate morphological development. However, other than the axial skeleton, the evolution of highly specialized limbs makes metamerism a transitory embryologic phenomenon in mammals.

During the second gestational week, the bilaminar (ectoderm and endoderm only) human embryo begins morphological differentiation comparable to gastrulation in other embryonic forms. This modified, but similar, process first involves the formation of a specialized cellular aggregate in the ectoderm, the primitive streak, which is located at the caudal end of the presumptive embryo. Circumscribed areas of the primitive streak spread out and invaginate between the ectoderm and endoderm, forming the mesoderm and establishing the trilaminar (ectoderm-mesoderm-endoderm) embryo. The area of invagination becomes the primitive pit

and is surrounded by a cellular aggregate—the primitive knot. In the midline, the primitive knot produces the first characteristic structure to form in chordates, the notochord (chorda dorsalis). Unlike the invaginating mesoderm, at first the notochord is not located between the ectoderm and endoderm, but becomes intercalated with the endoderm of the roof of the gut (archenteron). The elongation of both the notochord and mesoderm takes place in a craniocaudal sequence; the anterior end of the notochord is formed first and is progressively added to, with the coccygeal elements (or tail elements) being formed last. The dorsal half of the notochord then separates from the ventral half, which has been attached to the endoderm, and forms a tubular structure, and true notochord, which is separate from both the ectoderm and endoderm.[86]

Following differentiation of the notochord, further induction commences as the undifferentiated mesenchyme lateral to these two structures begins to form highly cellular, parallel

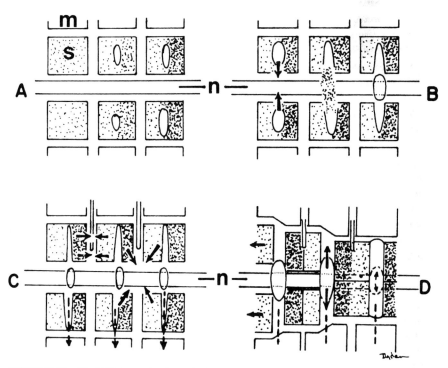

FIGURE 5-12 **(A–D)** *Schematic of vertebral segmentation and resegmentation. N = notochord, m = myotome, s = somite. (See text for details.)*

structures—the paraxial mesoderm. Further lateral proliferation of these two cell masses results in the elaboration of three distinct areas of the mesodermal plate—the medial paraxial columns, the intermediate columns, and most peripherally, the lateral plates. These plates give rise to the layers of the thoracic and abdominal cavities, whereas the intermediate columns will differentiate into the urogenital system. The paraxial columns will form the axial musculature.

Toward the end of the third week of gestation, somite formation commences in the paraxial mesoderm. Cells in the cranial region begin to proliferate and condense into paired segments. This cellular condensation-segmentation process continues caudad over the next 10 d until 42 to 44 somite pairs have formed (4 occipital, 8 cervi-

cal, 12 thoracic, 5 lumbar, 5 sacral, and up to 10 coccygeal pairs). However, only 33 to 34 pairs eventually will compose the adult spine, due to deletion of many of the coccygeal pairs. Some of the cranial somites are "deleted" by participation in the formation of portions of the skull and craniocervical articulations.

Initially, the mesenchymal cells of the somites are arranged radially around a central spherical cavity—the myocoele. As cellular proliferation and differentiation continue, the somites become triangular and develop discrete cell masses. The inner and outer cell masses first become evident, with the former becoming the dominant cell mass. The outer cell mass contributes to the tissue layers of the skin and subcutaneous tissue and is called the dermatome. The inner cell mass further differentiates to form two components. Dorsally, a cellular aggregation will become somatic (striated) muscle (the myotome), whereas ventrally, the cell mass will become skeletogenous tissue (the sclerotome).

The cellular aggregation of each sclerotome follows a pattern of loosely packed cells in the cranial half and densely packed cells in the caudal half (Fig. 5-12). Between these two cellular halves a fissure develops—the sclerocoele, or sclerotomic fissure of von Ebner. Cells juxtaposed to this fissure migrate to the notochord and encase it, forming the perichordal ring (which is the precursor of portions of the intervertebral disc). The sclerotome continues to develop, dividing completely into cranial and caudal cellular components. Concomitant with this division in a cranial-caudal sequence, there is cellular migration toward the notochord. This process of sclerotome differentiation appears to be mediated by the ventral half of the neural tube (probably in conjunction with notochordal inducers), whereas the neural crest–derived spinal ganglia appear to induce neural arch elements.

A second mass of cells of ectomesenchymal origin migrates dorsally, juxtaposed to the neural tube, to form the neural or vertebral arch (Fig. 5-13). Resegmentation of the arches does not occur to any significant degree. Further, the neural arch usually begins formation only after resegmentation of the centra is almost finished.

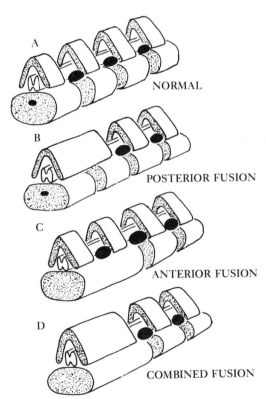

FIGURE 5-13 *Formation of the neural arch.* **(A)** *The posterior elements evolve relatively independently of the vertebral centra.* **(B)** *If a ganglion is removed experimentally, posterior fusion will develop, but contiguous central development is normal.* **(C)** *If the notochord is damaged, complete central and posterior fusion results.* **(D)** *Damage to the ganglion and the notochord causes anterior and posterior fusion.*

The neural arches alternate with the spinal ganglia and thus are situated intersegmentally with respect to the myotomes, so that each neural arch is connected to two successive myotomal segments. Thus, the vertebral bodies and the neural arches appear to be under different cellular induction controls and have relative independence in their early developmental patterns.

As the central cell migration occurs, the cranial cell mass begins to unite with the caudal cell mass of the next rostral sclerotome. This process is termed sclerotomic resegmentation. When the process is completed, the notochord is surrounded by a series of vertebral centra that are derived from adjacent somites. Failure to adequately divide or resegment represents possible mechanisms for the formation of congenital

scoliosis. Since the neural arch formation process evolves from a relatively separate cellular aggregation of the sclerotome, it may develop relatively independently of vertebral centrum structural failures, so that fused vertebral bodies may not necessarily be associated with fused posterior elements, and *vice versa*. More recently, some workers have suggested that the resegmentation concept is not completely valid, feeling that the vertebrae develop in their definitive positions from the loosely aggregated cellular zones, and the ribs and intervertebral discs arise from the more densely aggregated zones.[74] In some vertebrates, particularly *Cetacea*, resegmentation does not occur, leading to cervical fusions as a normal state of development (Fig. 5-14).

The formation of the atlas (C1) and axis (C2),

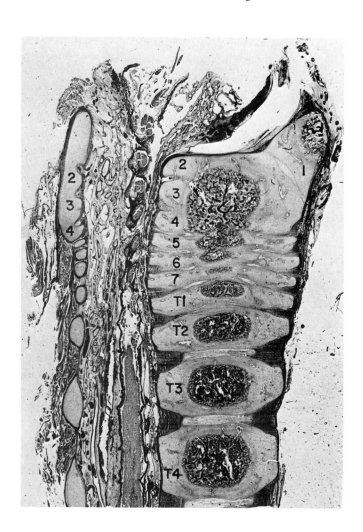

FIGURE 5-14 *In some animals vertebral fusion is normal. This spine from a cetacean embryo* (Globicephala) *shows early fusion of all the cervical vertebra.*

by virtue of their unique anatomy, differs significantly from the general vertebral formation pattern (Fig. 5-15). As previously mentioned, a number of occipital somites play an integral role in the structural formation of the basicranium. The caudal half of the fourth occipital somite fuses with the cranial half of the first cervical somite to form, in lower vertebrates, the proatlas. The ossiculum terminale of C2 (dens) may represent this structure in mammals (Fig. 5-16). In humans, this somite fusion also contributes to ligaments extending from the skull to the dens. The major cell mass of the dens is derived from the caudal half of the first and the cranial half of the second cervical somites. The same somite fusion also contributes to the anterior arch of C1 and some of the supporting ligaments between C1 and the dens. The centrum of C2 is derived from the caudal half of the second and the cranial half of the third cervical somites. The normal resegmentation process (sclerocoele formation) is incomplete in the second cervical somite and allows fusion of the centra of C1 and C2.

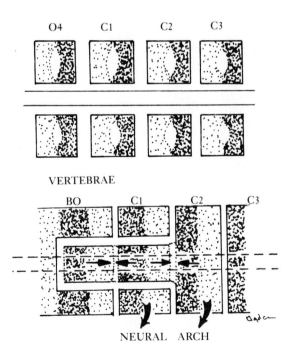

SOMITES

| O4 | C1 | C2 | C3 |

VERTEBRAE

| BO | C1 | C2 | C3 |

NEURAL ARCH

FIGURE 5-15 *Schematic of the modification of the development of the upper cervical spine to form the basiocciput-atlanto-axial motion segment.*

The notochord becomes totally encased by the migrating mesenchymal cells of the paired sclerotomes as they coalesce in the midline. As the vertebral column continues to differentiate, the contained notochord is gradually compressed and degenerates, although embryonic cells may transiently persist within the vertebral body as the mucoid streak (Fig. 5-17). However, between the vertebral bodies, the notochordal cells undergo mucoid change to form the gelatinous nucleus pulposus. Cells from the sclerocoele region form the perichordal ring, thus bridging the space between the resegmented somites. Eventually this perichordal tissue will become the annulus fibrosus.

The aforementioned processes of cellular differentiation, aggregation, migration, and reaggregation of the axial skeleton occur between the third and sixth weeks of gestation. During the sixth week, the mesenchymal anlagen begin to develop centers of chondrification.[43] Two centers appear on either side of the notochord and fuse around it to make a more completely unified chondrification center. Two other centers form in the neural arch and eventually fuse dorsally to establish a solid neural arch and begin spinous process formation. The final two centers appear at the junctions of the mesenchymal centrum and neural arches, and by lateral extension form the transverse processes. Concomitant with vertebral chondrification the perichordal ring condenses into a thick ring of nonchondrous cells that establish a dense annulus fibrosus around the differentiating nucleus pulposus. The cartilage model of the vertebra, by expansion of the chondrification centers, becomes a solid unit presenting no lines of demarcation between the body, neural arch, and ribs. However, when endochondral ossification commences later, the thoracic rib cartilage begins to separate from the centrum, whereas in the cervical, lumbar, and sacral regions, the costal processes will maintain continuity with the centrum throughout ossification.

Following completion of a completely cartilaginous axial skeleton, the next development stage is *primary* ossification. Three primary centers of ossification occur in each vertebra except C1 and C2. One ossification center appears in

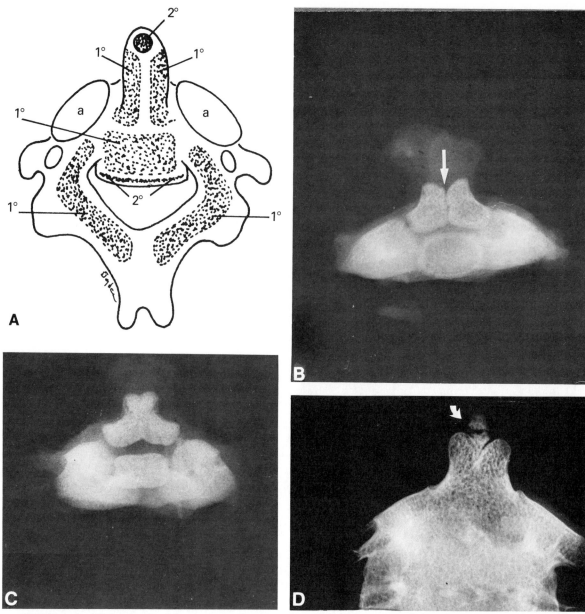

FIGURE 5-16 **(A)** *Schematic of development of various primary* **(1°)** *and secondary* **(2°)** *ossification centers in the atlas* *(C2). A = articulations.* **(B)** *Neonatal atlas showing bipartite ossification in the dens. Arrow indicates between bipartite centers.* **(C)** *By 6 mo postnatal, these ossification centers have fused, leaving a "cleft" at the tip.* **(D)** *By 5 to 7 yr the seconday ossification center appears in the tip of the dens. This is the ossiculum terminale* (*arrow*).

each body (centrum) and one in each side of the neural arch. As a prelude to ossification, the cartilage cells hypertrophy and calcify the matrix. Small vessels from the cartilage canal system reach this differentiated region, and the ossification process commences. Ossification initially begins in the vertebral bodies in the lower thoracic and upper lumbar regions and then proceeds craniad and caudad. However, in the cervical region, the primary ossification centers of the vertebral bodies may appear sequentially after the primary centers in the vertebral arches.

This vertebral body ossification process begins approximately in the 15th to 16th week of gestation and continues through the 24th week, when enlargement of the primary ossification center forms epiphyses and epiphyseal growth plates at the superior and inferior margins of the vertebra. These structures allow further vertebral growth by endochondral ossification, comparable to growth in the longitudinal bones. The cartilage plates are vascularized by a small cartilage canal system, although not as extensively as the epiphyses of the long bones. This vascular system is derived from the surrounding perichondrium and ligamentous tissue. However, these vessels do not penetrate the annulus fibrosus, which is avascular during development and remains so into adult life. The vascularity within the end-plate cartilage canal system will eventually support development of the secondary ossification center of the vertebral body—the ring apophysis. The ring apophysis is a C-shaped structure that commences ossification in adolescence and may persist into the twenties. It anchors the annulus to the vertebral body. Interestingly, ring apophyses are found only in large primates; other vertebrates have distinct plates at each end of the vertebral body (Fig. 5-18).

The ossification patterns of the atlas and axis (C1, C2) again differ markedly from the remainder of the vertebrae. The anterior atlas has three

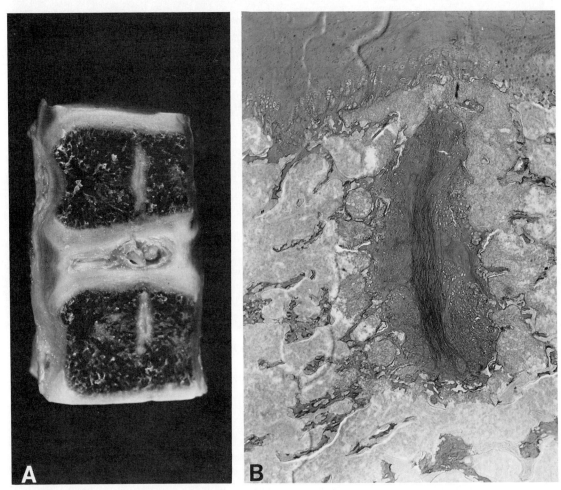

FIGURE 5-17 **(A)** *Thoracic vertebrae (sagittal section) from 5-mo-old child with chondrodystrophy. The notochord remnant is evident in each primary ossification center.* **(B)** *Microscopic section of notochordal tissue with surrounding cartilaginous remnants.*

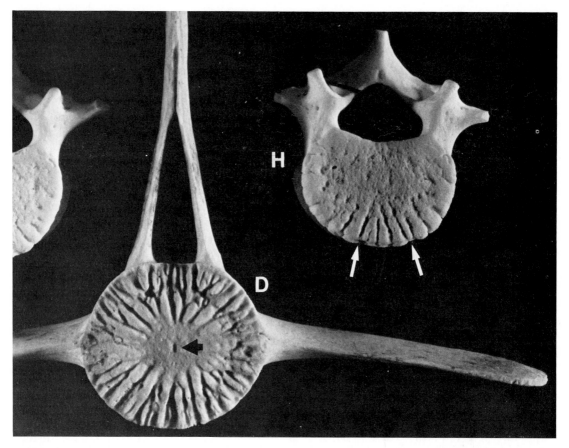

FIGURE 5-18 *Mammalian species differences in end-plate development between a dolphin (Tursiops-T;),* **D** *which develops a complete end-plate, and a human (Homo-H;),* **H** *who develops an incomplete ring around the lateral and anterior regions. Note the radial development of the end-plate undulations and the notochord "remnant" (black arrow) in the dolphin. In contrast the human shows irregular, asymmetric undulations (white arrows).* This incomplete epiphyseal-physeal development may be an anatomical predisposition to scoliosis, although other factors undoubtedly interact with the changing structure.

primary centers of ossification, whereas the neural arches have two centers. The axis develops five primary and two secondary centers of ossification. The centrum and neural arch centers form in the conventional manner (at about the 10th week), whereas the dens forms two laterally situated centers at about the 20th week. The two dens centers fuse near the end of gestation, although a superior cleft may still be present. By the second year, the secondary ossification center appears in the tip. The cartilage plate between the ossification centers of the centrum and dens may persist until the second decade (Fig. 5-19). When fusion of these centers does occur it may be eccentric and may mimic a fracture.

The vertebral arches begin primary ossification at about the eighth week. In contrast to the primary centers in the centra, these appear first in the cervical neural arches and appear progressively caudad. However, the ossified laminae and pedicles first unite with the ossification center in the centrum in the upper lumbar region and progress craniad and caudad. Secondary centers of ossification are formed in the spinous processes and transverse processes during adolescence. The cervical and, less frequently the lumbar, vertebrae may develop small secondary ossification centers in which the costal process has been incorporated into the centrum.

The pattern of formation of the primary ossification centers in the centra and neural arches varies significantly. The cartilaginous centra exhibit early development of a cartilage canal (vascular) system and begin endochondral ossification analogous to the development of a secondary ossification center of a long bone. Because of this pattern, there is no periosteum until the ossification center expands to the peripheral margins of the centra, and the centra are surrounded by perichondrium during the fetal period and early infancy. In contrast, the neural arches develop a primary bone collar, periosteum, and primary ossification center in a manner analogous to primary ossification center formation in tubular bones.

Fusion of the primary ossification centers of the centrum and arch occurs anterior to the anatomical pedicle at the site of the original neuro-

central synchrondrosis (Fig. 5-20). There is no pattern of ossification center development in the lumbar neural arches to suggest that the pars defect in spondylolisthesis or spondylolysis is congenital because of a fusion failure of ossification centers. The normal site of ossific fusion is well anterior to the pathologic defect. A definite problem that may result from improperly timed neurocentral fusion is spinal stenosis. There is endochondral growth in the fusion areas that undoubtedly contributes to diametric widening of the spinal canal, with additional widening occurring concomitantly by a similar posterior process. Premature osseous fusion, either anteriorly or posteriorly, would preclude further canal widening. Further, since these are endochondral processes, failure to grow at normal

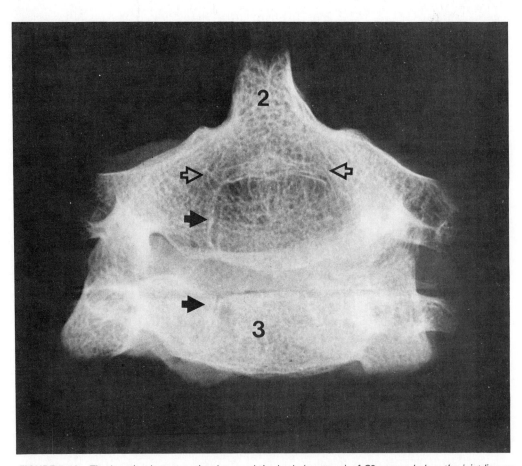

FIGURE 5-19 *The junction between the dens and the body (centrum) of C2 occurs below the joint line so that a fracture at the level of the C1-C2 joint would be through the dens ossification center. This junction may remain as an "epiphyseal ghost" roentgenographically, and should not be confused with a fracture (open arrows). The neurocentral synchrondrosis is still evident in C2 and C3 (solid arrows).*

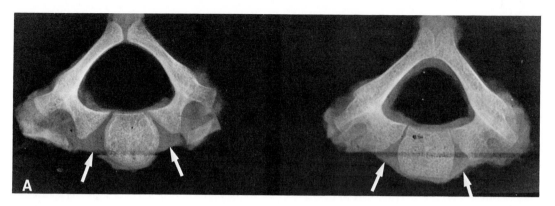

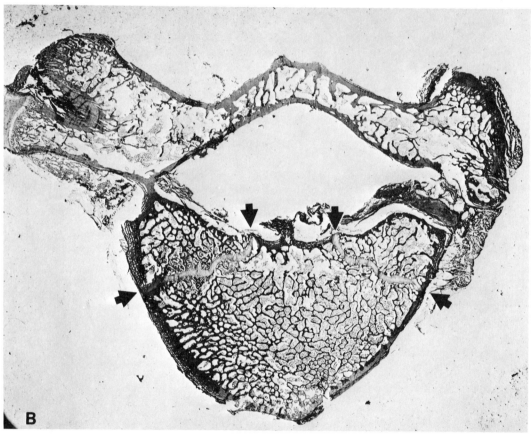

FIGURE 5-20 *Similar to the anatomy seen in Figure 5-19, the junction between the vertebral centrum and the posterior elements creates a neurocentral synchondrosis that is within the eventual vertebral body, anterior to the articulations. (A) Early neurocentral synchondroses at birth and 3 mo (arrows). (B) More mature stage showing beginning closure and incorporation of some of the posterior element bone with the central bone to form the mature vertebral body.*

rates also could impair proper diametric increase of the spinal canal. This may be the mechanism of spinal stenosis in achondroplasia.

As previously mentioned, the primary ossification center of each vertebral body is initially associated with a spherical growth plate. This growth plate enlarges toward the sides of the vertebral mass and the intervertebral discs. Gradually, the continuous growth region becomes separated into two separate growth plates located superiorly and inferiorly, creating a situation analogous to the tubular bones. Owing to ellipsoid enlargement of both the intervertebral disc and the ossification center, the central portions of the growth plate thin out, and the lateral and anterior portions become relatively thicker, creating the "ring" apophysis. Each of these apophyses appears, radiographically and histologically, to be set in a groove extending around the upper and lower borders of the developing vertebral bodies. By 11 yr of age, small foci of ossification usually develop in the ring apophyses. These multiple foci are similar to the early secondary ossification center of the trochlea. By 12 yr of age, these ossific foci have coalesced to form a C-shaped structure, the radiologic "ring," which is the analogue of the secondary ossification center of the tubular bones.[93] Fusion of the apophyseal ossification center with the primary ossification center of the vertebral body begins by 14 to 15 yr of age, but may not be completed until age 25 yr in the lumbar region.

Ribs

The ribs develop from the costal processes, which are derived from the caudad portion of the sclerotome along with the neural arch. The costal processes extend outward in the clefts between the myotomes, thus forming relationships with two successive myotomes. The primary center of ossification appears at about the ninth week, near the future angle of each rib. This ossification commences prior to the primary centers appearing in the corresponding vertebrae. The cartilaginous rib then ossifies progressively in proximal and distal directions, although the distal ends of the thoracic ribs always remain cartilaginous. Secondary centers of ossification appear during adolescence—two in the tubercle and one in the head. In the cervical region, the costal process usually regresses and forms the anterior half of the vertebral arterial arch. In the lumbar region, the costal processes eventually become part of the large transverse processes. In both regions, this process has the potential to continue development and form an accessory cervical or lumbar rib. In the sacrum, the costal processes participate in the formation of the alae.

Sternum

The sternum first arises as a pair of mesenchymal condensations that may be derived from the lateral mesodermal plates surrounding the thoracic cavity.[12] They are first evident at 6 wk of gestation and initially are independent of each other and of the developing ribs. However, once each band becomes associated with the corresponding ribs, the two lateral bands begin to unite in the ventral midline. This coalescence first occurs cranially, with the two bands also joining the presternal mesenchymal mass (which will become the manubrium) and the two lateral suprasternal masses (which will be involved in sternoclavicular development). Coalescence continues in a caudad direction, and by 9 wk of gestation the fusion is usually complete. If the process is incomplete, a cleft sternum, a perforated sternum, or a cleft xiphoid might result. Primary ossification begins at about 5 fetal mo, but not all ossification centers are present until early childhood. Although the early cartilaginous sternum is continuous, the ossification pattern is a reflection of metamerism (Fig. 5-21). The presence of two ossification centers in a sternal segment is not uncommon, reflecting the dual lateral origin of each segment.

Appendicular skeletal development

While the somites are forming and the neural tube is closing, the limb-forming area, or limb morphogenetic field, arises as a localized differentiation of the lateral plate mesoderm.[1,7,8,62,75,106-108] The somatic layer begins to thicken by cellular proliferation. These cells then lose their epithelial connections to the lateral plate and migrate away, reaggregating as a mesenchymal cell mass, the presumptive limb bud.[84] This mesenchymal mass is in continuity with a primitive capillary plexus. The mesenchyme becomes closely associated with the inner surface of the ectoderm. However, there are not major morphological changes in the ectoderm, which appears at this stage to be a mechanical barrier to more rapid proliferation of the mesenchymal aggregate. A very early relationship is established between the mesoderm and ectoderm

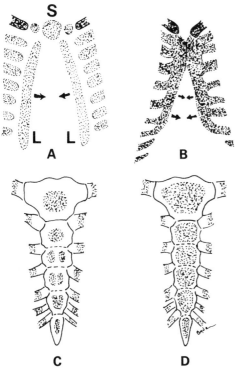

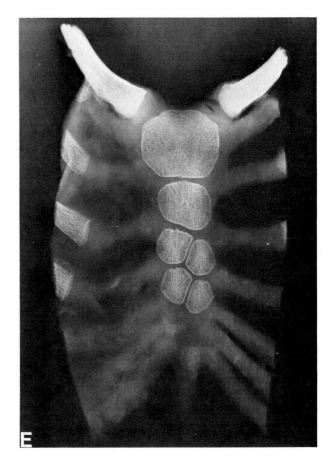

FIGURE 5-21 **(A–D)** *Schematics of sternal formation and ossification from initially separate presternal* **(S)** *and lateral band* **(L)** *anlagen.* **(E)** *Postnatal sternal specimen, showing the segmented ossification characteristic of immature sternebrae.*

of the presumptive limb. All subsequent differentiations will be controlled by these positional cell layer inter-relationships. Cellular condensation and matrix elaboration in the mesenchyme induces cellular thickening in the overlying ectoderm. Both processes (mesodermal and ectodermal) begin prior to the limb bud being externally evident.

Further proliferation of the ectoderm induces outgrowth of the underlying mesenchyme, establishing a definitive limb bud. This occurs adjacent to the fifth through seventh cervical somites, at the 21 to 29 somite stage for the upper limb bud, so that the arms begin formation not only before the leg anlagen, but even before the somite formation process—including those essential to the leg buds—has been completed. The lower limb similarly begins differentiation and bud formation before the most caudad somites have completely formed. The limb buds

become separated longitudinally from the dorsal and ventral body contours by the development of the sulcus dorsolateralis and the limb-bud ventral pit. Differentiation of the human limb occurs more slowly than does the mouse limb and shows some different patterns.[106] Extrapolation of experimental data, especially involving potential teratogens, must be done with great care.

Of the two blastemal components contributing to the formation of the limb bud, the mesodermal component appears more important. This presumptive limb mesenchyme is a genetically determined self-differentiating mass, in which type (forelimb, hindlimb), polarity (extensor-flexor or post- preaxial) and internal structure are determined independently of eventual somite-derived contributions.[64] Pieces of the lateral plate may be removed experimentally in the differentiating phase and transplanted anywhere

along the Wolffian ridge. The overlying local ectoderm at the transplant site soon will associate
with the mesodermal transplant, and the limb
bud will develop heterotopically into the appropriate structure, but the neural and vascular contributions instead will be derived from the
nearest available somite segments. In contrast,
the presumptive limb ectoderm does not possess
such self-differentiating capacity and, if transplanted alone, will not necessarily give rise to a
new limb bud. Ectoderm from any part of the
embryo may be transplanted near the appropriate region of the lateral plate and will cooperate
in the formation of the appropriate limb bud,
that is, the ectoderm overlying the upper limb
bud still develops. With further development,
the ectoderm will become an active, rather than
a passive, component of the limb bud.

The limb ectoderm establishes two layers or
metabolic zones.[96] The outer layer, which relies
on the amniotic fluid for much of its metabolic
interchange, becomes relatively inactive as a
major functional component in limb differentiation. This layer is termed the periderm. In contrast, the inner cell layer undergoes rapid cell
proliferation in a circumscribed area of the limb
bud to create the apical ectodermal ridge (AER)
or marginal streak.[97] The AER becomes primarily responsible for the continual outgrowth and
proximodistal differentiation of the limb bud,
functioning as a pacemaker that induces differentiation of the underlying mesenchyme in the
appropriate sequence. If the AER is experimentally removed, limb bud formation will cease at
the stage of development reached at the point of
removal, that is, early AER removal may stop
limb development at the humerus stage, whereas
later removal may disrupt development at the
forearm or wrist differentiation stage. However,
even though subsequent distal development is
disrupted, continued growth and differentiation
of the already differentiated structures can and
does occur. Many transverse hemimelic conditions may arise because of generalized damage to
a major segment of the AER-mesodermal interaction at the appropriate time (probably by
blocking essential biochemical pathways). Inter-
calary hemimelia or phocomelia, in contrast, are
probably due to more selective or localized dam-

age to the AER inductive capacity for a certain
skeletal component, but these conditions may
also be due to defective differentiation in later
stages (that is, transition from mesenchyme to
cartilage or from cartilage to bone). The AER
apparently mechanically induces mesodermal
outgrowth by providing a particular spatial configuration that allows the underlying mesenchyme to express innate differentiation capacities.[80,81]

The outgrowing mesoderm forms three
layers—(1) a superficial layer, which is always
the leading edge of the mesoderm and is very
active mitotically, (2) an intermediate zone, and
(3) a deep zone, where mitotic activity decreases,
intercellular matrix formation increases, and the
cells become more compacted. The deep layer
forms the first structural evidence of the mesenchymal skeleton, whereas the intermediate layer
will differentiate into periskeletal tissue (perichondrium, periosteum, joint capsules, musculotendinous units). The superficial layer
is the region subjected to AER induction. This
layer, in turn, forms both the intermediate and
deep layers, doing so in a proximodistal sequence. That is, the superficial layer forms a
musculoskeletal condensation that will begin to
undergo further differentiation, whereas the
superficial layer continues to form, in continuity,
each successive component of the limb bud. This
mesodermal anlage develops centrally within the
limb bud.

In order to remain inductively active, the
AER requires a maintenance factor that appears
to be derived from the differentiating mesoderm
(most likely from the active superficial zone).
Thus, the limb mesoderm and AER have reciprocal chemotactic relationships. Either relationship could feasibly be disrupted by a teratogen,
seriously impairing the reciprocal, inductive-
maintenance capacity, and adversely affecting
further limb development.[58,60,61,85]

The limb bud continues to flatten and broaden
into a paddle as it differentiates more distally,
with hand development preceding foot development. The edge of the hand (foot) plate is initially circular, but subsequently becomes penta-
gonal, with the projecting points indicating the
sites of future digits (Fig. 5-22). The AER in-

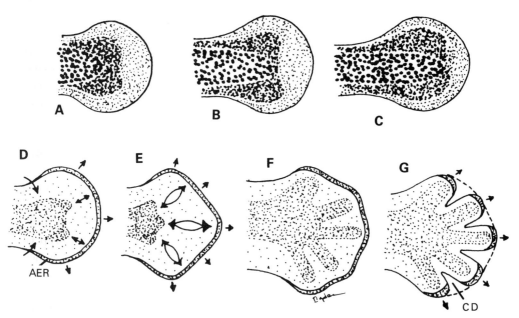

FIGURE 5-22 **(A–C)** *Progressive development of the hand or foot from an outgrowing "paddle." The mesen-chymal skeletomuscular anlagen progressively develop and interact with the apical ectodermal ridge* **(AER)**. *Cellular death* **(CD)** *in the interdigital areas leads to digital separation.*

duces the continuous mesenchyme to form five ray extensions that are still in continuity with the main cell mass. The spaces between the rays form depressions that continue to deepen, undergo cell necrosis, and finally form the inter-digital clefts (the web spaces are remnants of this process). Abnormal cleft formation can lead to the various types of syndactyly and would allow juxtaposition of ray anlagen (or AER) that could lead to symphalangism. The AER remains at the tip of each digit and induces further growth until all the phalanges have formed fully.

The limb blood vessels do not develop *de novo* as outbranchings from the main stem artery. Rather, larger blood vessels develop by hemodynamic selection from the extensive, pre-existent capillary network. Increased flow through certain capillary areas (a function of the particular metabolic demands of the differentiat-ing musculoskeletal blastema) leads to progres-sive enlargement of the one pathway, usually in a proximodistal sequence. Thus, it is not surpris-ing that vascular variation is common through the axial and appendicular musculoskeletal sys-tem. Failure to evolve a channel can lead to the lack of a vessel (e.g., no ulnar artery at the wrist), whereas development of a different channel can place an artery in an unexpected position (e.g., superficial radial artery at elbow or wrist). If a skeletal anlage fails to develop, vascular needs will be less, and certain arterial channels may not develop (Fig. 5-23).[27]

Concomitant with differentiation of discrete, innervated muscle masses, the mesenchymal cells become active and begin to elaborate an intercellular matrix, entering the precartilage stage and rapidly continuing transformation into cartilaginous anlage. Since the primary function of the skeletal system is structural support, this cellular transition may represent a response of the mesenchymal skeleton to the beginning func-tion in the adjacent muscles (i.e., mechanical in-duction). However, since this transition may also occur in tissue culture, the mesenchymal cells undoubtedly have an intrinsic capacity for trans-formation. The timed appearance of this intrin-sic capacity is inter-related with functional re-quirements. Once the cartilaginous anlage is formed, the cell clones become stabilized and are no longer capable of significant self-differentiation, but rather are more and more dependent upon adjacent tissue interactions (both biochemical and biomechanical).

The development of the limb progresses to a cartilaginous primordia in a proximodistal sequence over a 4-d period. The differentiation of the cartilage is preceded by progressive changes in cellular contacts at specific locations in the precartilage mesenchyme. The biosynthesis and diffusion through the extracellular matrix of a cell surface protein, such as fibronectin, could lead to spatial patterns of the molecule that serve as the chemical basis for the emergent cartilaginous primordia. As cellular differentiation proceeds, the size of the mesenchymal diffusion mass is reduced in discrete steps, leading to se-

quential reorganization of morphogen patterns. These successive patterns correspond to the eventual skeletal elements, whose emergence also depends on the maintenance of a unique boundary condition at the limb apex.[65]

Chondro-osseous development

Chondrification starts centrally and progresses toward the periphery of the mesenchymal anlage, at which point the intermediate and deep layers juxtapose. In this region, the perichondrium differentiates. The perichondrium surrounds the still-continuous anlage, crossing the sites of the presumptive joints. However, interzones soon begin to form at these sites. The

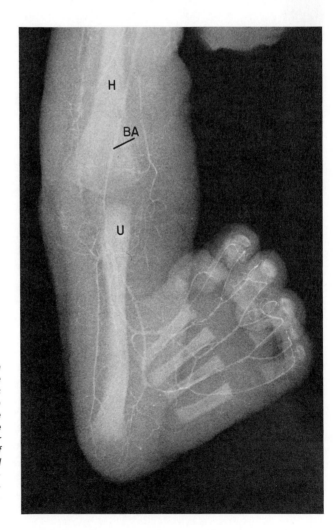

FIGURE 5-23 *Injection of radial hemimelia specimen, showing altered development of the vasculature distal to the elbow. Undoubtedly this is an interactive phenomenon. Failure to develop skeletal and/or muscular anlagen decreases the vascular demand of a developing area. Since the blood vessels become defined only after skeletogenesis, certain vessels will have little, if any, biologic stimulus to develop as major arterial or venous pathways. Therefore, vascular anomalies become a secondary concomitant to skeletal deficiencies.* H = *humerus.* U = *ulna.* BA = *brachial artery.*

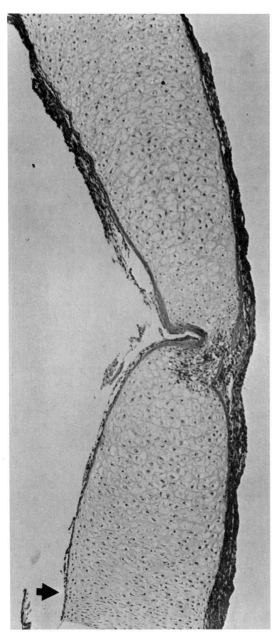

FIGURE 5-24 *Early cartilaginous femur from 80- to 90-mm (crown-to-rump) human fetus. The central cells have hypertrophied in anticipation of the next step—ossification. Cells further away do not exhibit hypertrophic change (arrow).*

perichondrium establishes continuity with the cartilaginous layers of the interzones and "loses" continuity across the joint as this tissue becomes fibroblastic and evolves into the joint capsule. Thus, the continuous mesenchymal anlagen

gradually are replaced by the discontinuous cartilaginous skeleton that resembles the final osseous skeleton in basic structural contours.

The cartilaginous skeleton grows by perichondral apposition (including the chondrogenic layer of the interzone) and interstitial enlargement (which is both cellular and matrical). Experimental evidence suggests that extrinsic mechanical stresses associated with normal function are necessary for normal interstitial growth of epiphyseal cartilage during postnatal development, strongly suggesting that functional activity may influence the rate of cell proliferation. Functional activity is the apparent stimulus for the differentiation of perichondral cells into chondroblasts. If a bone is transplanted, three major cartilage changes may ensue: (1) the rate of proliferative activity in the cell columns may decrease, (2) the cartilage may fail to maintain a satisfactory increase in transverse diameter, and (3) the cells of the perichondrium may differentiate into osteoblasts rather than chondroblasts.[59]

The cartilage cells within the anlage pass through five developmental stages that are comparable to the growth plate zones. Histologically and functionally, this zonal gradation resembles the characteristic zones of the growth plate. However, each of these early zones is thick (i.e., greater numbers of cells in the longitudinal direction), and the orientation within each zone is distinctly transverse (not longitudinal), which undoubtedly arises from the major growth pattern and direction of expansion of the cartilaginous anlage being progressively diametric (whereas the primary growth expansion pattern of the postnatal appendicular skeleton is longitudinal).

This transverse growth pattern results in a narrow midshaft and progressive widening toward the ends (Fig. 5-24). The narrowest portion contains the phase five cartilage cells. The surrounding perichondrium begins to thicken, becomes presumptive periosteum, and forms a thin layer of osteoid tissue adjacent to the phase five region. This osteoid tissue is quickly mineralized to become bone matrix, forming a discrete circumferential structure—the primary bone collar. The outer cell layer now becomes osteoblastic periosteum, although it is in continuity with the perichondrium. The primary bone collar becomes multilayered. As this collar is maturing, the phase five cartilage intercellular matrix calcifies. The bone collar is then penetrated at several points by cell masses and blood vessels (vasoformative irruption) that begin replacement of cartilage by bone (Fig. 5-25). This is the primary ossification center.

Primary ossification center formation occurs in the major long bones toward the end of the second gestational month. The humerus is usually the first to ossify, followed by the radius. The femur, tibia, and ulna all ossify at approximately the same time, whereas the fibula is usually the last to ossify.[72]

The multilayered bone collar contains a capillary network within the primitive trabecular spaces and is in continuity with the more extensive capillary network in the outer regions of the muscular anlage (muscle and bone require higher oxygen tissue levels than cartilage to undergo normal differentiation). The irruption capillaries and osteoblastic tissue are derived from this network within the bone collar. Although several vessels may enter and initiate ossification, usually only one will become dominant (hemodynamic selection). This vessel, the nutrient artery, initially enters the anlage at right angles to the longitudinal axis and maintains this orientation during most of prenatal development. The primary ossification center contains osteoblastic and angioblastic tissue.

Once the initial ossification center has been formed and the nutrient artery established, further ossification progresses rapidly toward each end as the cartilage of the four other zones begins more rapid maturation to phase five cartilage. This sequential replacement of cartilage by bone is characteristic of endochondral ossifica-

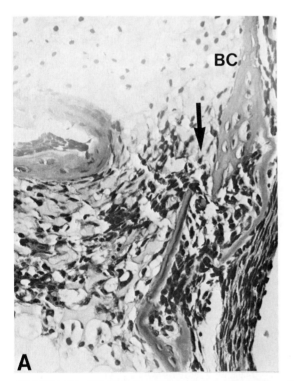

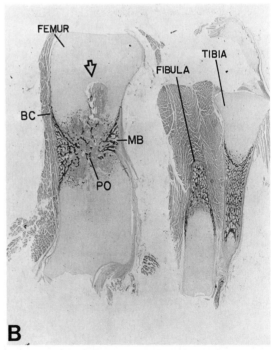

FIGURE 5-25 **(A)** *Early formation of bone collar* **(BC)** *and vascular irruption (arrow) to begin formation of the primary ossification center.* **(B)** *Early primary ossification in the monotreme (platypus) femur, tibia, and fibula. The femur shows evidence of the bone collar* **(BC)** *and the membranous bone derived from the periosteum* **(MB)** *surrounding primary ossification* **(PO)** *within the hypertrophic cells. Vascular irruption and ossification is proceeding rapidly into the proximal femur (arrow). In the tibia, periosteal bone and primary ossification center bone have already remodeled into a contiguous mass.*

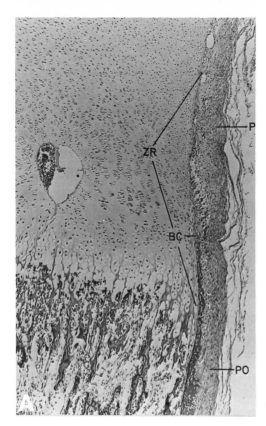

FIGURE 5-26 **(A)** *Early (prenatal) development of the zone of Ranvier* **(ZR)**. *This structure, a regional modification of the continuous periosteum* **(PO)** *and the perichondrium* **(PC)**, *plays a major role in the development of the physeal collar* **(BC)** *and the elaboration of peripheral physeal tissue.* **(B)** *Later fetal stage, showing a more defined zone of Ranvier indenting the margin of the physis and epiphysis. The bone collar extends to the germinal cells, but the zone of Ranvier extends further. The structure above the center of the physis in each section is a remnant of rapid upward expansion of the primary vascular irruption. This is the human analogue of the region shown in Figure 5-25***B**.

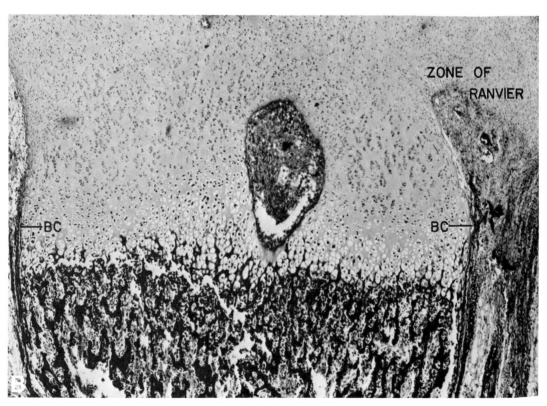

tion. The bone first formed is a loose trabecular network that fuses with the multilayered periosteal shell. The ossification process extends at relatively equal rates toward each end of the bone, with new cartilage formation also occurring at approximately the same rate for each end. Only postnatally does there appear to be a significant difference in the rates of growth for each epiphysis and physis. As the primary bone approaches each end, the cartilage begins to more closely resemble a growth plate. This usually occurs by the end of the third or early in the fourth gestational month. Concomitant with the primary ossification center progressing toward the cartilaginous ends is the primary periosteal collar also extending toward these regions, but it is always slightly ahead of endochondral ossification. Once the physis is established (usually after 70 to 80% of the cartilage has been replaced by primary ossification), the periosteal ring stops further extension toward the epiphysis and remains level with the zone of hypertrophic cartilage (with which it continues growth in an integral fashion), although it may extend further as osteoid tissue to reach the germinal zone. The cellular association of periosteal ring, peripheral physis, and fibrovascular tissue is referred to as the zone of Ranvier, which is an important area of diametric expansion of the physis (Fig. 5-26). The periosteal ring does not always extend to the zone of hypertrophy, especially in the smaller bones (metacarpals), and may not completely surround the physis in every bone.

As the individual bone elongates and widens in the metaphyses by the normal process of endochondral ossification, extensive remodeling begins during the fourth and fifth fetal months. When the trabecular bone and bone collar initially unite, they form a diaphyseal shaft of relatively uniform diameter. In contrast, the metaphysis must progressively widen to accommodate the diametrically expanding physis and epiphysis. Active remodeling occurs in two areas of the metaphysis—central and peripheral. Bone is removed from the peripheral cortical surface, whereas new bone is added to the endosteal surface. The endosteal bone will become contiguous with the diaphyseal cortical bone. Bone remodeling is so active that the metaphyseal cortex

is relatively porous (see Fig. 5-10). This "porous" bone is easily penetrated by an osteomyelitic abscess originating within the metaphysis, allowing it to reach the subperiosteal space (or joint if this region happens to be intra-articular, as in the proximal femur). The central part of the metaphysis also remodels, with primary spongiosa being replaced by secondary spongiosa.

While remodeling is occurring in the metaphysis, the diaphysis is readily increasing in diameter by appositional (intramembrous) bone deposition, endosteal remodeling, and formation of a nonosseous medullary (marrow) cavity. The endosteal surface is the site of both new bone formation and osteoclastic osteolysis.

Remodeling normally varies from bone to bone, and even within a bone. If it fails to occur properly, the bone ends become more and more flared or club-shaped, and the diaphysis becomes widened. This can be seen in several bone displasias (osteopetrosis, Gaucher's disease, Engelmann's disease).

By birth, the long bones consist of metaphyseal and diaphyseal trabeculae that are primarily oriented longitudinally and cylindrically, with secondary trabeculae intermittently spanning the intervening spaces (Fig. 5-27). These trabeculae contain coarse-fibered or woven bone. There is only a small marrow cavity. However, near term, lamellar (compact, osteonal) bone begins to develop, although extensive formation of this fine-fibered type of bone is principally a postnatal phenomenon. As this newer (lamellar) bone is forming, cortical thickness and trabecular orientation will be in accord with intraosseous stress patterns.[11] This is known as Wolff's law. Basically, this law states that bone formation will increase in areas of compression and decrease in areas of tension. Similarly, the trabeculae will orient along major stress lines and will eventually form secondary trabeculae that act as struts or tie beams.

Types of growth mechanisms

The growth plate or physis is the essential mechanism for endochondral ossification. It appears in rudimentary form as the five phases of the cartilaginous anlage, and assumes characteristic

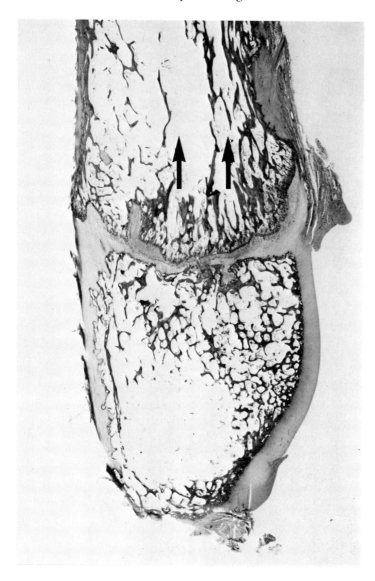

FIGURE 5-27 *Distal fibula, showing longitudinal orientation of juxtaphyseal metaphyseal bone. This pattern arises because of the rapid rate of longitudinal growth and the remodeling of primary spongiosa into secondary spongiosa. Arrows emphasize longitudinal direction of trabecular bone.*

cytoarchitectural patterns by the fourth month of gestation, when the ossification center has expanded to occupy approximately 70 to 80% of the anlage length.

Structurally, there are two basic types of growth plates—discoid and spherical, with each type having several variations.[69,70] Most primary growth plates (i.e., those arising as a consequence of the formation of the primary ossification center) of the long bones are discoid. They are characterized by a relatively planar area of rapidly differentiating and maturing cartilage that grades into but is distinct from the remain-

der of the hyaline cartilage of the chondroepiphysis. The primary function of a discoid physis is to allow rapid longitudinal growth. However, it also contributes to circumferential expansion. Discoid physes (i.e., an epiphysis primarily subjected to tensile rather than compressive forces). The tibial tuberosity is such a structure. Instead of the normal columnar cytoarchitecture, this type of physis is characterized by large amounts of fibrocartilage, which apparently reflects a structural adaptation of the physis to high tensile stresses.[68] Similar structural changes undoubtedly exist in other apophyses, such as the lesser trochanter, but certainly do not occur in the greater trochanter, which is misappropriately labeled an apophysis. Although there is tensile force through the glutei, there are also major compressive forces directed through the vastus lateralis and external rotators, so this structure is not purely responsive to tension, as fits the definition of apophysis. Thus, the cytoarchitecture of the greater trochanteric physis is the same as that of the capital femoral physis.

In the short tubular bones (phalanges, metacarpals, metatarsals), two discoid physes and an associated chondroepiphysis initially form, but with subsequent skeletal growth only one end forms a true chondroepiphysis and physis, which will be primary mechanisms for longitudinal growth in each bone (Fig. 5-28). In contrast, at the other end the hyaline cartilage is slowly replaced until only a small amount re-

mains between the articular surface and the physis. This growth plate will become a mechanism for continued contoured growth and will assume a spherical shape with decreased column length. The spherical physis makes only a small contribution to longitudinal growth. Because of the replacement of virtually all the hyaline cartilage, the preconditions for formation of an ossification center do not exist, and therefore the physis cannot be removed by physiologic epiphyseodesis. Instead, these physes enter a quiescent phase, just under the articular cartilage.

Another structural portion of the epiphysis sometimes encountered in the small bones of the hands and feet is the pseudoepiphysis (Fig. 5-29). Although often found in association with pathologic conditions, the pseudoepiphysis may represent the persistence or accentuation of an otherwise relatively normal structure.[37] The

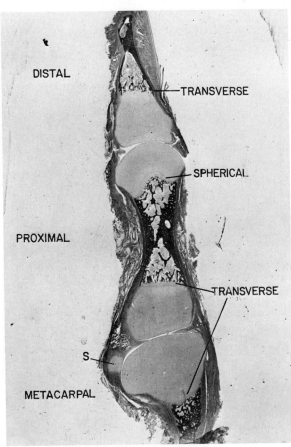

FIGURE 5-28 *Sagittal section of neonatal digit, showing distal phalanx, proximal phalanx, and metacarpal (including sesamoid [**S**]). Transverse physes develop at one end and eventually form a secondary ossification center. At the other end, either no epiphysis is present or a spherical physis forms, produced by the rapid replacement of the cartilage. Such a physis may form a pseudoepiphysis (see Figure 5-29).*

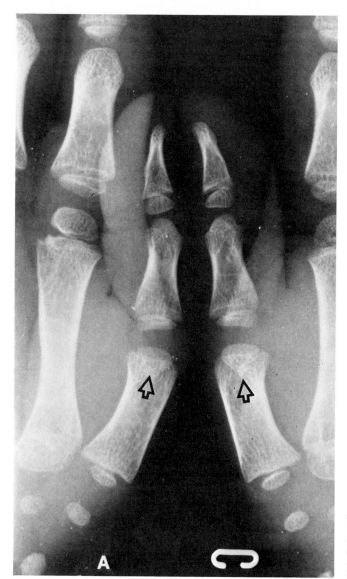

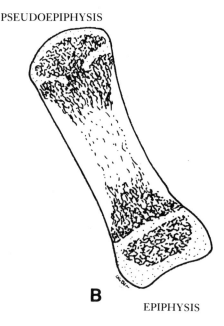

PSEUDOEPIPHYSIS

B

EPIPHYSIS

FIGURE 5-29 *A pseudoepiphysis may form normally or in pathologic situations (e.g., cretinism). It is formed by a "burgeoning" front of ossification from the metaphysis, a pattern of epiphyseal ossification that is characteristic of some amphibia.* **(A)** *Roentgenogram.* **(B)** *Schematic.*

bone that forms in the nonepiphyseal end is really an extension from the metaphysis and is not a true ossification center. Apparently the greatly increased vascularity and poorly formed matrix of the pseudoepiphysis enhances this irregular ossification, which begins centrally and extends centrifugally, creating a mushroom-shaped appearance in cross-section that appears as a separate ossification center radiographically.

A spherical growth plate, as well as the early secondary ossification center, is found in the small bones of the carpus and tarsus. By pro-

gressive centrifugal expansion the growth plate gradually assumes the contours of the bone or epiphysis, although it does not reach the margins until very late in skeletal maturation, so that a perichondrium rather than a periosteum is present. In the epiphysis, this enlargement of the secondary physis and ossification center leads to juxtaposition of part of the spherical growth plate against the primary discoid growth plate, creating a temporary bipolar growth zone. The epiphyseal contribution to the bipolar physis is eventually replaced by a subchondral bone plate, whereas the remainder of the spherical growth plate can still be found along the epiphyseal margins and under the articular surface, thus allowing continued expansion of the epiphysis commensurate with diametric expansion of the physis and metaphysis. The vertebral body initially also has a spherical growth plate but eventually develops parallel discoid physes.

The pelvis, since it evolves from three primary ossification centers, develops several physes (Fig. 5-30). The most prominent runs along the iliac crest—the iliac apophysis. This structure is the major growth mechanism for the large iliac bone. Like the greater trochanter, it is important to conceive that this is not a true traction apophysis, since the attachments of the abdominal muscula-

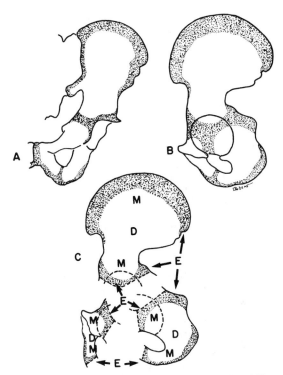

FIGURE 5-30 *Schematic of ossification-chondrification patterns in pelvis.* **(A)** *Anteroposterior view.* **(B)** *Lateral view; notice the confluence of the three component bones—ilium, ischium, and pubis—to form the triradiate cartilage.* **(C)** *Exploded view to show how each component bone may be viewed as an analogue of a longitudinal bone, with a diaphysis* **(D)**, *metaphyses* **(M)**, *and epiphyses* **(E)**. *The triradiate cartilage represents a fusion of the epiphyses of all three bones. The ischium and pubis also form a synchondrosis, and the pubic epiphyses also contribute to the symphysis pubis.*

ture are more than offset by the attachments of the gluteus maximus, tensor fascia lata, and iliac muscles, which must be considered as having a compressive effect upon the physis. The three ossification centers expand toward each other and form the triradiate cartilage at the level of the hip joint. This structure is composed of intersecting bipolar growth plates and represents a unique situation that allows acetabular growth.[54] The pubic and ischial ossification centers also meet near the midline and form a conjoint growth plate that parallels the contribution from the opposite side, with fibrocartilaginous tissue intervening—the symphysis pubis.

The physis has a characteristic and virtually unchanging cytoarchitectural structure from early fetal life until skeletal maturation (Fig. 5-31). The major differences among the growth plates can be found in the relative amounts of cells in each zone,[2] overall heights of the physis (these two factors being reflections of growth rates), and cellular modifications, such as replacement of the zone of hypertrophy with a zone of fibrocartilage.[2,18] These basic patterns can be analyzed as zones on the basis of either histologic or functional criteria.

The zone of growth is concerned with both longitudinal and diametric expansion of the bone. It is the area in which cellular addition and mitosis occurs. The resting cells are intimately associated with the blood vessels that supply this region (epiphyseal vessels). These small arterioles and capillaries may be instrumental in providing perivascular undifferentiated cells that can be added to the pool of resting chondrocytes. Additional resting cells are also elaborated peripherally through a specialized area of the perichondrium, the zone of Ranvier. The next stage in this zone is active cell division. This appears to occur in both longitudinal and transverse directions, although principally in the former, and leads to the earliest evidence of cell column formation. In an active growth plate, these cell columns can compose half the overall height of the physis. The randomly dispersed collagen of the resting and dividing regions becomes more longitudinally oriented between the columnar cells.

The next functional area is the zone of carti-

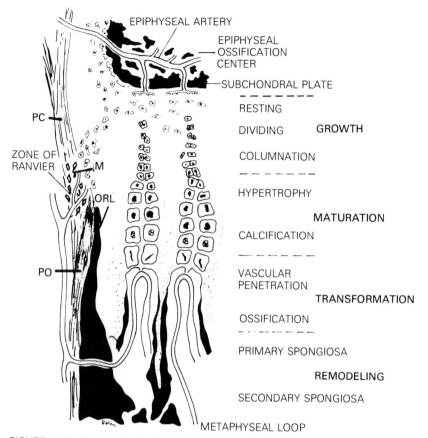

EPIPHYSEAL ARTERY

EPIPHYSEAL
OSSIFICATION
CENTER

SUBCHONDRAL PLATE

PC

RESTING

DIVIDING   **GROWTH**

ZONE OF
RANVIER

COLUMNATION

M

HYPERTROPHY

ORL

MATURATION

CALCIFICATION

PO

VASCULAR
PENETRATION

TRANSFORMATION

OSSIFICATION

PRIMARY SPONGIOSA

REMODELING

SECONDARY SPONGIOSA

METAPHYSEAL LOOP

FIGURE 5-31 *Schematic of the zones of the growth plate concerned with longitudinal and latitudinal ossification.* **PC** = *perichondrium,* **PO** = *periosteum,* **M** = *undifferentiated mesenchymal tissue,* **ORL** = *ossification ring of Lacroix. The various zones concerned with longitudinal growth are depicted on the right by anatomical and physiologic divisions. Latitudinal (appositional) growth occurs through the periosteum, perichondrium, and zone of Ranvier.*

lage formation. In this zone, increased intercellular matrix is formed and undergoes the significant biochemical changes necessary for eventual ossification. The matrix becomes metachromatic and calcifies. The chondrocytes become hypertrophic—a reflection of their increased metabolic activity. The fate of these chondrocytes at the end of this zone is controversial. Some authors feel that all the cells degenerate,[9] whereas others feel that some or all modulate to become osteoblasts under the influence of vascularization (changing oxygen tension).[15,50]

The last zone is that of cartilage transformation. The cartilage matrix (chondroid) is sufficiently calcified to allow vascular invasion by the metaphyseal sinusoidal loops. Electron micro-

scopic studies suggest that these vessels are a closed, not open, system.[10] They invade the hypertrophic cell columns by a breakdown of the transverse septae. This tissue is mineralized quickly to create bone matrix—the primary spongiosa. By remodeling, the initial bone (surrounding cartilage) is removed and replaced by a more mature secondary spongiosa that no longer contains remnants of the cartilaginous precursor.

The cytoplasmic components of the physeal chondrocytes change in the various zones. There is a progressive increase in the content of endoplasmic reticulum, mitochondria, lysosomes, and Golgi complexes from the zone of small-sized cartilage cells (germinal and resting cells) to the zone of hypertrophic cells. In contrast, the content of lipid bodies, vacuoles, and multivesicular bodies decreases progressively through these zones.[2,7,49] The zone of hypertrophy appears to contain cells that are metabolically very active.

The fate of the last cell in the cell column, the zone of provisional calcification, remains conjectural. Some studies have suggested that fragmentation of the cell membrane with the loss of all cytoplasmic components makes death the ultimate fate of the physeal chondrocyte.[7] Others have suggested that such cellular dissolution does not occur and that the hypertrophic chondrocytes ultimately become bone cells.[15,50]

The growth plate derives its blood supply from three regions—the epiphyseal circulation, the metaphyseal circulation, and the perichondrial circulation.[46,51] The epiphyseal circulation varies structurally with the growth of the ossification center. Vessels enter and are distributed to the chondroepiphysis within specialized structures termed cartilage canals. These canals course throughout the epiphysis and send branches to the resting cell region of the growth plate. Occasionally, these vessels may also communicate across the physis, anastomosing with the metaphyseal circulation. These transphyseal vessels may be found in the larger epiphyses, are usually more frequent at the periphery than central regions, and become less and less frequent as the secondary ossification center enlarges. By the time the subchondral plate is formed, transphyseal vessels are no longer evident. While they are present, they do give a potential route for the spread of infection from the metaphysis into the epiphysis, especially peripherally.

The cartilage canals contain a central artery and veins and a complex capillary network that surrounds the central vessels, but stays within the confines of the canal, and forms a "glomerular" tuft as the endarterial terminus of each canal system.[35,98] These canals have several important characteristics. First, and most important, they supply discrete regions within the epiphysis, with virtually no intraepiphyseal anastomoses between canalicular systems of adjacent regions (although anastomoses are relatively common in the perichondrial region). Second, the canals enter the epiphysis at fairly regular intervals along the growth plate periphery, but much

more irregularly in other regions of the epiphysis. Third, the canals probably serve as a source of chondroblastic cells for continued interstitial enlargement of the chondroepiphysis. Fourth, the canals are surrounded by a more dense area of hypertrophic cartilage and increased intercellular matrix that may render an internal structural support system to the chondroepiphysis. Fifth, the canals appear to play a primary role in the development of the secondary ossification center.

Once the ossification center begins to form and enlarge, the epiphyseal circulatory pattern changes. Several cartilage canal systems contribute to the enlarging ossification center, thus creating significant anastomoses between canal systems that were previously endarterial. When the subchondral plate forms, small vessels cross the plate and form vascular expansions that supply relatively discrete regions of the physis. The proximity of cells and vessels suggests that some of the resting zone cells may originate from undifferentiated perivascular tissue. These epiphyseal vessels never penetrate between the cell columns, so that the central zones of the growth plate are avascular. This creates a gradient of oxygen tension that undoubtedly plays a role in cellular differentiation. There are no anastomoses between these small arteries after they cross the subchondral plate. They are effectively endarterial to the particular segment of the physis that they supply.

The metaphyseal circulation is derived from two sources—the nutrient artery, which supplies the more central regions, and the perichondrial arteries, which supply the peripheral regions. The terminal portions of both systems form a series of loops that penetrate between the trabeculae to reach the lower limbs of the zone of hypertrophy. The venular side of the loop enlarges to form a sinusoid (several adjacent venules may contribute to each sinusoid). The rheology imposed by the capillary loop and the sinusoid apparently renders this area particularly susceptible to bacterial localization and subsequent osteomyelitis.

The perichondrial circulation is the vascular network coursing around each epiphysis, although with considerable anatomical variation.

Such variation is most pronounced in the limited vascular supply to the capital femoral epiphysis. This system is usually derived from major arterial and venous channels that are separate from those supplying the nutrient vessels. The smaller vessels derived from this circulatory system supply the epiphysis and selected areas of the metaphysis. However, the most important derivation appears to be the system of small vessels within the zone of Ranvier. The functional integrity of these vessels in the zone is essential to continued appositional growth at the periphery of the epiphyseal growth plate. The vessels in the zone of Ranvier may permit communication between the epiphysis and metaphysis, allowing the spread of a metaphyseal focus of osteomyelitis into the epiphysis in the older child.

Patterns of growth

Characteristically, the growth of long bones is considered as longitudinal phenomenon.[87] However, the physes may expand in other significant ways. The discoid physis must also expand in a diametric or latitudinal direction.[47,76,78] This occurs by cell division and matrix expansion within the physis (interstitial growth), but more importantly by cellular addition from the periphery at the zone of Ranvier (appositional growth).[56] These processes are depicted in Figure 5-32. The capacity for interstitial growth in the discoid growth plate appears directly related to epiphyseal ossification center enlargement. When there is a chondroepiphysis or a small, spherical ossification center, the pliable hyaline cartilage of the epiphysis does not present a significant mechanical barrier to interstitial expansion of the juxtaposed growth plate. In fact, both regions appear to undergo integrated interstitial expansion. However, with increasing development of the epiphyseal ossification center, a discrete subchondral plate forms, to which juxtaposed portions of the discoid physis, by virtue of vascular requirements, become "attached." Further interstitial (latitudinal) expansion of the physis is effectively precluded in those areas ap-

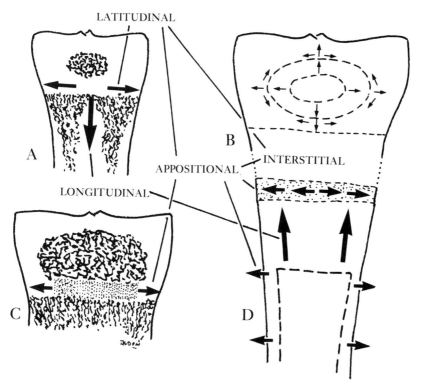

FIGURE 5-32 *Schematic of different patterns of growth from the epiphyseal-physeal end of a long bone.*

posed to the subchondral plate. When a secondary ossification center has attained the diametric size of the metaphysis, latitudinal expansion is possible only at the periphery through the zone of Ranvier. The spherical growth plate expands because of rapid interstitial expansion, but it also undergoes radially directed "longitudinal" growth that corresponds to the metaphyseal ossification process. Interstitial expansion of the spherical physis occurs virtually throughout the existence of the ossification center.

Metaphyseal-diaphyseal modeling

The initial cartilaginous portion of the endochondral skeleton is relatively pliable and can be deformed if stresses are applied normally, excessively, or pathologically. If the epiphyseal cartilage is deformed, the secondary ossification center will develop but not in a normal fashion, following instead the deformed cartilage contours that basically direct the capacity to ossify. Similarly, if the physeal contour is altered, the subsequent primary spongiosa pattern will be altered. In contrast, formed bone is a harder, relatively rigid material. Once formation of mature lamellar bone occurs in the postnatal state, it is very difficult for any changes in mass or shape to come about solely by interstitial expansion. Instead, metaphyseal and diaphyseal appositional growth must account for the bulk of new bone formation as the bone increases diametrically in overall size. Basically, the only normal mechanisms by which formed bone, particularly diaphyseal bone, can increase in size include (1) surface apposition of new bone and (2) surface resorption of old bone. During growth, continual changes are necessary to maintain the normal shape of the bone. There is a prevailing concept that the trailing edge of the metaphysis progressively decreases in diameter to that of the diaphysis (cutback zone). This is a misconception. Although occurring to some extent, the overall size of the metaphysis is a reflection of the eventual size that the diaphysis will eventually attain by subperiosteal new bone deposition (membranous) as the bone grows and matures in both a longitudinal and latitudinal manner (Fig. 5-33). Many of the early schematics, such as

those shown by Enlow,[21] have placed an accentuated flair to the metaphysis that does not realistically depict latitudinal growth of either metaphysis or diaphysis. In particular, if one looks at mammals that do not remodel (e.g., *Cetaceans*), it becomes very obvious that extensive amounts of periosteal new bone or membranous bone fill in the gaps created by the progressive growth of the endochondral cones (Fig. 5-34). In a terrestrial mammal with extensive remodeling at the periosteal and endosteal surfaces, as well as formation of a marrow cavity, the resultant effect leaves a multitude of architectural patterns in different parts of the diaphyseal cortex. These areas are further altered, in turn, by internal remodeling through the mechanism of Haversian system formation.

The apparent progressive decrease in metaphyseal diameter is accomplished by periosteal resorption and deposition, together with endosteal deposition. These processes cease once the diaphyseal diameter of skeletal maturity is reached. Since the diaphysis itself slowly increases in diameter as the bone grows in length, the separate and relatively independent process of periosteal new bone formation is found along the diaphysis. This periosteal bone typically contains longitudinal lamellae with numerous primary, longitudinal, nonhaversian canals. The different layers of bone deposited before and after growth reversal are usually separated by prominent reversal tidemarks.

At the same time that the diaphysis is changing in size and thickness, the cross-sectional shape of the bone is changing at each successive level, and the cortex is slowly shifting to allow for the normal curvature that is present along the longitudinal axis of the shaft. These changes are accomplished by deposition of bone on one side and resorption on the other, a process termed drift. Since the bone appears to have shifted its contours, osseous drift may be recognized on a cross-section of diaphyseal bone by asymmetry of the various layers, with an excess of periosteal bone on one side and endosteal on the other (Fig. 5-35).

The elaboration of metaphyseal woven bone and its eventual remodeling may be relatively less dependent on the normal control mecha-

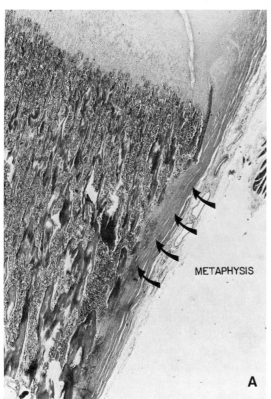

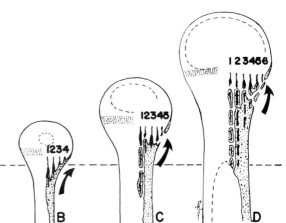

FIGURE 5-33 *Histologic section* **(A)** *and schematics* **(B–D)** *of the development of the metaphysis. As the peripheral endochondral cell column and bone formation proceeds diametrically (latitudinally) a "flare" of fenestrated cortical bone is produced (solid arrows) that must be incorporated into the more mature and more solid diaphyseal bone, which is primarily membranous (periosteal derivation).* This requires extensive remodeling.

nisms, including mechanical and endocrine stimuli, although it does respond to local factors such as increased or decreased blood flow, pH, and temperature. The lack of uniform orientation of collagen in woven bone may be a reflection of this altered responsiveness. The apparent changes in woven bone, such as the formation of Harris growth lines (Fig. 5-36), reflect a slowdown of the normal process of endochondral bone formation, probably by a slowing down of the rate of cartilage turnover rather than being an actual reflection of change in the newly formed primary spongiosa. Thus, bone that characteristically forms longitudinal trabeculae in the primary spongiosa when the rate of transformation is slowed down is oriented in a more latitudinal fashion. This again reinforces the concept that the elaboration of woven bone is primarily a reflection of rates of growth, rather than a response to chemical stimulation. As such it also is not as biomechanically protected an area; it is subjected to failure (fracture) through epiphyseal and metaphyseal regions. Such fractures occur quite frequently in the growing child.

The chondro-osseous skeleton is maintained by active cellular function produced by continuous internal change at microscopic as well as macroscopic levels. In order to carry out the two main skeletal functions, that of remodeling or maintenance (skeletal homeostasis) and that of mineral homeostasis, the osteocytes, which constitute over 95% of the total cells in bone, must have a dual role.[53] It is often difficult to distinguish one role from another, in fact, the two are reasonably integrated. Only by studying both as separate as well as integrated functions can we gain reasonable insight into the internal dynamics and structural changes of bone tissue. Within their natural environment, cells in different locations exhibit different levels of activities, so the overall effect on bone depends on the combined changes. Therefore, a change in the rate of cellular activity may or may not have an effect on

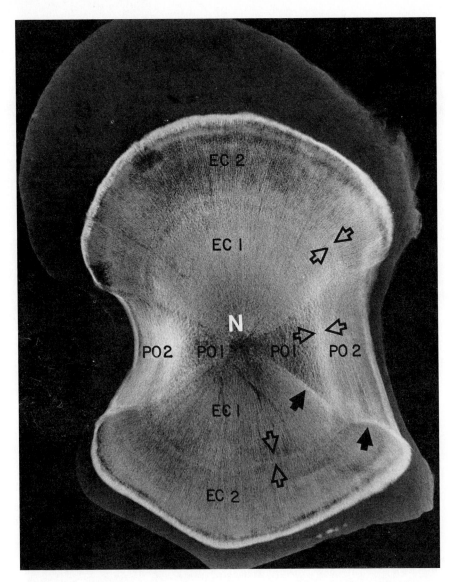

FIGURE 5-34 *Slab section roentgenogram of a young humpback whale (10-cm line drawn at top). This animal does not form a marrow cavity or significantly remodel the two types of bone, so that demarcation is readily evident. Later during growth, the margins will remodel sufficiently so that they are not sharply discernible. The bone "ghost" probably represents the size of the bone (metaphysis and diaphysis) at birth, whereas the additional bone is the growth occurring postnatally until the animal's death, probably during the first year of life.* **EC 1** = *endochondral bone formed fetally;* **EC 2** = *endochondral bone formed postnatally.* **PO 1** = *periosteal (membranous) bone formed fetally;* **PO 2** = *periosteal bone formed postnatally. Note how the bone in the endochondral cones radiates from the nutrient artery* **(N),** *the initial site of primary ossification, toward the physes. The solid arrows depict demarcation between the endochondral cone and the contiguous periosteal bone. The open arrows depict the margins of endochondral and periosteal bone formed at full gestation.*

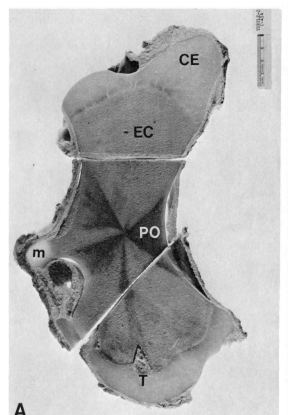

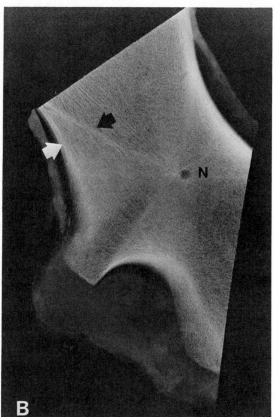

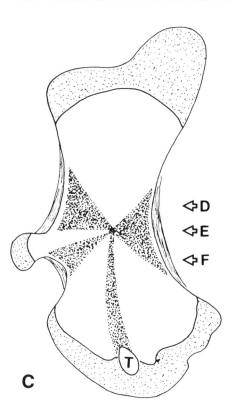

FIGURE 5-35 *Sections of the humerus in the leatherback turtle, an unusual, possibly endothermic reptile with many chondro-osseous characteristics that resemble marine mammals, rather than other ectothermic marine turtles.* **(A)** *Sagittal section, showing proximal and distal chondroepiphyses* **(CE)**, *endochondral cones* **(EC)**, *and deeply pigmented periosteal bone* **(PO)**. *Because of the presence of the medial epicondyle* **(M)** *and intraosseous tendon* **(T)**, *areas of bone formation are subdivided.* **(B)** *Radiograph of the middle section shown in* **A**. *The central nutrient artery, the site of initial ossification, is readily evident* **(N)**. *The various regions of endochondral and membranous bone may be demarcated, although there is a certain amount of blending. The arrows show a distinct laminar pattern in some of the bone derived from the periosteum. This may represent annual growth increments.* **(C)** *Schematic showing two types of bone and orienting the transverse sections,* **D–F**, *which also show variable contributions of endochondral and periosteal bone to diametric growth.*

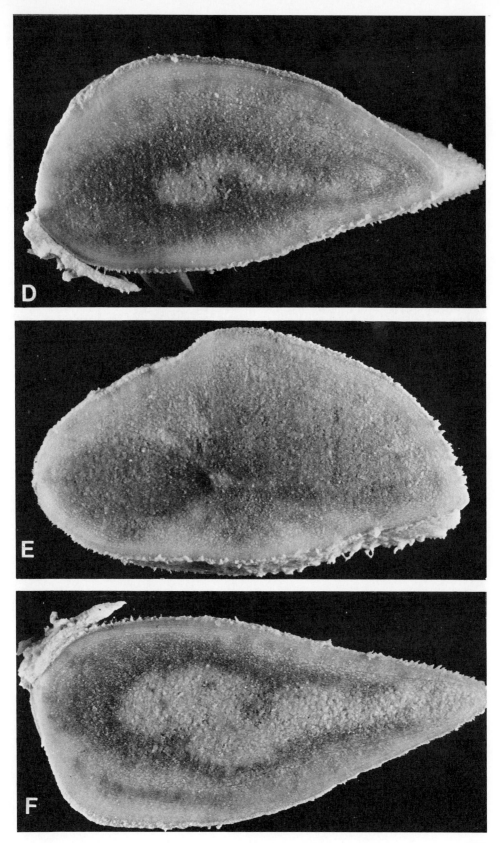

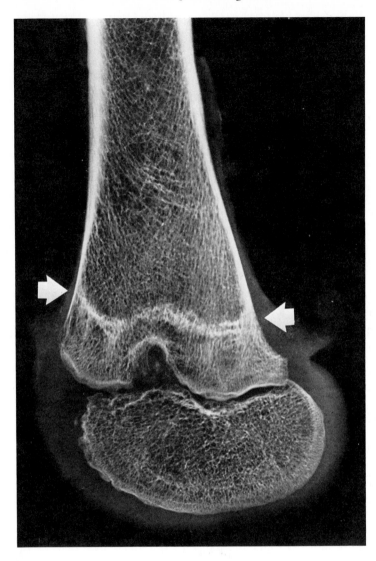

FIGURE 5-36 *Harris growth line (arrows). This occurs when a systemic disease, or sometimes even a major fracture, alters the skeletal growth dynamics sufficiently so that the primary spongiosa is oriented in a transverse, rather than a longitudinal, pattern. A similar line is forming at the physeal-metaphyseal interface.*

bone structure or on the quantity of bone present. Several functions have to be identified, but the two that are most important during growth and maturation of the child's skeleton are modeling and remodeling.

Modeling, in contrast to growth, with which it is commonly confused, refers to architectural modifications within the growing skeleton. This activity continually reshapes each bone throughout the growth period. It also terminates at maturity, although it can be reactivated locally in pathologic conditions. The slow enlargement in the diameter of long bones throughout life might also be considered a form of modeling.

Remodeling maintains and rearranges lamellar bone, once it is developed by modeling. Such maintenance-oriented activity during childhood differs from modeling. Remodeling has minimal effect on the size and ultimate shape of the bone. The rigidity of bone creates special circumstances not found in most other tissues. Cortical bone cannot grow by interstitial expansion, but only by new bone deposition on the surfaces. Therefore, in densely compact bone the remodeling process must begin with bone resorption in order to produce surfaces for the apposition of new bone. Remodeling occurs in packets of cellular activity termed basic multicellular units

(BMU). The sequence of resorption-formation appear valid for cortical bone remodeling, as well as for trabecular bone. In trabecular bone the cycle may be completed on an unrestricted bone surface, whereas in cortical bone the space slowly decreases in size to that of a relatively tiny canal.

Structurally, the skeleton is maintained through the activity of BMU (remodeling) located both on free bone surfaces and along the vascular channels. Although these are reasonably active in adults, they are extremely active in children in whom the skeleton is undergoing very dynamic processes of reorientation of weightbearing stress units. Remodeling events on all surfaces appear to have a common pattern, with similar life cycles in both trabecular and Haversian bone. The Haversian systems found in cortical bone represent the end result of previously active remodeling units. In long bones, these systems run parallel to the longitudinal axis of the bone and appear round or oval on transverse section. Their architecture and cellular relationships are best studied in longitudinal sections in which the cylinder will be seen to have a blunt end that contains osteoclasts (the cutting cone). A short distance along the canal, active new bone formation is apparent over a length about seven times greater than the length of the actual cutting cone.

The osteocytes within bone, together with the osteocytes lining external and internal surfaces and resting osteoblasts, form a continuous syncytium of cells lining all surfaces, including the larger trabecular spaces as well as lacunae and tiny canaliculae. The cellular continuum is organized into distinct functional subunits that do not always communicate directly with each other. For instance, metabolic interchange apparently does not take place across the cement lines that border subunits. Therefore, the cells in each subunit may respond independently from neighboring units. Each of these packets of cells may be termed a bone metabolic unit, which represents an organizational unit of metabolic activity that remains after a remodeling unit has completed its task. Rasmussen and Bordier[79] have suggested that the term bone remodeling unit be used during the remodeling phase and

BMU be used once remodeling has been completed (i.e., in the mature skeleton).

The concept that bone remodeling is carried out by packets of cellular activity indicates that bone formation is coupled to bone resorption, so that an increase or decrease of one causes a similar change in the other. Rarely does one increase while the other decreases. The abnormalities of remodeling activity found in disease states may be due to changes in the number of active BMUs, changes in the time needed to complete the remodeling cycle or component parts of it, or relative changes between the three functional envelopes (endosteal, periosteal, and intracortical).

Within the past decade, evidence for several distinct cellular-based systems has made it apparent that various parts of the skeleton within a given bone respond differently to systemic regulation, to pharmacologic agents and to disease processes. Three basic kinds of bone surfaces may be seen if a cross-section of a diaphysis is examined—periosteal, endosteal, and lamellar (Haversian). In the metaphysis, the three systems are periosteal, endosteal, and woven. These have been termed the triple envelope systems. Such a classification would be of little value if all areas showed the same response to a given stimulus, as one might expect since the cells appear identical histologically and histochemically. Each surface, however, appears to exhibit behavior that, to some extent, is independent from the others.

The cells in these three regions form a complex group of subsystems in which the behavior of the osteoblasts and osteoclasts in one area is distinctive from that in the others. Each envelope shows a typical pattern of changing with age, particularly during the early stages of skeletal maturation, until physiologic epiphyseodesis is reached: The periosteal envelope increases in size throughout the period of growth, but becomes progressively less active as skeletal maturation is reached. The haversian envelope includes intracortical spaces and shows diffuse changes at all ages before and after skeletal maturity and can be considered to be relatively constant in size. The endosteal envelope includes the endosteal wall of the diaphyseal cortex, which progressively loses bone throughout most of adult life, resulting in slow enlargement of the medullary canal.

Initiation of the remodeling cycle begins with activation of precursor (osteoprogenitor) cells in a localized area in bone. The stimulus produces mitotic division in the precursor cells, producing osteoclasts that gradually resorb bone. After resorption subsides, the reversal phase begins. New osteoblasts appear and lay down similar amounts of bone as previously resorbed. Once the cycle has been completed, cellular activity returns to its resting state, leaving the remaining osteoblasts as inactive lining cells or surface osteocytes.

Morphologically, the new bone made by a remodeling unit may be differentiated from adjacent bone by a cement or reversal line that remains as permanent evidence of previous activity. The cement line forms the outer limit of bone resorption just prior to new bone deposition and indicates the extent of resorption. Owing to the method of bone formation, the new unit of bone is, to some extent, an independent entity, since it does not communicate with adjacent bone across cement lines.

Bone resorption must precede new bone formation, and this is a function carried out by osteoclasts, although the possibility remains that surface osteocytes also may be able to resorb bone. In cortical bone, resorption cavity results from the tunneling action of a cutting cone

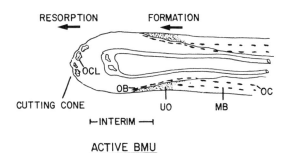

ACTIVE BMU

FIGURE 5-37 *Characteristic modeling-remodeling within haversian bone. The active bone modeling–metabolism unit* **(BMU)** *comprises three regions: an area of resorption with the cutting cone and osteoclasts* **(OCL)***; an interim phase with modulation of perivascular mesenchymal tissue (osteoprogenitor cells); and an area of formation, with osteoblasts* **(OB)** *initially forming unmineralized osteoid* **(UO)** *that subsequently forms mineralized bone* **(MB)***, incorporating osteocytes* **(OC)** *within interconnected lacunae.*

travelling along the vascular canal in line with but slightly oblique to the long axis of the bone. This sequence of events may be recognized most clearly in longitudinal sections. The cutting cone is a broad, cone-shaped osteoclastic front that leaves an elongated resorption cavity (Fig. 5-37). Although the resorption cavity progresses in a longitudinal direction, the individual osteoclasts resorb bone in a radial direction. The osteoclasts move from the central canal, peripherally covering the distance equal to the radius of the resorption cavity. The irregular cavities remaining after initial osteoclastic resorption are called Howship's lacunae. The cutting cone is followed by a zone of scattered osteoclasts that plane down the edges of Howship's lacunae, slightly increasing the diameter of the cavity. This cutting cone has little respect for cement lines, resting lines, or edge of bone.

A short distance behind the cutting cone, numerous osteoblasts may be seen producing new bone that progressively fills the cavity formed by osteoclastic activity. The new bone forms the shape of a cone (the filling cone) resulting from progressive narrowing of the central canal as the wave of cellular activity advances longitudinally through the bone. A longer period of time is needed to refill or close the resorption cavity than to form it initially. Bone formation, therefore, follows bone resorption, and the distance between the osteoclasts and osteoclasts represents the latent or reversal period between the two processes. Since there is a delay in the deposition of collagen and matrix until it is calcified, which may last 8 to 10 d, areas of active bone formation always contain a layer of unmineralized osteoid called the osteoid seam. This lag between matrix formation and mineralization has caused some disagreement over the definition of bone formation. Some define bone formation as matrix production, which is a cellular process, whereas others feel that mineralization, which is an extracellular process, represents a secondary event that usually, but not necessarily, follows.

Biomechanics

Studies of trabecular bone, particularly single trabeculae, indicate that the material properties of trabecular bone approximate those for cortical bone. Yet when considered as a tissue, the difference in relative porosity between trabecular bone, as in the vertebral body, and cortical bone, as in a tibia, produces a striking difference in the overall organ mechanical properties. The modulus of elasticity and the ultimate strength are roughly one order of magnitude greater in cortical as compared with trabecular bone.

This greater flexibility of trabecular bone allows it to dampen sudden stresses more effectively, a quality that might explain its pattern of distribution throughout the developing skeleton. The transition from trabecular bone in the metaphysis and epiphysis to cortical bone in the diaphysis provides an effective mechanism for load transmission through the joints. Through a progressively thickening cortex and a decreasing trabecular density, the forces are more uniformly distributed from all parts of the subchondral plate to the cortex.

The effects of force on growth cartilage and epiphyseal cartilage are incompletely understood. Physiologic stress appears necessary for the continued, orderly development of both discoid and spherical growth plates. These stresses may be either compression or tension, or a combination of both. It is important to realize that there is a biologic range of compression-tension responses for each growth plate and that each growth plate is not only responsive to one type of stress or the other. Within this physiologic range, increasing tension or compression accelerates growth, whereas decreasing tension or compression decelerates growth. Beyond the physiologic limits of either, growth may be significantly decreased or even stopped. These principles often are referred to as the Heuter-Volkmann law of cartilage growth, although they were originally proposed many years before by Delpech.[56] The rate of response to cause longitudinal growth is probably greater for compression than tension. Each growth plate, although being primarily responsive to compression or tension, may have regions within it that respond to the opposite force.

Besides the effects of mechanical forces on the growth plates, there is an anatomical restraint in the periosteum. The periosteum attaches directly and firmly into the zone of Ranvier at each end, but is only loosely attached to the diaphysis and metaphyses. Experimental circumferential resection of a portion of the periosteum will cause accelerated longitudinal growth. This phenomenon is well recognized in children's fractures. The elevation of the periosteum in osteomyelitis effectively lengthens it and lessens intrinsic tension, thus allowing a temporary increase in the growth rate, although the increased vascularity exerts a conjoint effect. Thus, the stimulus to growth caused by weightbearing compression forces is tempered by the intrinsic compression imposed by the periosteum.

The discoid growth plate is never completely planar, but rather is variably convoluted. This convolution may be caused in part because each physis tends to align its various regions perpendicularly to the absorbed forces in each region. This minimizes shear stresses within the physis. However, genetic factors may also play a role.

Chondro-osseous tissues are subjected to only four types of external forces: compression, tension, shear, and torsion, or to any combination of these. The organization of skeletal tissue and the overall organ structure of any given bone reflects the adaptation to the dynamic conditions normally produced by such constant external loading.

A relatively consistent relationship seems to exist between muscle mass and bone mass, with each adapting to changes in the other. This is further accentuated in the developing human in that the periosteal sleeve, which seems to exhibit a certain intrinsic control mechanism on rates of longitudinal growth, serves as the attachment of the developing muscle mass.[99] Therefore, the well-known influence of muscle strength and physical activity on bone development is merited in part by the integrated influence between bone and muscle, with the balance between the two constantly adjusted in response to some unknown control mechanism. During growth, skeletal mass increases 20 times from the newborn to the adult, whereas muscle mass increases forty times, indicating that the mechanical efficiency of the skeleton probably doubles as bone matures. Mechanically, a greater proportion of muscle is needed as the limb grows, since the work required to move a limb is proportional to the fourth power of its length, whereas the work achieved by muscle is proportional to the cube of its length.

Adaptation is achieved by alteration in the gross and microscopic shape of bone, the inner structure, and the material distribution along its length and over its cross-section. Although bone is not a homogenous material, an intact bone appears to be a body of uniform homogenous strength having an optimum construction. The laws that govern the adaptation of bone to mechanical stress, though poorly understood, are commonly known as Wolff's law, which states that a bone bent by a mechanical load adapts by depositing new bone in the concave side and resorbing the bone on the convex side. In a similar fashion the Heuter-Volkmann law describes responsiveness of cartilage to applied loads.

Haversian systems represent the primary mechanism by which cortical bone maintains its efficiency in resisting stress. A number of observations indicate that biologic stress triggers the development of Haversian systems. First, they develop secondarily, not as part of the primary bone formed during growth. Second, their number increases with increasing age. Third, within the bone they have a higher concentration in areas of greater stress. Fourth, in the absence of muscle pull as in poliomyelitis, myelomeningocele, and osteogenesis imperfecta, osteonal remodeling is delayed or absent.[53] For example, the mature femur that is subjected to weightbearing but never to muscle pull as a result of severe poliomyelitis has few or no secondary osteons.

Physiologic control mechanisms

Growth within the physis and its eventual closure are regulated by various hormones. Thyroxine is extremely important in early physeal and epiphyseal development. Lack of this hormone causes (1) loss of integrity of the articular cartilage, (2) extensive erosion of the hyaline chondroepiphysis by bone and fibrous tissue, (3) extensive vascularization of the chondroepiphysis (there may be twice as many cartilage canal systems, without the normal canal demarcation), (4) abnormal distribution of the matriceal acid mucopolysaccharides (glycosam-

inoglycans), and (5) decreased physeal width, affecting the zone of hypertrophy most extensively. Thyroid (or lack of same) appears to have little direct effect on ossification. The most severe form of hypothyroidism is cretinism, in which overall skeletal development is retarded, and pseudoepiphyses may develop. The effect of thyroxine on skeletal growth appears to be synergistic with growth hormone. Growth hormone affects the cells of the resting germinal zones to induce cell division and widen the physis. The mode of action is not completely understood, but probably occurs through a second hormone called sulfation factor. Sex hormones also affect physeal growth. Testosterone initially stimulates the physis to undergo rapid cell division and widening during the growth spurt (anabolic effect), but eventually manifests an androgenic effect that slows down growth and leads to consolidation of the cartilage. Estrogens suppress growth plate activity by two mechanisms: (1) an apparent indirect effect through suppression of sulfation factor (by peripheral antagonism), and (2) a direct effect to increase calcification of the matrix, which is a prerequisite to physeal closure.

Physiologic growth cessation

Once physeal growth has stopped, these structures disappear concomitantly with fusion of the secondary ossification center to the metaphysis. This process begins earlier in the female than in the male and, like the appearance of primary and secondary ossification centers, follows a reasonably predictable sequence from bone to bone.[33,63] The earlier closure in the female appears to be due to the estrogenic compounds that accelerate cartilage growth and matrix elaboration. Though the time of onset and completion of fusion is influenced significantly by the sex hormones, the chronological relationship among individual bones is similar for both sexes.

Physiologic epiphyseodesis (epiphyseal union) characterizes the growth maturation of the physis. This process begins with the formation of an ossified region (bridge) between the epiphyseal ossification center and the metaphysis and ends with the complete disappearance of the cartilaginous physis and its replacement by trabecular bone. Most concepts of closure are based upon radiographic studies, since histologic data is sparse. In fact, much of the hitherto available information has been based upon histologic descriptions of "lapsed union" in rats, in which the larger physes may remain cartilaginous and capable of further growth throughout adult life.[16,17]

Histologically, several important changes occur. The juxtaepiphyseal subchondral bone plate of the epiphysis thickens and may have areas of neocartilage formation.[38] A similar bony thickening occurs in the juxtaepiphyseal metaphysis, in such a way that parallel bone plates begin to form on either side of the physis (Fig. 5-38). However, this process may differ among bones, with the formation of the metaphyseal plate being more variable. The basic cellular arrangement of the physis does not change significantly while these plates are being formed. However, there are extracellular changes, with calcification and mineralization extending into the germinal and resting zones to form multiple tide lines. Similar multiple tide lines develop concomitantly along the cell columns, indicating progressive calcification and mineralization from the metaphyseal side also. This latter process leads to rapid replacement of the cell columns by the metaphyseal bone plate. The next step is perforation of the physis by extension of the bone plates behind the advancing margins of calcification. The coalescence of the epiphyseal and metaphyseal plates results in the formation of transversely oriented trabeculae that are evident both radiologically and histologically long after "closure."[14] The pattern of perforation varies. It seems that the larger bones are characterized by multiple perforations and a residual plate. Small segments of the physis may still be evident peripherally and may account for the persistent lucency on radiographs. The smaller bones usually have a single perforation that may be either central or peripheral, but that gradually enlarges to envelop the entire physis. This closure pattern has less tendency to leave a residual bone plate.

In addition to the problem of the histologic characteristics of closure, there is a similar paucity of information regarding the time elapsing

between cessation of physeal function and actual fusion.[3] An attempt to assess this temporal course in the hand phalanges using serial roentgenography showed a mean value of 13 mo (a range of 8 to 18 mo) between cessation of longitudinal growth of the phalanx and radiologically complete closure.

Joints

As previously discussed, the blastemal appendicular skeleton is initially formed as a continuous structure, with no spaces or joints separating the major anlagen from each other.[36,73,74] However, as the mesenchymal model begins chondrification, concomitant changes occur in the region of the presumptive joint to create the interzone (Fig. 5-39). This structure has three layers—two parallel chondrogenic layers and an intermediate, less dense layer. The primitive joint capsule begins to differentiate at the same time. It is derived from the interface of the intermediate and deep mesoderm that give rise to the perichondrium and periosteum, thus establishing continuity of the joint capsule with the contributing chondro-osseous structures. The more peripheral regions of the interzone intermediate layer form synovial tissue. Blood vessels penetrate the evolving joint capsule to reach the blastemal synovium, but they do not penetrate the central joint regions. The intra-articular structures (e.g., menisci and cruciate ligaments) appear as further cellular condensations in the intermediate layer mesenchyme. The remaining undifferentiated cells of the intermediate layer become associated with the two chondrogenic layers. Once the basic articular contours and intra-articular structures are established, minute spaces begin to appear in the intermediate zone. These spaces coalesce to form the joint cavity. Cavitation is probably an enzymatic process. The chondrogenic layers establish the contours of the opposing joint surfaces, taking along cells of the intermediate layer that will form synovium in the recesses. Cavitation quickly follows into these areas so that the joint spaces are firmly established by 10 wk of gestation.

Because of coexistent development of inner-

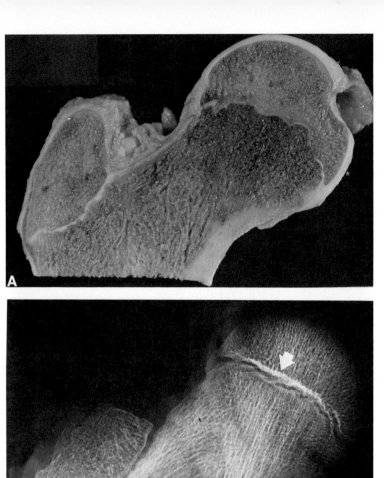

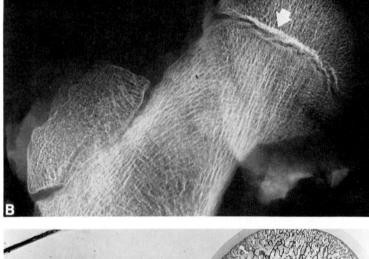

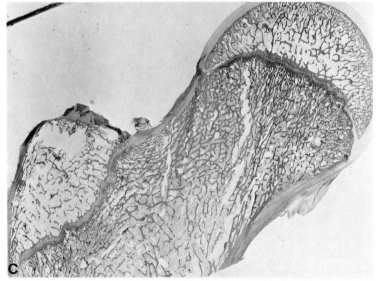

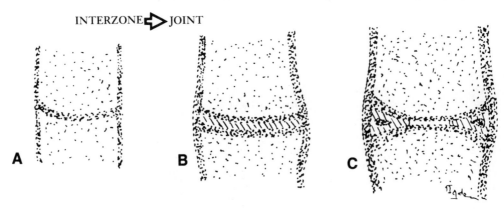

FIGURE 5-39 *Schematic of the formation of mesenchymal-cartilaginous interzone between skeletal anlagen, with subsequent cavitation to form the joint.*

vated muscle, some motion can begin early. This enhances joint remodeling to only a small degree *in utero.*[41] However, postnatally, joint motion and joint reaction forces are extremely consequential to the final adult joint contours.

Some diarthroidal (synovial) joints differ in the basic developmental patterns. Small joints in the hands and feet may show considerable delay between interzone formation and cavitation, sometimes proceeding to the primary ossification stage before a definitive joint is established. The distal interphalangeal joint and some carpal and tarsal joints may not go through the homogenous three-layer zone, instead forming a joint directly from the layer of dense cartilage between the developing bones. Synchondroses form in a fashion similar to that of diarthroidal joints, except that no intermediate zone develops (in the ribs), or the interzone becomes fibrocartilaginous (symphysis pubis).

Joints are relatively self-differentiating structures that can attain their basic form through factors presumably intrinsic to the interzone cells and possibly some inductive influence from juxtaposed skeletal blastema. If a joint primordium is removed from the limb bud and grown in culture, it has only a limited capacity for self-differentiation. That is, a joint-like structure will form, but will be morphologically limited in overall developmental potential. However, if a small amount of adjacent skeletal blastema is included in the explant, more complete differentiation does occur. When a presumptive joint region is excised from the mesenchymal skeleton, the remaining tissue can redistribute and re-form the interzone to create a normal joint. However, resection of the interzone after chondrification has commenced results in fusion of the juxtaposed anlagen and a complete lack of a joint (chondrification is equated with stabilization of independent self-differentiating capacity).

When the hyaline cartilage of the chondro-epiphysis first forms, there is no significant histochemical or histologic difference between the cells of the joint surface (derived from the chondrogenic layer of the interzone) and the remainder of the hyaline cartilage. However, at some point the articular cartilage also becomes stabilized and different from the epiphyseal cartilage. Although techniques are not yet available to detect any significant chemical differences, an interesting experiment has firmly established that these two cartilage types are different functionally (and, by implication, chemically). If a core of articular and underlying epiphyseal cartilage is removed, turned 180°, and reinserted, the transposed epiphyseal cartilage will form bone at the joint surface, but the articular cells

◄ FIGURE 5-38 *Physiologic epiphyseodesis.* **(A)** *The physis begins to thin.* **(B)** *A thickening of the subchondral plate occurs in the epiphyseal ossification center (arrow).* **(C)** *A similar thickening occurs in the juxtaposed metaphyseal bone. Tide lines form among the physeal cells. Finally, small bridges of bone begin to bridge the physis to coalesce these two areas of subchondral osseous proliferation.*

will remain cartilaginous and will be completely surrounded by the enlarging secondary ossification center.[57] This articular cartilage does not appear capable of calcification or ossification. As skeletal maturity is reached, a tidemark develops near the articular cartilage; this appears to be a boundary between these two cell regions.

The articular cartilage, like physeal cartilage, must be able to respond to joint reaction forces, both physiologic and pathologic. Pathologic increases in compression forces retard physeal growth. The reaction in articular cartilage differs. The compressed cells undergo histochemical modulation that dissolves the intercellular matrix and allows migration of cells away from the abnormal pressures, at which point they begin to re-form lacunae and matrix. However, migration of large numbers of cells yields lacunae containing multiple cells. The subchondral bone adjacent to these multicellular regions appears to increase, leading to osteophyte formation.

I would like to extend my sincere thanks to Drs. James Mead, Charles Potter, and Richard Thorington of the Smithsonian Institute for help in obtaining comparative skeletal material from immature animals, and to Gerald Conlogue, Gertrude Chaplin, Mary Bronson, Patti Milot, and Patricia Cosgrove for their help in producing this study.

This study has been partially funded by N.I.H. Grants ROI-HD-10854 and K04-AM-00300, the Easter Seal Research Foundation, and the Crippled Children's Aid Society.

References

1. Amprino, R.: Aspects of limb morphogenesis in the avian embryo. *In* Denhaan A., and Ursprung, H., editors: Organogensis, New York, Winston, 1965.
2. Anderson, C. E., and Parker, J.: Electron microscopy of the epiphyseal cartilage plate, Clin. Orthop. 58:225, 1968.
3. Bardeen, C.: Studies of the development of the human skeleton, Am. J. Anat. 4:265, 1905.
4. Bateman, N.: Bone growth: A study of the grey-lethal and microphthalmic mutants in the mouse, J. Anat. 88:212, 1954.
5. Becks, H., Asling, C., Simons, M., Evans, H., and Li, C.: Ossification at the distal end of the humerus in the female rat, Am. J. Anat. 82:203, 1948.
6. Belanger, L.: Osteocytic osteolysis, Calcif. Tissue Res. 4:1, 1969.
7. Bell, E., Kaighn, L., and Fessenden, L.: The role of the mesodermal and ectodermal components in the development of the chick limb, Dev. Biol. 1:101, 1959.
8. Berrill, N.: Morphogenetic fields, their growth and development, Dev. Biol. 7:342, 1963.
9. Brighton, C. T., Sugioka, Y., and Hunt, R. M.: Cytoplasmic structures of epiphyseal plate chondrocytes, J. Bone Joint Surg. 55A:771, 1973.
10. Brookes, M.: The Blood Supply of Bone: An Approach to Bone Biology, New York, Appleton-Century-Crofts, 1971.
11. Chamay, A., and Tschantz, P.: Mechanical influences in bone remodeling. Experimental research on Wolff's law, J. Biomech. 5:173, 1972.
12. Chen, J.: Studies on the morphogenesis of the mouse sternum, J. Anat. 86:387, 1952.
13. Cohen, J., and Harris, W. H.: The three-dimensional anatomy of Haversian systems, J. Bone Joint Surg. 40A:419, 1958.
14. Cope, Z.: Fusion-lines of bones, J. Anat. 55:36, 1920.
15. Crelin, E., and Koch, W.: An autoradiographic study of chondrocyte transformation into chondroclasts and osteocytes during bone formation in vitro, Anat. Rec. 158:473, 1967.
16. Dawson, A.: The age order of epiphyseal union in the long bones of the albino rat, Anat. Rec. 31:1, 1925.
17. Dawson, A.: A histological study of the persisting cartilage plates in retarded or lapsed epiphyseal union in the albino rat. Anat. Rec. 43:109, 1929.
18. Dodds, G.: Row formation and other types of arrangements of cartilage cells in endochondral ossification, Anat. Rec. 46:385, 1930.
19. Dodds, G.: Osteoclasts and cartilage removal in endochondral ossification of certain mammals, Am. J. Anat. 50:97, 1932.
20. Dodds, G., and Cameron, H.: Studies on experimental rickets in rats. I. Structural modifications of the epiphyseal cartilages in the tibia and other bones, Am. J. Anat. 55:135, 1934.
21. Enlow, D. H.: The Human Face, New York, Hoeber, 1968.
22. Fell, H.: The osteogenic capacity in vitro of periosteum and endosteum isolated from limb skeleton of fowl embryos and young chicks, J. Anat. 66:157, 1932.
23. Fell, H.: Skeletal development in tissue culture.

In Bourne, G., ed.: The Biochemistry and Physiology of Bone. New York, Academic Press, 1956.

24. Felts, W.: The prenatal development of the human femur, Am. J. Anat. 94:1, 1954.

25. Felts, W.: Transplantation studies of factors in skeletal organogenesis. I. The subcutaneously implanted immature longbone of the rat and mouse, Am. J. Phys. Anthropol. 17:201, 1959.

26. Frantz, C., and O'Rahilly, R.: Congenital skeletal limb deficiencies, J. Bone Joint Surg. 43A:1202, 1961.

27. Fraser, B. A., and Travill, A. A.: The relation of aberrant vasculogenesis to skeletal malformation in the hamster fetus, Anat. Embryol. 154:111, 1978.

28. Gardner, E.: The embryology of the clavicle, Clin. Orthop. 58:9, 1968.

29. Gardner, E., and Gray, D.: The prenatal development of the human femur, Am. J. Anat. 129:121, 1970.

30. Gardner, E.: Osteogenesis in the human embryo and fetus. *In* Bourne G., ed.: Biochemistry and Physiology of Bone, New York, Academic Press, 1970.

31. Gray, D., and Gardner, E.: Prenatal development in the human knee and superior tibiofibular joints, Am. J. Anat. 86:235, 1950.

32. Gray, D., Gardner, E., and O'Rahilly, R.: The prenatal development of the skeleton and joints of the human hand, Am. J. Anat. 101:169, 1957.

33. Greulich, W., and Pyle, S.: Radiographic Atlas of Skeletal Development of the Hand and Wrist, Stanford, University of California Press, 1959.

34. Gruneberg, H.: The Pathology of Development: A Study of Inherited Skeletal Disorders in Animals, New York, John Wiley & Sons, 1963.

35. Haines, R.: Cartilage canals, J. Anat. 68:45, 1933.

36. Haines, R.: The development of joints, J. Anat. 81:33, 1947.

37. Haines, R.: The pseudoepiphysis of the first metacarpal in man, J. Anat. 117:145, 1974.

38. Haines, R.: The histology of epiphyseal union in mammals, J. Anat. 120:1, 1975.

39. Hall, B.: Cellular differentiation in skeletal tissue, Biol. Rev. 45:455, 1970.

40. Hall, B. K.: Histogenesis and morphogenesis of bone, Clin. Orthop. 74:249, 1971.

41. Hall, B. K.: Immobilization and cartilage transformation into bone in the embryonic chick. Anat. Rec. 173:391, 1973.

42. Hall, B. K.: Evolutionary consequences of skeletal differentiation, Am. Zool. 15:329, 1975.

43. Hall, B. K.: Chondrogenesis of the somitic mesoderm, Adv. Anat. Embryol. Cell Biol. 53, Fasc. 4, 1977.

44. Hall, B. K.: Developmental and Cellular Skeletal Biology, New York, Academic Press, 1978.

45. Halstead, L. B.: Vertebrate Hard Tissues, New York, Springer-Verlag, 1974.

46. Harris, H.: The vascular supply of bone, with special reference to the epiphyseal cartilage, J. Anat. 64:3, 1929.

47. Hert, J.: Growth of the epiphyseal plate in circumference, Acta Anat. (Basel) 82:420, 1972.

48. Holtrop, M.: The origin of bone cells in endochondral ossification. *In* Third European Symposium on Calcified Tissues, New York, Springer-Verlag, 1966.

49. Holtrop, M. E.: The ultrastructure of the epiphyseal plate. I. The flattened chondrocyte, Calcif. Tissue Res. 9:131, 1972.

50. Holtrop, M. E.: The ultrastructure of the epiphyseal plate. II. The hypertrophic chondrocyte, Calcif. Tissue Res. 9:140, 1972.

51. Irving, M.: The blood supply of growth cartilage, J. Anat. 98:631, 1964.

52. Jaffe, H.: Metabolic Degenerative and Inflammatory Diseases of Bones and Joints, Philadelphia, Lee & Febiger, 1972.

53. Johnson, L.: The kinetics of skeletal remodeling. *In* Bergsma, D., ed.: Structural Organization of the Skeleton, Birth Defects Vol. II, No. 1, 1966.

54. Kember, N.: Patterns of cell division in the growth plates of the rat pelvis, J. Anat. 116:445, 1973.

55. Krook, L., Belanger, L., Henrikson, P., Lutwak, L., and Sheffy, B.: Bone flow, Rev. Can. Biol. 29:157, 1970.

56. Lacroix, P.: The Organization of Bones, Philadelphia, Blakiston, 1951.

57. McKibbin, B., and Holdsworth, F.: The dual nature of epiphyseal cartilage, J. Bone Joint Surg. 49B:351, 1967.

58. Medoff, J.: Enzymatic events during cartilage differentiation in the chick embryonic limb bud, Dev. Biol. 16:118, 1967.

59. Meikle, M. C.: The influence of function on chondrogenesis at the epiphyseal cartilage of a growing long bone, Anat. Rec. 182:387, 1975.

60. Milaire, J.: Histochemical aspects of limb mor-

phogenesis in vertebrates, Adv. Morphogenet. 2:183, 1962.

61. Milaire, J.: Etude morphologique et cyto-chemique du developement des membres chez la souris et chez le taupe, Arch. Biol. (Leige) 74:129, 1963.

62. Mitolo, V.: A model approach to some problems of limb morphogenesis, Acta Embryol. Exp. (Palermo) 3:323, 1973.

63. Moss, M., and Noback, C.: A longitudinal study of digital epiphyseal fusion in adolescence, Anat. Rec. 131:19, 1958.

64. Murray, P., and Huxley, J.: Self-differentiation in the grafted limb-bud of the chick, J. Anat. 59:379, 1925.

65. Newman, S. A., and Frisch, H. L.: Dynamics of skeletal pattern formation in developing chick limb, Science 205:662, 1979.

66. Noback, C.: The developmental anatomy of the human osseous skeleton during the embryonic, fetal and circumnatal periods, Anat. Rec. 88:91, 1944.

67. Ogden, J. A.: Changing patterns of proximal femoral vascularity, J. Bone Joint Surg. 56A:941, 1974.

68. Ogden, J. A., Hempton, R., and Southwick, W. O.: Development of the tibial tuberosity, Anat. Rec. 182:431, 1975.

69. Ogden, J. A.: Development of the epiphysis. *In* Ferguson, A. B., Jr., ed.: Orthopaedic Surgery in Infancy and Childhood, Baltimore, Williams & Wilkins Co., 1975.

70. Ogden, J. A.: Development and growth of the musculoskeletal system. *In* Albright, J. A., and Brand, R., eds.: Scientific Basis of Orthopaedics, New York, Appleton-Century-Crofts, 1979.

71. O'Rahilly, R.: Morphological patterns in limb deficiencies and duplications, Am. J. Anat. 89:135, 1951.

72. O'Rahilly, R., and Gardner, E.: The initial appearance of ossification in staged human embryos, Am. J. Anat. 134:291, 1972.

73. O'Rahilly, R., and Gardner, E.: The embryology of bone and bones. *In* Bones and Joints: IAP Monograph No. 17, Baltimore, Williams & Wilkins Co., 1976.

74. O'Rahilly, R., and Gardner, E.: The embryology of movable joints. *In* The Joints and Synovial Fluid, Vol. 10, New York, Academic Press, 1978.

75. O'Rahilly, R., Gardner, E., and Gray, D.: The ectodermal thickening and ridge in the limbs of

staged human embryos, J. Embryol. Exp. Morphol. 4:254, 1956.

76. Pratt, C.: The significance of the "perichondral zone" in a developing long bone of the rat, J. Anat. 93:110, 1959.

77. Pritchard, J.; A cytological and histochemical study of bone and cartilage formation in the rat, J. Anat. 86:259, 1952.

78. Rang, M.: The Growth Plate and Its Disorders, Baltimore, Williams & Wilkins Co., 1969.

79. Rasmussen, H., and Bordier, P.: The Physiological and Cellular Basis of Metabolic Bone Disease, Baltimore, Williams & Wilkins Co., 1974.

80. Saunders, J.: The proximo-distal sequence of origin of the parts of chick wing and the role of the ectoderm, J. Exp. Zool. 108:363, 1948.

81. Saunders, J., Cairns, J., and Gasseling, M.: The role of the apical ridge of ectoderm in the differentiation of the morphological structure and inductive specificity of limb parts in the chick, J. Morphol. 101:57, 1957.

82. Saunders, J., Gasseling, M., and Saunders, L.: Cellular death in the morphogenesis of the avian wing, Dev. Biol. 5:147, 1962.

83. Scammon, R., and Calkins, L.: The Development and Growth of the External Dimensions of the Human Body in the Fetal Period, Minneapolis, University of Minnesota Press, 1929.

84. Searls, R.: The role of cell migration in the development of the embryonic chick limb bud, J. Exp. Zool. 166:39, 1967.

85. Searls, R., and Janners, M.: The stabilization of cartilage properties in the cartilage forming mesenchyme of the embryonic chick limb, J. Exp. Zool. 170:365, 1969.

86. Sensenig, E.: The early development of the human vertebral column, Contrib. Embryol. 33:21, 1949.

87. Siegling, J.: Growth of the epiphyses, J. Bone Joint Surg. 23:23, 1941.

88. Sissons, H.: Experimental determination of rate of longitudinal bone growth, J. Anat. 87:228, 1953.

89. Sissons, H.: The growth of bone. *In* Bourne, G., ed.: The Biochemistry and Physiology of Bone, Vol. III, New York, Academic Press, 1971.

90. Streeter, G., Henser, C., and Corner, G.: Development horizons in human embryos, Contrib. Embryol. No. 230, Reprint II:166, 1951.

91. Swinyard, C.: Limb Development and Deformity: Problems of Evaluation and Rehabilitation, Springfield, Charles C. Thomas, 1969.

92. Symposia of The Society for Experimental Biology: Control Mechanisms of Growth and Differentiation, New York, Academic Press, 1971.

93. Taylor, J.: Growth of human intervertebral discs and vertebral bodies, J. Anat. 120:49, 1975.

94. Thompson, D. W.: On Growth and Form, Cambridge, University Press, 1942.

95. Tonna, E. A.: An electron microscopic study of osteocyte release during osteoclasis in mice of different ages, Clin. Orthop. 87:311, 1972.

96. Toole, B.: Extracellular events in limb development. *In* Bergsma, D., ed.: Skeletal Dysplasias, New York. Symposia Specialists, 1974.

97. Tschumi, P.: The growth of the hind limb bud of *Xenopus larvis* and its dependence upon the epidermis, J. Anat. 91:149, 1957.

98. Trueta, J.: Studies of the Development and Decay of the Human Frame, Philadelphia, W. B. Saunders Co., 1968.

99. Videman, T.: An experimental study of the effects of growth on the relationship of tendons and ligaments to bone at the site of diaphyseal insertion, Academic dissertation. University of Helsinki, 1970.

100. Von der Mark, K., and Von der Mark, H.: The role of three genetically distinct collagen types in endochondral ossification calcification of cartilage, J. Bone Joint Surg. 59B:458, 1977.

101. Wake, D. B., and Lawson, R.: Developmental and adult morphology of the vertebral column in the plethodontid Salamander *Eurycea bislineata*, with comments on vertebral evolution in the amphibia, J. Morphol. 139:251, 1974.

102. Warkany, J.: Congenital Malformations, Chicago, Year Book Medical Pubs., 1971.

103. Whalen, J., Winchester, P., Krook, L., Dische, R., and Nunez, E.: Mechanisms of bone resorption in human metaphyseal remodeling, Am. J. Roentgenol. 112:526, 1971.

104. Williams, L.: The later development of the notochord in mammals, Am. J. Anat. 8:251, 1908.

105. Wyburn, G.: Observations on the development of the human vertebral column, J. Anat. 78:94, 1944.

106. Yasuda, Y.: Differentiation of human limb buds in vitro, Anat. Rec. 175:561, 1974.

107. Zwilling, E.: Limb morphogenesis, Adv. Morphol. 1:301, 1961.

108. Zwilling, E.: Morphogenetic phases in development, Dev. Biol. (Suppl.) 2:184, 1968.

The structural framework of the body is provided by bone and cartilage. Continuous repair and development of this framework requires the constant function of enzymatic sequences for tissue degradation and reconstruction. The same general biochemical systems that exist elsewhere in the body are also active in these tissues to provide the structural intermediates and energy for repair and growth; however, the specialized structural arrangement and tissue constituents require the function of additional specialized enzyme systems.

Bone contains calcium phosphate as hydroxyapatite crystal deposited upon the collagen fiber, whereas cartilage is formed by the attachment of large amounts of proteoglycan to collagen. Bone not only serves a structural function but also serves as a storehouse for the inorganic minerals of the body. The rate at which these minerals can be mobilized for other requirements depends upon the manner in which they are deposited. It is the inter-relationship between the hydroxyapatite crystals and the collagen fiber that determines the unique mechanical property of bone. Details of the relationship between collagen and mineral are not completely understood, but the structural organization of the collagen fiber appears to act as a nucleation site for the deposition of hydroxyapatite crystal.

In contrast, cartilage is composed of collagen fibers upon which large quantities of polyglycans are deposited and associated. The polyglycans bind water and thereby provide elastic properties to cartilage. The collagen fiber is responsible for tensile strength and serves to confine the expanding nature of the attached proteoglycan. All of these substances are present in a highly ordered arrangement. Several different types of collagen have been shown to exist, but all types assume a triple helix structure as collagen fibrils are formed. The proteoglycans of cartilage also have an ordered structure that not only contributes to their own physical properties but also establishes their inter-relationship to the collagen fiber.

ROBERT E. KUHLMAN

6

functioning enzyme systems in skeletal tissue and their relationship to structure

Collagen synthesis

Collagen, the most abundant protein in mammals, is a fibrous protein accounting for 25% of the body weight and provides the structural framework for all organisms. It has the distinctive property of forming insoluble fibers that have very high tensile strength. The chemical bonds and molecular organization of collagen produce this tensile strength. As tissues age and mature, the character of their collagen content changes as it undergoes alteration of its molecular bonds. These changes produce modification in the physical properties of collagen and the tissues that it composes (Table 6-1). Collagen can be modified to meet the needs of specialized tissues, as, for example, when it forms the framework for bone, tooth, or tendon. Some types of collagen will calcify and others will not. All molecules of collagen are arrayed in parallel fashion, with all the amino acid ends pointing one way and all the carbonyl groups pointing the other to form fibrils. The amino acid sequence of collagen provides its basic architectural structure, and this framework produces its subsequent mechanical relationships and characteristics. To produce body structure, collagen is associated with other substances to form a composite material, and this association requires the production of several specialized types of collagen. Some types combine solely with proteoglycans to form cartilage, whereas others combine with mineral to form bone. The type of collagen formed is related to the composition of the three fibrillar strands that wind together to form the characteristic triple helix, the degree of secondary inter- and intramolecular cross-linking that exists, and the ex-

tent to which carbohydrate is attached to the collagen molecules.

A major difference between the collagen of bone and that of tendon is the extent and quality of covalent cross-linking that occurs between molecules. The formation of different types of collagen molecules is not unique to the protein synthesis of collagen. Several genetically distinct types of hemoglobin molecules, for example, are also known to be synthesized.

Since collagen metabolism is markedly altered in a variety of connective tissue diseases, knowledge of the control mechanisms normally operative in collagen metabolism can be expected to lead to an increased understanding of many disease processes and will serve in determining therapeutic measures.

The precise sequence of enzymatic events resulting in the biosynthesis of collagen encompasses all known biochemical events, and relies upon the general biochemical resources of the body. To achieve the specialized collagen structure, certain specialized enzyme sequences relate particularly to its synthesis, and they will be described in more detail. Collagen fibers are synthesized by the fibroblast or osteoblast intracellularly and are secreted as precursors (procollagen) that form monomer collagen fibrils to produce the basic unit of the collagen fiber—the so-called tropocollagen molecule. Three of the tropocollagen molecules associate together spontaneously in a left-handed helical arrangement to form the collagen fibril.

Since the collagen present in young animals has not yet established excessive inter- and intramolecular stabilization or so-called cross-linkages, it is possible to extract from this tissue

TABLE 6-1 TYPES, DISTRIBUTION, AND COMPOSITION OF DIFFERENT VARIETIES OF COLLAGEN

COLLAGEN TYPE	CHAIN STRUCTURE OF HELIX	DISTRIBUTION
Type I	α-1, α-1, α-2	Bone Dermis Tendon Dentin
Type II	α-1, α-1, α-1 [II]	Cartilage
Type III	α-1, α-1, α-1 [III]	Cardiovascular system
Type IV	α-1, α-1, α-1 [IV]	Basement membrane

intact tropocollagen in pure form for study. This material has a molecular weight of 285,000 and is formed by three polypeptide α-chains, each containing about 1050 amino acid residues wrapped to form a left-handed triple helix structure. Under the electron microscope these fibers have a visible periodicity along the fiber at 640 A. It is the longest known chain protein and is about 3000 A long and 15 A in diameter. The individual α-chains form a left-handed helical structure. Several types of α-chains have been demonstrated, each differing in amino acid composition, chain type, and carbohydrate content.

Several types of collagen have been described, but it is the first two types that have the greatest distribution. Type 1 collagen is found in bone, tendon, dermis, fascia, and aorta and is a coarse type of collagen composed of two α-1 and one α-2 chains. Type 2 collagen is found in hyalin cartilage, nucleus pulposus, and the vitreous and embryonal neural retina, and consists of three α-1 chains. These α-chains form a polypyroline-type helix that extends through the length of the molecule.

A particular amino acid composition is distinctive of the protein collagen. Glycine molecules occur at nearly every third position in the amino acid sequence, and so collagen contains one-third glycine. This compares with about 5% glycine in hemoglobin. Analysis of collagen from many areas and species has indicated that it invariably contains about 11 to 14% hydroxyproline. Hydroxyproline and hydroxylysine are unique to collagen, which contains more of these amino acids than does any other protein. The sequence glycine-proline-hydroxyproline has been found to recur frequently in the amino acid sequence of collagen. The only other known proteins to have a regular recurrent sequence are silk, fibron, and elastin.

The molecular arrangement of collagen produces the rod-shaped tropocollagen molecule, and three of these molecules spontaneously wind together to form a structure similar to a stiff cable. The three α-strands are held to each other by hydrogen bonds between peptide NH groups of glycine and CO groups on other chains. The helical form of the α-chain results from the repulsion of pyrrolidone rings of proline residues.

These relationships are responsible for the strength of the fiber. A 1-mm fiber has been shown by mechanical testing to withstand loads up to 10 kg. The structure produced by these cooperative inter-reactions is quite crowded, and this fact is responsible for the importance of glycine to the molecule, as its small size makes it the only molecule that can fit inside the helix. In contrast, the bulky ring structures of proline and hydroxyproline are accommodated outside of the helix. The small space occupied by glycine allows the three α-chains to come close together and wrap around each other. In nature generally, glycine has been shown to have a critical role allowing conformity of folding polypeptides.

The stability of the collagen helix depends upon its content of proline and hydroxyproline specifically as imino acids. The higher the imino acid content, the more stable the helix will be. It has been demonstrated that the imino acid content of collagen increases in the evolutionary trend from cold-blooded warm-blooded species, and it is the interlocking effect of proline and hydroxyproline residues that provides the stability of the helically formed strands of tropocollagen.

The hydrogen-bound attraction of tropocollagen fibers is not sufficiently stable, however, to hold collagen together by itself, and so following the association of tropocollagen fibrils that occur in a quarter-staggered array, molecular cross-linkages are formed. First, intramolecular cross-links occur between α-chains by a type of aldol condensation and then through intermolecular cross-links between fibers through Schiff base reactions, to be described later.

The geometry assumed by the association of tropocollagen molecules produces the characteristic 680 Å cross-striations exhibited by collagen and results from the arrangement of tropocollagen molecules in a quarter-staggered array. This arrangement results in a gap of 400 Å between the end of one tropocollagen molecule and the start of the next. The tropocollagen molecules therefore are not linked end to end. It is in this gap between molecules that the initial mineral is deposited during the earliest phase of bone formations. These gaps serve as nucleation sites for the formation of hydroxyapatite

([Ca$_{10}$PO$_4$]$_6$OH$_2$). The initial component deposited in these gaps appears to be phosphate.

There is a precise relationship between the axillary· inter-relationship of fibers with one-quarter staggers between molecules. The relationship of quarter-staggering is absolutely reproduced, and there is a hole at the point at which the end of one molecule fails to abut against the other.

The molecular synthesis of collagen

The formation of collagen occurs both intracellularly and extracellularly (Fig. 6-1). Inside the fibroblast (or osteoblast if bone is the final result

of collagen assembly) the amino acid composition of the particular type of collagen to be formed is dictated by DNA, and through transcription to messenger RNA located in the ribosomal structure of the cell sequential polymerization of amino acids then occurs to form polypeptide chains. Studies of the translation of messenger RNA for collagen synthesis have been limited, but those studies that have been made have used organ culture of mouse calvaria. These investigations indicated that chains are assembled throughout their length by the sequential addition of individual amino acids, and not by assembly of shorter polypeptide chains. Organ culture of rat calvaria indicated that these chains are assembled at a rate of about 200 residues/

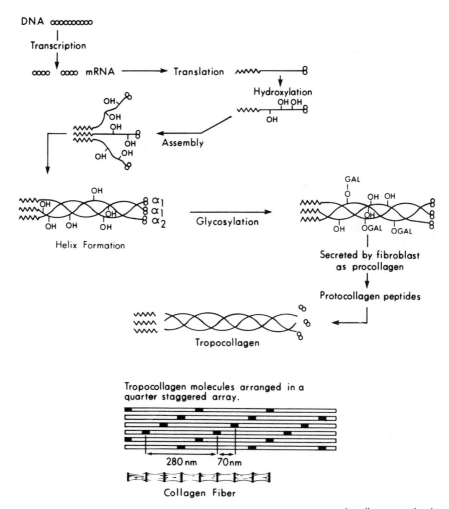

FIGURE 6-1 *Schematic representation of the steps of collagen synthesis.*

min, a translation rate of about one-third that previously observed for messenger RNA hemoglobin α- and β-chain formation. At present, no explanation exists for this difference in translational rate.

Information has been accumulated to show that subsequent to the assembly of the primary collagen structure and prior to its deposition in fiber form, the polypeptide chains of collagen are subjected to a number of post-translational chemical modifications.

Although hydroxyproline and hydroxylysine are characteristic amino acids of collagen, they are not incorporated into the protein as such but rather in unhydroxylated form. The assembled amino acid sequence then undergoes hydroxylation of most of its lysine and proline content by the enzyme protocollagen hydroxylase. This enzyme reaction fails to proceed without oxygen, ferrous iron, and α-ketogluterate as cofactors. Ascorbic acid (vitamin C) is essential for the reaction to occur and acts as a reducing agent. If anything serves to inhibit hydroxylation, the reactive triple helix cannot be assumed, and procollagen builds up in the cell until synthesis stops.

The actions of protocollagen hydroxylase are specific, and probably several enzymes exist for this function. Following their incorporation into the growing collagen α-chain, pyrol residues immediately preceding glycyl residues constitute the potential substrate for the hydroxylating enzyme peptidylproline hydroxylase. Certain lysyl residues generally located in the third portion of the collagen triplet are hydroxylated by a second enzyme—peptidyl lysine hydroxylase. Both enzymes are dependent upon the same cofactors (ascorbic acid, ferrous iron, α-ketogluterate, and molecular oxygen). Molecular oxygen serves as the source of oxygen for the hydroxyl group, and α-ketogluterate is an absolute requirement that undergoes stoichiometric decarboxylation in relation to the amount of hydroxyproline formed. The ferrous iron binds with the enzyme and probably serves as the site of attachment for molecular oxygen. These chemical reactions occur on nascent α-chains prior to their release from the ribosomes. It is possible to inhibit this hydroxylation process

either by withdrawing molecular oxygen or by introducing a chelating agent to bind ferrous iron. Collagen synthesized under these conditions remains substantially unhydroxylated. Furthermore, carbohydrate cannot be subsequently attached to hydroxylysine, and as a result defective procollagen molecules accumulate intracellularly. Hydroxyproline, hydroxylysine, and/or the carbohydrate appear necessary for the membrane transfer of the procollagen formed. Unhydroxylated collagen is insufficiently stable to maintain a triple helix configuration, as these are the residues that stabilize the helix.

The hydroxylation that occurs by this system is quite specific, and the enzyme does not work on free proline or lysine, but works only after they have been incorporated into a polypeptide sequence and when they are situated on the amino side of a glycine residue.

Since ascorbic acid is an essential requirement for hydroxylation, when it is unavailable, a disease state known as scurvy results. Collagen synthesized when ascorbic acid is not present lacks hydroxylation; it is unable to form fibers properly and therefore has inadequate mechanical strength, and the tissues it composes have very poor mechanical characteristics as a result.

A second post-translational modification that occurs is glycosylation of hydroxylysine. Collagen contains carbohydrate units attached covalently to hydroxylysine residues, commonly as a glucose-galactose disaccharide attached to the hydroxyl group. The extent to which carbohydrate is associated with collagen depends upon the type of collagen formed and the specialized nature of the tissue it forms. Tendon, for example, has less associated carbohydrate than does lens capsule.

Carbohydrate is attached to collagen intracellularly by glucosyltransferase and galactosyltransferase that functions in the rough endoplasmic reticulum.

As these post-transcriptional modifications occur, the triple helix configuration is assumed spontaneously by the charge repulsion of pyrrolidine rings of proline residues, of which there are three per turn, as dictated by the amino acid sequence.

Both glycosyltransferase and hydroxylation

steps stop after the triple helix is formed, and therefore the formation of hydroxylysine and hydroxyproline, as well as glycosylation, is self-regulating. About 100 modified residues/chain result, and the triple helix cable obtained is very stable at 37° C.

It is of interest to note that a hereditary disorder characterized by highly elastic skin, scoliosis, and hypermobile joints has been described (Ehlers-Danlos syndrome), in which the lysyl residues are not adequately hydroxylated because of defective lysyl hydroxylase function. The hydroxylation of lysine is of critical importance in establishing and maintaining the functional role of the collagen fiber.

After procollagen has been formed, it is transported across the cell membrane into the intracellular space. This biosynthetic precursor to tropocollagen exhibits the unusual solubility characteristic of remaining in solution under conditions in which collagen molecules ordinarily would spontaneously precipitate to form fibers. Evidence has accumulated that pepsin-susceptible amino acid sequences are located at both the amino and carboxyl ends of the pro α-chains thus formed. The amino terminal amino acid sequence appears to have a molecular weight of about 11,000, and the carboxyl terminal peptide has a molecular weight of 31,000 as compared with 145,000 for the pro α-chain itself. These chains also have a substantially different amino acid composition than does collagen. For example, they contain cysteine, no hydroxyproline, as far less than the expected amounts of glycine. These terminal peptides appear to be primarily responsible for the antigenicity of collagen.

Several physiologic roles have been postulated for these additional terminal peptide sequences of the procollagen molecules. It has been postulated that they account for the rapidity with which the collagen helix is formed during biosynthesis, that they may further facilitate accurate alignment of the α-chains into the triple helical structure, and that they may serve to expedite transportation across the cell wall.

In the extracellular space, these amino and carboxyl terminal extensions of procollagen are removed physiologically by a neutral protease—procollagen peptidase. It is necessary to excise these terminal peptides before normal collagen fibers can be formed. In this manner, collagen fiber formation is analogous to fibrin formation from fibrinogen. Specific amino terminal and carboxyl terminal procollagen peptidases have been demonstrated. These enzymes are localized extracellularly at the site of fiber formation.

Once the terminal peptides are removed from procollagen, insoluble tropocollagen precipitates in the form of rod-like fibers 3000 Å long and 15 Å wide. They spontaneously associate to form collagen fibers and do so in a special way. Each tropocollagen fiber is aligned into parallel and linear arrays with each amino terminus and carboxyl terminus pointing in the same direction. Each amino terminus is displaced by about a quarter-stagger of the molecular length. The tropocollagen molecules therefore do not abut end to end, but rather are separated by a space of about 400 A. Attachment between fibers occurs in a side-to-side fashion. These end gaps between tropocollagen fibrils form the nucleation site for bone hydroxyapatite crystal formation.

Abnormalities of procollagen peptidase functions have been reported associated with a congenital anomaly occurring in calves, called dermatosparaxis, in which diminished or lack of procollagen peptidase activity results in impaired fiber formation and a resultant very poor tensile strength of the dermis.

Once spontaneous tropocollagen molecular association into a quarter-stagger array has occurred, the formation of strong, properly functioning collagen fibers then depends upon the development of intra- and intermolecular covalent cross-links. This cross-linking occurs through an aldol-type condensation of lysyl- and hydroxylysyl-derived aldehydes and through the formation of Schiff bases. Bonding of this nature is unique to collagen and elastin (Fig. 6-2).

The intramolecular cross-links are those within the tropocollagen molecule and are derived from lysine side chains by the action of lysyl oxidase, which converts the amino terminus of lysine to an aldehyde. Two of these aldehydes then undergo the common aldol con-

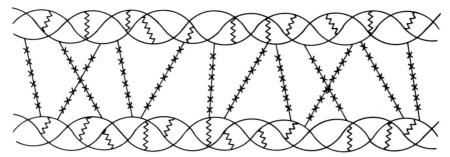

FIGURE 6-2 *A schematic representation of the intra- and intermolecular cross-linkages that are established between collagen molecules as aging changes occur. These cross-linkages result from aldol-type condensation between portions of the tropocollagen molecule and by Schiff base reactions between fibers.*

densation in which the enolate ion derived from one of the aldehydes attaches onto the carbonyl group of another aldehyde. Lysyl oxidase is a copper-requiring enzyme and appears dependent upon pituitary hormone. β-Amino propionitrile is an irrevocable inhibitor of lysyl oxidase, and its administration results in the formation of defective collagen, similar to that found in patients with Marfan's syndrome. Lathyrism, the experimental syndrome produced by nitrile administration, is in some ways similar to the clinical picture of Marfan's syndrome.

After the aldol cross-links are formed, they, in turn, can react with the histidine side chain to form a histidine-aldol cross-link, whereupon the aldehyde group of the aldol-histidine cross-link can form a Schiff base with another side chain such as hydroxylysine. Through this process, four peptide side chains may be covalently bonded together. The formation of the latter Schiff base bonds occurs intermolecularly between tropocollagen fibers.

The extent to which cross-linking of collagen fibers occurs varies with physiology, functions, and the age of the tissue. Achilles tendon from a mature rat is highly cross-linked, whereas flexible tail tendon is less so. The degree of cross-linking in any tissue generally increases with age.

In addition to these specialized systems, collagen protein synthesis uses the generally known pathways of peptide bond formation, which depend upon activation of the carbonyl groups of the amino acid to be added to the peptide sequence by adenosine triphosphate (ATP). Activated amino acid groups are bound through an adenosine monophosphate (AMP) bridge to an enzyme acting as an intermediate bridge to an enzyme acting as an intermediate amino acid transferring compound to the receptor protein:

$$\text{Amino A to be added} + \text{ATP} \xrightarrow{\text{Enzyme}}$$
$$\text{(Enzyme-AMP-amino A)}$$
$$+ \text{ inorganic pyrophosphate}$$
$$\text{Peptide} + \text{(enzyme-AMP-amino A)} \rightarrow$$
$$\text{Peptide-amino A} + \text{enzyme} + \text{AMP}$$

The synthesis systems, producing nucleic acids, and other synthesis systems as well, result in by-product accumulations of inorganic pyrophosphate that, if allowed to accumulate, will inhibit the mineralization of bone. It must be hydrolyzed to lower energy inorganic phosphate by inorganic pyrophosphate to restore phosphate economy and prevent inhibition of calcification. Inorganic pyrophosphatase activity is present in calcifying tissue at those sites at which active collagen synthesis is occurring.

Once formed, collagen provides a basic tensile strength and architectural framework to the tissue to be formed. Other materials are deposited upon and within the collagen fiber to form a composite material. As with any complex composite material, the final combination will have mechanical features quite different from each of its constituents.

When cartilage is formed, the collagen framework is combined with proteoglycans, which fills the structure with water and results in its elasticity and compressibility. An excellent example of this inter-relationship is the nucleus

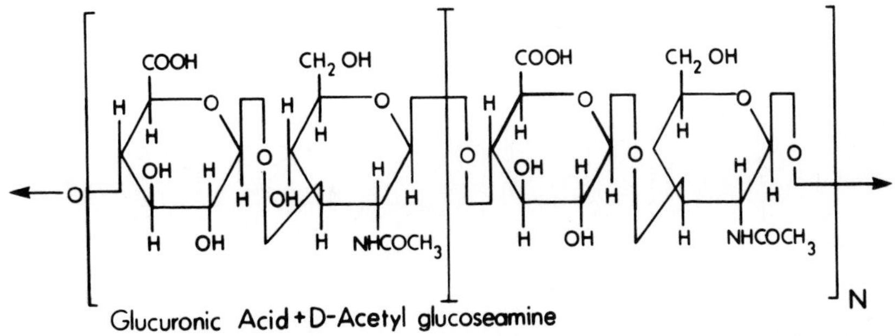

Glucuronic Acid + D-Acetyl glucoseamine

FIGURE 6-3 *Structural representation of the polymer hyaluronic acid; note the similarity to chondroitin (Fig. 6-3) and chondroitin sulfate (Fig. 6-4). Only two segments of a massive chain are illustrated.*

pulposus of the intervertebral discs. In contrast, bone fabric is stiffened by the deposition of mineral salts and proteoglycans into the precise spacing provided by the quarter-stagger arrangement of the collagen fiber.

Ground substance—enzymatic synthesis

The biochemical assembly of matrix substance occurs in cartilage and bone at a relatively rapid rate. The chondrocyte is responsible for matrix synthesis in both articular and epiphyseal cartilage. All stages of synthesis appear to occur intracellularly and may be divided into four steps: (1) synthesis of the protein core of the proteoglycan, (2) synthesis of glycosaminoglycans, (3) assembly upon the protein core, and (4) addition of sulfate to chondroitin or keratin. Several workers have demonstrated that synthesis of glycosaminoglycan can occur in cell-free preparations if appropriate enzymes and a protein

core are present; however, under physiologic conditions this synthesis occurs intracellularly.

Glycosaminoglycans are formed through the combination of hexuronic acid and an amino sugar. When unsulfated, these compounds are referred to as acid mucopolysaccharides. The most abundant such compound is hyaluronic acid (Figs. 6-3–6-5).

Hyaluronic acid
 = glucuronic acid–N-acetylglucosamine

(An unbranched polymer)

Chondroitin
 = glucuronic acid–N-acetylgalactosamine

When sulfated, these compounds are known as sulfated mucopolysaccharides. Different types of chondroitin sulfate are formed depending upon the location sulfated. Long-chain molecules containing 20 to 30 repeating disaccharide units and having a molecular weight of 15,000 to

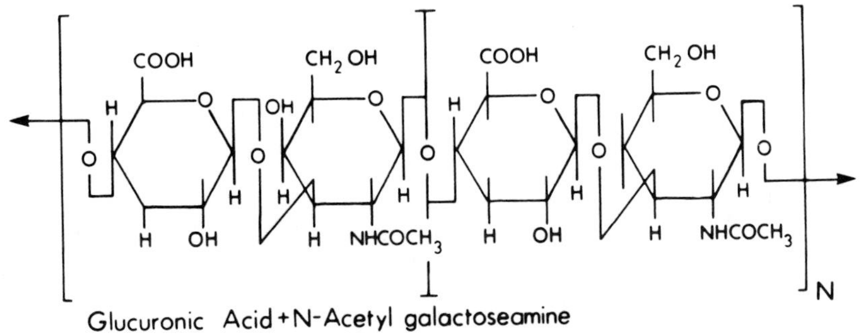

Glucuronic Acid + N-Acetyl galactoseamine

FIGURE 6-4 *Chondroitin, an unsulfated acid mucopolysaccharide.*

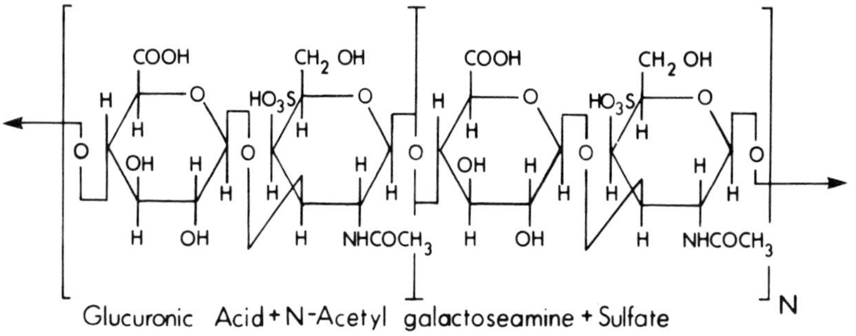

CHONDROTIN SULFATE A

FIGURE 6-5 *Chondroitin sulfate polymer is represented. Only two segments of a massively polymerized chain are demonstrated.*

20,000 result from the polymerization of these compounds (Table 6-2).

The formation of these —O—glycosidic bonds between sugars requires large free-energy changes and preliminary phosphate activation of the sugars involved by uridine triphosphate (UTP) or ATP is required for synthesis.

All substrates used for aminoglycan synthesis are derived from glucose (Fig. 6-6). A "primer" of core protein is required for chondroitin sulfate assembly that contains appropriate serine-glycine groups. Assembly is begun at the linkage region, and glycosaminoglycan is sequentially assembled. Uridine diphosphate (UDP)-xylose first attaches to serine by xylosyltransferase action, followed by two galactose molecules derived from UDP-galactose, which attach first glycosidically to xylose, and then to one another. The reaction is catalyzed by galactosyl trans-

ferases. Glucuronic acid is added, and finally UDP–N-acetylgalactosamine donates N-acetylgalactosamine. The sequence of linkage then repeats to form a polymer. All of these synthetic activities occur in the Golgi apparatus and seem independent of ribosomal structures.

After the chain reaches a satisfactory length, sulfation occurs by the addition of a high-energy sulfate group.

Pathway for chondroitin sulfation

$$\text{Sulfate} + \text{ATP} \xrightarrow{\text{Sulfate adenyltransferase}}$$
$$\text{Adenosine-5-phosphosulfate (APS)} + \text{PPi}$$

$$\text{APS} + \text{ATP} \xrightarrow{\text{Adenylsulfate phosphotransferase}}$$
$$\text{3 phosphoadenosine-5-phosphosulfate (PAPS)} + \text{ADP}$$

TABLE 6-2 COMPOSITION AND STRUCTURE OF IMPORTANT MUCOPOLYSACCHARIDES

MUCOPOLYSACCHARIDE	COMPOSITION		STRUCTURAL LINKAGE
	HEXURONIC ACID	AMINO SUGAR	
Chondroitin	D-Glucuronic acid	N-acetyl-D galactosamine	β-1—3; β-1—4
Chondroitin Sulfate A (Chondroitin 4-sulfate)	D-Glucuronic acid	N-acetyl-D galactosamine 4-sulfate	β-1—3; β-1—4
Chondroitin Sulfate C (Chondroitin 6-sulfate)	D-Glucuronic acid	N-acetyl-D galactosamine 6-sulfate	β-1—3; β-1—4
Chondroitin Sulfate B (Dermatan sulfate)	L-Iduronic acid	N-acetyl-D galactosamine 4-sulfate	α-1—3; β-1—4
Hyaluronic Acid	D-Glucuronic acid	N-acetyl-D glucosamine	β-1—3; β-1—4
Keratosulfate	D-Galactose	N-acetyl-D glucosamine 6-sulfate	β-1—4; β-1—3

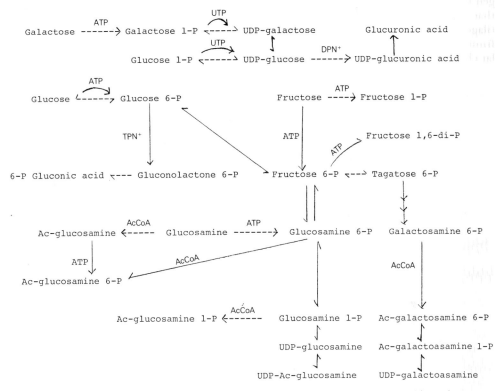

The enzymic interrelationships between hexoses and their derivatives in mammalian tissues. P - phosphate; AC - N-acetyl; AcCoA - acetyl coenzyme A; ATP, UTP - adenosine and uridine triphosphate; UDP - ester of uridine   diphosphate.

FIGURE 6-6 *The pathways for the enzymatic derivation of the intermediates required for the synthesis of glycosaminoglycans from glucose are illustrated.*

Chondroitin + PAPS $\xrightarrow{\text{Sulfotransferase}}$
        Chondroitin sulfate + phospho AMP

An active sulfate is formed by ATP, which, in turn, is donated to the fourth carbon of chondroitin to form chondroitin sulfate A, or to the sixth carbon to make chondroitin sulfate C. The attachment is mediated by a specific sulfotransferase. Keratosulfate presumably is similarly formed.

In some way the cell extrudes the proteoglycan molecule extracellularly. The proteoglycan

molecule is then linked in an ordered arrangement to a core protein (Figure 6-7), as postulated by Rosenberg,[29,30] to form a highly ordered molecular structure.

Rosenberg[29,30] has also postulated the ordered structure that results when the proteoglycan subunits aggregate extracellularly and arrange along a core of hyaluronic acid (Figure 6-8). The proteoglycan subunit binds to the hyaluronic acid core at the protein-rich terminal end. Two-link proteins have been identified that have molecular weights of 45,000 to 50,000 and serve to

PROTEOGLYCAN SUBUNIT

FIGURE 6-7 *Dr. L. Rosenberg has postulated this ordered arrangement and attachment of the proteoglycan subunit to a core protein. (Protein by Dr. L. Rosenberg, Montefiore Hospital, New York)*

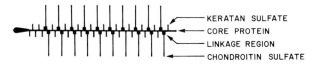

KERATAN SULFATE
CORE PROTEIN
LINKAGE REGION
CHONDROITIN SULFATE

attach the proteoglycan aggregates to the hyaluronic acid core and stabilize the union.

Cartilage is the structural tissue that results from the combination of proteoglycan and collagen fiber. The complex molecular arrangements that result have specific properties that give cartilage its resiliency and lubrication. Extending from the long filamentous proteoglycan molecular chain are multiple, negatively charged sulfate and carbonyl groups. Large amounts of water are hydrogen-bound to the molecule, and repulsion of negative charges distributed in enormous numbers around the proteoglycan molecular side chains forces the molecule to expand. The attachment of the expanding proteoglycan molecule to collagen, whose tensile strength serves to confine this expansion, provides strength and rigidity to the complex structure that results. At

PROTEOGLYCAN AGGREGATE

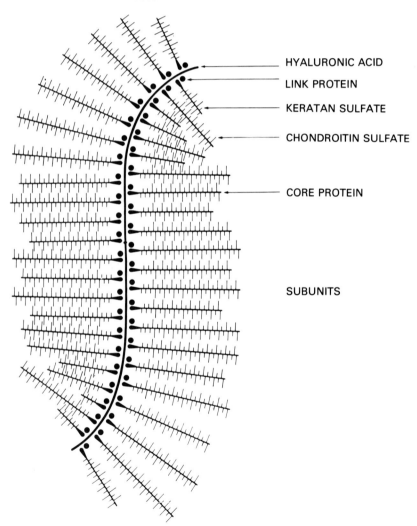

HYALURONIC ACID

LINK PROTEIN

KERATAN SULFATE

CHONDROITIN SULFATE

CORE PROTEIN

SUBUNITS

FIGURE 6-8 *The multiple proteoglycan subunits attach as described in the text to a long hyaluronic acid molecule. The attachment is stabilized by a link protein. (Provided by Dr. L. Rosenberg, Montefiore Hospital, New York)*

the same time, resilience occurs from its capacity to release bound water under pressure and regain it when pressure is released.

The anionic nature of the proteoglycan molecule allows combination with cationic dyes such as alcain blue, toluidine blue, crystal violet, and so forth. The highly ordered nature of the molecule, however, binds these dyes in strict spatial relationships and causes their polymerization. This action results in a shift of their absorption spectra, and the well-known metachromatic staining characteristic results. Safranin-O has been shown by Rosenberg[29,30] to bind only to proteoglycan and not to collagen, and so it may be used to determine proteoglycan distribution. It is interesting to note that heparin, a polymer of glucosamine-N-sulfate and glucuronic acid, is similar in structure to chondroitin.

Significant differences exist among fetal, adolescent, and adult cartilage. The immature animal has more chondroitin 4-sulfate than the older animal, in which chondroitin 6-sulfate predominates. Chondroitin 4-sulfate (type A) is the principal mucopolysaccharide present in growing bone. Chondroitin sulfate B (dermatan sulfate) is the predominate proteoglycan of skin, tendon, and heart valve. Keratosulfate is found principally in the cornea.

Proteoglycans play a major part in the formation of all tissues, but the content of cartilage exceeds that of any other tissue. The collagen fiber of cartilage is imbedded and bathed in these molecules, which attach in a specific manner to the collagen fiber. They play a role in the process of endochondral ossification and accumulate in the hypertrophic cartilage cell area during this process. They must, however, be removed from the collagen fiber before mineralization of bone can occur, and consequently, the loss of metachromatic-staining characteristics always precedes mineralization.

Collagen and Proteoglycan degradation

Collagenase

Prior to 1959, there was no direct evidence that mature mammalian collagen was affected by any enzyme under physiologic conditions. However, there exist several biologic situations that seem to require function of a physiologically active collagenase system. Most notable of these is the resorption of collagen that occurs in the postpartum uterus. During this process, large amounts of collagen are removed from this enlarged structure and excreted as hydroxyproline in the urine. Another situation dramatically demonstrating collagenase function is the disappearance of the tadpole tail during metamorphosis. Collagenase systems are also necessary for remodeling of long bones during growth and are responsible for the appearance of trophic ulcers and the very rapid cartilage destruction characteristic of rheumatoid arthritis. These systems also serve to explain the facility of tumor to invade normal tissue.

It has been known since the work of Phemister that staphylococcal enzymes and general proteases would degrade collagen only if it was first denatured by heating to temperatures greater than 55° C. Denaturation of collagen cannot occur until its temperature is raised above 55° to 60° C. It is unlikely that even the most severe febrile illnesses could result in *in vivo* collagen denaturization.

By definition, collagenase is an enzyme capable of degrading native collagen in its helical form under physiologic conditions. Gross[9,10] was the first to demonstrate the presence of such a physiologically active collagenase. He did so by tissue culture of tadpole tails, which disappear under the influence of such a system. From tissue culture preparations he was able to isolate and prove the existence of a physiologically active collagenase system. To date, a number of such enzyme systems have been isolated from a number of normal and pathologic tissues using tissue culture techniques.

Native collagen is resistant to general body animal tissue protease, as it must be to survive as a body framework. The structural resistance of collagen is based upon its triple helix structure, which results from the presence of glycine at each third amino acid sequence and the characteristic presence of hydroxyproline and hydroxylysine. Cross-linkages between fibrils within the helix further enhance molecular stability. It is the presence of the hydroxyproline and the associated structural arrangements that determine the resistance of collagen to degradation by general body proteases. Certain areas of the collagen molecule are susceptible to attack and cleavage. Although mammalian proteases have a minimal effect on native collagen, trypsin in high concentration will slowly attack collagen from the carbonyl end. Chymotrypsin and pepsin cleave the short nonhelical region of native collagen found at the amino terminus in such a way as to render the molecule soluble in aqueous extracts and yet preserve its native helical form. Under ordinary circumstances, however, these activities result in negligible collagen degradation, and before they can exert an appreciable effect, the collagen structure must be modified.

Bacterial collagenase systems derived from *Clostridium histolyticum*, in contrast to mammalian collagenases, cleave collagen into multiple small peptides by action at many sites, and slip off segments sequentially from each end of the molecule.

The physiologically active collagenase Gross[9,10] described was inhibited by ethylenedianinetetraacetic acid (EDTA) and cysteine but not by diisopropyl fluorophosphate (DFP), and it required calcium. It was necessary to use organ culture of the tadpole tails to demonstrate the enzyme, as only very small amounts of enzyme are free in tissue at any one time. He demonstrated that native collagen is cleaved by this enzyme into two pieces: an amino terminal end composed of 75% of the fibril, and a carboxyl terminal composing the other 25%. The triple helix structure is retained, and further degradation continues to be resisted. The smaller helical structure formed, however, is more susceptible to trypsin cleavage through the C-terminal glycine and the end-terminal leucine or isoleucine.

Every other mammalian collagenase cleaves native collagen in the same manner. Gross has further suggested that once the collagen molecule within the fibril has been attacked in the extracellular space, the fibril frays, and more soluble reaction products disperse within the surrounding tissue fluids as they become more soluble. With dispersion comes increased denaturation at lower temperatures, and the helical structure is lost. Once this happens, other proteases that can degrade gelatin are able to function.

Collagenase has been derived from several sources. Gross[9,10] has demonstrated that only tadpole epidermal tissues could produce collagenase, whereas most normal skin collagenase is produced in the dermis. Whole tissue from cholesteatoma of the middle ear produced large amounts of collagenase.[1] It also has been obtained from granulation tissue and tissue cultures of rheumatoid synovium. Collagenase activity has not been found in association with tissues that are highly differentiated, as, for example, in cells of the endocrine glands or lymphocytes. Free collagenase activity has been demonstrated in the synovial fluid of rheumatoid arthritic patients but not in that of osteoarthritic patients.

Evidence suggests that collagenase is secreted as an inactive precursor zymogen. Enzymes from lysozymes at pH 5.7 and trypsin at pH 7.6 will activate zymogens to release an active collagenase. These factors indicate that there is a controlled regulation of tissue collagenase activity. For example, cyclic adenosine monophosphate (AMP) will stimulate collagenase production. Agents that inhibit collagenous function also exist. Collagenase is released into tissue as a procollagenase with a molecular weight of 120,000, which decreases as the active component appears.

Mechanism of action of collagenase

Much debate exists as to the mechanism of action of collagenase. One theory suggested that the initial step involved some sort of depolymerase function. Depolymerase enzymes that have been described are active only at a pH of 4.0, and never above pH 6.0. Cuervo and Howell,[2] using elegant microtechniques, were able to demonstrate that the lowest pH present in avascular articular cartilage was 6.8. The pH of purulent synovial fluid, with its lowered oxygen tension, has been reported at 6.8. Conditions of pH seem to prevent the physiologic function of any known polymerase enzyme.

Pure collagenase cleaves the collagen triple helix generally at one locus only, the 39-40 interband. The helical nature of the collagen seems related to its binding by the collagenase enzyme, and it appears that collagenase cleaves the triple helix at one or possibly a few loci without definite specificity. General proteases are then more active in cleaving the products formed from the primary cleavage. It may also be that the primary cleavage of collagen is sufficient for the dissociation of small fragments from the fibril, which they are more easily degraded by general protease systems.

Poorly cross-linked fibers have increased susceptibility to collagenase activity. The process of aging, with its introduction of stable intramolecular cross-links, may result in the accumulation of collagens that are resistant to breakdown and retard remodeling of these tissues. This factor may explain some of the differences in healing characteristics in youth and age.

Collagen degradation in bone is influenced by the mineral content in and around the collagen fiber, and the presence of hydroxyapatite mineral confers protection to bone collagen to both enzymatic and thermal denaturization. Bone mineral must be removed before collagenase can degrade matrix. Proteoglycan aggregates similarly afford protection to collagen fibers against enzymatic breakdown.

The assay of native collagenase requires a substrate of native collagen in soluble helical form. Collagen substrate containing a radioactive residue is prepared in tissue culture, and when acted upon by collagenase the radioactivity is released into solution and can be measured.

Physiologically, active collagenase has been obtained from the synovium of rheumatoid patients, synovial fluid, skin, healing wound, and bone, polymorphonuclear leukocyte and cholesteatoma, and other tissues associated with tumors.

Collagenase functions during the growth and development of bone. During periods of growth, the overall rate of collagen formation is in excess of that being resorbed. Local areas of difference in the rate of resorption and formation result in changes in shape. Remodeling will continue to take place during this process even into adult life. It becomes apparent that some regulation of the collagenase system is important to the normal remodeling and growth of bone. Increased col-

lagenase activity has been demonstrated in Paget's disease and in the hyperparathyroid state. In both situations rapid bone resorption occurs, and an abundance of osteoclasts have been observed in bone tissue.

Chronic heparin treatment has been demonstrated by Griffith[7] to be associated with an osteoporosis. The addition of heparin to organ culture media of mouse calvaria will produce a substantial increase in the amount of bone resorption that occurs, with suboptimal concentrations of parathyroid hormone. Paralleling bone resorption in these experiments a hydroxylproline-containing peptide was released into solution, indicating actual collagen destruction took place. These observations indicate that in some manner heparin serves to activate or potentiate collagenase activity.

The laboratory of Glimsher[34] has described the isolation, purification, and mechanism of action of mouse bone collagenase. They observed a pH optimum for culture enzyme of 8.0 and estimated its molecular weight at 41,000. Heparin appeared to enhance the specific activity of the enzyme when collagen was used as a substrate. This effect of heparin is interesting in view of the documented occurrence of heparin osteoporosis.[7] A possible role in the regulation of collagen turnover by heparin has been suggested, but further study is indicated.

The occurrence of a cholesteatoma as a sequel to chronic mastoiditis appears as a mass of accumulated, well-organized epithelium with granulation tissue that invades the middle ear. It has an unusual capacity for bone invasion. Abrahmson[1] has demonstrated an unusual amount of collagenase enzyme to be produced by this tissue, and it is felt that this enzyme is responsible for the invasive nature of the lesion.

The work of Vaes[35,36] discussed the precursors of bone collagenase and their mechanisms of activation. Bone explants in tissue culture release into surrounding medium a collagenase that attacks native collagen in solution at about neutral pH using either reconstituted or insoluble fibrils, and fragments representing 75% and 25% of the molecules, respectively, are produced by the action of the enzyme. This collagenase, however, was also found to be present in a latent state in culture fluids, which could be activated by treatment with trypsin. This treatment decreased the molecular weight of the latent collagenase from 110,000 to 90,000. The latent nature of collagenase can be explained in two ways: (1) the collagenase is released from the cells as an inactive proenzyme or zymogen that is activated by a limited proteolysis of its molecule or (2) the collagenase forms an inhibitor enzyme complex with some protein inhibitor that is thereafter dissociated by the activation process, either because of partial proteolysis by trypsin or because the trypsin has a higher affinity for the inhibitor than does the collagenase. Vaes' experiments indicated the latter to be very unlikely, and he believes latent procollagenase is excreted as a zymogen.[34,35,36]

There appears to be a control mechanism for the extracellular activation system of the procollagenases, and work is now being focused on these mechanisms. Vaes[35,36,37] further has established that bone explants that release procollagenase also release in a closely parallel manner a distinct neutral proteinase that is active not only on casein but also on the protein core of proteoglycans and on denatured collagen. He found this proteinase to be present in a latent state in culture fluids surrounding mouse bone explant. Upon activation, it degrades cartilage proteoglycans, denatured collagen, and casein. The activity demonstrated upon proteoglycans is interpreted as resulting from the lysis of the protein core of the proteoglycans micromolecule and is significant in the degradation process for proteoglycans. These enzymes were different from the two proteoglycan-degrading neutral serine proteinases—elastase and the chymotrypsin-like enzyme cathepsin B present in human polymorphonuclear leukocytes.

These studies of Vaes[35,36,37] pertain to a neutral proteinase as distinct from the collagenase excreted into the tissue media as a procollagenase. These neutral proteinase systems function to degrade proteoglycans and are also subject to control mechanisms. There has been no explanation established as to the mechanism of this latency of these neutral proteinases. The addition of heparin to culture media causes a progressive accumulation of these enzymes in a parallel manner.

The simultaneous secretion of both enzymes allowed Vaes to suggest the hypothesis that both enzymes participate in the same general physiologic process, presumably extracellular matrix degradation. The collagenase may initiate the fragmentation of the collagen molecule by allowing its denaturation and fragmentation, followed by further degradation by other neutral proteinases. Moreover, the same neutral proteinases that act on denatured collagen appear to have a closely related proteinase function in the degradation of proteoglycans. Thus, the two main components of the extracellular framework of connective tissue could be degraded into soluble fragments by these enzymes at a neutral pH. The size of the fragments formed by their action could then be further degraded and digested by enzymes of the lysosomal system.

Although several lysosomal acid proteinases are able to degrade proteoglycans, evidence for their participation in extracellular degradation is debated, and it seems necessary that a latent neutral proteinase first degrade the proteoglycan before lysosomal systems can become operative. Vaes[34,35,36] and coworkers have described a metal-dependent neutral proteinase that can degrade the core of cartilage proteoglycan. The enzyme is found in a latent form in culture media and is probably activated by a limited proteolysis with trypsin.

Lysozyme in cartilage

Lysozyme was first observed by Sir Alexander Fleming,[5] who described its presence in tears, saliva, and nasal secretion. He demonstrated it characteristically to be bacteriolytic. Lysozyme is an enzyme that has been shown to hydrolyze the $\beta1,4$ link between N-acetylneuraminic acid and N-acetylglucosamine. Lysozyme will hydrolyze chitin, which is the linear polymer of N-acetylglucosamine. It therefore has some $\beta1,4$ N-acetylglucosamidase activity. It has further been demonstrated that chitodextrans, as well as some other oligosaccharides derived from chitin, will act as substrates. None of these substrates, however, are present in mammalian tissues.

In mammalian systems, lysozyme has been demonstrated to be present in secretions of organs exposed to airborne bacteria, as, for example, tears, saliva, milk, and sputum. For some reason, patients with monocytic leukemia excrete large amounts of lysozyme in their urine and may secrete as much as 2.6 g/d. The enzyme may, in fact, be crystallized from their urine. Lysozyme ordinarily is held intracellularly within lysosomal structure, but in cartilage it exists exclusively extracellularly.

Lysosomal structure can be demonstrated intracellularly by acid phosphatase staining mechanisms. The lysosomal structure has a lipid membrane that envelops a series of enzymes, of which lysozyme is only one. Additionally, acid phosphatase and several acid proteases are held within the lipid envelope. It is the characteristic association of nonspecific acid phosphatase systems with the lysosome that permits acid phosphatase staining techniques to demonstrate their presences.

Fleming,[5] in his initial studies, demonstrated unusually high concentrations of lysozyme in cartilage and synovial fluid for reasons that are not understood. Lower concentrations were demonstrated in skin. Healing tissue that had been chronically inflamed or in which large amounts of granulation tissue were present contained large amounts of lysozyme.

Although lysozyme is cationic and forms salt-like complexes with cartilage proteoglycans and chondroitin sulfate *in vitro*, it is not seen bound to proteoglycan in the native tissue.

Wolff[40] in 1927 found that lysozymes were very strongly bound to lipid and that it was impossible to extract lysozyme back into an aqueous solution unless lipid was first extracted from the tissue.

Some patients that exhibit a lysozymuria also have an associated higher rate of renal potassium loss and an osteoporosis complicated by the occurrence of fractures. Wolinsky and Cohen[41] have demonstrated lysosomal activity in rabbit bone and have observed variation of its distribution throughout the bone. The administration of parathyroid extract will produce a striking fall of tissue lysozyme activity of the femur and all other tissues (except for some reason the lung) while simultaneously increasing blood levels of the enzyme. Fleming pointed out that articular cartilage contained the highest concentration of lysozyme of all tissues, organs, and secretions studied.

Lysosome activity is present in synovial fluid, and substantial elevations of it in fluid from rheumatoid arthritic patients has been demonstrated. The activity was further increased in rats with polyarthritis, a condition in some ways quite similar to rheumatoid arthritis in humans. Low synovial levels of lysozyme have been demonstrated in post-traumatic arthritic tissue and in serum-negative polyarthritis and arthritis associated with plasmocytic dyscrasias. High lysozyme activities are observed in gout, infectious arthritis, and other nonspecific arthritides, but its level is not generally correlated with the number of polymorphonuclear or monocytic cells present in the synovial lining. Kuettner[17] has speculated that lysozyme intra-articularly may exert a polysaccharidase activity, especially on N-acetylglucosamine, and it results in the breakdown of polysaccharides having glucosamine in their structure. Some correlation exists between the changes in mucopolysaccharide metabolism and serum lysozyme activity in rheumatoid arthritic patients.

Studies of cartilage lysozyme have indicated that its content varies with age, and there is a higher concentration of it at a time when active growth is occurring. In epiphyseal cartilage, the highest concentration present is in the hypertrophic cartilage area and in the zone of provisional calcification. Ricketic epiphyseal areas contain less lysozyme, and the epiphyses of rats with hypervitaminosis D contain more lysozyme than do normal animals. Aortas, which normally do not calcify, do so when large amounts of vitamin D are given, and as calcification occurs, large amounts of lysozyme are observed to accumulate in the vessel wall. Although lysozyme is uniquely located extracellularly in cartilage, there is no known physiologic function for lysosome in cartilage.

The highest levels of lysozyme in cartilage are in those areas of epiphysis undergoing the transition to bone. Kuettner[17] has provided a hypothesis for the role of lysozyme in cartilage physiology. It is his feeling that this cationic protein promotes calcification by inducing the disaggregation of cartilage proteoglycan aggregates, which themselves are inhibitors of calcification. Its distribution contributes to the precisely governed phenomenon of cartilage calcification. The columnar cells of the epiphysis contain the enzyme extracellularly on the lacuna, and it is presumably bound in this location by hyaluronic acid. In the calcifying zone, hyaluronic acid can be extracted and lysozyme then released to the extracellular matrix, where it would serve to disaggregate the polyglycans and contribute to calcification. These theories, however, have little confirmation.

The relation of phosphatases to cartilage and bone

Robinson in 1923[28] first established the association of alkaline phosphatase to bone production and fracture repair. Despite 50 yr of study, no definite causal relationship has been established between these activities. The exact role that alkaline phosphatase may play in bone production and fracture repair remains ill defined. Attempts have been made to explain calcium phosphate precipitation as a result of focal phosphate ion accumulation resulting from the action of alkaline phosphatase, but these efforts have failed. Alkaline phosphatase, furthermore, is found in large quantities in the kidney and in biliary ducts of the liver as well as in other locations in which calcification normally does not occur. Cells of articular cartilage also have been demonstrated to contain alkaline phosphatase. In the epiphysis, alkaline phosphatase becomes much more prominent in the transition regions between the hypertrophic cartilage cells and the zone of provisional calcification. Periosteum and deer antler velvet contain large amounts of alkaline phosphatase.

Calcification, however, seems to occur only when alkaline phosphatase is present. Newman

and Logan in 1953, using x-ray crystallographic analysis of bone salt, showed that the structure of bone mineral is compatible with hydroxyapatite, and they pointed out that a solid phase of apatite could not possibly form spontaneously by precipitation of calcium with local accumulations of phosphate ions but could form only by crystallization, either by stepwise additions of ions to a nucleation center or by some similar process involving the hydrolysis of a secondary calcium phosphate. They pointed out that the highly oriented crystal structure of bone could not be formed by calcium phosphate precipitation alone. Further evidence that mineralization does not occur by alkaline phosphatase acting to accumulate local phosphate ion concentration rests in the observation that active oxidative metabolism must be present for calcification and bone formation to occur. Furthermore, any metabolic inhibitors or poisons that interrupt the function of the Embden-Meyerhoff pathway and tricarboxylic acid cycle will prevent active calcification and bone formation. ATP is necessary for bone formation and cartilage calcification in embryonic sheep epiphysis. Evidence has accumulated from Danilli and Fell[3] and others that alkaline phosphatase appears in some way related to collagen fiber formation.

Of interest is the observation of Huggins in 1933, who found that pieces of urinary and gallbladder epithelium, which both contained large amounts of glycerol phosphatase, produced bone when transplanted into muscle. Attempts to produce heterotrophic bone formation by injection of alkaline phosphatase in the muscle, however, have been uniformly unsuccessful. Sobel believes that the process of calcification *in vivo* can and probably does take place without the intervention of phosphatase and adds further support to the concept that alkaline phosphatase is somehow connected to the production of organic matrix and the elaboration of the collagen fibril.

Large numbers of phosphatase-positive polymorphs are seen in areas around fracture and skin wounds within 24 hr of injury. They are accompanied by phosphatase-positive fibroblasts that appear to produce a mass of phosphatase-positive fibers. Loss of the phosphatase activity occurs as healing progresses. The appearance of phosphatase-positive fibers occurs during the healing process of skin wounds as well as at the site of fracture healing. All of these factors would seem to indicate that alkaline phosphatase probably plays some role in collagen fiber formation.

Vaes[35,36] has investigated the relationships of alkaline phosphatase, inorganic pyrophosphatase, protein phosphatase, and acid phosphatase in bone. More sophisticated investigative techniques have shown the problem to be increasingly complex, as there appear to be multiple alkaline phosphatases of different substrate specificities and pH optimum.

Acid phosphatase is an even more complex problem. Early studies of acid phosphatase were carried out histochemically using α.glycerol phosphate as substrate and tissue sections that in some cases had been fixed, as it was then thought that alkaline and acid phosphatase were fairly stable and easily preserved in tissue for study. In fact, however, acid phosphatase has been shown to be an extremely unstable, labile enzyme easily destroyed by careful efforts of preservation. Closer biochemical study revealed that multiple acid phosphatases exist throughout tissues. All acid phosphatase, however, does appear to be localized in lysosomal structures and is contained within the lipid envelope of the lysosome. It is this fact that has allowed identification of lysosomal structures through specific staining of acid phosphatase contained within the lipid envelope of the lysosome.

Differential centrifugation of bone homogenate has resulted in preparations of phosphoprotein phosphatase, acid inorganic pyrophosphatase, acid β-glycerol phosphatase, and various other less-well-defined acid phosphatases. Vaes[35,36,37] observed the highest specific activity of all these enzymes to be in the light mitochondrial fraction. The highest specific activity of alkaline inorganic pyrophosphatase and of various other alkaline phosphatase activities was found in the microsomal fraction.

Cytoplasmic extracts prepared in this manner from bone demonstrated the various acid phosphatase activities to exist in a latent form and as much as one half of the total acid phosphatase activity in bone is in fact latent. The latent enzyme can be unmasked by a number of treatments, which include surface tension agents, low osmotic pressure, and freezing and thawing. The same agents unmask lysosomal β-glucuronidase activity in a parallel manner. These results are consistent with the concept that phosphoprotein phosphatase, acid inorganic pyrophosphatase, β-glycerol phosphatase, and other acid phosphatases as well are all contained within the lysosomal structure. Microsomal fractions obtained by differential centrifugation of bone homogenates exert alkaline phosphatase activity upon many different substrates, including inorganic pyrophosphate, phosphoprotein (casein), paranitrophenylphosphate and β-glycerol phosphate. Particle-bound alkaline phosphatase sediments at a lower rate than does acid phosphatase and becomes more concentrated in the so-called P fraction. These factors strongly suggest that acid phosphatase activites are associated with the lysosomes, and alkaline activities are bound to the rather poorly characterized "microsomes," a group of particles that in liver contain rough and smooth membranes of the endoplasmic reticulum as well as fragments of the plasma membrane.

Inorganic pyrophosphatase does appear to have a known specific function and serves to break down inorganic pyrophosphate that accumulates as a result of tissue growth to low-energy inorganic phosphate (Fig. 6-9).[21] Using quantitative microchemical techniques, an enzyme has been demonstrated to be localized in the epiphyseal line to the proliferating cartilage cell zone that will hydrolyze inorganic pyrophosphatase at pH 8.0. Localization of inorganic pyrophosphatase in the proliferating cartilage cell zone of the epiphysis is of interest, as this is the major location of tissue synthesis required for epiphyseal growth. Virtually all metabolic sequences thus far demonstrated to synthesize protein use ATP-activated amino acids and liberate inorganic pyrophosphate as they are incorporated into peptide chains. Similarly, synthesis of DNA has been demonstrated to follow a similar pattern. These and other related reactions produce several molecules of pyrophosphate for every molecule of activated complex.

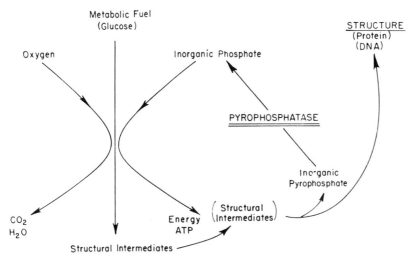

FIGURE 6-9   *Inorganic pyrophosphatase appears to be the only phosphatase occurring in skeletal tissue for which a specific role can be postulated. The probable functional inter-relationships of this enzyme are schematically illustrated.*

The inorganic pyrophosphatase system serves to prevent the accumulation of these inorganic pyrophosphate complexes and to permit cyclic utilization of inorganic phosphate. Furthermore, inorganic pyrophosphate acts to inhibit mineralization and calcification of bone by disruption of the crystal structure and must be removed before mineralization can occur. It is not clear, however, why the primary spongiosa, also an area of intense cellular proliferation, has not demonstrated large amounts of inorganic pyrophosphate activity. Indeed, it appears that inorganic pyrophosphatase is needed to reduce inorganic pyrophosphate in energy level to inorganic phosphate in order to prevent interference with the calcification process.

The biochemical events associated with the transition of cartilage to bone

The process of endochondral ossification

The growth of long bone occurs at the epiphysis by the process of endochondral ossification. During this process the sparsely placed unorganized cartilage cells proliferate and become rigidly aligned in the form of columns containing flattened cells (Fig. 6-10). The columns are separated by parallel bands of matrix and collagen fibers. These cells become swollen and appear to hypertrophy as they approach the zone of ossification. The adjacent matrix loses its proteoglycan content and therefore its metachromatic staining characteristic and becomes calcified. Abrupt transition of the collagen fibers from a noncalcified to a calcified state occurs at the zone of provisional calcification in the primary spongiosa. Histochemically, alkaline phosphatase becomes increasingly active as the organization of these cellular areas progresses, and it is particularly active at the zone of ossification.

The development of quantitative microchemical techniques has made it possible to study the enzymatic and physical alterations that accompany the process of endochondral bone formation, and it has become possible to quantitatively study cell clusters from each of these areas of the epiphyseal line.

The epiphysis overall contains large amounts of phosphorus, but as the cellular process of endochondral calcification advances, phosphorus content increases from a negligible fraction of the weight of the free and proliferating cell cartilages area to 4.25% of the hypertrophic cartilage cell and to 7% of the dry weight of the zone of provisional calcification and primary spongiosa (Table 6-3). Measurement of the enzyme content in these areas has demonstrated the presence of glucose 6-phosphate,[19] and lactic, isocitric, and malic dehydrogenases as well as alkaline phosphatase, phosphoglucosomerase, acid phosphatase, and inorganic pyrophosphatase. Lactic dehydrogenase has the greatest activity of the enzyme studies and was most active in the proliferating cartilage cell zone.

In the epiphyseal line, enzymes are present that are mediating carbohydrate metabolism not only through the Embden-Meyerhoff pathway and the citric acid cycle but also through the hexosmonophosphate shunt (Figs. 6-11 and 6-12). The cellular areas of the epiphyseal plate resemble those of the brain and retina by having lactic and malic dehydrogenase and phosphoglucosomerase as three of their most active enzymes.[25,26] Peak lactic dehydrogenase content in the proliferating and hypertrophic cell area reflects their avascularity, with subsequent low oxygen tension in that area and the reliance of these cellular areas on anaerobic glycolysis for energy production. Areas closer to blood supply, particularly the primary spongiosa, have higher levels of malic dehydrogenase and glucose 6-phosphate dehydrogenase. This observation reflects the growing importance of aerobic metabolism through the citric acid cycle and direct

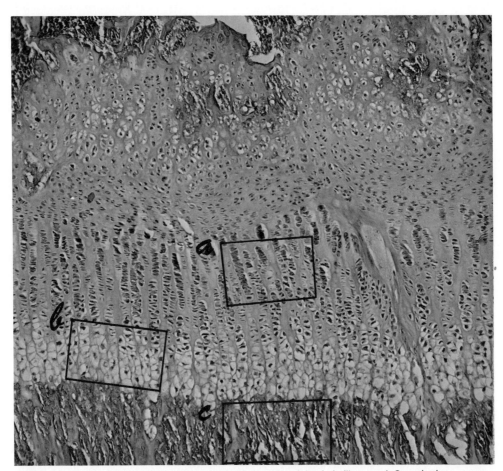

FIGURE 6-10 *Endochondral bone formation in the rabbit epiphysis is illustrated. Quantitative measurement of tissue enzyme and substrate content in selected areas from* **(a)** *the proliferating cartilage cell and* **(b)** *the hypertrophic cartilage cell.* **(c)** *Provisional calcification zones have been made using quantitative microchemical techniques, hematoxylin-eosin stain × 85.*

TABLE 6-3 PHOSPHORUS, ACID-SOLUBLE SOLID AND TOTAL SOLID CONTENT OF THE INDICATED AREAS OF THE DOG EPIPHYSEAL PLATE

LOCATION	TOTAL PHOSPHORUS CONTENT (mol/kg)	TOTAL SOLID CONTENT (g/liter)	ACID-SOLUBLE SOLID CONTENT (g/kg dry weight)
Unorganized cartilage cells	0.015	534	227
Proliferating cartilage cells	0.122	472	205
Hypertrophic cartilage cells	1.51	413	571
Primary spongiosa	2.15	849	689

oxidative pathways as oxygen is made increasingly available by invasion of blood supply into the epiphysis.

Activity of alkaline phosphatase in the epiphyseal plate is most noteworthy.[23] On a dry weight basis it is the only enzyme that is more active in the epiphyseal plate than in the cellular areas of the brain. A study of the phosphatase distribution using dinitrophenylphosphate as a substrate and measuring at pH 10.5 and pH 3.75 has demonstrated similar distributions of acid and alkaline phosphatase through the epiphyseal line. Inorganic pyrophosphatase through the epiphyseal line. Inorganic pyrophosphatase measured at the optimum pH 8.0 demonstrated that this enzyme has activity only in the zone containing proliferating cartilage cells. The more familiar nonspecific alkaline phosphatase, with its ability to split phosphate esters at alkaline pH, is present in the hypertrophic cartilage cell zone and in the primary spongiosa. Increasing activity of this system and that of the nonspecific acid phosphatase is associated with an increased inorganic phosphate content. Previous work, however, has failed to link this phosphatase activity with the phosphate accumulation required for mineralization. As pointed out previously, although acid phosphatase and alkaline phosphatase in these quantitative microchemical studies are considered single enzyme systems, they probably represent a composite activity of several systems.

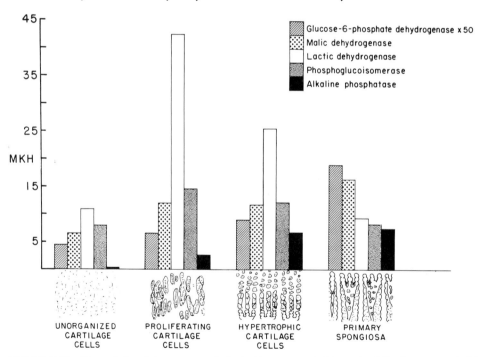

FIGURE 6-11 *The activity of the enzymes indicated is represented in each of the four recognizable areas of the epiphyseal line. Activity is expressed in terms of moles of substrate split or converted per kilogram dry weight of tissue per hour.*

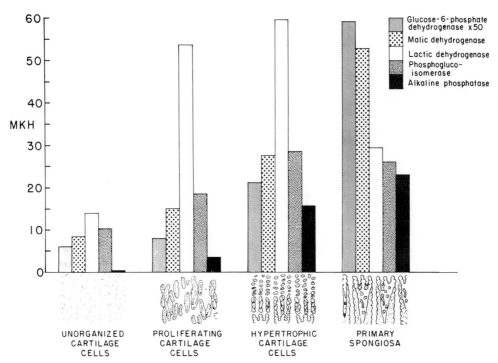

FIGURE 6-12   *The results demonstrated in Fig. 6-11 have been recalculated on the basis of nonacid extractable solid, and illustrate enzyme activity present in these tissue areas in a manner that can be more realistically compared with that of other tissues.*

Inorganic pyrophosphate has been identified in articular and epiphyseal cartilage, and localization of inorganic pyrophosphatase in the proliferating zone of epiphysis is of interest in view of the role pyrophosphate plays in biologic synthetic systems.[19] Inorganic pyrophosphate is a unique compound in biologic systems and has been demonstrated to be the by-product of several different types of structural syntheses.[15] All metabolic sequences thus far demonstrated to synthesize protein use ATP-activated amino acid intermediates that are incorporated into peptide chains with formation of free inorganic pyrophosphate. The synthesis of important DNA has been demonstrated by Kornberg[15] to follow similar patterns. These and other reactions produce several molecules of pyrophosphate for every molecule of activated complex. It seems reasonable that some enzymatic mechanism must prevent the accumulation of inorganic pyrophosphate and permit cyclic reutilization of inorganic phosphate.

It is not clear why primary spongiosa, also an area of intense cellular proliferation, does not demonstrate inorganic pyrophosphatase activity. Krane and Glimsher[16] have demonstrated that ATP is extensively bound by apatite crystals and that this binding is prevented and reversed by the presence of inorganic pyrophosphate. One might speculate that the accumulation of pyrophosphate in the primary spongiosa is prevented by the association of pyrophosphate with apatite crystals in this area and that this association exerts a protective effect. An attempt to schematically illustrate the role that inorganic pyrophosphatase may have in the cyclic metabolic sequences affecting bone growth is given in Fig. 6-9.

The hypertrophic cartilage cell zone

During endochondral ossification the proliferating cartilage cells, supported in columns by tubular channels of matrix and collagen fibers, swell and enlarge to form the hypertrophic car-

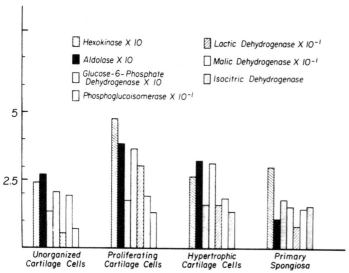

FIGURE 6-13 *The distribution of glycolytic enzymes through the rabbit epiphyseal line is demonstrated. Values are reported as moles of substrate converted per kilogram dry weight of tissue. Note the substantial activity present in the hypertrophic cartilage cell area.*

tilage cell area. Contemporary views of histology hold the cellular constituents of the hypertrophic cartilage cell zone to be in a dying and disintegrating state. Near its edge, the cartilaginous matrix lying between the cellular columns undergoes calcification to become the zone of provisional calcification and primary spongiosa (Figs. 6-13 and 6-14).

Study of the glucose, lactate, ATP, inorganic phosphate, and hydroxyproline content, as well as the enzymes mediating carbohydrate metabolism and their localization, have indicated that

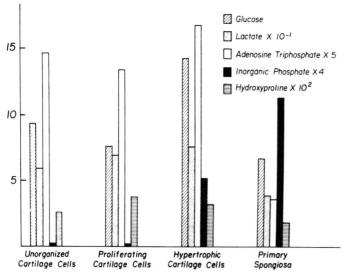

FIGURE 6-14 *The quantitative distribution of important constituents through the rabbit epiphyseal line is illustrated. Results are reported as micromoles per gram dry weight of tissue.*

active oxidative metabolism occurs in the epiphyseal line, and the high levels of these parameters of cellular metabolism in the hypertrophic cartilage cells appear inconsistent with the concept that it is composed of dying, deteriorating cells.[22] Although inorganic pyrophosphatase is contained almost exclusively in the proliferating area, there is also some activity in the hypertrophic cartilage cells, indicating that synthetic activity is occurring there also. Acid phosphatase activity, which must be considered an indication of all lysosomal enzymes, is quite active in the hypertrophic cartilage cell area. Its presence is probably related to the revision of cartilage matrix occurring in this area and reflects the importance of the lysosomal enzymes to this process. The hypertrophic area, despite its supposedly dying state, has the highest ATP and glucose content present in the epiphyseal line.

The epiphyseal structure has the remarkable capacity of providing functioning structural support and at the same time allowing longitudinal growth to occur. Although the active area of the plate has been illustrated to undergo active biochemical synthesis, the metabolic cost of maintaining a given volume of cartilage is low as compared with other tissues. For example, the brain contains 1.5 M of glucose/kg of tissue, 2.3 M of lactate/kg of tissue, and 2.4 M of ATP/kg of tissue, and upon devitalization, these metabolic substrates are used within minutes, whereas epiphyseal cartilage retains its considerably smaller content of these structures for a prolonged time, as illustrated in Figures 6-15 and 6-16.

The epiphyseal mechanism functions with nearly identical morphological structure throughout many phylogenetic species. Investigation of the enzyme distribution through the epiphyseal line in several mammalian species indicates that they are biochemically similar also. Morphologically, although the hypertrophic area appears to contain dying cells, biochemically it acts as a living and growing tissue. The discrepancy between microscopic and chemical findings may well represent a fixation artifact. Uptake studies using tritiated cytidine have indicated that active RNA synthesis and hence protein synthesis occurs in the hypertrophic areas of the epiphyseal line. The most sensitive index to high oxygen tension is transitory, increased length of the zone of hypertrophic cells with persisting high oxygen tension; the cartilaginous portions of the epiphyseal line show narrowing and pro-

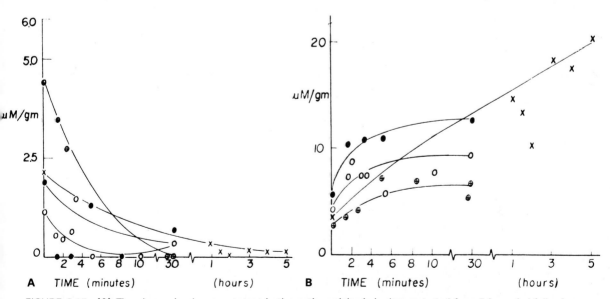

FIGURE 6-15 **(A)** *The change in glucose content in the entire epiphysis is demonstrated for a 5-hr period following death. Results are reported as micromoles per gram wet weight of tissue.* **(B)** *The change in lactate content of the entire epiphysis is demonstrated for a 5-hr period following death.*

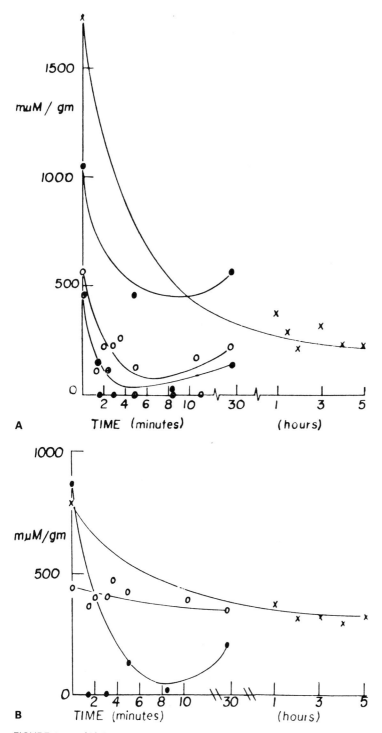

FIGURE 6-16 **(A)** *Phosphocreatine content of whole rabbit epiphysis and its change after death. Results reported as millimicromoles per gram of wet tissue.* **(B)** *ATP content of the whole rabbit epiphysis and its change after death.*

196

gressive loss of acid mucopolysaccharides and eventual loss of the hypertrophic cartilage cell zone.

The biochemical relationships of deer antlerogenesis and endochondral bone formation

Bone formation occurs not only as a structural element to support the body but also as an appendage when it forms antler structure in reindeer. It is formed in this structure by a process that has both similarities and differences to that of endochondral ossification (Fig. 6-17).

Previous workers (Wislocki)[39] have demonstrated that the process of antlerogenesis results in the production of a true bone structure complete with a canalicular system. What makes this process particularly remarkable in the deer antler is the rapid rate of bone formation that occurs. Our studies have demonstrated that antler length increases at an average rate of ¼ in/d. The rate of true bone formation is much more rapid than that observed in any other body location or animal regardless of its age or species. This unprecedented rate of bone formation results in the production of a structure in a 3- to 4-mo period of time equivalent to one sixth of the entire total skeletal bulk of the animal. This structure is shed annually and must be regrown each year. The demands upon the calcium reserves of the animal during this period of rapid bone manufacture do not produce any change in blood levels of calcium, phosphorus, or protein. These observations reflect the extensive compensatory activity of the parathyroid system in these animals with renal regulation of phosphate level. Of

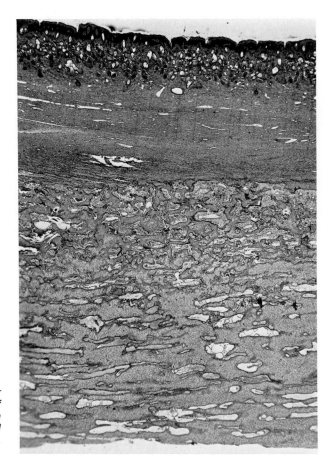

FIGURE 6-17 *Histologic preparation of deer antler velvet during active bone formation. Samples of tissue taken from representative areas have been assayed for their enzyme content and compared with those present in developing epiphysis, hemoxylin-eosin stain × 10.*

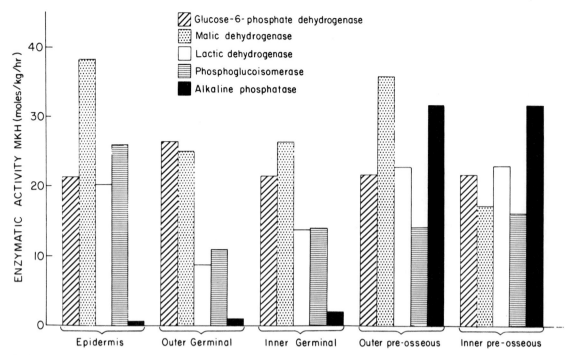

FIGURE 6-18   *The measurement of carbohydrate-metabolizing enzymes in the functional areas of the deer antler velvet is represented. The results are presented in terms comparable to those used previously in the study of enchondral bone development (moles of substrate split or converted per kilogram dry weight of tissue per hour).*

particular importance to this process of bone formation, again, is the enzyme alkaline phosphatase, whose activity in serum was demonstrated to rise as much as five times over resting levels at periods of active antler formation. The marked fall in circulating enzyme after amputation of the growing antler indicates that the source of the enzyme is the active proliferating cellular areas of the antler, and that the escape of the enzyme from these areas into the venous blood is the source of the high levels circulating in the body.[6]

Using conventional staining techniques, Wislocki[39] has demonstrated basophilic proteoglycan ground substance and characteristic metachromatic staining features present in the preosseous areas of the deer antler tine prior to actual ossification. His studies have demonstrated that these very active bone-forming areas contain large amounts of lipid material, and he has illustrated histologically the distribution of elastic tissue, calcium, phosphate, and nonspecific

phosphatase in the antler structure. He further has provided detailed descriptions of the histologic features of the progressive stage of bone growth in the deer antler.

Briefly, antler growth begins each spring from a pedicle overlying the frontal bone. The pedicle is covered with a newly formed hairless skin that is filled with highly vascular immature proliferative fibrocellular tissue. A narrow intermediate zone of spongy osseous trabeculae later develops, which resembles the frontal bone. Growth of the antler, however, proceeds outward from this site, and antlerogenesis occurs from the tip. The soft skin covering the antler consists of an epidermis resting on a well-demarcated corium. The corium can be divided into an inner and outer layer and has long parallel collagenous bundles that are interspersed with numerous vascular channels. The corium rests on a lamella of fibrocellular tissue, the so-called preosseous zone, which undergoes calcification and arrangement into bone. The fibrocellular cap is similar to periosteum, as it has the property of producing bone, and it is the fibrocellular layer over the pedicle that commences the deposition of spongy bone into irregular delicate columns beneath the preosseous zone. Growth occurs from the tip downward, whereas calcification of newly formed bone takes place at the base of the antler upward toward the tip. Antler growth, however, is dependent upon and controlled by the formation of the germinal layer from skin—an ectodermal derivative.

Enzymes mediating carbohydrate metabolism were found distributed in similar amounts through the different stages of maturation present in the antler tine (Fig. 6-18). Its content of lactic dehydrogenase is substantially less than in the epiphyseal line. In contrast, much higher levels of aerobically functioning enzymes of malic, glucose 6-phosphate dehydrogenase, and phosphoglucosomerase are observed.[18] Their presence reflects the excellent blood supply and high oxygen tension present. These enzymes are approximately twice as active as they are in dog epiphyseal line, for example. Lactic dehydrogenase levels are somewhat lower than anticipated from other studies. It seems likely that the very rapid bone growth present in the deer antler is the result of greater energy availability provided by the more efficient function of aerobic metabolic pathways. The level of phosphate in the antler tine is substantially less than it is in epiphyseal cartilage. In contrast, alkaline phosphatase sharply increases in the preosseous zones, and in these locations rises to an extremely high level. There is, however, little bone salt deposited in these locations, and this observation supports the hypothesis that alkaline phosphatase probably does not function to provide a local increase in phosphate ion concentration, but rather is important in matrix synthesis. The level of alkaline phosphatase is four times greater than the highest level in the epiphyseal plate of the dog, and it is felt that the extremely high levels of alkaline phosphatase present in the preosseous areas of the antler tine are responsible for the circulating enzyme of the blood (Fig. 6-19).

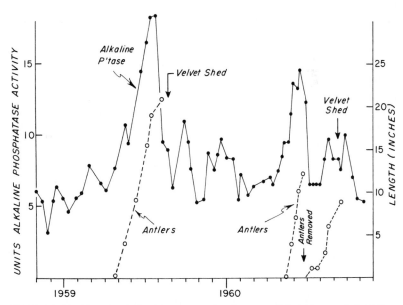

FIGURE 6-19   *The correlation between antler tine growth in inches and circulating alkaline phosphatase levels measured in Bodansky units is demonstrated. Note the precipitous alkaline phosphatase drop that occurs when the velvet is shed. One year later, 4 wk after growth began, the tine was amputated. Note the decline of alkaline phosphatase circulating in the blood.*

The biochemical response of the cartilaginous epiphysis to devitalization

The alterations of tissue biochemistry that occur in epiphyseal cartilage during the immediate postmortem period are largely unknown. It is of interest that several epiphyseal disorders appear to be the result of *in vivo* death. In general, histologic studies have been unable to illustrate the subtle biochemical changes that precede morphologically recognizable tissue necrosis. Lowry[25,26] has developed highly sensitive specific methods for the assay of metabolic intermediates in extremely small tissue samples and has applied these techniques to investigate the sequence of events biochemically that occur in the brain following death. This advance in methodology has permitted us to delineate some of the immediate postmortem biochemical sequences that occur in connection with epiphyseal cartilage death. The *in vivo* contents of glucose, lactate, ATP, and phosphocreatine of the rabbit epiphyseal cartilage have been measured and their rates of change following devitalization documented.[19,21] This information has provided us with some estimate of (1) the normal rate of carbohydrate metabolism present in the areas of the epiphyseal line, and (2) the time required for biochemical death and disruption of epiphyseal cartilage and the associated biochemical sequence of events. Initial studies using whole epiphyseal homogenates demonstrate that soon after interruption of nutritional supply, the normal metabolic arrangement of the epiphysis is altered. Lowry[25,26] demonstrated that brain loses substantial amounts of ATP and phosphocreatine during the first minute after decapitation. We were unable to demonstrate biochemical changes in the whole epiphysis during the first 90 sec after death because of technical problems. However, 10 min following tissue isolation, the glucose content fell to low levels and remained there throughout the period investigated. These observations indicated that primarily anaerobic glucose catabolism occurred in the isolated epiphysis, and it was demonstrated that the resultant end product was lactate, which accumulated to substantial levels after devitalization. ATP levels fell immediately after devitalization

to about one half of the *in vivo* level and then remained stable for long periods. In general, more variability was encountered in the measurement of epiphyseal substrate content, and it is believed that these observations reflected their labile nature. In general, little or no difference could be detected in the response of samples that were devitalized and allowed to remain in contact with air, as compared with those that were maintained under oil. Presumably the large sample size, which comprised the entire epiphysis, prevented significant atmospheric diffusion. Although substantially less active metabolically than the brain, in which similar studies have been carried out, epiphyseal cartilage is demonstrated to be living, metabolizing tissue that undergoes immediate biochemical modification following interruption of the blood supply. Initially, glucose reserves are depleted anaerobically with simultaneous accumulation of lactate. Phosphocreatine content drops sharply, recovers somewhat, and then remains essentially stable. ATP levels fall to about one half of their resting level, then stabilize, and remain stable for more than 5 hr. Epiphyseal cartilage depletes its reserve of high-energy compounds at a considerably slower rate than does brain. Lowry[25,26] has estimated adult rat brain use of ATP at 2.2 μmol/g/min of tissue, which is several order of magnitudes greater than that indicated for epiphyseal cartilage. The considerably lower content and utilization rates of high-energy phosphate compounds in the epiphysis with respect to the brain could be easily expected on the basis of its contrasting physiology. Presumably the lack of neutral and contractile elements in cartilage make extensive, immediately available high-energy phosphate reserves unnecessary.

Maintenance of high-energy phosphate levels occurs by the metabolic conversion of glucose to lactate and through the transfer of high-energy phosphate from phosphocreatine. These observations explain the clinical fact that unlike the central nervous system, epiphyseal cartilage nutrition may be interrupted for a considerable period of time during surgical procedures without influence upon further growth potential or function.

After gross study of the entire epiphysis, it

became apparent that the information obtained represented the reaction of devitalization of many composite structures. Application of quantitative microchemical methods were undertaken to study the biochemical effects of devitalization in the individual cellular constituents of the epiphyseal line. In general, similar results occur, but significant quantitative differences are shown in the proliferating and hypertrophic cartilage cell areas and the primary spongiosa, which are much more responsive to a lack of nutritional supply. During the first hour of avascularity a significant decline in glucose content occured only in the primary spongiosa. ATP declined significantly only in the morphologically active zone of proliferating cartilage cells. Lactate increased significantly only in the primary spongiosa. After 2 hr of avascularity the glucose content of all the epiphyseal zones had fallen to barely detectable levels. ATP content was well preserved in the more dormant, unorganized cell zone and to a lesser extent in the primary spongiosa, but was reduced in the other epiphyseal areas to almost nothing. Lactate increased throughout the epiphyseal areas (Figs. 6-20–6-23).

Concomitant studies of skeletal muscles were undertaken to compare the responses of these two tissues to devitalization. The rate of change in the substrate concentration during complete ischemia was much more rapid in skeletal muscle than in the epiphyseal line. During the first 10 min, the only statistically significant drop in skeletal muscle was in the phosphocreatine content; however, after the first 10 min, the content of ATP and phosphocreatine dropped off significantly with simultaneous lactate accumulation. Glucose levels remained constant or increased compared with the control levels. Phosphocreatine had nearly disappeared at the end of the first hour. ATP, although reduced by some 80% or more from the control level, was still detectable up until the fifth hour of study (Figs. 6-24 and 6-25).

These observations demonstrated that tissue metabolism continues in an isolated system and that the metabolic activity in the presence of ischemia of skeletal tissue proceeds almost entirely in an anaerobic fashion, as it would have to without oxygen. In general, the modification in the substrate content of the epiphyseal plate and the surrounding skeletal muscle occurs in a much less dramatic fashion than it does in the brain, which has been studied by previous investigators. Epiphyseal cartilage responds much

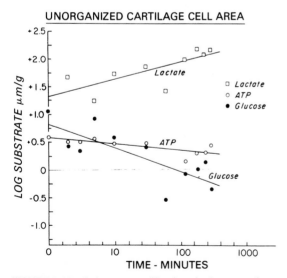

FIGURE 6-20 *Substrate modifications in the zone of unorganized cartilage cells of the epiphyseal line after devitalization. The log substrate concentration (micromole per gram) is plotted against time.*

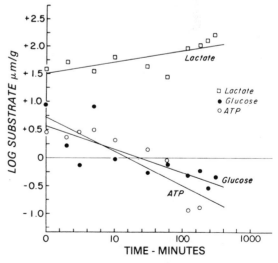

FIGURE 6-21 *Substrate modifications in the zone of proliferating cells of the epiphyseal line after devitalization. The log substrate concentration (micromole per gram) is plotted against time.*

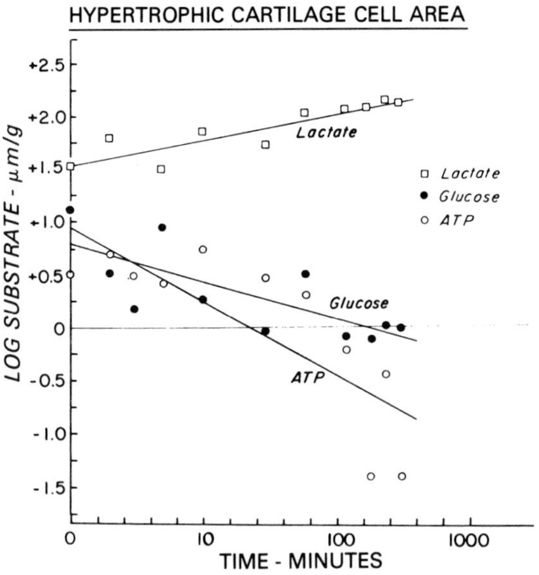

HYPERTROPHIC CARTILAGE CELL AREA

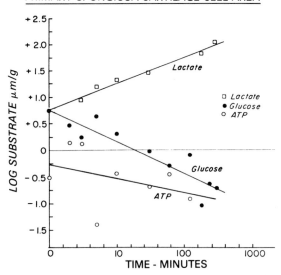

FIGURE 6-22 *Substrate modifications in the zone of hypertrophic cells of the epiphyseal line after devitalization. The log substrate concentration (micromole per gram) is plotted against log time.*

PRIMARY SPONGIOSA CARTILAGE CELL AREA

FIGURE 6-23 *Substrate modifications in the primary spongiosa of the epiphyseal line after devitalization. The log substrate concentration (micromole per gram) is plotted against time.*

TISSUE CONSTITUENTS OF SKELETAL MUSCLE

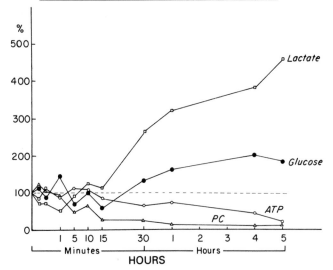

FIGURE 6-24 *Changes in tissue constituents of skeletal muscle after devitalization expressed as percentages of the in vivo levels: glucose = 1.57 mμ/mg, lactate = 11.8 mμ/mg, ATP = 5.16 mμ/mg, and phosphocreatine = 7.38 mμ/mg.*

202

more slowly to devitalization than the skeletal muscle, and there is a qualitative difference between the response of cartilage and muscle. Interestingly, skeletal muscle actually accumulates a small amount of glucose during the initial 5 hr of avascularity, whereas in epiphyseal cartilage the glucose is used, and drops to a low value early.

The question of when the precise biochemical event of death occurs in epiphyseal cartilage and muscle has not been answered by these studies. Presumably, however, biochemical death supervenes when all reserves of ATP have been depleted from the tissue. If this supposition is correct, these data indicate that the structural components of the epiphyseal line, and to a lesser extent of skeletal muscle, exhibit substantial reserve following devitalization. This observation correlates well with the known successful transplantation of epiphyseal structures and the recently described successful reimplantation of extremities after their severance from the body. A sequence of events can be postulated to occur following ischemia of epiphyseal cartilage, and it would seem that at first epiphyseal areas use all reserves at hand to maintain ATP levels. Tissue

EPIPHYSEAL CARTILAGE

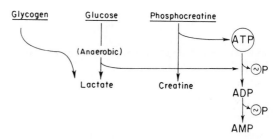

FIGURE 6-26 *Based upon the study of substrate depletion that occurs in the areas of the epiphysis following devitalization, this sequence of events can be postulated to immediately precede tissue death. When all reserves of high-energy phosphate have been depleted, death supervenes.*

metabolism in an isolated system continues exclusively anaerobically with extensive lactate accumulation and simultaneous glucose depletion. As these systems begin to fail, AMP accumulates (Figs. 6-26 and 6-27). In contrast, skeletal muscle maintains ATP by the anaerobic use of its substantial glycogen stores, again with lactate accumulation. Previous workers have demonstrated that the accumulation of AMP acts as a strong vasodilator. All of these observations indicate that epiphyseal cartilage and muscle of an extremity have considerable resistance to devitalization and serve to substantiate the feasibility of extremity transplantation and reimplantation.

TISSUE CONSTITUENTS OF MUSCLE

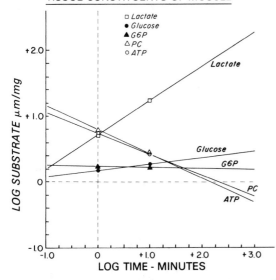

FIGURE 6-25 *Early changes in tissue constituents of muscle after devitalization. The logarithm of concentration (millimicromole per milligram) is plotted against time.*

SKELETAL MUSCLE

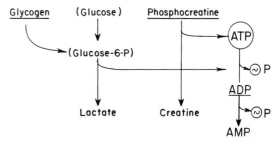

FIGURE 6-27 *Based upon the pattern of substrate depletion following devitalization of skeletal muscle, the biochemical sequence of events shown in this figure occurs in skeletal muscle until its ability to maintain a high-energy phosphate level is lost, at which time death occurs.*

The biochemical events associated with the transition to bone

The process of fracture healing

Prior study of fracture repair has been limited to the histologic description of the process. These studies have attempted to establish the roles of the periosteum and endosteum to the process. Supplementation of audioradiographic techniques have defined the importance of these structures and the origin of the vast number of cells involved in the process of fracture repair.

Limited biochemical information is available regarding the metabolic characteristics of the various tissues that constitute fracture callus and that participate in fracture healing, and most of it has resulted from histochemical staining methods. Robison[28] described the relation of alkaline phosphatase to fracture healing, and Stirling and Murray have attempted to relate acid and alkaline pH shifts in fracture hematoma to the process of fracture healing. Direct biochemical study of fracture callus has been limited, but the recent advances in technique have made it possible through the application of quantitative microchemical methods.

Biochemical analysis of some 3000 samples obtained from morphologically isolated uniform areas of fracture callus has been reported.[23] Many of these areas have morphological similarity to the cell zones of the epiphyseal line, and it is possible to identify in fracture callus areas of undifferentiated and hypertrophic-appearing cartilage cells. In other areas of fracture callus, rapidly proliferating fibrous tissue is recognizable. When these individual tissue areas were dissected out from fracture callus and their chemistry was compared with what appeared to be similar areas in the epiphyseal line, interesting observations were obtained. As would be expected, the results were substantially more variable, as the architecture of these areas was more irregular and difficult to define than in the more neatly arranged epiphyseal line (Table 6-4).

Levels of hexokinase, lactate, malic and isocitric dehydrogenase, as well as the phosphatase studies, closely approximated those previously demonstrated to exist in the proliferating and hypertrophic cartilage cell zones of the epiphyseal plate. No significant variation in enzyme content of the cellular constituents of fracture callus appeared to occur from the time that they were morphologically recognizable until the repair sequence was concluded. Little alkaline phosphatase was noted in the undifferentiated cartilage cell areas surrounding active fracture callus. However, as fibrous elements proliferated, more than a tenfold increase was observed, and the greatest content of alkaline phosphatase was observed in the hypertrophic cartilage cell areas adjacent to new bone formation. The localization of alkaline phosphatase in fracture callus was demonstrated to be similar to that present in epiphyseal cartilage. However, on a dry weight basis, fracture callus contains sub-

TABLE 6-4   ENZYME AND CONSTITUENT CONTENT OF 3-WK-OLD RABBIT FRACTURE CALLUS

| | FRACTURE CALLUS AREA | | | |
ENZYME	UNDIFFERENTIATED	PROLIFERATIVE FIBROUS TISSUE	HYPERTROPHIC CARTILAGE	NEWLY FORMED BONE
Malic dehydrogenase	37.2	19.7	20.0	10.1
Hydroxyproline	0.014	0.024	0.016	0.013
Hexokinase	0.27	0.30	0.20	0.13
Lactic dehydrogenase	210.0	85.6	28.6	21.2
Alkaline phosphatase	0.16	7.33	11.7	7.27
Glucose-6-phosphate dehydrogenase	0.03	0.16	0.15	0.15
Acid phosphatase	0.4	1.75	3.58	1.92
Isocitric dehydrogenase	5.92	3.91	1.51	1.29
Inorganic pyrophosphatase	2.63	2.96	3.75	2.64
Inorganic phosphate	0.05	0.38	0.40	3.75

Results are reported as moles of substrate split or converted per kilogram dry weight of tissue per hour.
Inorganic phosphate and hydroxyproline are reported as moles of phosphate present per kilogram of tissue dry weight.

FRACTURE HEALING

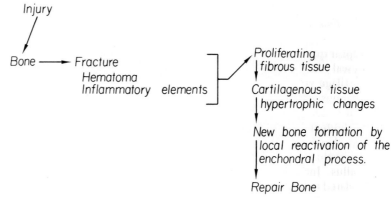

FIGURE 6-28 *Fracture healing may be considered a reactivation of the process of enchondral bone formation.*

stantially greater amounts than noted in the epiphysis.

Acid phosphatase distribution was quite similar to that of alkaline phosphatase and again was most active in hypertrophic zones. Inorganic pyrophosphatase activity was noted predominantly in proliferating fibrous tissue and cartilage area, and its activity appeared related to enzymic steps of tissue synthesis. Inorganic phosphate content increased from very low levels in the undifferentiated cells to high levels as bone was deposited. Hydroxyproline content was quite low in the undifferentiated zone, as would be expected by the complete lack of supportive structural elements in these undifferentiated cell

areas. However, little difference was noted in the hydroxyproline content of fibrous tissue and of the cartilaginous areas of callus. It would appear, therefore, that the major difference between these areas was the accumulation of proteoglycans interspersed between the collagen fibers of these tissues.

Enzymes mediating oxidative carbohydrate metabolism are present in considerable amounts in fracture callus, which indicates that the process of bone repair relies upon oxidative carbohydrate metabolism to obtain structural intermediates and energy. As soon as the cellular elements of fracture callus become defined, the quantitative relationships of their enzyme con-

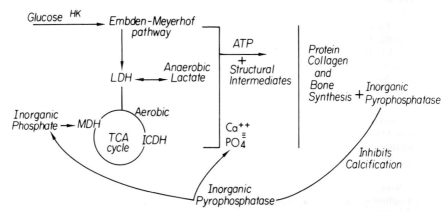

FIGURE 6-29 *Oxidative metabolism of glucose through known pathways produces structural intermediates for fracture repair. Inorganic pyrophosphate, produced as structural elements are assembled, is reduced to inorganic phosphate to prevent inhibition of calcification should the inorganic pyrophosphate accumulate.*

tent appear quite similar to the previously studied epiphyseal line hypertrophic and proliferative cartilage cell areas. Although the quantitative amount of each particular tissue element may vary during the process of fracture healing, the individual tissue areas, when they can be isolated, have essentially identical biochemical characteristics regardless of the age of the fracture callus. Inorganic pyrophosphatase appears to be related to structural synthesis and occurs in relation to the proliferating fibrous tissue and cartilaginous areas of callus. The decline of its activity as fracture union approaches seems to reflect a slow-down of tissue construction as repair nears completion. This enzyme plays an important role in removing the pyrophosphate accumulated from protein DNA and RNA tissue synthesis, which would otherwise serve to inhibit mineralization of newly formed bone (Figs. 6-28 and 6-29).

References

1. Abramson, M.: Collagenolytic activity in middle ear cholesteatoma. Ann. Otol. Rhinol. Laryngol. 78:112–124, 1969.
2. Cuervo, L. A., Howell, D. S., and Pita, J. C.: Role of carbonic anhydrase in maintaining a high PH at the calcifying site of epiphyseal plates. J. Clin. Invest. 50:23a, 1971.
3. Danielli, J. F.: Phosphatases and other enzymes considered in relation to active transport and the function of fibrous protein structures. Proc. Roy. Soc., Series B, 142:146–154, 1954.
4. Eisen, A. Z., Jeffrey, J. J., and Gross, J.: Human skin collagenase: isolation and mechanism of attack on the collagen molecule. Biochim. Biophys. Acta 151:637–645, 1968.
5. Fleming, A.: On a remarkable bacteriolytic element found in tissues and secretions. Proc. Roy. Soc., Ser. B. 93:306, 1922.
6. Graham, E. A., Rainey, R., Kuhlman, R. E., Houghton, E. H., and Moyer, C. A.: Biochemical investigations of deer antler growth. Part I., Alterations of deer blood chemistry resulting from antlerogenesis. J. Bone and J. Surg. 44A:482–488, 1962.
7. Griffith, G. C., Nichols, G. and Asher, J. D.: Heparin osteoporosis. J.A.M.A. 193:91–94, 1965.
8. Gross, J., and Lapiere, C. M.: Collagenolytic activity in amphibian tissues. A tissue culture assay. Proc. Natl. Acad. of Sci. U.S.A., 48:1014–1022, 1962.
9. Gross, J.: How tadpoles loose their tails. J. Invest. Dermatol. 47:274–277, 1966.
10. Gross, J., and Shoshans, S.: Biosynthesis and metabolism of collagen and in tissue repair processes. Israel, J. Med. Sci. 10:537–561, 1974.
11. Harris, E. D., Jr., and Krane, S. M.: An endopeptidase from rheumatoid synovial tissue culture. Biochem. Biophys. Acta. 258:566–576, 1972.
12. Harris, E. D., Jr., and Krane, S. M.: Collagenases, New Eng. J. Med. 291:558–563, 1974.
13. Hauser, P., and Vaes, G.: Synthesis and secretion of rabbit bone marrow macrophages in culture of a neutral proteinase that degrades cartilage proteoglycans. Biochem. Soc. Trans., 569th Meeting, Sussex, pps. 1091–1093.
14. Howell, D. S., Pita, J. C., Marquez, J. G. and Madruga, J. E.: Partition of calcium, phosphate, and protein in the fluid phase aspirated at calcifing sites in epiphyseal cartilage. J. Clin. Invest. 47:1121, 1968.
15. Kornberg, A.: Reversable enzymatic synthesis of diphosphopyridine nucleotide and inorganic pyrophosphate. J. Biol. Chem. 182:779, 1950.
16. Krane, S. M., and Glimcher, M. J.: Transphosphorylation of nucleoside di- and triphosphophate by apatite crystals. J. Biol. Chem., 237:2991–2998, 1962.
17. Kuettner, K. E., Eisenstein, Reuben, and Sorgente, N.: Lysozyme in calcifing tissues. Clin. Orthop., 112:316–339, 1975.
18. Kuhlman, R. E., Graham, E. A., Rainey, R., Houghton, E. H. and Moyer, C. A.: Biochemical investigation of deer antler growth, II. Quantitative microchemical changes associated with antler bone formation. J. Bone Joint Surg. 45A:345–350. 1963.
19. Kuhlman, R. E.: A microchemical study of the developing epiphyseal plate. J. Bone Joint Surg., 42A:457–466, 1960.
20. Kuhlman, R. E. and Miller, J. A.: The initial postmortem biochemical changes that occur in epiphyseal cartilage. Clin. Orthop. 42:191–195, 1965.
21. Kuhlman, R. E.: Phosphatase in epiphyseal cartilage. Their possible role in tissue synthesis. J. Bone Joint Surg., 47A:545–550, 1965.

22. Kuhlman, R. E. and Miller, J. A.: The biochemical changes proceeding tissue death in rats. J. Bone Joint Surg. 49A:90–101, 1967.

23. Kuhlman, R. E., and McNamee, M. J.: The biochemical importance of the hypertrophic cartilage cell area to enchondral bone formation. J. Bone Joint Surg., 52A:1025–1032, 1970.

24. Kuhlman, R. E. and McNamee, M. J.: The biochemical activity of fracture callus in relation to bone production. Clin. Orthop., 1975. 107:258–265.

25. Lowry, O. H.: The quantitative histochemistry of the brain. Histological Sampling. J. Histochem. and Cytochem., 1:420–428, 1953.

26. Lowry, O. H., Passonneau, J. V., Hasselberger, F. X., and Schulz, D. W.: Effect of ischemia a known substrates and cofactors of the glycolytic pathway in brain. J. Biol. Chem., 239:18–30, 1964.

27. Miller, E. J. and Matukas, V. J.: Biosynthesis of collagen., Fed. Proc. 33:1197–1204, 1974.

28. Robison, R. A.: The possible significance of hexosephosphoric esters in ossification. Biochem. J. 17:286, 1923.

29. Rosenberg, L., Choi, H., Pal, S. and Tang, L.: Carbohydrate, protein interactions in proteoglycans. *In* ACS Symposium Series, No. 88. Carbohydrate—Protein interaction. Ed. I. J. Goldstein. Am. Chem. Soc., 1979.

30. Rosenberg, L.: Structure of cartilage proteoglycans. In. dynamics of connective tissue macromolecules. Ed. P. M. C. Burleigh and A. R. Poole, North-Holland Publishing Company, pp. 105–128. Amsterdam.

31. Sakamoto, S., Goldhaber, P., Glimcher, M. J.: The further purification and characterization of mouse bone collagenase. Calcif. Tissue Res. 10:142–151, 1972.

32. Sakamoto, S., Sakamoto, M., Goldhaber, P., and Glimcher, M. J.: Mouse bone collagenase. Arch. Biochem. and Biophys., 188:438–449, 1978.

33. Schwartz, E. R., Ogle, R. C. and Thompson, R. C.: Arylsulfatase activities in normal and pathologic human articular cartilage. Arth. and Rheum. 17:455–467, 1974.

34. Shimizer, M., Glimcher, M. J., Tranis, D. *et al.*: Mouse bone collagenase: isolation, partial purification, and mechanism of action. Proc. Soc. Exp. Biol. Med. 130:1175–1180, 1969.

35. Vaes, G.: Lysosomes and cellular physiology of bone resorption, *In* Lysosomes in Biopby and Pathology. Ed. J. T. Dingle and H. B. Fell. Vol. 1., North-Holland Publishing Company, Amsterdam, 1969, pp. 217–253.

36. Vaes, G., and Eeckhout, Y.: The precursor of bone collagenase and its activation from protides of biological fluids. Vol. 22, Ed., H. Peeters, 1975, Pergamon Press, Oxford.

37. Vaes, G., Eeckhout, Y., Lenaers-Claeys, G., Francois-Gillet, C., and Duretz, J.: The simultaneous release by bone explants in culture and the parallel activation of procollaginase and of a latent neutral proteinase that degrades cartilage proteoglycans and denatured collagen. Biochem. J. 172:261–274, 1978.

38. Vreven, J., Lieberherr, M., and Vaes, G.: The acid and alkaline phosphatases inorganic pyrophosphatases and phosphoprotein phosphatase of bone. Biochem. et Biophys. Acta, 293:170–177, 1973.

39. Wislocki, G. B.: Studies on the growth of deer antlers. Am. J. Anat. 71:371–406, 1942.

40. Wolff, L. K.: Untersuchungen über das lysozyme. Z Immunitäetsforsch. 50:88, 1927.

41. Wolinsky, I. and Chon, D. V.: Bone lysozyme: partial purification, properties and depression of activity by parathyroid extract. Nature (London) 210:413, 1966.

Our understanding of skeletal physiology and pathology has dramatically improved since 1955 and is continuing to do so. This chapter surveys selected areas of that new understanding that concern orthopedists, both in passing specialty boards and in fulfilling ongoing clinical responsibilities. Although the editor assigned the task of describing bone remodeling processes, and that description does constitute the largest single section in this chapter, the subject must fit into perspective with other skeletal phenomena equally important to skeletal physiology and clinical practice. The bulk of this chapter supplies some of that important overview, and in doing so it concentrates upon the tissue mechanisms that underlie clinical affections, anticipating that a description of such mechanisms will endure longer as useful text than a description of current—and sometimes evanescent—concepts of what regulates those mechanisms. The text assumes familiarity with skeletal anatomy, histology, and pathology as current medical school curricula provide them, and it will define many of its terms—some new to anatomical sciences and others given arbitrary new meanings.†

First the text outlines a conceptual way to analyze the histologic composition of skeletal organs and then describes some important processes encountered in those organs.

The basic composition of skeletal organs

As the cell constitutes a fundamental unit of life, *simple tissues* form the fundamental unit of organs. A simple tissue contains one or more types of

H. M. FROST

7

skeletal physiology and bone remodeling *

* The writer is indebted to the medical illustration department of Henry Ford Hospital and to A. M. Parfitt, M.D. for most of the illustrations in the text, and also to P. Meunier, M.D. for the stair graph concept. The staff of the Southern Colorado Clinic generously made available the time and facilities needed to produce this manuscript, whereas analytical discussions held with many colleagues in the past plus their shared experience and knowledge played an essential role in developing the insights found herein. Those colleagues include J. S. Arnold, D. Baylink, H. Duncan, D. Enlow, B. N. Epker, B. Frame, C. A. Hanson, Z. F. G. Jaworski, W. S. S. Jee, C. Johnston, P. Meunier, A. M. Parfitt, E. Radin, R. Recker, E. Sedlin, H. Takahashi, A. R. Villanueva, K. Wu, and W. Zinn.

† The explosion of knowledge in this field since 1955 has rendered the terminology of 1955 in some respects hopelessly inadequate. This has made it necessary to create or borrow new terms and to redefine older ones.

specialized cells, extracellular substances, and provisions for nourishing the cells, all organized into a fundamental complex that may have a short-range structural order (over domains <.5mm). Examples of simple skeletal tissues in this sense include hyaline and fibrocartilage, lamellar bone, woven bone, and fibrous tissue, all of mesodermal origin. The text will not discuss marrow, fibrocartilage, the musculature, or the nervous system.

If each simple tissue represents a letter in an anatomical "alphabet," it becomes apparent that nature uses such letters to construct anatomical "words," and the latter to construct sentences, paragraphs, and so on. Within this point of view, the diversity of skeletal anatomy, function, and disease in vertebrate species depends upon entities combining a few kinds of simple tissue elements or letters, each capable of a limited range of higher order structures, of behavioral activities, and of reactions to endogenous and external factors. The process resembles that found in a digital computer, which, using only zero and one as its basic alphabet, can combine, array and move these numbers around in ways that type books, do business accounting, play chess, and trace the evolutions of atoms, suns, and galaxies.

The simple skeletal tissues include the following, each appended by an identifying letter of our own alphabet:

Lamellar bone (L)	Fibrocartilage (C)
Woven bone (W)	Fibrous tissue (F)
Hyaline cartilage (H)	Bone marrow (M)

When spatial organization of one or more simple tissues occurs, usually over domains >.5mm, *complex tissues* arise. A complex tissue can consist of one or several simple tissues. The complex tissue composition of gross anatomical structures could then be represented as shown in Figure 7-1, the letter signifying the simple tissue(s) lying above, the name of the complex tissue made out of it lying below.

In the present sense, the embryonic epiphysis and articular cartilage contain the same single simple tissue element, as do spongy and compact bone and tendon and fascia. Their differences lie not in composition but rather in the *spatial organization* of the component tissues, differences that represent spatially acting effects on the growth process of a sculpting process to be described later.

The text now lists briefly some salient properties of four of the basic skeletal tissues. As a group, these four tissues compose extracellular gels made up of collagen and proteoglycans, the chemical and physical nature of which is to some degree specific to the specific tissues. These inherently elastic and compliant gels can mineralize, and if they do they then become rigid.[8,9,21,26,34,35,41,54,57,60]

Lamellar bone (mature bone)

Chemically, this simple tissue contains an organic matrix ($\approx$40% by volume) elaborated by osteoblasts in which mineral salts are deposited, the predominant ions including calcium and phosphate, with lesser amounts of magnesium, carbonate, hydroxyl, and sodium. By volume the matrix contains about 95% collagen and 5% mucopolysaccharides, and fully mineralized bone (excluding its canaliculae and lacunae) normally contains $\approx$3% water. Histologically, the collagen organizes into parallel layers or lamellae readily visible under polarized light (Fig. 7-2, left). Lacunae within this material contain osteocytes, flattened between the lamellae, that communicate with each other[74] and with

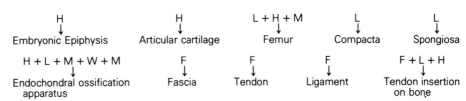

FIGURE 7-1 *The complex tissue composition of gross anatomical structures.*

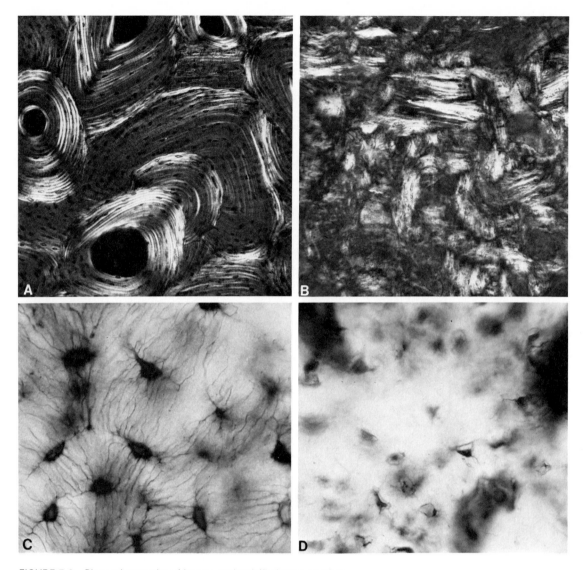

FIGURE 7-2   *Photomicrographs of human undecalcified bone sections.*

(A) *Cross-section of lamellar compact bone between crossed polars. The bright anisotropic lamellae alternate with dark isotropic lamellae with an average separation of ≈ 7μ. A secondary haversian canal lies near the lower border of the figure, × 100.*

(B) *Fuchsin-stained section, showing the osteocyte lacunae (oval dark shadows averaging about 8 × 15 μ) and some of their canaliculae. Both short- and long-range order appear in these photomicrographs. Some form of mineral exchange with the blood and a form of matrix turnover (oncosis) probably occur in the bony halo enveloping the lacuna, the "halo volume" as described by this author,[21] as indicated by varied studies done by Leonard Belanger and associates, L. C. Johnson, M. Heller-Steinberg, P. Meunier, R. Courpron, D. Baylink, B. Engstrom, L. Matthews, R. Talmage and the writer. However, of this story much remains undisclosed, × 700.*

(A and B). *Comparable views of woven bone, but at about 30% lower magnification than **(C)**. The warp and woof pattern between crossed polars shows a lack of long-range order (see also Fig. 7-14**A**). **(D)** the lacunar geometry shows a lack of short-range order, using a length of approximately 0.5 mm as the criterion of distinction. We know little of the functions of osteocytes in lamellar bone, however; we know nothing of the functions of those in woven bone.*

adjacent vascular spaces by way of a pervading spatially ordered network of fine canaliculae (diameter $\approx.4\ \mu$) that usually pass perpendicularly through the lamellae (Fig. 7-2, left). This tissue is innervated, and the possible functions of that innervation in a "fail-safe" mechanism are discussed elsewhere.[25,26]

Because of both long- and short-range order (over domains less and more than 0.5 mm in length) in the alignment of its collagen fibers and the disposition of its osteocytes, lamellar bone has a grain, with respect to both its structure and its mechanical properties. That grain parallels the directions of the maximum tension-compression stress and strain arising in the bone under normal daily usage. Like a rug on a floor, layers of new lamellar bone conform to the underlying surface, one that is often shaped by prior osteoclastic activity. Lamellar bone appears in the gross forms of *circumferential lamellae*, *primary osteons* (an osteon is a haversian system), *secondary osteons, compacta,* and *trabeculae.*[73]

Behaviorally speaking, lamellar bone generates microvolt-level electromotive force (EMF) potentials on its surfaces, and streaming potentials within, when strained in flexure.[6,16,30] Also, with continued use it develops mechanical microdamage, a phenomenon analogous to the fatigue of metals and other synthetic structural materials (Fig. 7-3, left).[23,28] The osteocytes in lamellar bone have a half-life on the order of a decade. Differentiated, nondividing cells called osteoblasts make new lamellar bone and other cells named osteoclasts resorb it. Lamellar bone apparently cannot deposit *de novo* in tissues; it always deposits upon pre-existing bone, of either the lamellar or woven kind. No malignant lamellar-bone-forming tumor has been recognized.[66]

Woven bone (primitive bone, reactive bone, fibrous bone)

Chemically, this material has the same composition as lamellar bone. Structurally, using 0.5 mm as a dimensional reference, it lacks long-range and short-range order and oriented mechanical properties. It usually deposits as a disorganized clump of trabeculae that conform to the geometry of the capillary loops that precede and nourish their osteoblasts. The canaliculae and lacunae within woven bone lack uniform shape or alignment with respect to more distant ones (see Fig. 7-1, right).

Behaviorally, whereas lamellar bone deposits relatively slowly, woven bone can deposit relatively quickly and in massive amounts; it can also deposit *de novo* where no previous hard tissue existed. All known types of osteosarcomas form woven rather than lamellar bone as part of the neoplastic process.

In both healthy and diseased skeletons, living woven bone probably stimulates its own replacement by lamellar bone, for it does not usually endure for long without such replacement, a fact often useful when interpreting pathologic sections. Woven bone participates in the endochondral ossification process that replaces chondral structures by lamellar bone, in the formation of some bone anlage *in utero*, and in skeletal repair and defense reactions.[3,23,34]

Hyaline cartilage

Elaborated by chondroblasts, chemically this simple elastic tissue, a gel, has an extracellular phase made of about 25% organic matrix and 75% water. About 40% of that matrix is collagen; the remainder is mucopolysaccharide. Histologically, the tissue lacks an innervation; it forms the anlage of most bones during embryonic development, and after birth it provides the basic tissue composing *epiphyses, articular cartilage,* and *epiphyseal* and *apophyseal plates* (see Fig. 7-3, right). During growth it intervenes as a plate across bony tendon, ligament, and fascial attachments. It participates in the bone repair process. Mineralization converts it to calcified cartilage, which then probably stimulates its own resorption and replacement by woven bone, which, in turn, is usually replaced by lamellar bone. An inhibition of chondral mineralization in adult life* allows articular cartilage to retain

---

* Inhibition of resorption and replacement of mineralized cartilage also characterizes the adult state. This inhibition disappears in the macrorepair process and in many neoplasms.

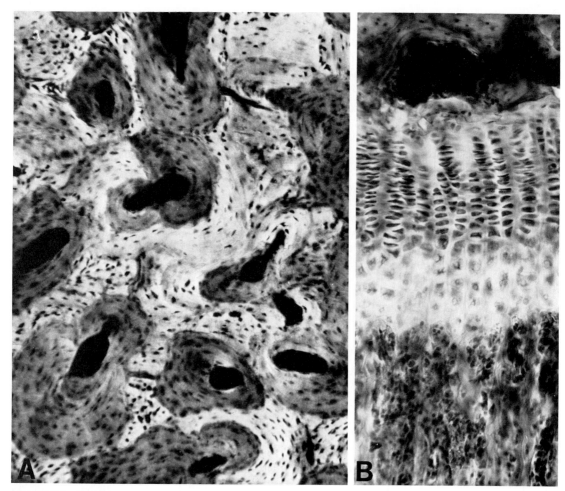

FIGURE 7-3 **(A)** *Photomicrograph of undecalcified cross-section of human femoral calcar, stained with basic fuchsin. Nine haversian canals lie surrounded by their dark osteons. In the interstitial lamellae between them most of the original osteocytes died, and their canaliculae filled completely with mineral, preventing in vitro staining (and percolation in vivo) and causing affected portions of the bone to appear clear. This condition is known as* **micropetrosis.** *Several dark-staining lines appear, connecting adjacent osteons. These lines comprise physical cracks in the interstitial lamellae. The result of mechanical fatigue, these* **microcracks**[28] *(one form of mechanical* **microdamage** *known to arise*[23]*) develop during life and weaken the intact bone in which they reside. The greatly increased frequency with which such cracks appear in micropetrotic bone (compared with health bone) has suggested that one of the functions of osteocytes consists of somehow detecting microdamage and initiating a new BMU to repair it. If so, a lack of osteocytes should lead to accumulating microdamage, as here, × 70. (Frost, H. M.: Bone Remodeling Dynamics, Springfield, Charles C Thomas, 1963)*

(B) *Photomicrograph of a longitudinal section decalcified and stained by hematoxylin-eosin through an epiphyseal plate, a complex tissue derived from hyaline cartilage by imposing upon it long-range order and an organized apposition to other tissues. The dark epiphyseal spongiosa occupies the top sixth of the figure, the plate itself occupies the next half, and the underlying secondary spongiosa occupies the lower third. The vertical columns of chondrocytes appear clearly, produced above by the plate's germinal layer and merging below into the clearer zone of calcified cartilage. This figure illustrates in microcosm the endochondral ossification process that plays a central role in skeletal genesis, growth, modeling, and repair.*

Replacement of that cartilage, and of both types of bone as well, involves the same sequence: first mineralization of the organic matrix, then (and apparently only then) its resorption, then deposition of the next type of tissue, which usually conforms to the following rule of thumb—woven bone on mineralized cartilage, lamellar bone on mineralized woven or lamellar bone. Work in the laboratories of H. DeLuca, T. Norman and R. McIntyre and L. Avioli among others has done much to unravel the roles of vitamin D metabolites in regulating these mineralization processes, particularly that in hyaline cartilage. But that story still unfolds, × 200.

its structural and functional properties over the human life span, and when disease does lead to such mineralization a seriously compromised joint usually results (i.e., as in chondrocalcinosis).

Like woven bone, hyaline cartilage can form *de novo* in soft tissues, and in many anatomical locations it is the first hard tissue elaborated. Several kinds of malignant chondral tumors—chondrosarcomas—as well as benign tumors and lesions occur. The endocrine control of chondral growth plays a major role in skeletal growth generally, because the adult's bony architecture reflects largely biomechanical factors (related to neuromotor activity) plus chondral growth affecting bone length and configuration. When bone replaces cartilage, the bone macroarchitecture conforms to the previously established chondral macrostructure.

Fibrous tissue

Elaborated by cells termed fibroblasts, chemically, this simple tissue embeds collagen in a compliant hyaluronic acid gel that contains relatively large amounts (i.e., $\approx75\%$) of water. This collagen differs slightly in composition and ultrastructure from that in cartilage and bone. Histologically, the collagen forms readily visible bundles in the light microscope, the tissue contains a resident population of flattened, elongated fibrocytes as well as nourishing blood vessels, and it has an innervation. Possible roles of that innervation in a fail-safe mechanism are discussed elsewhere.[22,26]

Mechanically, collagen serves as nature's thread, fashioned into an unorganized mass in *scar*, into three-dimensional supporting lattice works in *connective tissue*, into two-dimensional sheets of fabric in *fascia*, and into rope-like bundles in *tendon* and *ligament*, all of which represent complex tissues. Mechanically, the basic function of collagen probably lies in its strength and stiffness under tension loading only. It remains compliant in compression and shear and, therefore, under flexure too.

Both benign and malignant tumors and related lesions of fibrous tissue occur (fibrosarcomas, desmoids, fibromas, Dupuytren's contracture). A whole additional group of benign and malignant skeletal lesions occur that contain elements of two or more simple tissues.[1,66]

The text now considers some major processes affecting the aforementioned tissues—specifically, growth, modeling, remodeling, repair, and blood-bone exchange. These processes prove essential to the growth, development, and the very survival of both species and individuals.[59] Each of these processes follows its own special game rules.

Five basic skeletal processes

Growth

As arbitrarily defined herein, growth acts primarily to increase a tissue's *volume*.

UNMODIFIED GROWTH does not produce organized structures. Rather, unmodified tissue growth would produce basically spherical, unorganized lumps of tissue lacking the macroarchitecture, organization, and long-range order (over domains $>.5$ mm) found in normal anatomy.

Growth lies partly under the control of endocrine agents that are synthesized remote from but are brought to the growing tissue by the blood.[5] Other factors can modify the endocrinologic effects in the sense of both retarding and accelerating them. Such factors include systemically acting ones such as nutrition, phenotype, sex, and climate, and locally arising ones such as physical forces, mechanical strains, and alterations in perfusion and in the local chemical and electrical environment, alterations often reflecting special effects of other tissues juxtaposed to the growing tissue.

As to disorders primarily of skeletal growth (as defined previously) and of orthopedic concern, *such disorders seem confined to entities affecting the growth of hyaline cartilage*, and they represent various forms of dwarfism.[1,3,5,60,73] In some dwarfs the failure of cartilage to grow properly derives from a lacking or qualitatively abnormal endocrine agent or agents in the presence of potentially normal cartilage (i.e., pituitary dwarfism). In other dwarfs, an inherently defective cartilage cell cannot respond properly to normal agents (achondroplasia, Morquio's disease). In yet other dwarfs, acquired disease (most forms of rickets) impairs the response of potentially normal cartilage to normal endocrine agents.

Intriguingly, the writer does not know of any similar *growth* disorders affecting bony or fibrous tissues; certain disorders classified as such by others in fact represent disorders of the *modeling* processes, to be described. One suspects that if such disorders did exist, their profound effects on the organism would prohibit the very survival of the embryo *in utero*.

The name of the game in growth is achievement of adult body size.

Modeling

As in sculpting in clay, this term means local influences that alter the growth pattern and organization of a tissue or organ and thereby produce macroarchitectural features.[17,18,22]

LONG RANGE ORDER and/or organization always reflect the action of modeling influences upon underlying histogenetic and growth activities. In skeletal tissues, modeling usually reflects precise spatial patterns of local augmentations and retardations of the basic growth process, to which bone adds the resorptive drift, unique to that tissue. Although modeling begins in the embryo, this text is concerned with only the postnatal activity. Thus, the shapes of the adult distal femoral epiphyses, the cranium, the cruciate ligaments, and the intervertebral disc complex reflect various modeling influences shaping the otherwise randomly acting growth of the basic simple tissue or tissues involved. The structure and long-range order imposed thereby on simple tissues create complex tissues and our normal anatomical features.

The modeling influences described include local mechanical pressure and deformation, local electrical and related effects, and local variations in blood flow, ionic diffusion, and the composition of the local extracellular fluid. Many classic anatomists accepted as an article of faith that "function dictates structure." Modeling, in modifying growth, constitutes the means and provides the game rules that realize that article.

Modeling affects lamellar bone, fibrous tissue, and hyaline and fibrocartilage as well as the macrorepair processes, and it proceeds most rapidly in the infant, declines during subsequent growth, and approaches zero for clinical purposes after skeletal maturity. It appears in all known vertebrates, including extinct species. Table 7-1 lists a few representative modeling disorders, all of which represent abnormalities in macroarchitecture.

The name of the game in skeletal modeling is architecture and we presume its basic purpose is biomechanical.

Remodeling*

In the new bone lexicon this redefined term signifies the turnover of a tissue in microscopic packets in such a way that the tissue's overall composition and total mass or volume can remain unaffected. Within this arbitrary definition, differentiated cells produce remodeling and they organize into special functional units[19] which, in bone, constitute the basic multicellular unit (BMU) of Frost,[23] also named by some the bone remodeling unit or BRU.[57] An analogous but poorly studied packaged turnover also occurs in fibrous tissues,[19] but hyaline and fibrocartilage lack that particular kind of remodeling, although they do undergo a molecular level turnover.[9] Remodeling appears at appreciable levels of activity primarily in large and long-lived vertebrates that display the phenomenon of skeletal maturation. Small and short-lived animals such as mice, rats, hamsters, and chicks lack appreciable remodeling as defined herein and so cannot provide valid models of disorders of human remodeling. At least one role of the remodeling modality constitutes the repair of mechanical microdamage.[23,26] Table 7-2 lists some represen-

* Bone histomorphometry—the microscopic measurement of varied static and kinetic tissue parameters—has developed considerably since 1955,[29,38,39,47,70] in the process providing information that is more accurate by one or more orders of magnitude than previously available, as well as new kinds of information. This development played a major role in improving our understanding of skeletal physiology and disease. The development remains incomplete, however, and further fundamental progress in the field seems assured.

TABLE 7-1 EXAMPLES OF TISSUE MODELING DISORDERS

TISSUE		REPRESENTATIVE AFFECTIONS
CARTILAGE	Normal*	Limb torsions, clubfoot, metatarsus varus, tibial and femoral torsions, genu valgum and varum, pes planus, rocker bottom foot.
	Abnormal*	Chondrodystrophies, chondrodysplasias, rickets, achondroplasia, scoliosis, Jansen's disease.
BONE	Normal*	Coxa valga, bony deformities of club foot.
	Abnormal*	Osteogenesis imperfecta, osteopetrosis, Pyle's disease, deficiency rickets, hyperphosphatasia.
FIBROUS TISSUE	Normal*	Inguinal hernia.
	Abnormal*	Osteogenesis imperfecta, fibroelastic diathesis, collagen diseases (i.e., the rheumatoid hand), Ehlers-Danlos syndrome.[7]

* In the "normal" category the inherent modeling potential of the tissue in question remains normal, but it responds to an abnormal mechanical force environment. In the "abnormal" category an inherently abnormal modeling potential of the tissue in question produces disturbed architecture even in the face of a normal mechanical force environment.

tative disorders arising from bone and fibrous tissue remodeling affections.

The name of the game in remodeling is maintenance of previously established mechanical and physiologic competence.

Repair

The complex repair process heals gross physical injury to a tissue and/or organ, thereby restoring adequate function. It occurs in bony, cartilaginous, and fibrous tissue structures, and other local noxious stimuli besides simple fracture and/or incision can evoke it. In bone, in fibrous tissue, and probably in cartilage, two separate repair mechanisms exist, each with its own properties. One, the remodeling process, repairs *microscopic* damage of the tissue; the other, conventionally termed the repair process, repairs macro or *gross* injury to the tissue and/or organ.[19] Once unleashed, the macrorepair processes resist hindering influences better than do most other normal bodily activities, which seems sensible: any species lacking an imperative and dominating

macrorepair mechanism could not survive the evolutionary testing process. The macrorepair processes also serve to isolate and/or confine a variety of local threats such as infection, foreign bodies, and many tumors.

Thus the name of the game in repair is healing and defense.

Blood-bone exchange

Both electrolyte and acid-base substances exchange between the blood and the bone tissue.[4,33,36,48,50,57,58,63,65] The mineral content of the bone tissue provides a large sink-and-reservoir function that, by way of the blood flow through bone, allows the body's homeostatic mechanisms to meet otherwise potentially lethal challenges. Such challenges include acute and chronic alkalosis and acidosis and acute deficits and surfeits of some mineral ions in the extracellular fluid. It has become evident that this process requires adequate supplies of healthy osteocytes within the bone lacunae in order to function effectively.

So the name of the game here is homeostasis.

Having briefly characterized five of the major processes recognized so far in the skeletal system, the text now considers four of them in more detail; it omits further discussion of growth. Each discussion includes a brief listing of some diseases arising from malfunctions of the process in question.

TABLE 7-2 TISSUE REMODELING DISORDERS

TISSUE	REPRESENTATIVE AFFECTIONS
BONE	Spontaneous fractures, adult-acquired osteoporoses, osteomalacias, the bone RAP.
FIBROUS TISSUE	Spontaneous tendon ruptures, spontaneous ligament ruptures, spontaneous fascial herniations.

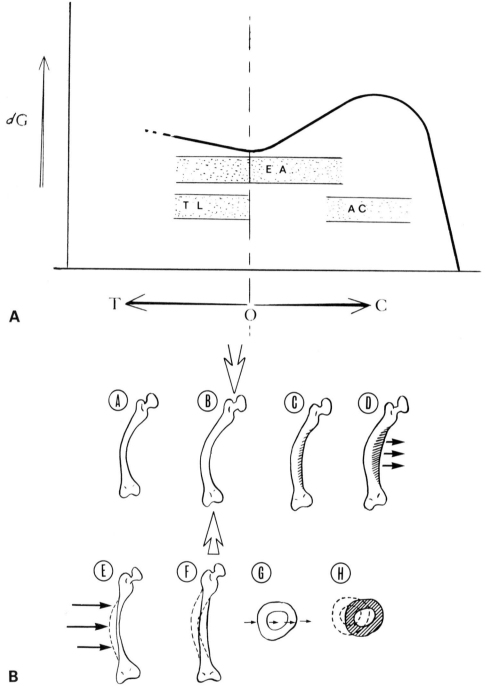

A

B

FIGURE 7-4 **(A)** *The chondral growth force response characteristic, or CGFR curve.[17] The vertical axis plots the speed of growth of a hyaline cartilage layer, against the time-averaged nontrivial loads it carries on the horizontal axis. Increasing tension lies to the left of the zero load point shown by the dashed vertical line, increasing compression lies to the right. The range of loading on the abscissa normally found for particular tissues is indicated by the shaded rectangles for tendon, ligament, and fascia* **(TL)**, *epiphyseal and apophyseal plates* **(EA)**, *and articular cartilage* **(AC)**. *The curve to the left of the zero point is its tension*

The modeling processes

Chondral modeling

Cartilage forms one of the most important tissues of the vertebrate skeleton, and nature appears to have assigned it many different roles that become evident upon examination of the ontogenetic, phylogenetic, and developmental processes.[34,59,73] Only one of those roles, modeling, will be characterized subsequently.

Like bone and fibrous tissue, the growth of hyaline cartilage responds to local mechanical factors, although doing so according to its own game rules.[17,22] The effects of such responses upon anatomical configuration underlie much normal skeletal architecture, including that of its articulations. This matter has been reviewed elsewhere recently,[17] and it suffices here to record a few highlights.

Figure 7-4, top, plots the growth speed of a hyaline cartilage layer (such as an articular surface, an epiphyseal plate, an apophyseal plate, or the cartilage plate lying across the attachment of a tendon or ligament to bone) on the ordinate, against changes in its mechanical loading during a normal life on the abscissa. That latter axis plots tension and compression loads on the plate as a continuum, zero loading lying in the middle, and both tension (toward the left) and compression (toward the right) increasing with increasing distance from the zero point. The inscribed curve (the CGFR curve) graphically portrays some of the game rules of chondral modeling and describes quite well the clinically known chondral growth responses to changing mechanical forces, although no knowledge exists at present as to their cellular and physicochemical determinants. A brief discussion of three chondral modeling phenomena follows.

EPIPHYSEAL PLATES

According to the parent algorithm,[17] growing epiphyseal plate cartilage normally loads on the curve's ascending compression limb, and both sides of a given plate normally carry identical unit loads. As a result, any minor limb malalignment at a hinge joint would augment the unit loading on the right side of the plate, for example, while decreasing it on the left, as in Figure 7-5. This increases subsequent growth on the right side of the plate and decreases it on the left. These changes restore the previous alignment, an elegant negative feedback response mode of growth with respect to limb alignment. This behavior automatically corrects minor malalignments of ginglymoid articulations having epiphyseal plates on at least one side. Conversely, should the malalignment become severe, unit loading on the right side of the plate moves over and down the steeply descending compression limb of the curve, to fall below that on the left side of the plate. Now the deformity increases with further growth, a positive feedback mode of response.

ARTICULAR CARTILAGE

According to the parent algorithm, articular cartilage normally loads on the peak of the curve's compression limb. Consequently, a high spot on

---

limb; the steeper ascending compression limb lies to the right of the zero load point and the most steeply descending compression limb lies to the right of that (Frost, H. M.: Calc. Tissue Res., 1979 [in press].

(B) Bone modeling activity responds in a stereotyped way to abnormal flexural strains and stresses in long bones. Given a femoral malunion as part **A**, normal activities and muscle body weight loads accentuate the femoral angulation with each load application, as shown in part **B**. As parts **C** and **D** illustrate, the right periosteal surface develops an osteoblastic drift, the left periosteal surface develops an osteoclastic drift, as shown in part **E**, which corrects the deformity as shown in part **F**. Parts **G** and **H** illustrate that directionally similar but, cellularly speaking, complementary drifts occur simultaneously on the inner walls of the cortex. Hence, one can formulate a clinically useful rule of thumb to characterize such behavior—the flexure drift tenet discussed in the text. Surface electrical phenomena may represent the natural transducing mechanism that relates bone surface drifts to such mechanical strains. The writer's proposal that the behavior discussed accounts for much normal bony architectural and modeling features[18] is currently under study by others. (Frost, H. M.: Bone Modeling and Skeletal Modeling Errors, Springfield, Charles C Thomas, 1973)

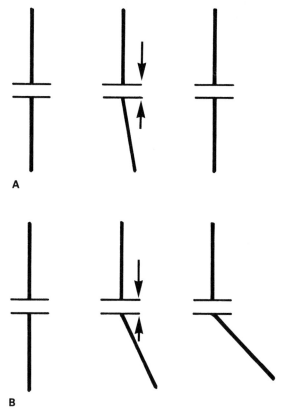

A

B

FIGURE 7-5   *A diagram of the femoral and tibial epiphyseal plates at the knee, as seen from the front, to illustrate two kinds of chondral modeling responses observed clinically in epiphyseal plates.*

(A) On the left, the normal alignment is demonstrated. In the middle is seen a slight malalignment—perhaps the result of a fracture malunion, which now slightly increases the unit loads on the right sides of the plates and decreases them on the left sides. Inspection of the ascending compression limb of the CGFR curve in Figure 7-4 reveals that this should increase growth on the right and decrease it on the left. This negative feedback response corrects the malalignment, as on the right.

(B) A severe malalignment in the middle moves the unit loads on the right side of the plates onto the descending limb of the CGFR curve, where its growth speed falls below that on the left side. Consequently this malalignment becomes worse with time, a positive feedback response. (Frost, H. M.: The Physiology of Cartilaginous, Fibrous and Bony Tissue, Springfield, Charles C Thomas, 1972)

any growing articular surface creates large unit compression loads geographically confined to the high spot. This depresses its growth, allowing the surrounding articular cartilage to rise with further growth and level the surface again, thereby restoring an even distribution of load.

This property has the higher order effect of causing a growing articular surface to adopt a shape compatible with the patterns of load and motion to which the neuromotor apparatus subjects it.[17]

TENDON ATTACHMENTS

In children, tendon attachments to the bony skeleton traverse a layer of hyaline cartilage lying on the bone surface, a layer that responds to the endocrine growth factors in the same way as all other hyaline cartilage. But the tension limb of the CGFR curve has a less steep slope than the ascending compression limb. Consequently, both the absolute and the axial (i.e., longitudinally directed) growth of tendon attachments regularly fall behind that of epiphyseal plates. The same properties apply to ligament and fascial attachments to bone.

The parent algorithm explains many other effects of the described properties that clinicians treating children's musculoskeletal disorders cannot afford to ignore. In brief, however, limb alignment, articular surface contour and alignment, and the growth of bony tendon, ligament, and fascial attachments, each reflects chondral modeling responding according to simple rules to forces generated by muscles and controlled and patterned by the nervous system. Only in the axial skeleton and the lower extremities does gravity significantly affect those modeling processes, and even there the neuromotor factor probably remains the dominant one. Thus, function dictates form.

DISEASES OF CHONDRAL MODELING

Two classes of chondral modeling diseases exist.[19] First and most common, the inherent modeling potential of the tissue remains normal; it produces abnormal structures in response to an abnormal mechanical force environment. Examples of such relatively common conditions appear in Table 7-2. Second, growing cartilage can model abnormally when an inherent abnormality exists in the cartilage itself and/or in its cells, either because of acquired disease (e.g., the varied forms of deficiency rickets) or because of genetic abnormality (e.g., the inherited rickets,

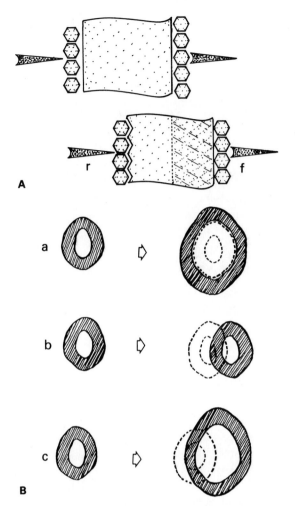

A

B

chondrodystrophies, and chondrodysplasias). The abnormal long bone and articular configurations observed in such diseases represent in large part a malfunctioning chondral modeling process but also represent in part the effects of mechanical creep in shear of thickened layers of cartilage that often have abnormal mechanical properties.

Bone modeling

DRIFTS

A collection of osteoclasts on a given bone surface, whether acting continuously or in successive waves without intervening bone formative activity, progressively erodes that surface much like a melting ice surface. Termed a resorptive drift, this process can move a surface through tissue space.[14,22] Its complement, the osteoblastic drift, causes a progressive buildup of a bone surface due to continuous or wave-like new bone deposition without intervening osteoclastic activity. These two drifts form the basic behavioral alphabet of bone modeling activity (Fig. 7-6). Osteoclastic and osteoblastic drifts normally occur in precise patterns on the periosteal and cortical-endosteal surfaces of the bony skeleton, stereotyped and reproducible from one individual to another of the same species, and their sum forms the process termed bone modeling herein (see Fig. 7-6, bottom).

FIGURE 7-6 **(A)** *The hexagons represent collections of osteoclasts or osteoblasts on periosteal and endosteal bone surfaces. Given a resorptive drift* **(r)** *on the left of a bone cortex (the stippled area) and an osteoblastic drift* **(f)** *on the right, an entire cortex can drift towards the right in tissue space (as seen on an x-ray). Later microscopic examination would reveal that the crosshatched material in the lower part would represent new circumferential lamellar bone. (Frost, H. M.: The Laws of Bone Structure, Springfield, Charles C Thomas, 1964)*
  (B) *In bone modeling, drifts occur in coordinated patterns, two cross-sectional patterns being shown here. In part* **a** *the periosteal envelope expands uniformly in all directions (an osteoblastic drift effect), as the marrow cavity (an osteoblastic drift effect). This occurs below the metaphyses during growth and does not displace the bone's original centroid and neutral axis at the level of the section in question. In part* **b** *the drift patterns move the whole diaphysis laterally through tissue space, which moves both the bone's original centroid and its neutral axis. The two types often combine, as is seen in part* **c.**[14] *(Frost, H. M.: Bone Modeling and Skeletal Modeling Errors, Springfield, Charles C Thomas, 1973)*

Properties

Bone modeling occurs primarily during growth, subsides to trivial levels after skeletal maturity, modifies primarily the periosteal and endosteal envelopes, and, unlike the remodeling process, does not greatly modify the trabecular and haversian envelopes. It establishes and maintains the characteristic macroscopic shapes of bones as they grow from infant to adult size. *We assume its architectural effects have biomechanical purposes.*[26,43,44,75] It forms the particular process that corrects the postfracture long bone deformities often occurring in children (see Fig. 7-13). It must by its nature change the local architecture and amount of bony tissue present.[19] As Koch[43] and Wolf[75] proposed long ago, its behavior implies that mechanical factors play at least a major role (and possibly an exclusive one) in evoking and patterning its geographic distribution in the growing skeleton.

As to those mechanical factors, the flexural deformations of malunited, angulated bones under *in vivo* loads correlate strikingly with the corrective drifts observed in such bones.[15,19] The *flexure-drift tenet* states the correlation thus:[18]

Under repeated nontrivial and uniformly oriented flexural strains, all bone surfaces drift toward the direction of the increasing concavity as flexural strain develops.

Figure 7-4, bottom, expands on this matter, currently under study by experimentalists and recently summarized elsewhere in some depth.[18] The writer suspects that strains on the order of .002 probably separate trivial from nontrivial levels for the case of lamellar bone.

DISEASES OF BONE MODELING

Bone modeling activity produces abnormal macroarchitecture under two different conditions.[19] In the first, an inherently defective modeling capacity exists, as in osteopetrosis, Pyle's disease, and osteogenesis imperfecta, in many kinds of severe rickets and, in adults, in Engelmann's disease and Paget's disease. The specific causes differ. In osteopetrosis and Pyle's disease, the skeleton cannot produce adequate numbers of functionally competent osteoclasts,[72] so that although resorptive drifts occur at the proper places and times on the skeleton's envelope geography, they cannot act quickly enough to keep pace with the osteoblastic drifts or the growth in length of the bone.

Current research in osteogenesis imperfecta[45,56] supports the proposal by Ramser and colleagues[56] that because of an abnormal collagen, a defective mechanically generated bone surface signal (the one that probably accounts for the flexure drift tenet) causes bone drifts to proceed too slowly to meet local mechanical and architectural needs. Thus, one hallmark of the imperfecta skeleton is gross architectural distortions of long bones—the consequence of multiple uncorrected fracture malunions.[1]

In rickets, retarded mineralization of new lamellar bone osteoid plus an increased fraction of bone surfaces covered by osteoid retard surface drifts, leading to longitudinal distortions of bones. Although surface signals have not yet been studied in rickets, the rachitic skeleton can produce adequate numbers of osteoclasts and osteoblasts.

In the second, and far more prevalent, class of bone modeling disorders, inherently normal modeling activity responds to an abnormal mechanical force environment and/or to abnormal chondral tissue growth patterns.[19] Examples include coxa valga, tibial torsion, and the tarsal bone abnormalities observed in pes equinovarus.

Fibrous tissue modeling

Under pure flexural, shearing, and/or compression loads, living fibrous tissue structures do not appear to respond specifically. However, under repeated nontrivial tension loads that stretch the tissue beyond some as-yet-undetermined limit (probably a unit strain on the order of $\approx .02$), some of the resident fibrocytes activate and make additional collagen, which increases the cross-section and thus the total tensile strength and stiffness of the structure.[19,22] This process continues until the structure's increasing strength reduces stretching by the original loads below that level that activates the resident fibrocytes. Collagen elaborated by this means aligns parallel to the axis of the elongation. Called the stretch-hypertrophy tenet,[19] the physicochemical basis for this behavior remains unknown. However, it has clinically useful and reliable effects upon the cross-section sizes of tendons and ligaments and upon the thickness of fascial sheets: the thickness, and thus the total strength, of such structures reflects the mechanical loads they carry rather than any direct action of the endocrine mechanisms that control skeletal growth. In other words, again, function dictates structure. Parenthetically, and as a general rule, when nature requires more strength in some skeletal structure, modeling provides it by commensurately increasing the amount of load-bearing tissue, without altering significantly the tissue's unit strength properties.

The remodeling processes

Bone remodeling and the BMU theory

This section discusses the BMU, the skeletal envelopes, the properties named Δ B.BMU and σ, the osteoporoses, and the idea of manipulating coherent BMU populations.

By way of background, lamellar bone provides virtually all of the human being's supply of compacta and spongiosa, and it has at least two basic functions. It provides rigid and strong physical support for the body and its articulations and for its musculature to act upon. And it provides a large sink-reservoir capacity to the blood to minimize threats to extracellular fluid homeostasis and acid-base balance.

With regard to their effectiveness over the human life span, with aging both the mechanical and homeostatic functions of a given moiety of lamellar bone deteriorate.[4,25,27] Although the deterioration probably does not become harmful over a year or less, it does become serious after a decade and more, because during normal life the typical unremodeled lamellar bone moiety progressively accumulates physical microdamage from continued straining, while a progressively increasing fraction of its osteocytes die simultaneously (see Fig. 7-3, left). The former phenomenon weakens and so predisposes a bone to fracture following minimal trauma or during normal mechanical usage (i.e., "spontaneous" fractures), whereas the latter phenomenon reduces the effective area of the physical interface across which rapid bone-blood fluxes of acid-base and electrolytes can occur.

By constantly removing old bone and replacing it with new, bone remodeling repairs these deleterious changes while they are still microscopic in geographic extent and trivial in their effects upon the mechanical (and homeostatic) competence of whole bones. This maintains a healthy intact skeleton over the human life span in spite of the fact that its material substance can retain functional competence for only a limited time. The text describes this remodeling process next.

THE BMU

Histologists knew well over 100 years ago that osteoclasts dissolve mineralized bone, returning its organic and inorganic components to the blood, whereas osteoblasts make new bone, first synthesizing its organic matrix and then causing that matrix to mineralize. Studies of human bone remodeling have revealed these two cellular activities to occur in "packets" and in a stereotyped sequence,[64] forming a basic multicellular unit of bone remodeling, the BMU, the properties of which follow.[10,11,12,23,52,53]

Activation

A new BMU begins somewhere on a skeletal surface when a competent local stimulus sets the biologic wheels in motion. Termed activation, this initiating process then leads to the following processes.

Resorption

Osteoclasts appear at the site in question and proceed to remove bone,[40,51] usually parallel to the local tension-compression strains. Probably derived from monocytes in the blood,[32,40,51] the batch of osteoclasts in a BMU tend to remove a fixed total quantity of bone, whereupon they disappear, to be followed by formation.

Formation

Osteoblasts arise from the local mesenchymal cells,[54] array on the previously resorbed bone surface, and begin to deposit the new organic matrix of lamellar bone that, after an 8-d delay or so, begins to mineralize. In both woven and lamellar bone this delay interposes a layer of unmineralized organic bone matrix between osteoblasts on one side and mineralized matrix (i.e., bone) on the other. That unmineralized layer is called osteoid or an osteoid seam.[10,12] The new lamellar bone deposit tends to achieve a constant final amount, approximately equal to that previously resorbed.[19]

When concluded these three processes have replaced a semimicroscopic "packet" of old bone with an equal amount of new bone (Fig. 7-7), circumscribed by a *cement line* ($\approx$ .2mm³ per

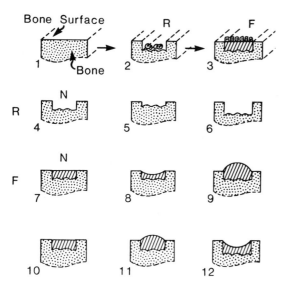

FIGURE 7-7 *Diagram of the remodeling BMU effects on the amount of bone present at some locus on a bone envelope. At No. 1, histologically inactive bone appears. At No. 2, following an activation event, the resorptive phase of a BMU has eroded a trough, and later, at No. 3, the following formation phase has filled it back up. This forms the basic A-R-F sequence of lamellar bone remodeling.*

The resorptive trough might be normal, too shallow (No. 5), or too deep (No. 6), and the amount put back into it might be normal (No. 7), too little (No. 8), or too much (No. 9).

The normal combinations found in humans appear to be as seen in No. 10 for the haversian envelope, No. 11 for the periosteal envelope, and No. 12 for the cortical-endosteal and trabecular envelopes. These situations represent, respectively, $\Delta B.BMU = 0$, $\Delta B.BMU > 0$ (or +), and $\Delta B.BMU < 0$ (or −). (Frost, H. M.: Clin. Orthop., 1980, in press)

BMU). The new bone moiety then serves as a bone structural unit (the BSU of Jaworski),[38,68] performing its mechanical and homeostatic functions until removed and replaced by an even later BMU. Average BSU lifetimes in humans range from 3 to 20 yr, depending on the local bone turnover rate.[23,29] This replacement process removes any microdamage affecting the replaced bone packet, and restores a full local supply of osteocytes.

The activation-resorption-formation sequence characterizes bone remodeling on all four skeletal envelopes throughout the human adult life,[19] as well as in all other long-lived bony vertebrates. It can turn bone over without altering its macroarchitecture or the total quantity of tissue present,[19] unlike the bone modeling process,

which must alter both. During human growth, it mixes with the surface drifts of bone modeling, and a gradual shift in proportions during growth causes most bone turnover to arise from modeling in young children, but from remodeling in the adult.

In an alphabetical shorthand, these events become A → R → F.

Tissue time-marking studies reveal that the total time taken by the ARF processes in a typical human BMU approximates 3 mo for haversian and endosteal remodeling, and somewhat less for trabecular remodeling.[29,39,46] This problem is currently under study. The text discusses this time period later. The individual and collective properties of the BMU make it possible to define a variety of parameters, the control of which in life have diverse and sometimes quite unexpected effects on the intact skeleton. The following text will describe some of these parameters and their effects.

The BMU concept has changed some of our ideas of bone physiology and pathophysiology,[52,53,57,68] and it has also engendered a new body of theory—called BMU theory—which, although still crystallizing out of its melt, has already received impressive observational support. However, back to remodeling and a characterization of four functionally separate collections of human remodeling BMU.

Skeletal envelopes

As Sedlin stated while working in the writer's laboratory, bone remodeling occurs on four functionally, as well as anatomically, distinct skeletal surfaces or envelopes,[23,61] each of which encloses or envelops a tissue volume that represents in part the mathematical integral of the envelope's past resorption and formation. Named the periosteal, haversian, endosteal, and trabecular envelopes, their anatomical features require no comment to this audience. Functionally, however, over the human life span there exists a positive bone balance on the periosteal envelope, an essentially zero balance on the haversian envelope, and a negative balance (i.e., progressive bone loss) on the endosteal and trabecular envelopes.[31,42,61] Although these balances vary characteristically in magnitude during growth and adult life, their signs normally do not, although in disease sign reversals can occur. Also, in both health and disease the balance parameters on the separate envelopes can alter independently of the others, and some agents seem to "focus" their effects upon a given envelope more than on others. The tissue mechanisms responsible for those balances receive attention next.

BONE BALANCE IN THE BMU (ΔB.BMU)

During growth, the largest net losses and gains of bone on the periosteal and endosteal envelopes result from the drifts involved in bone modeling activity. However, this activity subsides essentially to zero after age 20 yr or so in humans,[25] and thereafter, until death, 95% or more of the bone tissue turnover on all envelopes derives from BMU-based remodeling.[23] The small but definite annual positive periosteal balance found in human adults apparently reflects less bone removal than deposition per typical periosteal BMU. The adult's essentially zero haversian balance reflects deposition equal to resorption per typical haversian BMU (actually a minute negative balance exists here), whereas the negative endosteal and trabecular balances reflect more resorption that deposition per typical BMU. Figure 7-7 illustrates these phenomena. The term ΔB.BMU (read it thus: delta B per BMU) signifies the nature and size of any resorptive-formative excess per typical BMU. A positive value signifies an incremental gain, a negative one signifies a loss.

Given the properties of BMU-based remodeling known at present, and the fact that no significant modeling activity exists, the relative amounts of bone resorbed and formed per typical BMU determine wholly whether bone progressively disappears or accumulates at a given surface locale. When the amount resorbed exceeds that formed in the typical BMU (i.e., when ΔB.BMU < 0) a progressive loss occurs, whereas if the contrary situation holds (if ΔB.BMU > 0) a progressive accumulation occurs.

Two separate factors affect the rate of any

such gain or loss: the aforesaid size of any excess per BMU and the number of BMU activated on an envelope in unit time.[20,23,70] Figure 7-8 illustrates these important effects. To repeat an earlier point, the observed behavior of these balance-determining factors on the four envelopes reveals that although they tend to respond similarly on all envelopes to some factors, to other factors one envelope can respond independently of the others. This functional independence of the envelopes has some deep implications relative to pathogenesis, diagnosis, and treatment of skeletal disease, implications discussed elsewhere.[10,11,23,52,53,61] Before discussing the role of these factors in the genesis and treatment of human osteoporoses, some temporal properties of the ARF sequence deserve comment.

THE PROPERTY NAMED σ

The total period taken by the ARF process in a typical BMU, known as σ, has two subperiods. The first, the *resorption period*, equals the time the resorption process needs to evolve and finish; σ_r designates it. At the "switchover time" the resorption period ends, and new bone deposition and the *formation period* commence, designated as σ_f.[23,29] Thus $\sigma = \sigma_r + \sigma_f$ (see Fig. 7-8, left top). Subdivisions of these subperiods have begun to receive attention by experimentalists.

Among the clinically important properties of σ lies the fact that after any kind of competent challenge to the BMU parameters (whether experimental or natural, therapeutic or unintentional) an obligatory time must elapse before the steady state effects of that challenge can appear. (The steady state designates any condition maintainable indefinitely, such as zero bone balance = equilibrium, or an annual loss of -0.2% of the pre-existing bone; a transient represents any change in the system behavior that, because of the system's nature, *must* appear and then, equally, *must* disappear before the steady state can appear). Since steady state effects can cure skeletal disease, but transient effects cannot, usually this distinction has clinical value.

In sum: BMU theory staates that transient changes must *always* arise following an effective

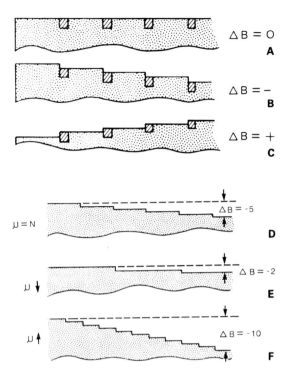

$\Delta B = 0$

A

$\Delta B = -$

B

$\Delta B = +$

C

$\mu = N$ $\Delta B = -5$

D

$\mu \downarrow$ $\Delta B = -2$

E

$\mu \uparrow$ $\Delta B = -10$

F

FIGURE 7-8 *"Stair graphs" after P. Meunier, illustrating the effect of some BMU parameters on bone balance. At the top left of each diagram lies a locus on a bone envelope. The shaded material beneath it represents the underlying bone. As time proceeds (toward the right) a new BMU arises at this locus, removes its packet of bone and replaces it with new bone. At yet a later time another BMU arises, and then another. The horizontal length of the figures might equal two years.*

(A): Here the bone removed equals that deposited, so no net change in bone quantity occurs and $\Delta B.BMU = 0$ as on the normal haversian envelope. (B) The bone removed exceeds that deposited, so a net loss occurs, in increments, and $\Delta B.BMU < 0$, as on the normal endosteal and trabecular envelopes. (C) The deposit of bone exceeds the withdrawal as on the normal periosteal envelope, so $\Delta B.MU > 0$.

The conclusion is that the sign of the $\Delta B.BMU$ parameter (i.e., +, 0, or −) determines whether the remodeling process adds or removes bone from an envelope over time.

Now hold the $\Delta B.BMU$ constant; D, E, and F illustrate the effect of a constant negative value. Under these conditions the annual bone loss will depend upon how many BMU pass over a bone surface locus in that time span. (D): A normal situation for the trabecular envelope. (E) Fewer BMU (i.e., decreased activation of new BMU) reduces the annual bone loss. (F) More BMU increase the annual loss. The μ on the left signifies the activation of new BMU.

The conclusion is that both $\Delta B.BMU$ and activation affect the rate of bone gain or loss in adult life, though only the $\Delta B.BMU$ parameter can convert an adult's bone balance from positive to negative, or conversely. Incidental to this message, the activation function provides virtually the sole BMU parameter, which regulates the steady state

challenge to the BMU system, *must* precede any steady state effects of that challenge, then must disappear in spite of continued treatment;*[24] *only then can the steady state effects appear.*

Now, as for the place of σ in the aforementioned:

σ represents precisely the obligatory time—the "lag time"—separating a challenge from the onset of its steady state effects.[24]

Any changes in the system arising before that σ period elapses should in theory—and so far invariably have in fact—prove to be transients.

Although the value of σ for a human in normal health approximates 3 mo for haversian remodeling and 2 mo for trabecular remodeling, values of several years regularly occur in some osteoporoses, osteomalacias, and other diseases. Also, each skeletal envelope can display its own unique value and changes, at least in some diseases, and drugs and hormones can alter both normal and abnormal values, although only scanty information exists on such matters at present.

The text next considers briefly two groups of diseases that arise from malfunctions of the human remodeling process: osteoporoses and osteomalacias.

Bone remodeling and the osteoporoses[1,2,11,23,37,41,49,53,55,61,67,71,76]

As an observation implying no criticism at all, almost as many definitions of osteoporosis exist as there are authorities who pontificate on the subject. The writer's views follow a lead first proposed by Urist in the early 1960s:[69] In the *disease* osteoporosis, an underlying *causative pathophysiologic state* associates with a skeleton

---

* Numerous, ingenious, and very diverse past attempts to perpetuate skeletal transients support this statement by having failed invariably to do so.

---

histologic bone turnover speed (any role of the oncosis phenomenon described by Johnson[41] is ignored here). Although utterly incomprehensible in terms of 1955 skeletal physiologic concepts—and an example of the unexpected effects of collective BMU activities referred to in the text—this prediction of BMU theory has successfully passed a decisive test of observation, done some years ago by Villanueva and Frost.[70] (Frost, H. M.: Clin. Orthop., 1980, in press) that displays both a *tissue volume deficit* and clinical disability caused by *mechanical incompetence* (i.e., unusual fragility and/or bone pain). Others discuss the underlying medical causes of osteoporoses;[1,52,53] this text focuses upon the volume deficit, the mechanical incompetence, and their mechanisms. Regardless of any current disagreements as to the biochemical, endocrine, and nutritional *regulation* of skeletal physiology, and such disagreements abound, the true regulatory agencies—whatever the ultimate agreement as to their nature—must exert their skeletal effects by acting on the tissue *mechanisms* described herein.

As to the volume deficit, absolute bone volume (ABV) defines a skeletal volume as the bone tissue remaining after subtracting marrow cavity and vascular space volumes from the intact skeleton (or bone).[21] Normally, the ABV augments during growth, peaks at about age 25 yr and thereafter declines, so that a normal 70-yr-old person may have about 60% as much bone as he did at age 25 yr.[23,31,61] Evaluating ABV deficits requires normal standards for the age, bone, race, sex, body size, and habitus in question. Note that the ABV deficit in an osteoporosis does not depend at all upon the quality of the bone tissue, which can remain normal or not.

The tissue volume deficit

As to its skeletal location, and as one reflection of the functional independence of the skeletal envelopes, ABV deficits in osteoporotic skeletons can occur in different anatomical patterns, according to the skeletal envelope or envelopes on which the deficit exists.[20,23] Figure 7-9 illustrates several of the possible kinds of such patterns. Relative to its pathogenesis, the osteoporotic volume deficit can arise by at least two fundamentally different mechanisms.

First, *disordered bone modeling can cause an osteoporosis*. Such an osteoporosis usually develops during childhood as a failure to accumulate a normal ABV during growth because of insufficient osteoblastic drifts or excessive osteoclastic drifts, or both.[19] Such childhood osteoporoses, which can affect all or only parts of the skeleton, occur in muscular dystrophy, biliary stenosis, osteogenesis imperfecta, Gaucher's disease, malnutrition, and paralysis arising early in life.

Second, *disordered bone remodeling also can cause an osteoporosis*, in part through an excessively negative ΔB.BMU in endosteal, haversian and/or trabecular BMU, and/or by way of a subnormally positive or an actually negative periosteal ΔB.BMU.[19] A normally negative endosteal-trabecular ΔB.BMU can also cause an osteoporosis, given increased activation, as shown in Figure 7-8, bottom.*[19] For example, in thyrotoxicosis BMU activation can increase by a factor of $\approx$15, so that the BMU take 15 times as many annual "bites" out of trabecular and cortical-endosteal bone as they do in the euthyroid state. Some of this bone loss repre-

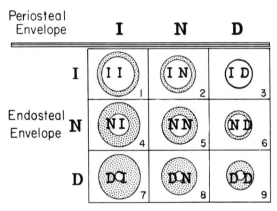

FIGURE 7-9 *Diagrams of a "standard" bone diaphysis as seen in cross-section, illustrating the periosteal and cortical-endosteal envelopes. The 3 × 3 matrix plots their size as increased (I), normal (N), or decreased (D). Nine possible anatomical envelope combinations of bone tissue volume result from this scheme, the one in No. 5 represents normal. These theoretical situations fit observation quite well, for example, senile, postmenopausal, and Cushing's osteoporoses fit into No. 2; The appearance of acromegaly goes from No. 5 to No. 4, and then to No. 1; Early osteogenesis imperfecta looks like No. 9 and as it matures its appearance is more like No. 6 and then like No. 5.*

This drawing omits the haversian and trabecular envelopes, and therefore is a simplification, although an instructive and useful one. (Frost, H. M.: Bone Dynamics in Osteoporosis and Osteomalacia, Springfield, Charles C Thomas, 1966)

---

* A modeling-derived osteoporosis represents a failure to accumulate adequate bone stores; a remodeling-derived osteoporosis represents a supranormal loss of previous and usually adequate bone stores.

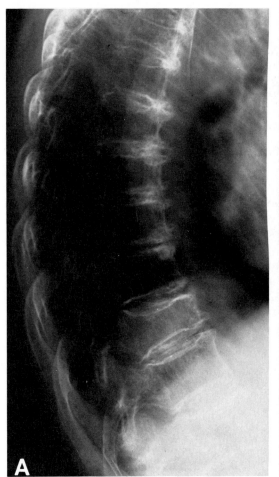
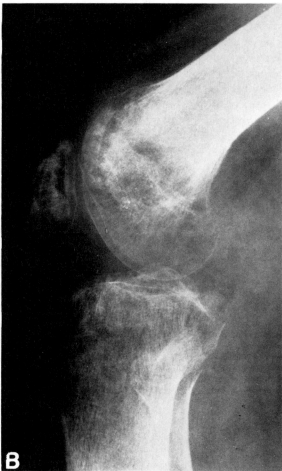

FIGURE 7-10 *Two quite different osteoporoses appear here.*

(A) Senile osteoporosis. A bone tissue volume deficit exists in the vertebral centrae where bone contacts marrow tissue—that is, on the endosteal and trabecular envelopes. It has existed for years, and one vertebra partially collapsed in the past but now is healed. This patient's skeletal symptoms are mechanical in origin, relating partly to the bone pain mechanism described in the text and partly to the altered posture, which accentuates the normal lumbar lordos and thoracic kyphos. Such symptoms respond regularly to the regimen outlined elsewhere (Orthop. Clin. North Am. 3:561–569, 1972). The bone deficit proves naturally irreversible (which does not imply that we cannot learn to cure it).

(B) So-called migratory osteoporosis.[13] Here, a naturally arising, very large increase occurs in BMU activation, but it remains confined to the region of a joint, which is a knee in this example. This greater BMU activation commensurately increases remodeling and turnover of the affected bones. The increase affects all four envelopes, and can cause 50% of the local spongiosa to disappear in as little as 6 wk. The bone pain in these patients regularly arises only during weight-bearing, and probably represents perception by the normal innervation of bone of excessive mechanical strains in the reduced amount of tissue. A suppressor of BMU activation (in this case a drug, oxyphenbutazone [Tandearil]) can reduce the hyperactivation. All of the then-active BMU go on to completion, but no new ones replace them. Therefore, as their holes fill up with new bone the osteoporotic tissue volume deficit "mysteriously" heals. Hence a naturally reversible osteoporosis. Similar patterns of loss and recovery appear in all high-turnover osteoporoses, whether regional or generalized.

sents an increased *remodeling space*, a temporary bone loss found in all high turnover states of the bony skeleton and caused by the presence of large numbers of resorption bays and cavities and incompletely filled up formation sites. This bone loss—seen also in the Regional Accelera-

tory Phenomenon[13,17,68]—regularly proves reversible.[20,68] Another part of this bone loss proves irreversible in nature—that representing the sum of all of the negative ΔB.BMU bites removed by completed endosteal and trabecular BMU.

Most (but not all) osteoporoses based on disordered remodeling develop during adult life.[19] Assured examples include the osteoporoses of Cushing's syndrome, of ageing, of thyrotoxicosis, of hyperparathyroidism, of hematologic conditions associated with an expanding bone marrow (myeloma, mast cell disease, certain lymphomas, and leukemias), and of the RAP. As already indicated, some of these osteoporoses remain naturally irreversible, others are reversible, and some fall in between those extremes (Fig. 7-10). The tissue deficit in adult-acquired generalized osteoporosis usually proves greater in the axial than in the appendicular skeleton and greater in the proximal than in the distal bones of a limb, and relatively greater deficits occur in spongiosa than in compacta. The greater surface : volume ratio of spongiosa probably accounts for the latter feature, whereas the concentration of hematopoietic marrow toward the axis of the body may have something to do with the first and second features.

Mechanical incompetence

Mechanical competence means the resistance of a skeleton to fracture and freedom from bone pain under normal usage. Clearly, a reduced amount of structural material will raise the stress levels generated in that tissue by normal loads, making fracture more likely. However two other factors also affect that competence: (1) bone turnover speed—reduced values (as occur in a majority of the symptomatic osteoporoses) associate with increased fragility, very likely because of accumulated microdamage,[19,20,23] and (2) a prolonged σ—values in excess of 5 yr occurring in some osteoporoses.[19,76] This prolongation probably allows individual microdamage foci to propagate faster than individual BMU can replace them with new bone,[20,23] causing microdamage accumulation.

The two commonest osteoporoses known to human medicine—senile osteoporosis and postmenopausal osteoporosis—lie in limbo regarding their pathogenesis, for it remains unknown whether they result from supranormal adult losses of originally normal bone stores or from normal adult losses of originally inadequate stores, or from both.[20] Their prolonged σ values also remain unexplained.[76]

Such problems aside, most adult-acquired and naturally irreversible osteoporoses present bone deficits largely confined to the endosteal and trabecular envelopes, both of which lie in contact with marrow tissue, which implies a cause-effect relationship discussed elsewhere.[23] These losses seem to derive from changes in the BMU parameters, BMU that normally—and irreversibly—shed bone lying in contact with marrow tissue. In addition, prolonged σ values and reduced tissue turnover speeds occur—although variably for the latter—in most established osteoporoses.

To summarize—a tissue volume deficit and mechanical incompetence characterize the bony skeletons of patients with symptomatic osteoporoses. The deficit may exist on any or all of the four skeletal envelopes (depending upon the causative pathophysiology); it may arise during growth as a modeling disorder or in adult life as a remodeling disorder, and both naturally reversible and irreversible deficits occur. The mechanical incompetence accompanies decreased structural material and reduced annual bone turnover,[55] and prolonged σ values (which imply "lazy" osteoclasts and osteoblasts). Although awaiting clear proof of the matter, the available data inescapably imply that *accumulating mechanical microdamage* links these otherwise seemingly unrelated associations.[19] Table 7-3 provides a mechanistic classification of some of the better known osteoporoses.

Clinical notes

The macrobone healing process proceeds normally in almost all osteoporoses, so that fractures, bone grafts, and surgical osteotomies pose few problems to orthopedists in that regard. The osteoporotic skeleton, because of its increased fragility, provides a weaker than normal anchorage for orthopedic hardware, which include screws, pins, plates, nails, and total joint replacement components. By suitable choice of procedure, device, and postoperative management one can usually avoid any disasters traceable (otherwise) to that fragility. The osteoporotic state *per se* poses no known unusual threats of homeostatic, electrolyte, acid-base, or nutritional disasters in operative, postoperative, or post-traumatic management. The writer

TABLE 7-3 MECHANISTIC CLASSIFICATION OF OSTEOPOROSES

| OSTEOPOROSIS | A RESULT OF | | NATURALLY REVERSIBLE | ENVELOPES AFFECTED | CLINICAL PREVALENCE (ON A SCALE OF 10) |
	MODELING	REMODELING			
Senile	0	+	0	E,T	10
Postmenopausal	0	+ (?)	0	E,T	8
Acromegaly	+	+	0	P,E,T	1
Cushing's disease	0	+	0	E,T	1
Cushing's syndrome	0	+	0	E,T	2
Osteogenesis imperfecta	+	0	0	P,E,T	1
Biliary Stenosis	+	0 (?)	?	P,E,T	1
RAP	0	+	+	P,H,E,T	9
Hyperthyroidism	0	+	+	P,H,E,T	1
Hyperparathyroidism	0	+	+	P,H,E,T	1
Metabolic acidosis	0	+	?	P,E,T	1
Muscular dystrophy	+	0	0	P,E,T	1
Myeloma	0	+	0	E,T	1
Gaucher's disease	+	?	0	P,E,T	1
Postparalytic	+	+	0	P,E,T	2

strongly suspects that the bone pain (without gross fracture) seen in many osteoporoses and in osteomalacia arises from supranormal bone strain, in turn caused by insufficient mechanical rigidity of the intact bone, in its turn caused by the factors already identified (the volume deficit and accumulated microdamage) plus, in the osteomalacic skeleton, the presence of significant amounts of incompletely mineralized, abnormally compliant bone matrix.[19] These factors may also account for the bone pain seen in some cases of active Paget's disease.[1]

Clearly, curing an established bone tissue volume deficit in an osteoporosis (only one of several ways of resolving the disability) requires somehow putting the adult skeleton into a positive (or in the case of children, a more positive) bone tissue balance, which means causing annual bone formation to exceed resorption. A few words about a promising idea in that regard appear next.

Coherence treatment of bone balance problems

BMU theory has led to the idea of creating and then manipulaing coherent BMU populations in order to change a bone balance for some therapeutic end. Recently reviewed elsewhere,[20] this section of the text abstracts the basis of that idea.

In Figure 7-11, left, a ladder graph diagrams the temporal history of the BMU collection in a bone sample. For present needs, the BMU collection portrayed by that figure has the property of *temporal incoherence*, because the R and F phases of each BMU function "out of step" relative to the others on the graph. In the bone populated by those BMU, as much resorption as formation occurs at any typical moment so that although the bone turns over, its tissue content remains essentially constant.

In Figure 7-11, right, however, a sudden activation "pulse" causes many BMU to begin at essentially the same moment throughout the bone, so they remain "in step" or *temporally coherent* subsequently, all performing resorption and switching to bone formation at nearly the same time. The durations of the resorption and formation periods, measurable by histomorphometric means,[29,38,47] are already known approximately for normal bone.

One value of this situation lies in the implications of an observed fact: all efforts to date to create a positive bone balance in human adults by treating the *incoherent* skeleton *continuously* with assorted agents have failed.* BMU theory suggests that failure could derive from two factors: (1) in humans, the agents in question exert similar kinds of effects on both osteoclasts and

---

* Example: In *in vitro* animal models calcitonin supposedly suppresses bone resorption but not bone formation. Yet, treating humans with it for long periods does not in fact progressively store bone in the adult skeleton.[20]

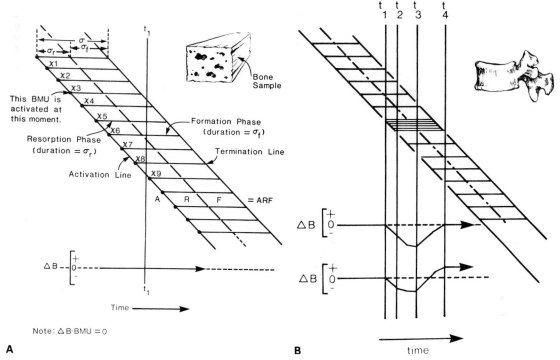

A   **B**   time

FIGURE 7-11   *Two ladder graphs.*

(A) *In the bone sample at the upper right, new BMU continually begin and others finish their ARF sequences. Let time lie on the horizontal axis. Then at x_1 a new BMU begins, resorbs its packet of bone over the σ_r period, and switches over to formation (the dotted diagonal "switchover" line), deposits bone for the σ_f period and becomes a new functional unit of bone at the "termination" line. Later another BMU (x_2), and then another (x_3), and so on, arise. Thus the BMU history of this sample extends up and to the left, its future down and to the right, just as one reads this paragraph. The vertical line t_1 corresponds to a biopsy done at that time. Serial sections of such a biopsy would reveal different BMU in all stages of their ARF sequences, depending on how long before the biopsy their activation occurred. Since any one BMU begins and evolves independently of all others, it displays* **temporal incoherence,** *the natural state of the unchallenged and unprepared human skeleton. Note that the BMU lines show only how long things last, not how much happens. Since as much resorption as formation occurs at any instant, the bone balance here (and $\Delta B.BMU$ too) = 0.*

(B) *In this simplified ladder graph a sharp pulse of activation suddenly initiates many new BMU, between t_1 and t_2. Starting at essentially the same time, they evolve through the subsequent resorptive, switchover, and formation stages at (nearly) the same times. Thus they display the property of* **temporal coherence.**

The bone balance (ΔB) curves at the bottom of the graph expose the long-range effects of two BMU "manipulations" on the total amount of bone tissue present. In the top curve only a BMU activation pulse occurs. As a result, a transient loss of bone arises and then recovers, so no permanent change in bone quantity develops. However, in the bottom curve, after the activation pulse the subject received an agent that reduced the size of the resorbed packets. At the switchover time the agent was stopped to free the subsequent osteoblasts so that they would deposit normal-sized packets of new bone in the subnormal-sized resorption cavities. This adds an increment of new bone to the pre-existing bone, a permanent one, that is, $\Delta B.BMU$ has been made to adopt a positive value. In principle one could repeat this sequential process as often as the therapeutic need requires, hence the "coherence treatment" of bone balance problems, and the ADFR type of such treatment for use in osteoporoses. (Frost, H. M.: Clin. Orthop., 1980, in press)

osteoblasts, and (2) the agents also depress the activation of new BMU, that dries up the future supply of osteoclasts and/or osteoblasts needed to produce a continuing therapeutic effect.[20]

In that light, the "coherence concept" suggests that by (1) pulsing the activation modality with one agent to suddenly create a large number of new temporally coherent BMU, (2) then giving the subject a second agent that depresses osteoclastic activity while that activity lasts, and (3) at the "switchover time" allowing the BMU formation phases to function free of depressor agent, a positive $\Delta B.BMU$ should develop. Since this *sequential treatment* embraces activating, then depressing, then freeing, and then repeating the sequence, it becomes in alphabetical shorthand the ADFR treatment. Encouraging early results of this scheme obtained by Meunier[46] have stimulated many investigators to try to develop a workable clinical technology out of it. Although proof of success in this endeavor remains in the offing at this writing, genuine optimism and enthusiasm now infuse a field that, in the past, has proved frustratingly refractory to our therapeutic efforts.

Finally, simply by altering the treatment sequence, for example to AFDR, one could accelerate loss of bone, and by developing a means to confine the effects to selected parts of the body it should become possible to treat regional ABV abnormalities while leaving the healthy parts of the skeleton unaffected.

Osteomalacias

Here again, as many defintiions of osteomalacia exist as there are authorities, one reason lying in the fact that although osteomalacias occur much less frequently than osteoporoses, research has revealed an unexpected variety and complexity in the group as a whole. Another reason lies in the differing biases of the clinicians, biochemists, radiologists, pathologists, and anatomists who have studied these diseases. It is probably fair to say that we do not yet have on hand the data required to classify these diseases with finality. For the present needs therefore an empirical and orthopedically biased approach to the matter must serve.[23]

Let us define osteomalacia the disease as one in which an underlying and causative *medical pathophysiologic syndrome* associates with an *osteomalacic skeleton*. Other authorities have discussed the former at length elsewhere.[1,3,9,41,52,53,57,66] As to the osteomalacic skeleton, it displays two major abnormalities (again within the context of the writer's clinical bias): a supranormal amount of osteoid exists, which displays characteristic kinetic cellular level abnormalities, and an impaired bone healing process exists. A few words about each of these changes follow.

OSTEOID ACCUMULATION

In the osteomalacic skeleton two changes arise, both affecting bone remodeling. First, the mineralization of new osteoid slows down so that mineralizing the organic matrix in a new packet of bone may take from 6 months to more than 10 yr to complete. The deposition of new matrix also slows down (implying lazy or compromised osteoblasts), usually in proportion to the retardation of mineralization. Thus, the osteoid seams can become thickened in some medically distinctive osteomalacias, and not become thickened in others.

Second, normal osteoblasts in lamellar bone spend perhaps 90 to 95% of their existence making new bone and only 5 to 10% of that time in a state of inactivity. Called "ON" and "OFF" states, in some osteomalacias the OFF states consume half of the osteoblast's total lifetime and in others may consume 85 to >95% of that time.

Both of these effects cause a given osteoid seam to persist in bone far longer than normal, so that if, as usually occurs, continued activation of new BMU goes on, osteoid accumulates in the skeleton, with respect to both its total quantity and its total surface. Hence the *hyperosteoidosis* of the osteomalacic skeleton, in which other kinds of mineralization defects also occur.

At present, histomorphometric analysis of tetracycline doubly and *in vivo* labeled bone biopsies provides the best method of recognizing and quantitating the features described.

IMPAIRED BONE HEALING

The impaired bone healing process in most osteoosteomalacias displays the following characteristics. After gross fracture, adequate invasion by granulation tissue occurs, followed by the appearance of osteoblasts (and chondroblasts), which then elaborate the organic matrices of woven bone and hyaline cartilage. However, those matrices cannot mineralize sufficiently to become rigid and strong, nor can they mineralize sufficiently to permit internal replacement by BMU-based lamellar bone. This arrests the fracture healing process at this stage. Hence, a delayed union or a nonunion arises. Upon correcting the underlying chemical defect or defects characteristic of the osteomalacia in question, mineralization of the new matrices resumes and the healing process can then proceed to its natural conclusion.

Clinical notes

When the impairment described occurs in a traumatic fracture or surgical osteotomy, a delayed or nonunion results. When it occurs after a bone grafting procedure a graft failure results. When it occurs following a stress fracture it is termed a Looser's zone or pseudofracture. Osteomalacic bone provides a weaker than normal anchorage for orthopedic hardware, and total joint replacement components tend to "walk" or migrate through underlying osteomalacic bone with time and load-bearing.

Most osteomalacias that impair bone healing are associated with depressed serum calcium values (assuming normal renal function) and low 24-hr urine calcium excretions and urinary calcium : creatinine ratios. Radiographically evident osteoporosis often accompanies the osteomalacic process. Table 7-4 lists the salient features of a few osteomalacias.

Some osteomalacias, if untreated, pose distinct threats to the operative and postoperative patient and to the severely traumatized patient, with respect to homeostasis, endocrine function (particularly parathyroid and adrenal cortical), perhaps the clotting mechanism, and nutrition. Since these situations seldom arise in North American and European practice (so that little awareness of the problem exists in the respective surgical communities), they can readily catch a clinician both unaware and unprepared. The writer estimates that in the average North American orthopedic practice one sees 30 to 100 osteoporotic patients for every osteomalacic one.

Fibrous tissue remodeling

The turnover mechanisms of human fibrous tissue structures have received far less study in the laboratory and clinic than those of bone and cartilage. However, and regardless of any molecular level turnover that may occur, a BMU-style remodeling mechanism also exists in human tendon, ligaments, and fascia.[19,22,26] Its histologic manifestations reveal the same ARF structure found in bone remodeling, its σ value probably approximates that of the bone remodeling process, and it manifests the same "packet" property. The major function of this remodeling mechanism probably constitutes repair of mechanical, fatigue-like microdamage while it is still microscopic in extent. Decreased activation and/or prolonged σ values of these fibrous tissue BMU, by impairing repair of such microdamage, probably underlie most spontaneous tendon ruptures and muscle herniations and ligament relaxations (as in rheumatoid arthritis) encountered in clinical orthopedics.

The macrorepair processes

Chondral healing

Older medical texts stated that hyaline cartilage (as in articular cartilage) could not heal an incision or a defect, and this idea remains wide-

TABLE 7-4 OSTEOMALACIAS

TYPE	ABNORMAL BONE HEALING	PSEUDO FRACTURES OCCUR	24-hr URINE CALCIUM	SERUM CALCIUM	SERUM PHOSPHATE	SERUM ALKALINE PHOSPHATASE	VALUE
D-Deficiency	+	+	D	D	D	I	I
Hypophosphatemic, acquired	+	+	D	V	D	I	I
Hypophosphatemic, familial	0	0	N	N	D	N	N
Baker-Dent disease	0	0	D	D	D	I	N
Malnutrition	+	+	D	D	V	V	I
Renal Osteodystrophy	+	+	D	N	I	I	I
2° Hyperparathyroidism	+	+	D	D	V	I	I
Metabolic acidoses	+	+	D	V	D	V	I

Code: D = decreased, N = normal, V = variable, I = increased.

spread. Yet many instances of an effective repair mechanism of human hyaline cartilage have passed before this author's eyes.[19] A commoner example: the osteochondritis dissecans defect in the articular cartilage of the medial femoral condyle in a 12-yr-old is regularly resurfaced by good hyaline articular cartilage 6 yr later when one reopens the knee to remove a meniscus or repair an acute cruciate rupture. Time led to the original and assuredly mistaken conclusion that this tissue cannot heal. Effective chondral healing probably requires 20 to 40 times longer than the relatively rapid healing of a skin incision, and investigators interested in the problem, being unaware of its sluggishness, did not observe it over sufficiently long periods to perceive it.

Experimentalists have now begun to study this matter, but lacking an adequate body of experimental data, this text will not discuss it further.

Fracture healing

A gross fracture of a living bone initiates a series of events that culminate when normal mechanical function and competence return, usually many months later.* Known collectively as fracture healing, these macroevents also affect healing of bone grafts and osteotomies, but discussion of such matters belongs elsewhere. For present needs these events, in order of their appearance in time, include the following:[1,26,35,66,73]

GRANULATION TISSUE PROLIFERATION

Granulation tissue proliferates into the fracture, bringing with it capillaries, fibroblasts, and progenitor cells. This requires producing popu-

lations of new cells and their differentiating into the required types and excretion of the appropriate intercellular substances. Although some texts list the fracture hematoma as an essential initial event, it probably is not, because both stress fractures and Looser's zones (neither of which develops a hematoma) heal well,[19] the latter of course following correction of the underlying chemical defect.

PRODUCTION OF NEW OSTEOBLASTS

Osteoblasts are produced by the cells in the granulation tissue, which then make the organic matrix of woven bone and initiate its mineralization. New chondroblasts and hyaline cartilage also often arise, particularly when motion occurs during the fracture healing process. When this phase ends, function usually resumes; the healing mass of new tissue is called *callus,* and its mineral deposits render it both mechanically rigid and strong and visible radiographically.

REPLACEMENT BY LAMELLAR BONE

The architecturally disorganized callus is replaced by lamellar bone, the consequence of invasion by haversian-type remodeling BMU. This replacement typically takes some 2 to 4 yr to finish; it parallels the strains developed in the tissue and at its culmination, normally oriented lamellar bone both bridges the fracture and lies continuous with the pre-existing lamellar bone on either side of the original fracture (see Figure 7-14, top).

---

* Intriguingly, clinical situations exist in which the biologic mechanisms that usually detect *micro*damage of bone and initiate its repair by a BMU seem to become "deaf," so that accumulation of unrepaired microdamage ultimately leads to a spontaneous gross failure or fracture. This now constitutes *macro*damage, and a perfectly normal macrorepair process then ensues, a situation regularly encountered in idiopathic aseptic necrosis of the femoral head, for example.[23,26] The converse also occurs: although the macrorepair process proves "deaf," the microrepair process does not, and the biologic failure illustrated in Figure 7-12 shows an example of this phenomenon. Such "behavioral dissociations" imply fundamental differences in regulation.

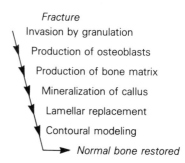

FIGURE 7-12   *Schematic of the macrorepair processes.*

MODELING ACTIVITY ARISES

Modeling activity arises concurrently with replacement by lamellar bone on the periosteal and endosteal surfaces of the bone, tending to convert the bulbous periosteal and endosteal contours of the fracture callus to the contours characterizing the bone prior to its fracture. This modeling proceeds rapidly and effectively in young children (see Fig. 7-11, left) but becomes very sluggish after skeletal maturity. Figure 7-12 summarizes the sequences described.

Diseases of fracture healing

Impairment of any stage in the healing complex can delay or prevent union, creating a need to interfere to restore union, cosmesis, and optimal function. Such nonunions divide reasonably well into two major groups, which the writer names the "technical failure" and the "biologic failure" of the bone healing process.[19]

TECHNICAL FAILURES

When technical failure occurs, the potential biology of the whole bone healing process remains inherently normal, but some aspect of the fracture management blocks the healing process. Such blocks can result from excessive distraction or otherwise poor reduction, from excessive motion (particularly in shear or pistoning) during the healing process, from interposition of soft tissues between the fragments, from local infection that destroys the granulation tissue (Fig. 7-13), and the like. Correcting a technical failure only requires identifying and correcting the particular impediment to bone healing, which will then go on to its normal conclusion. Virtually any kind of bone graft (autogenous or not, onlay or inlay, massive, or in many small chips), as well as simple drilling and related nongrafting procedures, usually lead to successful healing of a technical failure.[19,26] The typical hallmark of the technical failure represents adequate amounts of radiographically visible callus around each major fragment but separated by a mobile gap between them. The callus proves the inherent competence of the underlying biologic factors.

BIOLOGIC FAILURES

Biologic failures form a distinct minority group, probably less than 10% of all clinical nonunions in the United States.[19,26] Nevertheless, they can create troublesome and challenging problems. Here, in spite of proper management, some biologic defect in the local tissues causes defective union. Several types of biologic defects occur, including those contained in the following paragraphs.

Impaired ability to elaborate primary callus

Most biologic failures are caused by an impaired ability to elaborate primary callus, which can stem from deficient generation of the new cells (capillaries, fibroblasts, osteoblasts) required to make the callus, or from differentiation of new cells into fibroblasts rather than osteoblasts (and chondroblasts) in that stage of the healing process. This group develops little or no radiographically or histologically evident callus around the major fracture fragments, even after many months have passed (see Fig. 7-13, right).

Achieving reliable union in this group usually requires a procedure *that bypasses the callus stage of healing,*[19] and that allows BMU-based bone remodeling to bridge and repair the fracture line directly. As Schenk[62] has noted, this requires close-fitting contact of the fracture surfaces, maintained for many months by a rigid fixation technique that allows less than $\approx 100\ \mu$ of relative motion of the fragments at the fracture plane. A variety of techniques can serve these requirements adequately, given that one understands the facts. Far more often than not, simple onlay grafts, multiple chip grafts, homogenous and heterogenous grafts, and/or simple drilling across the fracture line fail to evoke union of these problems.[19] The role of electrical stimulation of impaired bone healing appears promising, but its kinds, effects, and indications lie unresolved at present, although it is under intensive study around the world.[6,9,16,30]

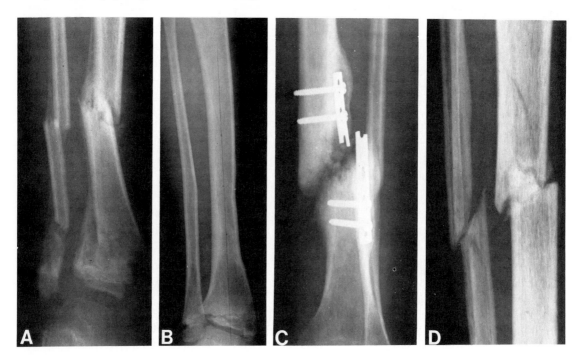

FIGURE 7-13 **(A)** *A complex malunion of tibia and fibula in a young child.* **(B)** *The modeling-corrected bones several years later. This is bone modeling in action.* **(C)** *A "technical failure" of bone union. An infection resulting from the initial operative procedure prevented the adequate consolidation into a single mass of the abundant callus generated around each major fragment. Adequate drainage, antibiotics, and removal of the hardware led to subsequent union in spite of imperfect apposition of the fragments. No bone graft was needed.* **(D)** *An example of a "biologic failure." In spite of adequate reduction and immobilization and the passage of many months, only trivial amounts of callus appear. Poor blood supply did not cause the phenomenon because the longitudinal tunneling shown in the compacta represents dramatically supranormal BMU-based remodeling, which, in turn, demonstrates commensurately supranormal perfusion. Union was achieved with a securely fixed sliding graft, only one of a variety of ways that could have proved equally successful. Union was produced by many new remodeling BMU traversing the nearly absolutely immobile and closely fitted interfaces between the fragments and between the graft and the fragments. This takes longer than healing by the "callus route," typically 2 to 3 times longer.*

Impaired remodeling of the primary callus

On rare occasions—the writer's personal cases all occurred in children—the callus forms in normal time and amount, function resumes whereupon, disconcertingly, the fracture then progressively angulates, typically some 2 to 5 mo after the original injury. Here the initial resorptive phase of the BMU that ultimately will replace the callus with lamellar bone does occur, and riddles the callus with holes. However, a long delay arises in the subsequent deposition of new lamellar bone in these BMU, thereby temporarily weakening the riddled mass of somewhat "plastic" callus.[19,26]

Because of its rarity, the clinicians caring for it usually have not understood this entity. Little hard information exists as to the bone and calcium physiology of these subjects, although in the writer's personal series no consistent abnormalities existed in their serum and urine chemistries.

Treating this entity has proved simple: remanipulate (under anesthesia) to correct the angulation, recast, and leave the cast on *three times longer than normally indicated* for an uncomplicated fracture. This extra time seemingly allows the sluggish formation side of the ARF sequence a head start, for no subsequent problems arose in patients so treated by the writer. Several autogenous chip-type onlay grafts of such malunions known to the writer proved disastrous; the graft plus both ends of the major fragments subsequently resorbed, leaving a large bone defect filled with fibrous tissue. A few such situations have led to malpractice actions.

Impaired mineralization of callus

This problem can arise in an osteomalacia in adults,[1,52,53] and in many (but not all) forms of rickets in children.[5,53] Here the osteoblasts (and chondroblasts) appear and make the appropriate organic matrix, but because of the biochemical disorders associated with the osteomalacia the callus does not mineralize sufficiently to provide a rigid union. Note that rickets associated with perfectly normal bone healing occurs in the familial hypophosphotemic (i.e., familial vitamin D resistant) form.

When a mineralization defect of this kind exists, correcting the underlying biochemical abnormalities usually restores normal bone healing. With increasing experience and knowledge of osteomalacias, this group of patients—not often encountered in the United States and Canadian practice—becomes increasingly complex and diverse.

Impaired modeling

When a fracture heals with some angulation and/or a local sharp change in periosteal contour, and function resumes, local surface stress concentrations arise at the changes in contour, predisposing to refracture following otherwise minimal trauma. A competent modeling modality normally and specifically corrects such situations. Consequently, if modeling cannot proceed normally, the persisting fracture deformity will predispose the affected bone to later refracture. An incompetent modeling faculty occurs in osteogenesis imperfecta, in many cases of osteopetrosis, and in Pyle's disease, and of course modeling proceeds very slowly, even at best, in healthy adult humans.[25]

Fibrous tissue healing

Fibrous tissue healing displays striking parallels to the bone healing process.[35] Thus, following an incision or rupture of a fibrous tissue structure, granulation tissue first invades the gap, and then differentiated fibroblasts deposit an unorganized feltwork of collagen called the scar and

analogous to the fracture callus. This tissue lacks strength (Fig. 7-14).

Function usually resumes at this time, as does also a BMU-type internal remodeling process that, over a period of ≈ 1 yr, replaces the structurally disordered scar with highly ordered fibrous tissue, the collagen fibers of which parallel the tension loads carried by the structure.

CLINICAL NOTE

The initial healing process seems to require 6 to 8 wk to "mature" the scar to the point of biomechanical competence, because if gradually progressive loading of a repaired ligament (as an example only) begins after that 6- to 8-wk period, proper replacement of the scar or callus occurs, and the ligament does not stretch out in the process. However, if loading resumes much before that time the repair does stretch out, leaving the ligament lax and the repair therefore ineffective.

As with fracture callus, the scar (a simple tissue) lacks the tensile strength of the mature, fully oriented complex tissue. Figure 7-14 diagrams at least one of the reasons. The processes described underlie all tendon, fascial, and ligament healing.

The blood-bone exchange process

Although an awareness of blood-bone exchange of electrolytes and acid-base substances goes back many decades, it has only been about since 1965 that the basic tissue mechanisms responsible for it began to emerge in reasonable detail and perspective, and some controversy (and probably considerable ignorance) still plagues the matter.* The text will try to meld the differing views into a 1980 judgement of their roles. To begin then:

Numerous clinical and experimental facts reveal that electrolyes and acid-base substances do

---

* A general surgeon colleague of the writer, Dr. Rodney Dwyer, applies an expression to the challenging and baffling, an expression that seems peculiarly apt to the present subject matter: "I wish I understood everything I know about this problem."

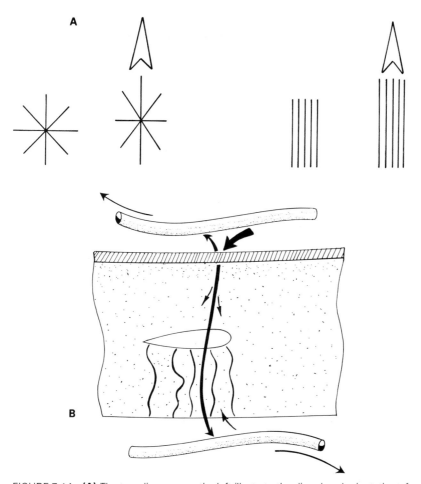

FIGURE 7-14 **(A)** *The two diagrams on the left illustrate the disordered orientation of the trabeculae and collagen fibers, characterizing woven bone and scar, respectively. A tensile load applied to such a structure is carried by only a small fraction of such a tissue's fibers, which therefore makes it weak. The two diagrams on the right illustrate the long-range order of the fibers in lamellar bone and tendon. When the tension load aligns parallel to the fiber grain (in nature the modeling and remodeling processes cause this to be so) the same volume of tissue has significantly increased strength and rigidity. (Frost, H. M.: Orthopaedic Biomechanics, Springfield, Charles C Thomas, 1973)*

(B) *The Arnold-Frost model of blood-bone exchange is diagrammed here. A capillary at the top carries blood into the bone from right to left. Its water and electrolytes leave the capillary (large arrow) and contact the bone surface below. Here in the thin-shaded surface layer a very rapid turnover of bone salt and water occurs in exchange with solute ions in the adjacent extracellular fluid. Some of the solution in the surface layer then reenters the capillary (small left arrow) while some of it "percolates" more slowly through the deeper mineral to leave the bone at a different location below (long vertical arrow). The "bone cell lining layer" discussed by some authors may "drive" the rapid surface turnover (electron microscopic work in the laboratories of Les Mathews and Roy Talmage lend support to this idea), whereas the osteocytes, and possibly the lining cell layer too, may drive the percolation process. (Frost, H. M.: Bone Modeling and Skeletal Modeling Errors, Springfield, Charles C Thomas, 1973)*

exchange between bone and blood, and that both rapidly acting (within 20 min or so) and slowly acting (within several weeks and years) modes of exchange exist. Controversy and inquiry surround not those facts but rather the mechanisms that account for them. A preoccupation with calcium homeostasis, to the virtual exclusion of other aspects of homeostasis, has biased the directions of that controversy. This text will present the *Arnold-Frost model* of blood-bone exchange, one that incorporates features of many other models.[4]

Clearly, since osteoclasts solubilize bone, including its inorganic phase, augmenting their activity should release additional bone salt to the blood, and suppressing them should produce the converse effect. Osteoblasts have complementary but less-well-studied activities, and probably hour-to-hour and day-to-day modulation of these activities under endocrine and other forms of regulation does contribute to the regulation of bone-blood exchange in response to homeostatic need.[57] However, and although these effects formerly were considered the major or even the only ones regulating blood-bone exchange, an increasing belief arises that they may instead play only minor roles.

The percolation hypothesis

The percolation hypothesis is a facet of the Arnold-Frost model that proposes two separate phenomena (see Fig. 7-14); one is essentially a *volume phenomenon*, the other is a *surface* phenomenon, speaking in the domain of the millimeter and using some of John Marshall's terminology. As to the former, extracellular water percolates through myriad ultramicroscopic channels (which do exist) in mineralized lamellar bone and that tend to parallel its microscopic grain.[4] The canalicular network lies ideally disposed to cut across these channels, and thus to feed and drain them both.[74] This exposes at any one instant an enormous surface—many hundreds of square meters—of bone mineral to a relatively small volume of extracellular fluid. This fluid (according to this model) enters the bone at numerous discrete surface locations and leaves it at numer-

ous others. The cells lining bone surfaces and osteocytes probably both drive this percolation and control its direction and speed. Groups of these cells may even alternate between "pushing" and "pulling" states. Exchange experiments imply that a given water molecule makes its passage through the percolation bed in about 20 min or less, implying a linear length of passage through the bed on the order of 1 mm. The percolation bed has the properties of a molecular sieve, admitting small molecules and ions but not large ones.

Given these facts, even minor changes in the extracellular fluid could equilibrate with the bone mineral by percolating through bone. Passage through this percolation bed probably provides the chief mechanism for the "slow exchange" fraction known to occur between bone and blood. Figure 7-15 shows an example of a mineralization phenomenon that could arise as a consequence of this volume exchange process, reacting over years to a particular homeostatic challenge.

As to the surface phenomenon referred to, at any typical instant, numerous but discrete regions of the bone surface very rapidly turn over and exchange with the blood their chief mineral ions and water. The turnover extends several microns into the subsurface material, it occurs in an hour or less, and it probably accounts for much of the "fast exchange" fraction. One infers, reasonably, that the metabolic state and activity of the lining cell layer on these surfaces somehow controls this turnover, as Robinson[58] and Talmage[65] have suggested. These lining cells may alternate between "ON" and "OFF" states, so that this week's active surface locus may become next week's inactive one.[19] Figure 7-16 summarizes the material just given.

The four factors described appear in their order of decreasing importance as the writer views the matter, and at this writing many authorities might disagree with that order. Indeed, elaborate models exist that assign most of the homeostatic activity only to osteoclasts, as summarized by Rasmussen and Bordier,[57] or primarily to the rapid surface exchange, as proposed by Talmage and colleagues.[50,65] Time, and a sharing

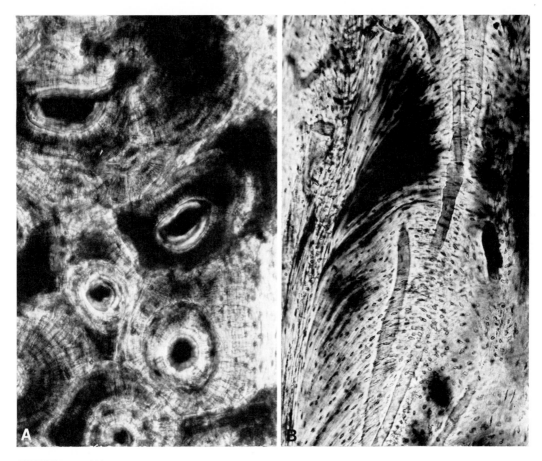

FIGURE 7-15 **(A)** *Undecalcified cross-section of compact human bone, stained with basic fuchsin. Five haversian canals appear, surrounded by their osteons. The dark areas, representing incompletely mineralized bone matrix, would appear radiolucent on microradiographs. Called* **feathering,** *this sample came from a youngster who had chronic hypoxia and hypercarbia due to congenital heart disease, and the changes in mineralization shown here probably reflect the effects of a long-duration drain by the blood on the skeletal mineral reservoir. Other morphologically distinct forms of mineralization abnormalities appear in some diseases but have received little study,* × *80.* [4,23,25]

  (B) *Longitudinal undecalcified section of a severely bowed tibia from a youngster with rickets. Same magnification and stain as the section in* **B.** *However, here the dark-staining zones reflect not deficient mineralization but rather a prefailure change, probably due to mechanical creep in shear, on the part of a bone loaded near to its limit of tolerance in flexure. This constitutes another observed form of microdamage, one found primarily in children in the writer's experience. Trabecular microdamage of several kinds has also been observed, by J. S. Arnold, the writer, E. Radin, and others.*

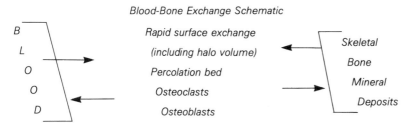

Blood-Bone Exchange Schematic

B
L   Rapid surface exchange   Skeletal
O   *(including halo volume)*   Bone
O   Percolation bed   Mineral
                     Osteoclasts
D   Osteoblasts   Deposits

FIGURE 7-16. *The process of blood-bone exchange.*

of data, experiments, and ideas should ultimately resolve any conflicting views on the subject.

CLINICAL NOTE

Unfortunately, little study has been made of the role of the skeletal homeostatic function in clinical situations, and the writer can only append a persisting suspicion that some of the serious problems—and mortality—seen in multiply injured patients and in some elderly patients following major surgical procedures derive from acute malfunctions of that homeostatic modality. Of possible significance here: solubilizing bone mineral consumes acid and the converse consumes base. Beyond that, some transformations in the physicochemical state of bone mineral can do likewise. Here probably lies a virtually untouched but potentially fertile field for clinical investigation. This subject has many other fascinating aspects but the time has come to conclude this discussion.

Conclusion

This chapter necessarily ignored many matters, some small and some large, and has focused all too briefly upon others for which the writer has some special competence but that receive short shrift in most current basic science texts. The intent was to sketch an outline on a broad canvas, with the aid of which a student, through other studies, could draw in the missing detail and make the adjustments in line required by more complete information. The fields and the concepts considered herein remain under intensive study, and thus are still fluid and evolving. Even more fluid are our ideas of what the facts available to us mean, that is, our understanding of the roles and purposes nature intends for skeletal activities, from the level of organization of the cell to that of the intact human. However, if only as from a distance through a dense fog, one can see struggling to rise out of the soil of such concepts a new being, one long awaited and hoped for by orthopedists of the writer's vintage: a truly scientific and fundamental basis for what

now constitutes primarily an empirical art, the practice of clinical orthopedics. It comes, it will and must change things, and we must and will accept and adapt to that change.

References

1. Aegerter, E., and Kirkpatrick, J. A.: Orthopaedic Diseases, 4th ed., Philadelphia, W. B. Saunders Co., 1975.
2. Aitken, J. M., Hart, O. M., and Lindsay, R.: Oestrogen replacement therapy for prevention of osteoporosis after oophorectomy, Br. Med. J. 3:515–518, 1973.
3. Anderson, W. A. D., and Kissane, J. M.: Pathology, 7th ed., St. Louis, C. V. Mosby Co., 1977.
4. Arnold, J. S., Frost, H. M., and Buss, R. O.: The osteocyte as a bone pump, Clin. Orthop. 78:43–55, 1971.
5. Barnett, H. L., and Einhom, A. H.: Pediatrics, 15th ed., New York, Appleton-Century-Crofts, 1972.
6. Becker, R. O.: Electrical osteogenesis—pro and con, Calcif. Tissue Res. 26:93–97, 1978.
7. Beighton, P., and Moran, H.: Orthopaedic aspects of the Ehlers-Danlos syndrome, J. Bone Joint Surg. 51B:444–453, 1969.
8. Biltz, R. M., and Pellegrino, E. D.: The chemical anatomy of bone, J. Bone Joint Surg. 51A:456–466, 1969.
9. Bourne, G. H.: The Biochemistry and Physiology of Bone, 5th ed., New York, Academic Press, 1976.
10. Bressot, C., Courpron, P., Edouard, C., and Meunier, P.: Histomorphométrie des Ostéopathies Endocriniennes, pp. 1–260, Lyon, University Claude Bernard, 1976.
11. Courpron, P.: Données Histologiques Quantitatives sur le veillissement Osseux Humain, pp. 1–213, Thesis, Lyon, University Claude Bernard, 1972.
12. Dhem, A.: Le Remainiement de l'Os Adulte, Brussels, Eds. Arscia, 1967.
13. Duncan, H., Frame, B., and Frost, H. M.: Migratory osteolysis of the lower extremities, Ann. Intern. Med. 66:1165–1173, 1967.
14. Enlow, D. H.: Principles of Bone Remodeling, Springfield, Charles C Thomas, 1963.
15. Epker, B. N., and Frost, H. M.: Biomechanical control of bone growth and development: a histologic and tetracycline study, J. Dent. Res. 45:364–371, 1966.

16. Eriksson, C.: Electrical properties of bone. *In* Bourne, G. H. (ed.), The Biochemistry and Physiology of Bone, 5th ed., pp. 329–384, New York, Academic Press, 1976.

17. Frost, H. M.: A chondral modeling theory. Calcif. Tissue Res. 28:181–200, 1979.

18. Frost, H. M.: A lamellar bone modeling theory. Proceedings, Japan Orthop. Res. Society, in press, 1980.

19. Frost, H. M.: An original observation.

20. Frost, H. M.: Treatment of osteoporoses by manipulation of coherent bone cell populations, Clin. Orthop. 143:227–244, 1979.

21. Frost, H. M.: Bone Remodeling Dynamics, Springfield, Charles C Thomas, 1963.

22. Frost, H. M.: Physiology of Cartilaginous, Fibrous and Bony Tissues, Springfield, Charles C Thomas, 1972.

23. Frost, H. M.: Bone Remodeling and its Relation to Metabolic Bone Disease, Springfield, Charles C Thomas, 1973.

24. Frost, H. M.: The origin and nature of transients in human bone remodeling dynamics. *In* Frame, B., Parfitt, A. M., and Duncan, H. (eds.): Clinical Aspects of Metabolic Bone Disease, pp. 124–140, Amsterdam, Excerpta Medica, 1973.

25. Frost, H. M.: Bone Modeling and Skeletal Modeling Errors, Springfield, Charles C Thomas, 1973.

26. Frost, H. M.: Orthopaedic Biomechanics, Springfield, Charles C Thomas, 1973.

27. Frost, H. M.: Micropetrosis. J. Bone Joint Surg. 42A:144–150, 1960.

28. Frost, H. M.: Presence of microscopic cracks *in vivo* in bone, Henry Ford Hosp. Med. Bull. 8:25–35, 1960.

29. Frost, H. M.: Tetracycline based analysis of bone remodeling, Calcif. Tissue Res. 3:211–217, 1969.

30. Fukada, E., and Yasuda, J.: On the piezoelectric effect of bone, J. Physiol Soc. of Japan 12:1158–1167, 1957.

31. Garn, S.: The Earlier Gain and Later Loss of Cortical Bone, Springfield, Charles C Thomas, 1970.

32. Gothlin, G., and Ericsson, J. L. E.: The osteoclast: review of ultrastructure, origin and structure-function relationship, Clin. Orthop. 120:201–228, 1976.

33. Groer, P. G., and Marshall, J. H.: Mechanism of calcium exchange at bone surface, Calcif. Tissue Res. 12:175–192, 1973.

34. Haines, R. W., and Mohiuddin, A.: Handbook of Human Embryology, Baltimore, Williams & Wilkins Co., 1965.

35. Ham, A. W.: Tratado de Histologia, 7th ed., Mexico City, Interamericana, 1975.

36. Heller-Steinberg, M.: Ground substance, bone salt and cellular activity in bone formation and destruction, Am. J. Anat. 89:347–379, 1951.

37. Jackson, W. P. V.: Osteoporosis of unknown cause in younger people, J. Bone Joint Surg. 40B:420–441, 1958.

38. Jaworski, Z. F. G. (ed.): Proceedings of the First Workshop on Bone Histomorphometry, pp. 1–395, Ottawa, Ottawa Press, 1976.

39. Jee, W. S. S., and Arnold, J. S.: Rate of individual haversian system formation, Anat. Rec. 118:315, 1954.

40. Jee, W. S. S., and Nolan, P. D.: Origin of osteoclasts from the fusion of osteocytes, Nature 200:225, 1963.

41. Johnson, L. C.: The kinetics of disease and general biology of bone. *In* Frost, H. M. (ed.): Bone Biodynamics, pp. 543–654, Boston, Little, Brown & Co., 1964.

42. Johnston, C. C., Smith, D. M., Nance, W. E., and Bevan, J.: Evaluation of the radial bone mass by the photon absorption technique. *In* Frame, B., Parfitt, A. M., and Duncan, H. (eds.): Clinical Aspects of Metabolic Bone Disease, pp. 28–36, Amsterdam, Excerpta Medica, 1973.

43. Koch, J. G.: The laws of bone architecture, Am. J. Anat. 21:177–292, 1917.

44. Lanyon, L. E., and Baggott, D. G.: Mechanical function as an influence on the structure and form of bone, J. Bone Joint Surg. 58B:436–443, 1977.

45. Lee, W. R.: A quantitative microscopic study of bone formation in a normal child and in two children suffering with osteogenesis imperfecta. Calcified Tissues, pp. 451–463, Belgium, University Liege, 1964.

46. Meunier, P.: Personal communication, 1978.

47. Meunier, P. (ed.): Bone Histomorphometry, Paris, Armour-Montagu, 1977.

48. Neuman, W. F., and Neuman, M. W.: Chemical Dynamics of Bone Mineral, Chicago, University of Chicago Press, 1958.

49. Newton-John, H. F., and Morgan, D. B.: The loss of bone with age, osteoporosis and fractures, Clin. Orthop. 71:229–252, 1970.

50. Norimatsu, H., Vander Wiel, C. J., and Talmage, R. F.: Morphological support of a role for cells lining bone surfaces in maintenance of plasma calcium concentration, Clin. Orthop. 138:254–262, 1979.

51. Owen, M.: Histogenesis of bone cells, Calcif. Tissue Res. 25:205–207, 1978.

52. Parfitt, A. M.: The actions of parathyroid hor-

mone on bone. Relation to bone remodeling and turnover, calcium homeostasis and metabolic bone disease, Metabolism 25:809–844, 1976.

53. Parfitt, A. M., and Duncan, H.: Metabolic bone disease affecting the spine. *In* Rothman, R. H., and Simeone, F. A. (eds.): *The Spine*, pp. 599–720, Philadelphia, W. B. Saunders Co., 1975.

54. Pritchard, J. J.: The osteoblast. *In* Bourne, G. H. (ed.): The Biochemistry and Physiology of Bone, 2nd ed., pp. 21–44, New York, Academic Press, 1972.

55. Ragab, A. H., Frech, R. S., and Ketti, T. J.: Osteoporotic fractures secondary to methotrexate therapy of acute leukemia in remission, Cancer 25:580–585, 1970.

56. Ramser, J. R., Villanueva, A. R., Pirok, O. J., and Frost, H. M.: Tetracycline-based measurement of bone dynamics in three women with osteogenesis imperfecta, Clin. Orthop. 49:151–162, 1966.

57. Rasmussen, H., and Bordier, P. J.: The Physiological and Cellular Basis of Metabolic Bone Disease, Baltimore, Williams & Wilkins Co., 1974.

58. Robinson, R. A.: Observations regarding compartments for tracer calcium in the body. *In* Frost, H. M. (ed): Bone Biodynamics, pp. 423–439, Boston, Little, Brown & Co., 1964.

59. Romer, A. S.: Vertebrate Paleontology, 3rd ed., Chicago, University Chicago Press, 1966.

60. Rubin, P.: Dynamic Classification of Bone Dysplasias. Chicago, 1964. Year Book Medical Publishers, 1964.

61. Sedlin, E. D.: Uses of bone as a model system in the study of aging. *In* Frost, H. M. (ed.): Bone Biodynamics, pp. 655–666, Boston, Little, Brown & Co., 1974.

62. Schenk, R. K.: Die Histologie der primaren Knochenheilung im Lichte neuer Konzeptionen uber den Knochenumbau, Unfallheilkunde 81:219–227, 1978.

63. Seliger, W. G.: Tissue fluid movement in compact bone, Anat. Rec. 166:247–255, 1970.

64. Takahashi, H., Epker, B. N., Hattner, R., and Frost, H. M.: Evidence that bone resorption precedes bone formation at the cellular level, Henry Ford Hosp. Med. Bull. 12:359–364, 1964.

65. Talmage, R. V.: Calcium homeostasis—calcium transport—parathyroid action, Clin. Orthop. 67:210–224, 1969.

66. Teitelbaum, S. L.: Metabolic and other nontumerous disorders of the bone, *In* Anerson, W. A. D., and Kissane, J. M. (eds): Pathology, 7th ed. St. Louis, The C. V. Mosby Co., 1977.

67. Tseng, T. C., Daeschner, C. W., Singleton, E. B., Rosenberg, H. S., Cole, V. W., Hill, L. L., and Brennan, J. C.: Liver disease and osteoporosis in children, J. Pediat. 59:684–709, 1961.

68. Uhthoff, H. K., and Jaworski, Z. F. G.: Bone loss in response to long term immobilization. J. Bone Joint Surg. 60B:420–429, 1978.

69. Urist, M.: Personal communication, 1961.

70. Villanueva, A. R., and Frost, H. M.: Evaluation of factors determining the tissue-level haversian bone formation rate in man, J. Dent. Res. 49:836–846, 1970.

71. Wakamatsu, E., and Sissons, H. A.: The cancellous bone of the iliac crest, Calcif. Tissue Res. 4:147–161, 1969.

72. Walker, D. G.: Osteopetrosis cured by temporary parabiosis, Science 180:875, 1973.

73. Weinman, J. P., and Sicher, H.: Bone and Bones, 2nd ed., St. Louis, The C. V. Mosby Co., 1955.

74. Whitson, S. W.: Tight junction formation in the osteon, Clin. Orthop. 86:206–213, 1972.

75. Wolff, J.: Die Lehre von der Funktionellen Knochengestalt, Virchov's Archiv. 155:256–315, 1899.

76. Wu, K., and Frost, H. M.: Bone formation in osteoporosis-appositional rate measured by tetracycline labelling, Arch. Pathol. 88:508–510, 1969.

Historical background

The possible relationship between vitamin D and bone has been apparent for centuries. Francis Glisson, FRCP* (1597–1677) prepared a 200-page treatise entitled De Rachitide, which provided the first comprehensive and medically accurate description of rickets. Virtually simultaneously and quite independently D. Whistler in Rotterdam, The Netherlands published in 1645 his Ph.D. dissertation on Morbo puerli anglorum, quem patrio idiomate indigenae vocant *the ricketts*. Both these publications describe the puzzling relationships between bone abnormalities, dietary states, and "outdoor exposure." These intuitive relationships were further supported by the scientists and physicians of the 17th century who found a correlation between the incidence of the bone disease rickets and the lack of sunshine. These observations ultimately led to the brilliant studies by Sir Edward Mellanby of London, England who devised the first experimental diet that was capable of producing rickets in puppies. An important, but at that time unappreciated, aspect of Mellanby's experimental protocol was that his puppies had no access to sunlight or ultraviolet light. His observations were soon followed by the demonstration of the existence of the antirachitic vitamin D calciferol by Hess and Gutman in New York and McCollum and colleagues in Baltimore, Maryland. Shortly thereafter, Goldblatt and Soames in London, England, as well as Steenbock and Black in Madison, Wisconsin, demonstrated the critical role of ultraviolet light in producing vitamin D from a provitamin present in the skin.

Once the connection between antirachitic activity, ultraviolet light, and $\Delta 5,7$-unsaturated sterols, such as 7-dehydrocholesterol and ergosterol, was appreciated, it was possible for Askew and coworkers in England, and Windaus and his colleagues in Germany to carry out a chemical characterization of vitamin D_3, which is a secosteroid, formally known as 9(10)seco-cholesta-5,7,10(19)-dien-3β-ol. Seco-steroids are those in which one of the rings has undergone fission by

ANTHONY W. NORMAN

8

bone and the vitamin D endocrine system

* FRCP = Fellow of the Royal College of Physicians, (United Kingdom)

breakage of a carbon-carbon bond; in the instance of vitamin D_3 this is the 9,10 carbon bond of ring B of 7-dehydrocholesterol.

Vitamin D_3 or cholecalciferol is the naturally occurring form of the vitamin and is normally derived by exposure to sunlight of the precursor 7-dehydrocholesterol, which is present in the skin. Vitamin D_2 or ergocalciferol is produced synthetically through ultraviolet irradiation of the sterol ergosterol. The minimum daily requirement for humans of either vitamin D (calciferol) is 400 IU; 1.0 IU is equivalent to 25 ng or 65 pmol. The primary biologic functions of vitamin D are to mediate intestinal calcium absorption and to permit normal skeletal development.

A formal definition of a "vitamin" is that it is a trace dietary constituent required to effect normal functioning of a physiologic process. Emphasis here is on *trace* and the fact that the vitamin *must* be supplied dietarily; this implies that the body is unable to synthesize the vitamin in question. Thus calciferol is a vitamin only when the animal does not have access to sunlight or ultraviolet light. Under normal physiologic circumstances all mammals, including humans, can generate adequate quantities of vitamin D through ultraviolet photolysis. It is largely due to a historic accident that calciferol was classified as a vitamin rather than as a steroid hormone. Although chemists have certainly appreciated the strong structural similarity between vitamin D and other steroids, this correlation has not been widely acknowledged until recently in the biologic-clinical or nutritional sciences.

In fact, the unusual prominence that vitamin D enjoys in a clinical setting is a result of the effects of a deficiency of the steroid on bone metabolism. When sunlight is lacking, a dietary requirement for vitamin D develops, and it is in this sense that the steroid vitamin D gains prominence as a vital nutritional substance. As long as people lived or worked primarily outdoors and had access to minimal levels of ultraviolet light, their needs for vitamin D could be largely met by the generation of this steroid in the skin. However, in the 1800s, with the industrial revolution and the expansion of urban life (when exposure to ultraviolet light was greatly reduced), the deficiency aspects of vitamin D in relation to the bone became strikingly apparent. Rickets and osteomalacia were found in virtually epidemic proportions in factory workers in many cities in England in the middle to late 1800s.

Any discussion of the actions of vitamin D on bone tissue is complex. This is due in part to the fact that despite our unraveling of the pathway for the metabolism of vitamin D by the kidney into 1,25-dihydroxyvitamin D_3 [1,25$(OH)_2D_3$] and our current understanding of the proposed steroid hormone mode of action of vitamin D metabolites in intestinal tissue, there are as yet no definitive answers to questions regarding the specific effects of vitamin D or its metabolites on bone tissue. A second reason has to do with the inherent complexity of the morphology of bone tissue. Although it might be argued that the cellular anatomy of bone is no more complex than that of other body organs, such as the kidney or brain, it is certainly obvious that the intrinsic physical properties of bone have not lent themselves to ready manipulation by the physiologist and biochemist who may wish to probe in detail aspects of various subcomponents.

The vitamin D endocrine system

Metabolic pathway

Until the 1960s little progress was made in understanding the mode of action of calciferol. Much work focused on the nutritional and putative cofactor functions of the molecule. However, since 1965 there has emerged a new model for the mechanism of action of this important seco-steroid. The model is based on the concept that in terms of both chemical structure and mode of action, vitamin D is similar to other steroid hormones such as estradiol, progesterone, testosterone, hydrocortisone, aldosterone, or ecdysone.

In fact, it is now recognized that there is an extensive metabolic pathway for converting the prohormone vitamin D into its hormonally active form or forms (Fig. 8-1). To date, there are eight known daughter metabolites of calciferol. The principal metabolites in the blood are 25$(OH)D_3$

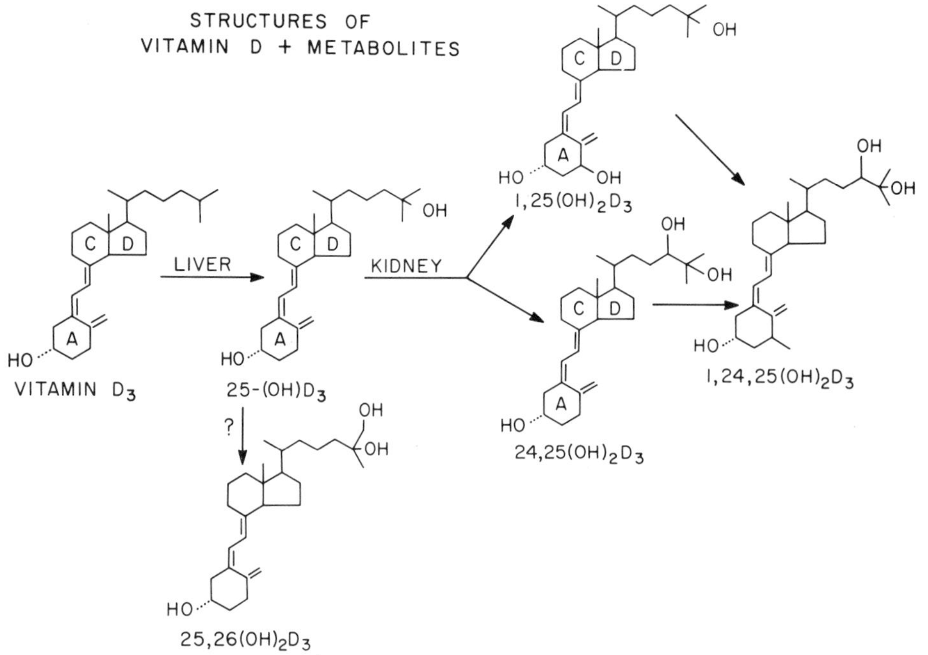

FIGURE 8-1 *Metabolic pathway for vitamin D transformation.*

(15–30 ng/ml), 24,25(OH)$_2$D$_3$ (1–3 ng/ml), and 1,25(OH)$_2$D$_3$ (30–40 pg/ml). The plasma concentrations and biologic function of the other five metabolites are not yet known. In this system, the biologically active form of vitamin D, particularly in the intestine and also probably in the bone, is the steroid 1,25-dihydroxyvitamin D$_3$ [1,25(OH)$_2$D$_3$]. There is some preliminary evidence supporting the actions of 24,25(OH)$_2$D$_3$ at the parathyroid gland and bone. The endocrine gland that produces these two dihydroxylated biologically active forms of vitamin D is the kidney. After metabolic conversion of vitamin D$_3$ into 25-hydroxyvitamin D$_3$ [25(OH)D$_3$] by a liver mitochondrial enzyme, this circulating form of the seco-steroid serves as substrate for either the renal 25(OH)D$_3$-1-hydroxylase or the 25(OH)D$_3$-24-hydroxylase. Both enzymes are located in the mitochondrial fraction of the kidney cortex. In fact, the 1-hydroxylase has been shown to be localized in the kidney of members of every vertebrate class from teleost through amphibians, reptiles, and avians to many mammals including primates. The 1-hydroxylase is a cytochrome P-450 containing enzyme that involves an adrenodoxin component and that in-

corporates molecular oxygen into the 1α-hydroxyl functionality. In this respect, the 1-hydroxylase enzyme system is a classic mixed function steroid hydroxylase similar to the steroid hormone hydroxylases located in the adrenal cortical mitochondria.

Regulation of production of 1,25(OH)$_2$D$_3$

Extensive evidence has been presented supporting the view that the steroid hormone 1,25(OH)$_2$D$_3$ is produced only in accord with strict physiologic signals dictated by the calcium "demand" of the organism; a bimodal mode of regulation has been suggested (Fig. 8-2**A,B**). On a time scale of minutes, changes in the ionic environment of the kidney mitochondria resulting from the accumulation or release of calcium or inorganic phosphate may alter the enzymatic activity of the 1-hydroxylase; on a time scale of hours parathyroid hormone (PTH) has been found to be capable of stimulating the production of 1,25(OH)$_2$D$_3$, possibly by stimulating the biosynthesis of the 1-hydroxylase itself. Recent studies using primary cell cultures of chick kidney cells have conclusively shown that the presence of 1,25(OH)₂D₃ also induces the formation of the 24-hydroxylase enzyme system and the production of 24,25(OH)₂D₃. Thus, the kidney is clearly an endocrine gland capable of producing in a physiologically regulated manner appropriate amounts of 1,25(OH)₂D₃ and 24,25(OH)₂D₃.

There is both physiologic and biochemical evidence of a "short" feedback loop between the

kidney and the parathyroid gland, wherein the dihydroxylated vitamin D metabolites modulate PTH secretion. It has long been known that the release of PTH is governed by a "long" loop feedback of ionized calcium concentration in the blood. Recently it has been shown that direct infusion into the parathyroid gland of both 1,25(OH)₂D₃ and 24,25(OH)₂D₃ can inhibit the secretion of PTH. There is also direct biochemi-

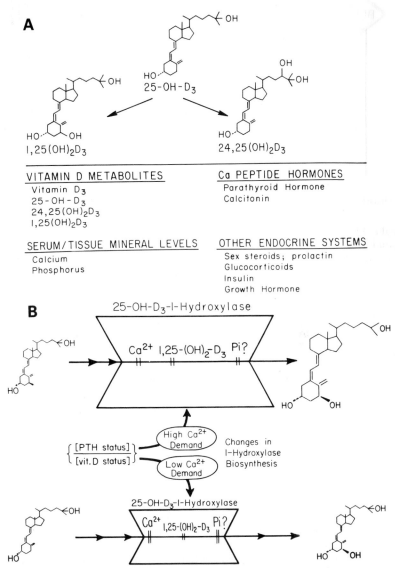

FIGURE 8-2 *Regulation of the renal 25-hydroxyvitamin D₃-1-hydroxylases.* **(A)** *Summary of the factors that under* in vivo *conditions can modulate the production of 1,25(OH)₂D₃.* **(B)** *Summary of the biochemical components of the 1-hydroxylase system and agents that under* in vitro *conditions can inhibit the production of 1,25(OH)₂D₃.*

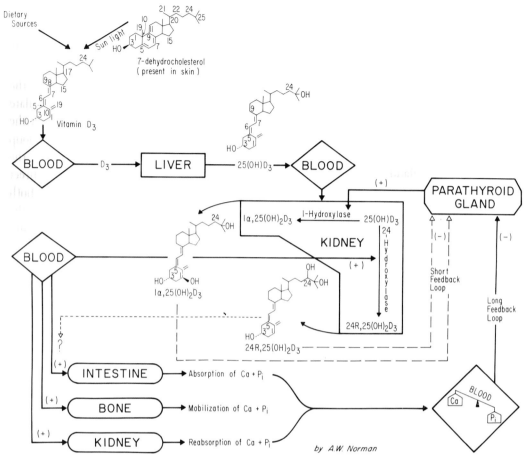

FIGURE 8-3 *Flow chart of the vitamin D endocrine system.*

cal evidence for the existence of both cytosol and nuclear receptors for 1,25(OH)₂D₃ in the parathyroid gland (see later discussion). Thus, the hormonally active forms of vitamin D can apparently modulate the secretion of parathyroid hormone; this is similar to the action of the classic steroids such as the glucocorticoids or estrogens that "feed back" directly on the hypothalamus and pituitary to inhibit secretion of adrenocorticotropic hormone (ACTH) and follicle-stimulating hormone (FSH). There is also increasing evidence that a number of other hormones besides PTH can modulate the production of 1,25(OH)₂D₃. These include growth hormone, prolactin, estrogens, and possibly glucocorticoids. The biochemical basis of these effects is not yet clearly delineated (see Fig. 8-2B).

Figure 8-3 summarizes our current understanding of the vitamin D endocrine system; in this system the kidney serves as an endocrine gland to produce 1,25(OH)₂D₃ and 24,25(OH)₂D₃ subject to modulation by a number of physiologic signals including PTH.

Steroid hormone mode of action of 1,25 (OH)₂D₃

The mode of action of 1,25(OH)₂D₃ in the target organ—the intestinal mucosa—to stimulate calcium absorption has been conclusively shown to be analogous to that of other steroid hormones (Fig. 8-4). Definitive biochemical evidence supports the existence of a two-step process: first, the steroid hormone 1,25(OH)₂D₃ associates with a 3.7S cytosol receptor (65,000 daltons), which then migrates to the intestinal nuclear chromatin fraction, in which there are specific acceptor sites. As a consequence of the presence of the steroid-receptor complex in the nucleus, there ensues a stimulation of template activity including the biosynthesis of a messenger RNA for a calcium-binding protein (CaBP). The amount of intestinal CaBP has been shown to be exactly proportional to the amount of 1,25(OH)$_2$D$_3$ localized in the intestinal mucosa and the specific activity of the renal 25(OH)D-1-hydroxylase as well as to the level of vitamin D–mediated intestinal calcium absorption.

Calcium and phosphorus homeostasis

Background

Any consideration of the inter-relationships between vitamin D and other hormones must take into account the known physiologic effects of vi-

tamin D as well as the two peptide hormones—PTH and calcitonin—on calcium and phosphorus metabolism. Table 8-1 summarizes the physiologic effects of the three principal hormones of calcium and phosphorus metabolism. The intertwining actions of the three hormones of calcium and phosphorus homeostasis clearly reflect the crucial roles of both calcium and phosphate in the biologic processes of higher animals. It is of utmost importance to maintain the extracellular calcium ion concentration within narrow limits; accordingly, the higher the phylogenetic order, the greater the complexity of sophisticated endocrinologic inter-relationships and mechanisms developed to ensure ion homeostasis.

Calcium is essential to a great number of cellular processes. One need only recall the important role of calcium in muscle contraction, its key role in the process of blood clotting, its obligatory association with a number of enzyme activities,

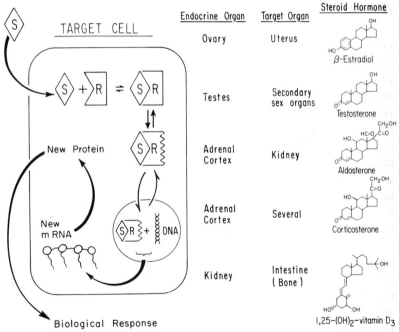

FIGURE 8-4 *Generalized two-step model of the action of steroid hormones in their target tissues. The left panel indicates how steroid hormones (including 1,25-(OH)$_2$D$_3$) are believed to interact in their target tissue (the target tissue for 1,25(OH)$_2$D$_3$ is the intestinal mucosa).* **R** = *a protein receptor localized in the cytoplasmic portion of the cell.* **SR** = *the steroid-receptor complex, which undergoes a temperature-dependent activation step prior to its entry into the nucleus of the cell. The right panel illustrates the structural similarities of many steroid hormones, including 1,25(OH)$_2$D$_3$.*

TABLE 8-1 PHYSIOLOGIC EFFECTS OF CALCITONIN, PTH, AND VITAMIN D (AND METABOLITES) RELATED TO MINERAL METABOLISM

EFFECT	CALCITONIN	PTH	VITAMIN D
INTESTINAL			
Calcium absorption	↓?	↑	↑
Phosphate absorption	?	?	↑
RENAL *			
Phosphate excretion	↑	↑	↓
Calcium excretion	↑	↓	↓
Hydrogen excretion	→	↓	?
Potassium excretion	Slight ↑	↑	?
Sodium excretion	↑	↑	?
Adenyl cyclase activity	→	↑	?
SKELETAL			
Calcium mobilization	↓	↑	↑
Mineralization of bone matrix			↑
OTHER			
Plasma levels of calcium	↓	↑	↑
Plasma levels of phosphate	↓	↓	
Body weight	?	?	Increases

* (After H. Rasmussen: *In* Williams, R. H. (ed.): Textbook of Endocrinology, 5th edition, Philadelphia, W. B. Saunders Co., 1974.

its possible role as a "second messenger" in many cyclic AMP–mediated responses, and its obvious contribution to the skeleton as well as to the formation of eggshell in birds to gain insight into the *raison d'être* of its stringent regulation.

The three prime target tissues related to calcium and phosphorus homeostasis are the intestine, in which these ions enter into the physiologic milieu, the bone, in which they are stored and made available for minute-by-minute regulation of the serum levels of these ions, and the kidney, in which their principal rate of excretion can be affected. The maintenance of calcium and phosphorus homeostasis thus involves the delicate inter-relationships of absorption by the intestine, accretion and reabsorption by bone tissue, and urinary excretion by the kidney.

Calcium in plasma exists in three forms: free or ionized, complexed to organic ions such as citrate, and protein bound. The total concentration of calcium in plasma is normally 2.5 mM, or 10 mg/dl. Under normal circumstances approximately 46% of the total plasma calcium is bound to protein (primarily to serum albumin), the remaining 54% being ultrafilterable. Thus, there are two basic mechanisms for generating free or ionized calcium in the plasma—that which can be manipulated by endocrine mecha-

nisms and that which can occur by changing the concentrations of plasma protein. It is assumed that the useful and therefore regulated portion of calcium is the ionized type, since there is no evidence that endocrinologic changes affect the protein binding of calcium.

The plasma concentrations of the several ionic types of phosphate are not so stringently regulated; rather, they are manipulated in concert with the endocrine perturbation, which may have effected changes in calcium concentration. Under normal circumstances, phosphate is present in plasma at a level of 1.2 mM, or in the range of 2.5 to 4.3 mg/dl (of phosphorus). Approximately 10% of the plasma phosphate is protein bound; the remainder exists as free phosphate, either as HPO_4^{2-} or $H_2PO_4^-$. The relative proportions of these two ionic types are dependent on plasma pH. There are many biologic uses of phosphate that extend from its role as an inorganic ion to its multiple involvements as organic phosphate in a plethora of both enzymatic and structural proteins as well as in nucleic acids.

It is apparent from Table 8-1 that vitamin D plays a dominant role in increasing the intestinal absorption of calcium and phosphorus; however, it should be appreciated that this uptake process is regulated according to the needs of the animal and is dictated by certain physiologic signals. Once calcium and phosphate are made available in the plasma, a delicate balancing operation occurs between accretion and mobilization in the bone and excretion by the kidney. In the event that the dietary intake or availability of calcium and phosphorus is diminished or increased, it is possible to tip the balance in favor of increased bone mobilization or increased bone accretion to meet the stringent prerequisite of a constant serum calcium level. Thus, serum calcium may become elevated through stimulation of bone calcium mobilization or through PTH stimulation of the tubular reabsorption of calcium at the kidney. Concomitantly, PTH stimulates phosphate excretion, so that as serum calcium concentration increases there is usually an associated fall in the plasma phosphate level. In contrast, if serum calcium levels become too elevated, the action of calcitonin may come into play. Simply speaking, calcitonin is believed to block many of the actions of PTH at the skeletal level, thereby preventing further elevation of serum calcium levels. Also associated with increased secretion of calcitonin is an increase in calcium excretion by the kidney, which can contribute to a reduction in circulating levels of serum calcium.

Figure 8-5 is a schematic diagram illustrating calcium and phosphorus metabolism in a normal adult male. Calcium and phosphorus are both absorbed into the body primarily in the duodenum and jejunum. In addition to the calcium ingested in the diet (for a normal male, the dietary requirements range from 400 to 1200 mg/d), approximately 600 to 700 mg is added to the intestinal contents by way of intestinal secretions. Thus, of the approximate total of 1600 to 1700 mg of calcium present in the lumen of the intestine, shown in the model in Figure 8-5, approximately 700 mg is reabsorbed into the bloodstream, leaving the remaining 900 to 1000 mg to be excreted in the feces. After calcium has

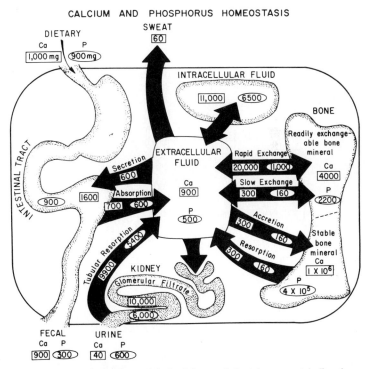

FIGURE 8-5 *A schematic model of calcium and phosphorus metabolism in an adult man having a calcium intake of 1.0 g/day and a phosphorus intake of 0.8 g/day. All numerical values are milligrams per day. All entries relating to phosphate are calculated as phosphorus. Entries for calcium are given in the rectangles, whereas entries for phosphorus are given in the ovals.*

entered the extracellular pool, it is in constant flux or exchange with the calcium already present in the extra- and intracellular fluids and in certain compartments of the bone and the glomerular filtrate. The entire extracellular pool of calcium turns over between 40 and 50 times/d. On a daily basis, the glomerulus filters some 10,000 mg of calcium, but the renal tubular reabsorption of this ion is so efficient that under normal circumstances only between 100 and 150 mg appear in the urine. In the event of hypercalcemia, the urinary excretion of calcium rises in a compensatory fashion. However, it rarely exceeds a value of 400 to 600 mg/d. The renal tubular reabsorption of calcium is stimulated by PTH and possibly by vitamin D or one of its metabolites. The increased urinary excretion of calcium is also stimulated by phosphate deprivation, acidosis, adrenal steroids, and saline diuresis. It should also be noted that an additional 30 to 100 mg of calcium is lost per day through the skin through sweating.

The term readily exchangeable bone pool is not definable explicitly in anatomical terms. It simply represents that fraction of calcium in bone that is in rapid equilibrium with calcium in plasma, in which "rapid" implies the capability

of exchange on a minute-by-minute basis. Of the total bone calcium of 1000 to 1200 g in a 70-kg man, approximately 0.4%, or 4000 mg, is present in the readily exchangeable bone pool compartment.

The dynamics of phosphate metabolism are not particularly different from those of calcium. Under normal circumstances, approximately 70% of the phosphate in the diet is absorbed. Absorption of phosphate is inter-related in a complex fashion with the presence of calcium and can be stimulated by a low-calcium diet as well as by vitamin D or its metabolites. The intestinal absorption of phosphate is inhibited by high dietary calcium levels, aluminum hydroxide injection, and beryllium poisoning. Phosphate in the body is also partitioned among three major pools: the kidney ultrafiltrate, the readily exchangeable fraction of bone, and the intracellular compartments in the various soft tissues.

As indicated in Figure 8-5, the major excretory route for phosphate is by way of the kidney. The handling of phosphate by the kidney is determined by the rate of glomerular filtration, tubular reabsorption, and possibly tubular secretion. Thus, the glomerulus filters some 6000 to 10,000 mg/d of phosphorus. A normal man given

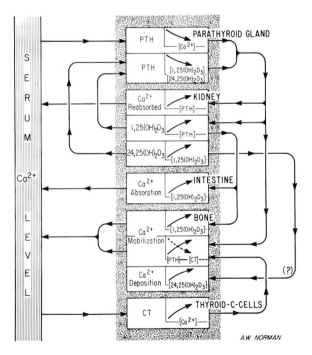

A.W. NORMAN

FIGURE 8-6 *Flow chart of the regulatory relationships that effect calcium homeostasis.*

a diet of 900 mg of phosphorus excretes approximately 600 mg/d in the urine. As already indicated, the major endocrine function of PTH is to regulate the tubular reabsorption of phosphate. Thus, high circulating levels of PTH stimulate the urinary excretion of phosphate by blocking the tubular reabsorption of the inorganic ion present in the glomerular filtrate. The urinary excretion of inorganic phosphate may be decreased by kidney failure, hypoparathyroidism, phosphate deficiency, and Addison's disease.

Role of the bone

Any discussion of the integrated control of calcium and phosphorus homeostasis must include a detailed consideration of the contributions of bone to this process. The average adult human being contains approximately 1200 g of calcium and 500 to 600 g of phosphorus (present as inorganic phosphate). Nearly 90% of both of these ions resides in the hydroxylapatite crystals of bone, with the remainder being present in extracellular fluids and other cellular compartments. Thus, bone tissue provides an enormous reservoir of both calcium and phosphorus and, in view of the dynamic movement of these ions into and out of bone, it is apparent why this organ can play such a prominent role in calcium and phosphorus homeostasis.

Central to the consideration of calcium and phosphorus homeostasis is the fact that the endoskeleton of higher organisms serves two important functions: (1) a metabolic role concerned with the maintenance of a dynamic steady state not only of calcium and phosphorus but also of many other ionic constituents for the body's extracellular fluids, and (2) a mechanical or supportive function integral to locomotion and protection of the organism. A characteristic feature of bone that enables it to fulfill both these functions is that the skeleton normally undergoes a process of continual remodeling throughout life. This remodeling process is governed by changes in the mechanical stresses on the skeleton as well as by effects of metabolic regulators. Bone tissue is responsive to the following hormones: PTH, calcitonin, $1,25(OH)_2D_3$, $24,25(OH)_2D_3$, growth hormone, gonadal hormones, thyroxine, and glucocorticoids.

Figure 8-6 presents a summary of our current understanding of the inter-relationships of the three primary regulators of calcium homeostasis. The purpose of this chapter is to review our current understanding of the interactions of vitamin D with bone tissue.

Vitamin D and bone

The problem

In view of the multiple steps that are associated with bone morphology, physiology, and metabolism, it is a challenging prospect for the experimentalist to identify precisely the specific site of intervention of vitamin D and/or its metabolites. Historically, the problem has been simplified to involve one of two questions: (1) does vitamin D and/or its metabolites affect bone matrix formation and mineral deposition? or (2) does vitamin D and/or its metabolites effect bone mineral mobilization and matrix degradation? In view of the complex inter-relationships between vitamin D and its metabolites and PTH hormone and calcitonin, an additional challenge is to assess whether any putative vitamin D "effect" is permissive in that it allows other essential regulators to act, or whether it is direct, that is, is mediated solely by the steroid molecule itself.

The two chief changes in bone tissue that occur concomitantly with a severe vitamin D deficiency are (1) a failure of normal mineralization of bone matrix, ultimately leading to an increased accumulation of unmineralized osteoid, and (2) a decrease in bone resorption activity and the number of osteoclast cells present.

In rickets, the primary deficiency is caused by a defective calcification process. Figure 8-7 shows a photograph of the rachitic dogs that Mellanby used in his classic studies that produced for the first time experimentally the state of rickets. Since calcification along the column of hypertrophied cartilage cells in the bone does not occur, there is a disorderly invasion by blood vessels, and the usual zone of provisional calcification is not resorbed. With time, the cartilage

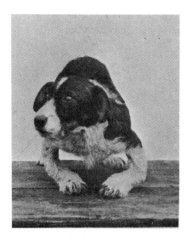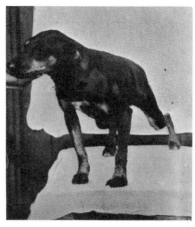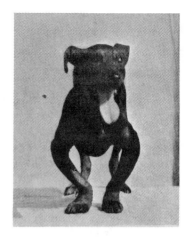

FIGURE 8-7 *Photographs of rachitic dogs raised by Sir Edward Mellanby in his classic studies that led to the first experimental production of rickets. (Mellanby, E.: Medical Research Council Special Report, No. 61, London, 1921)*

cells continue to proliferate into the zone of provisional calcification; therefore, the cartilage plate becomes wider than normal. Elsewhere in the skeleton, new osteoid or collagen tissue is laid down on bone surfaces, but it too fails to calcify.

In the young child with active rickets, two very discernible attributes are the bowing of the legs (Fig. 8-8) and the enlargement of the costochondral joints of the rib cage (Fig. 8-9). The characteristic "bowing of the legs" in rickets is due to the inability of the malformed skeleton to properly support the weight of the soft tissues. For the adult with osteomalacia, endochondrial growth has been completed and the epiphyseal abnormalities characteristic of rickets already discussed are not apparent. In adult osteomalacia, however, there is an excess of osteoid seams, and bone surfaces along the osteoid are not resorbed. Also, the remodeling of the bone that normally occurs is greatly diminished.

When either vitamin D_3 or its metabolites $25(OH)D_3$ or $1,25(OH)_2D_3$ are administered to a vitamin D–deficient animal, one of the earliest changes seen at the morphological level in the bone is the re-establishment of a normal calcification front in the osteoid surfaces. The fact that vitamin D treatment may lead to a re-establishment in the osteoid surface of a normal calcification front before there is any detectable change in the circulating concentration of calcium and phosphorus has been taken by some investigators as unequivocal evidence that vita-

min D and/or its metabolites act directly on bone. Preliminary evidence supports the existence of a specific high-affinity binding protein for $1,25(OH)_2D_3$ in the cytosol of fetal rat bone that may be related to the biologic effect. The assumption is that vitamin D, or more likely one of its metabolites, is acting in bone tissue as a steroid hormone in a manner analogous to that documented to occur in the intestinal mucosa cells.

The following sections review the various aspects of bone morphology and metabolism in which vitamin D or its metabolites are reported to have effects.

Effects on bone collagen

The primary connection between vitamin D and collagen is the disease state rickets. The rachitic state is characterized in growing animals by an accumulation of cartilage matrix, which not only fails to mineralize but also is resorbed only with difficulty. A vitamin D deficiency results in less organic matrix, which is less heavily mineralized than normal bone; associated with this in the rachitic tissue is a modest accumulation of water. As a result, vitamin D–deficient bone appears to be more porous than that obtained from normal animals.

However, the primary question is whether vitamin D has any effect on the many steps associated with collagen biosynthesis. There is as yet

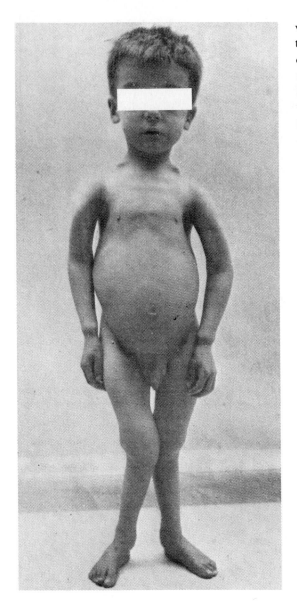

FIGURE 8-8 *Classic appearance of rickets in a child. (Norman, A. W.: Vitamin D: The Calcium Homeostatic Steroid Hormone, New York, Academic Press, 1979)*

was not found to occur in the skin obtained from the same animals. These results suggested that one of the early consequences of vitamin D administration to rachitic chicks might be a stimulation of synthesis of bone collagen, which would serve as a new matrix for the deposition of mineral made available by increased intestinal absorption of calcium. On the basis of radioisotope findings it was found in other studies that collagen synthesized in the shaft of bones from rachitic rats was similar in chain composition to collagen normally synthesized by bone samples obtained from vitamin D–replete, normal rats. A major problem of interpretation in studies of this type is whether the observed change is caused simply by the immediate consequences of a vitamin D or metabolite deficiency at the molecular level or whether the effect is produced by a change in calcium metabolism. That is, perturbations of calcium metabolism at the osteoclast level might also produce the reported changes.

Several laboratories have studied the relationship of vitamin D status to the "cross-link pattern" in the various chains of mature bone collagen. They found changes in the proportions of the major reducible cross-links—dihydroxylsinonorleucine and hydroxylsinonorleucine; this could affect the rate of maturation of bone collagen. Again, it was not possible to determine unequivocally whether the observation was attributable to the hypocalcemia associated with vitamin D deficiency or to an absence of vitamin D or its metabolites *per se*. However, these workers proposed that in the absence of vitamin D or its metabolites, more immature collagen is synthesized and the organization, packing, and structure of the resulting matrix is insufficient to support normal bone mineralization and related turnover activities. They further proposed that the structure of the collagen matrix must mature by a series of metabolic turnover steps, which are essential to ensure normal mineralization, and that vitamin D is essential for this process.

Even more recent studies have measured directly the activity of lysyl oxidase, an enzyme responsible for the production of aldehydic precursors for lysine-derived collagen cross-links in

no definitive answer to this question; undoubtedly due to the many separate steps associated with collagen biosynthesis, secretion, and maturation. There have been reports suggesting an effect of vitamin D in increasing the incorporation of tritiated proline into bone collagen measured *in vivo* in chicks. This increased rate of proline incorporation mediated by vitamin D

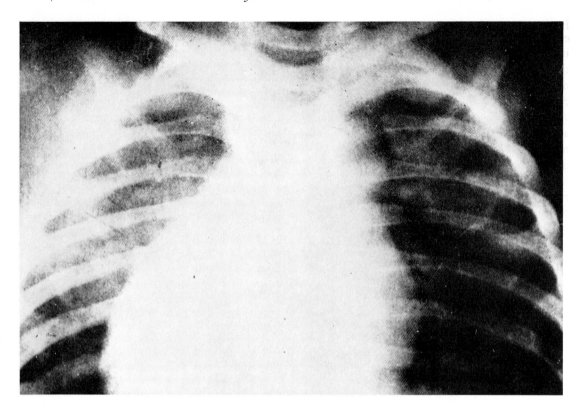

FIGURE 8-9   *X-ray appearance of the rib cage of a child with a classic rachitic "rosary." The beaded appearance results from enlarged costochondral regions of the bone.*

tibial metaphyses from either vitamin D–replete or vitamin D–deficient chicks. This study reported that lysyl oxidase activity was increased twofold in the vitamin D–deficient chicks as compared with activities measured in birds receiving physiologic doses of vitamin D_3. It was further noted that an increased dietary level of calcium in the vitamin D–deficient state had no effect on the measured lysyl oxidase activity.

It is possible to envision a steroid hormone–like action of $1,25(OH)_2D_3$ or another vitamin D metabolite, possibly $24,25(OH)_2D_3$, acting directly in the bone osteoid, stimulating the production of key enzymes related to the production of procollagen. Observations consistent with this suggestion are the reports that the experimental generation of uremia and consequent renal osteodystrophy produces a pattern of bone collagen reminiscent of a vitamin D deficiency without any changes being manifested in the collagen present in the skin of the same animals. These

data indicate that the osteodystrophy associated with chronic renal insufficiency is characterized by an alteration of the quantitative relations between cross-links and aldehydic precursors of bone collagen.

Effects on bone mineral metabolism

An early review of the possible role of vitamin D in bone formation was given by Nicolaysen and Jansen.[22] By that time it was well appreciated that vitamin D played a prominent role in stimulating absorption of calcium from the intestine. However, no definitive data had been put forth concerning possible effects of vitamin D on bone formation. An important point is that most workers in the field at this time (1930s–1940s) were impressed by the potent effects of vitamin D in preventing the characteristic lesions of rickets. In fact, it had already been reported that vitamin D added to an *in vitro* suspension of hypertrophic cartilage cells had no effect on calcification. Another interesting experiment was carried out by cultivating osteogenic tissue *in vitro* and it was observed that in a medium containing plasma from a normal chick, calcified bone was formed but that a similar tissue grown in a medium containing plasma from a vitamin D–deficient chick formed only abnormal osteoid tissue and additional cartilage. Furthermore, the addition to the growth medium of both calcium and phosphorus salts, either separately or together, did not fully compensate for the vitamin D deficiency. Thus, one is faced with the important question of whether the effects of vitamin D on bone accretion are the result of direct intervention of the steroid or its metabolites or whether the effects are caused by a secondary effect produced indirectly by changes in peripheral calcium and/or phosphorus metabolism. Accordingly, investigators carried out a series of experiments in which efforts were made to elevate the serum calcium and phosphorus levels of vitamin D–deficient animals so that measurements could be made on bone accretion; these results were then compared with bone accretion resulting from the dietary administration of vitamin D.

In similar studies, other workers carried out incubations with rat tibia obtained from either normal or rachitic animals in a "calcifying medium" that was either devoid of or contained supplemental vitamin D. They could show no *in vitro* effect of vitamin D in promoting calcification of the rat tibia obtained from either rachitic or normal animals. However, rachitic bones from animals previously administered vitamin D *in vivo* but not exhibiting any calcification *in vivo* did show a much greater calcification *in vitro*. The calcifying capacity of the rachitic bones appeared to increase with the increase in time after vitamin D administration. In fact, these investigators reported that the maximal effect *in vitro* coincided with the first evidence of calcification having commenced *in vivo*.

Still other workers studied the effects of dietary vitamin D levels on the *in vitro* mineralization of chick and rat metaphyses. The experiments were based on the premise that formation of bone calcium hydroxylapatite can be determined by the solubility product (K_{SP}) for calcium and phosphorus; when this constant is exceeded, crystallization may occur. The primary purpose of these studies was to determine whether vitamin D and/or normal serum calcium levels are necessary for the formation of bone matrix that is competent for mineral deposition. Undermineralized metaphyseal slices from rachitic chicks that were incubated for 5 d *in vitro* in media with four different $Ca^{2+} \times HPO_4^{2-}$ ion products had significantly less mineral deposited than slices from vitamin D–replete chicks or, more importantly, from chicks that had a rachitogenic diet supplemented with high levels of dietary calcium. These data support the concept that hypomineralization of rachitic bone *in vivo* is caused mainly by a reduced serum calcium level and thus suggest that vitamin D does not have a direct effect on bone mineral accretion.

In a notable series of papers, Nicolaysen and coworkers[22,23] compared the effects of dietary vitamin D versus manipulations of both dietary and blood calcium and phosphorus levels. The primary conclusion was that vitamin D was required for normal calcium metabolism at all ages, not only in the rat but also in humans. Furthermore, it was clearly established that the intestinal absorption of calcium throughout life is subject to regulation and adaptation and is a process in which vitamin D was postulated to be integrally involved. They also concluded that there is a continuing requirement for vitamin D to effect normal bone accretion and remodeling throughout life. Thus, they implied that vitamin D has a direct effect on bone mineral formation.

One important consequence of the work of Nicolaysen was the postulation of the existence of an "endogenous factor," which in some way transmitted from the bone to the intestine a signal that indicated a need for increased intestinal absorption of calcium. It now appears that the isolation and chemical characterization of $1,25(OH)_2D_3$ likely represents the identification of the "endogenous factor" of Nicolaysen. Clearly, the steroid $1,25(OH)_2D_3$ has many of the properties of the "endogenous factor" that pertain to adaptation of intestinal calcium absorption; what remains to be elucidated are pos-

TABLE 8-2 RELATIVE EFFECTS *IN VIVO* OF VITAMIN D METABOLITES AND ANALOGUES ON CHICK TIBIA ASH WEIGHT*

METABOLITE	DOSE FOR 50% INCREASE† (NG/CHICK/D)	RELATIVE POTENCY
$1\alpha,25(OH)_2D_3$	8	7.5
$1\alpha,(OH)D_3$	11	5.5
$25(OH)D_3$	30	2.0
D_3	60	1.0
$1\alpha,24(R),25(OH)_3D_3$	70	0.8
$24(R),25(OH)_2D_3$	120	0.5
$25(OH)-5,6-trans-D_3$	160	0.4
$1\alpha,24(S),25(OH)_3D_3$	440	0.1
$5,6-trans-D_3$	720	0.08
$24(S),25(OH)_2D_3$	1300	0.05

* After A. Boris *et al.*: J. Nutr. 107:194, 1977.
† Oral dose in nanograms/chick/day required to produce over a 21-d test period 50% of the maximum attainable tibia ash content. Ash content of vitamin D–deficient control tibia was 85 mg and this was increased maximally to 211 mg by vitamin D_3 or $1\alpha,25(OH)_2D_3$ treatment.

sible direct effects of the steroid on bone mineral accretion.

The next stage in the development of bone-vitamin D relationships came with the routine availability of radioactive ^{45}Ca. After administering either oral or intramuscular doses of $^{45}Ca^{2+}$ (to obviate effects of vitamin D on intestinal calcium absorption), it was concluded that vitamin D increases the rate of calcium accretion into bone. However, it was not determinable whether this increased movement of calcium into bone was a primary and direct effect of the vitamin or its metabolites or whether it was due to an increased flow of calcium to the bone.

Table 8-2 summarizes the relative potencies of various vitamin D metabolites and analogues in supporting bone ash development *in vivo* in the chick. Although it cannot be concluded from these data that vitamin D or the relevant analogue participated directly in bone accretion events, it is apparent that some analogues are strikingly more effective than others in providing "the optimal environment" for mineralization.

It would be expected that if vitamin D or its metabolites have direct effects on bone, the relevant cells would have stereospecific receptors for binding of the steroids. Several laboratories have reported the presence of a $1,25(OH)_2D_3$-binding protein in fetal rat bone. Thus, it ultimately should be possible to define the architecutre of bone cell receptors for vitamin D metabolites and to compare their specificities with the intestinal receptor for $1,25-(OH)_2D_3$. There is no *a priori* reason why intestinal and bone receptors for $1,25(OH)_2D_3$ should have identical functional group requirements.

Certainly the most clearly demonstrable effect of vitamin D on bone is its ability to carry out calcium mobilization. This effect can be documented *in vivo*, where it is usually assessed by elevation of serum calcium, and *in vitro* through release of ^{45}Ca from bone that has been prelabeled with the isotope *in vivo*. It is now apparent that not only the parent vitamin but also the metabolites $25(OH)D_3$, $1\alpha,25(OH)_2D_3$, and $24R,25(OH)_2D_3$ have a capability of mobilizing bone calcium. In this regard, $25(OH)D_3$ and the parent vitamin D are approximately equally potent, and $24R,25(OH)_2D_3$ has one half the activity of the parent vitamin; $1\alpha,25-(OH)_2D_3$, however, is the most active of all compounds that have been studied to date.

The most quantitative method for evaluating bone calcium mobilization is through the use of an *in vitro* system. Pregnant mice or rats or newborn mice are injected with a massive dose of $^{45}Ca^{2+}$, and several days later paired half-calvaria are explanted and placed in organ culture medium. These half-calvaria are then either treated with the test steroid at the required dose level for 48 hr or are not treated, and the release of ^{45}Ca into the medium is measured and compared with its control (Fig. 8-10). One interesting observation is that the parent steroid, vitamin D, is inert in these *in vitro* systems; it has no capability of mobilizing bone calcium. This is the most direct evidence that a metabolite of vitamin D, rather than the parent vitamin, is active in bone events. In a variation of the assay protocol, the test substance can be injected *in vivo* into the animal prior to explanting the calvaria to the organ culture medium. When vitamin D is administered *in vivo*, and the bone calvaria are evaluated under *in vitro* conditions for bone calcium mobilization, there is definitive evidence for mobilization activities, and this is assumed to result from the metabolism of the parent vitamin to the appropriate metabolites. Figure 8-10 presents a comparison of relative biologic potencies of $1,25(OH)_2D_3$, $25(OH)D_3$, and $1(OH)D_3$. The most striking observation is that the structural feature that enhances the activity of vitamin D_3 with regard to bone calcium mobilization is the simultaneous presence of both a 1-hydroxyl and a 25-hydroxyl group. It has been stated that "the most potent bone mobilizer known to man is $1,25(OH)_2D_3$."

There are definitive morphological changes in bone tissue in a vitamin D deficiency as compared with a normal vitamin D–replete state. However, it is difficult to gain specific insight into the molecular mechanism of action of vitamin D and/or its metabolites in bone tissue from an evaluation of these morphological changes. Nonetheless, such observations may provide information as to the appropriate areas of focus for biochemical studies. Certainly the most characteristic lesion of vitamin D deficiency is the wide epiphyseal growth plates that are associated with increased numbers of hypertrophic cartilage cells. It should be noted that in the rat these lesions occur only if the vitamin D–deficient animal has been raised on a low-phosphate diet; the morphological changes can be largely ameliorated by administration of dietary phosphate alone. Accordingly, this morphological defect may be related to perturbations in mineralization and subsequent failure of bone resorption or of the growth plate rather than to the specific presence or lack of vitamin D and/or its metabolites.

Several laboratories have studied the early

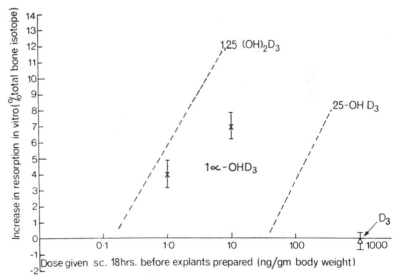

FIGURE 8-10 *Comparison of the bone mobilizing actions of 25(OH)D₃ and 1,25(OH)₂D₃ added* in vitro *to bone explants. Paired half-calvaria from 6-d-old mice prelabeled with ⁴⁵Ca were either treated with the indicated steroid at the indicated doses for 48 hr or not treated. The response is plotted as the increase in resorption expressed as the difference (treated half and control half) in percent release of bone isotope into the medium. The points are mean ± S.E.M. (Reynolds, J. J., Holick, M. F., and DeLuca, H. F.: Effects of vitamin D analogs on bone resorption, Calcif. Tissue Res. 15:333, 1974)*

morphological changes occurring at the epiphysis of rachitic chicks following vitamin D administration *in vivo*. They followed the presence and changes in content of neutral polysaccharides and sulfated mucopolysaccharides. Their work suggests that alterations in the metabolism of carbohydrates, specifically bone mucopolysaccharides, are under the influence either directly or indirectly of vitamin D. Still other workers have found that vitamin D altered the total lipid, phospholipid, total and free fatty acid, and free and esterified cholesterol contents of the long bones of rats. If vitamin D has the capability of altering sulfate as well as phospholipid metabolism, it is possible to envision how histologic and morphological changes may subsequently ensue. These observations are supported by a careful histochemical study of rachitic epiphyseal cartilage during healing in the rat that resulted from the administration of vitamin D_3. This study included an evaluation of changes in glycogen, lipid, nucleoproteins, alkaline phosphatase, and the glycoproteins of the matrix. The principal observation was that the administration of vitamin D brought about a marked increase in the glycogen content of the proliferative zone of the cartilage plate immediately prior to the onset of calcification. This suggested that the failure of rachitic cartilage to calcify was caused by a disturbance in glycogen metabolism. This work provides the foundation for further exploration of glycogenolysis and organic acid metabolism in bone tissue (see following section).

Until 1960 only decalcified bone specimens were used for routine histologic studies. Since that time it has been possible to evaluate sections of undecalcified bone and to quantitate several additional parameters including the resorptive surface, amount of osteoid, decalcification front, and osteocytic osteolysis. Bordier and colleagues[4] have made pioneering contributions to the understanding of the quantitative histology of bone. It is from such studies that the current understanding of bone dynamics and its associated morphological changes have resulted. They reported that in osteomalacia related to vitamin D deficiency there are certain quantitative changes in several histologic parameters, which are summarized in Table 8-3. It is clear that a vitamin D deficiency causes major morphological changes in bone tissue.

An additional development in technique is that of microradiography. Bone sections are prepared and from the microradiographic appearance, bone resorption surface and new bone formation can be quantitated. The technique is somewhat difficult to apply because unusually thin sections (5–10 μm) are necessary.

Effects on bone organic acid metabolism

The relationship between vitamin D and citrate metabolism in bone was first observed in 1941 in studies in cats; it was found that the citrate content of bones from vitamin D–deficient animals was approximately 50% that of normal animals. It should be recalled that 90% or more of the

TABLE 8-3 QUANTITATIVE HISTOLOGIC CHANGES OCCURRING IN VITAMIN D DEFICIENCY OSTEOMALACIA*

PARAMETER MEASURED	NORMAL CONTROLS (28 CASES)	SEVERE OSTEOMALACIA (28 CASES)
Osteocytic osteolysis (% of total osteocytic lacunae)	3.9 ± 0.6	9.3 ± 0.6
Bone resorption surface (% of calcified bone surface)	12.2 ± 4.0	33.8 ± 5.6
Calcification front (% of osteoid surface)	83.0 ± 10.0	19.2 ± 8.3
Osteoid surface extent (% of total bone surface)	14.6 ± 6.0	67.6 ± 13.7
Amount of osteoid (% of cancellous bone tissue)	5.7 ± 2.0	20.9 ± 7.7
Amount of cancellous bone tissue (% of total bone volume)	19.3 ± 4.0	27.8 ± 3.8

* After P. Bordier and S. Tun Chot: Clin. Endocrinol. Metab. 1: 197, 1972. Values are the mean + S.D.

TABLE 8-4 EFFECTS OF VITAMIN D STATUS ON RAT TISSUE CITRATE LEVELS*

TISSUE EXAMINED	VITAMIN D STATUS†		INCREASE (%)
	−D	+D	
Blood (μg/ml)	13.0	21.0	61.0
Heart (μg/g)	43.0	53.0	23.0
Kidney (μg/g)	18.0	38.0	111.0
Small intestine (μg/g)	61.0	76.0	25.0
Liver (μg/g)	13.0	12.0	
Bone (mg/g)	3.59	5.23	54.0

*After H. Steenbock and S. Bellin: J. Biol. Chem. 205:985, 1953.
† Both groups of rats were fed a vitamin D−deficient diet; + D rats received 6.5 nmol (100 IU) of D_3 three times weekly.

body citrate is found in the skeleton, in which it is associated with the mineral fraction. There had been some previous nutritional data that suggested that citrate might be capable of functioning as an antirachitic agent. It was noted that dietary citrate seemed capable of preventing rickets in rats fed a high calcium cereal diet. Subsequently it was found that these apparent "antirachitic actions" were mediated by citrate stimulating an increased hydrolysis of phytic acid in a noncereal, high-calcium diet so that more inorganic phosphate was available to the animals.

In other work it was shown that dietary vitamin D increases the citric acid content of many body tissues (Table 8-4) as well as inducing a citraturia.

Two hypotheses were put forward to explain possible actions of vitamin D on citric acid metabolism. On the one hand, it was felt that since rachitic tissue had reduced levels of citrate, vitamin D must enhance the biosynthesis of citric acid. On the other hand, it was proposed that in the presence of vitamin D there was a diminished rate of further metabolism or oxidation of citric acid with a concomitant increase in steady state levels.

In studies carried out with rat kidney tissue homogenates or mitochondrial preparations DeLuca and coworkers[6] clearly showed that administration of vitamin D *in vivo* lowered the oxidation rate of citrate and isocitrate but not that of any other tricarboxylic acid cycle intermediates. Surprisingly, this observation could be repeated by the addition *in vitro* of vitamin D to kidney mitochondria preparations. Further electronmi-

croscopic evaluation of isolated rat kidney mitochondria revealed that dietary vitamin D had a marked protective effect on the structural integrity of these organelles. It was then felt that the diminished oxidation of citrate observed previously could be explained in terms of a physical inhibition of citrate penetration into the mitochondria. In confirmation of this, Norman and DeLuca[9] found that the *in vivo* administration of vitamin D to rachitic animals resulted in an increase in the amount of (^{14}C) acetate converted to citrate by isolated bone segments *in vitro*. Also there was a corresponding decrease in the amount of radioactivity in the other organic acids of bone. Most importantly, in bone fragments obtained from vitamin D–treated animals, there was a decrease in the amount of $^{14}CO_2$ produced. These results demonstrate that vitamin D does not increase the synthesis of citrate from acetate in bone and are consistent with the view that the vitamin decreases the rate of conversion of citrate to subsequent intermediates in the tricarboxylic acid cycle in bone tissue as well as in kidney.

The observation of a relationship between vitamin D and bone citric acid levels suggested to some investigators that increased bone citrate levels might facilitate bone calcium mobilization, probably through the chelation of the calcium ion by citrate. Thus, there was a possibility that citric acid was the mediator of vitamin D action on bone. However, it has been possible to dissociate the effects of vitamin D on citric acid metabolism from those on bone in rats by administering cortisol. Although the tibias of vitamin D–deficient, cortisol-fed rats gave evidence of an increased calcification in response to administration of the vitamin, there was no corresponding elevation in either serum citrate levels or bone citrate levels.

In view of the prominent role of energy metabolism in the growth and development of cartilage, several laboratories have initiated a study of the effects of vitamin D and dietary phosphorus on oxidative enzymes in the epiphyseal cartilage of rachitic rats. It has been demonstrated that the development of rickets in rats resulted in an increased rate of lactate production by cartilage slices and that there was an increased level of the enzyme lactate dehydrogenase in rachitic cartilage extracts. Thus, there are biochemical data that support the previously discussed evidence for vitamin D–mediated histologic changes in cartilage tissue. However, at present there is no clear understanding of the molecular basis of the actions of vitamin D or its metabolites in mediating these changes. These effects, however, are reminiscent of those of some steroid hormones in terms of differentiation and proliferation of various tissues.

Certainly, one of the major problems in evaluating the biochemical actions of any hormone, including vitamin D metabolites, is the multiplicity of cell types present in this tissue. From animal experiments *in vivo* or bone organ culture experiments *in vitro* it is not always possible to discern which bone cell type is producing the response under study. Clearly, what is required is the development of appropriate tissue cell culture techniques that will make it possible to study selected bone cell populations. The recent biochemical characterization by several laboratories of bone cells grown in tissue culture that are differentially responsive to parathyroid and calcitonin hormones may represent an important methodological breakthrough in this regard.

The interaction of other hormones with the vitamin D endocrine system

Parathyroid hormone (PTH)

It has been clearly established that PTH stimulates bone resorption and that it is essential not only for bone growth and remodeling but also for calcium homeostasis. The effects of PTH on the formation of bone are not as clearly delineated. After large doses of PTH *in vivo*, collagen synthesis is initially inhibited. But repeated doses of PTH can ultimately lead to increased collagen synthesis and excessive amounts of metaphysical bone. PTH *in vivo* has been shown to inhibit proline and glycine incorporation into bone matrix; yet at the same time amino acid and nucleoside transport is stimulated in bone calvaria and bone cells, respectively. Also, PTH *in vivo* has been shown to transiently stimulate the incorporation of hexosamine into bone. Thus, PTH has both inhibitory and stimulatory effects on pathways involved in bone matrix synthesis.

Underlying all these "direct actions" of PTH on bone is the network of vitamin D–PTH interactions—both at the bone sites and in distal extraskeletal locations. There appear to be at least two mechanisms by which the output of $1,25(OH)_2D_3$ by the kidney can be modulated: (1) a short-time-scale regulatory process in which, on a minute-by-minute basis, changes in the ionic environment of the mitochondria effect a change in the activity of the $25(OH)D_3$-1-hydroxylase, and (2) a regulatory scheme involving hours during which changes occur in the absolute level of active 1-hydroxylase molecules in the mitochondria. It is entirely probable, but has not yet been proved, that the effects of PTH may be manifested on both general regulatory processes. That is, if PTH has the capability of changing the concentration of a critical ionic type in the renal cortical cells, it could inhibit or stimulate the production of $1,25(OH)_2D_3$.

The proposed inter-relationships between vitamin D and PTH are not new ones. The first hints of such relationships actually came from a consideration of phosphate metabolism rather than calcium metabolism. In particular, investigators were concerned with physiologic mechanisms regulating the renal excretion of inorganic phosphate. It was apparent from earlier studies on rickets, both in humans and in experimental animals, that there were certain perturbations in phosphate excretion. However, it was not until Nicolaysen[20] reported that vitamin D could promote the intestinal absorption of both calcium and phosphate metabolism that it became possible to postulate the first tentative types of inter-relationships between vitamin D, ion metabolism, and hormones that might also affect these ionic substances.

Rasmussen and coworkers[29,34] have studied the effect of parathyroidectomy and PTH administration on the concentration of plasma calcium and phosphorus in vitamin D–deficient and vitamin D–fed animals. Their studies emphasize that the response of the vitamin D–deficient, parathyroidectomized animal to the infusion of PTH differs from that of the vitamin D–fed controls. Qualitatively similar changes occurred in plasma phosphate levels as well as in the urinary excretion of calcium, phosphate, magnesium, sodium, and potassium, but in the vitamin D–deficient animals there was a sustained phosphaturia and secondary hypercalciuria and a hypercalcemia, which did not develop in the vitamin D–treated animal. It was concluded that vitamin D was necessary for the physiologic actions of PTH to mobilize calcium and phosphate from bone, but that vitamin D was not required for the action of PTH on the renal tubule.

Hypertrophy and hyperplasia of the parathyroid glands have been recognized since the late 1920s. More recent studies have been carried out to investigate the relationship among dietary calcium, vitamin D, and gland size and activity. It has been reported that there is an inverse relationship between dietary calcium and parathyroid gland size and gland "activity" as measured by the uptake of α-aminoisobutyric acid. However, all the chicks in that study were fed vitamin D, so it was not possible to independently assess the effect of the steroid or its metabolites on the gland size. In a later study, it was demonstrated that vitamin D increases serum calcium levels and decreases parathyroid gland weight, regardless of the dietary calcium or phosphorus level. There was, however, no evidence of an inverse relationship between gland weight and serum calcium levels when the data with and without vitamin D_3 were considered separately.

In retrospect, it is only fair to indicate that all of these workers carried out their studies without the knowledge we have today of vitamin D metabolism and the putative role of PTH in stimulating $1,25(OH)_2D_3$ production. In view of

the model of regulation of $1,25(OH)_2D_3$ production proposed (see Figs. 8-3 and 8-4), which emphasizes the interaction of vitamin D status and PTH status in the determination of the level of this enzyme, there are many possible points at which the interaction might occur. One possibility is the parathyroid gland itself, wherein the final metabolite $1,25(OH)_2D_3$ might exert a feedback effect, decreasing PTH secretion. This would have at least two consequences: (1) a decrease in the stimulatory actions of PTH on the renal $25(OH)D_3$-1-hydroxylase, and (2) a decrease in the entry of calcium into the blood from the intestine [stimulated by $1,25(OH)_2D_3$] and from bone (stimulated by both the steroid and PTH). Thus, a major advance was made in 1975 by Henry and Norman.[12] Using high-specific-activity radioactive preparations of $1,25(OH)_2D_3$, they were able to report the uptake of this steroid hormone by the parathyroid gland of vitamin D–deficient chicks. The parathyroid glands were capable of concentrating $1,25(OH)_2D_3$ at least fourfold over the circulating levels in the plasma. Further support for the existence of specific binding of $1,25(OH)_2D_3$ by the parathyroid gland came with the demonstration of the existence of a 3.1S receptor in the cytosol for the steroid. The discovery of a unique $1,25(OH)_2D_3$-binding component in the parathyroid gland is consistent with a steroid hormone action for this vitamin D metabolite at this site and its possible involvement in the regulation of PTH synthesis and/or secretion.

It should be recalled, however, that $1,25(OH)_2D_3$ is not the only metabolite produced by the kidney; a second metabolite produced in some physiologic circumstances is $24,25(OH)_2D_3$, a steroid that is not particularly biologically active in terms of stimulation of intestinal calcium transport or bone calcium mobilization. Henry and Norman[12] reported the possible combined actions of $1,25(OH)_2D_3$ and $24,25(OH)_2D_3$ in parathyroid gland activities. Their studies involved the feeding, either separately or in combination, of these two steroids to vitamin D–deficient chicks (for which there is no assay for the circulating levels of PTH) and evaluating the regression of enlarged chick parathyroid glands. These workers concluded that parathyroid gland regression, possibly in-

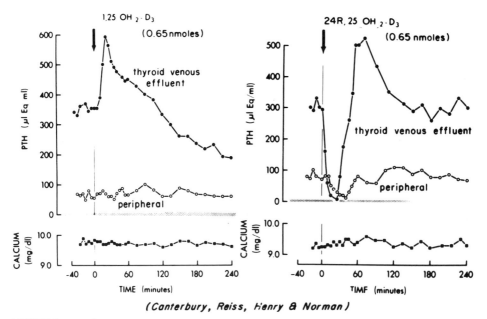

(*Canterbury, Reiss, Henry & Norman*)

FIGURE 8-11 *Effects of the administration of 1,25(OH)₂D₃ and 24,25(OH)₂D₃ on secretion of PTH in the normal dog.*

volving loss of cells, occurs within a few days of treatment with vitamin D metabolites and that this regression does not obligatorily follow an increase in serum calcium levels. Under circumstances in which $1,25(OH)_2D_3$ is present in low concentration, the presence of $24,25(OH)_2D_3$ is required to mediate gland reduction. These results suggest that vitamin D metabolites, in particular $1,25(OH)_2D_3$ and to a lesser degree $24,25(OH)_2D_3$, may play a role in modulating parathyroid gland functions as well as intestinal function.

With the development of our understanding of

the role of the endocrine system in processing vitamin D and a demonstration of its intimate inter-relationship with PTH and calcium metabolism, the intriguing prospect has arisen that vitamin D or one of its metabolites may modulate the secretion of PTH by the gland. Classic feedback actions of hypercalcemia in diminishing the secretion of PTH have been repeatedly documented. However, only more recently has it been speculated that there may be more than one feedback regulator, that is, both the calcium ion itself and the product of the kidney, $1,25(OH)_2D_3$.

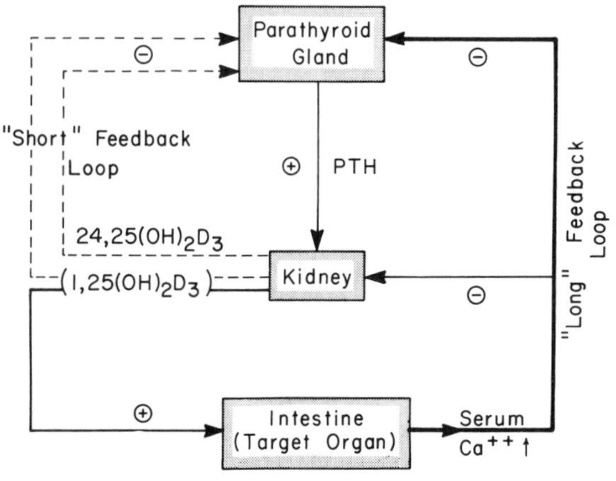

FIGURE 8-12 *Postulated feedback loops for the parathyroid-kidney calcium endocrine system. This is modeled on similar systems related to the neurohypophysis.*

Figure 8.11 presents the results of Canterbury and coworkers,[30] who studied the effects of either $1,25(OH)_2D_3$ or $24,25(OH)_2D_3$ infusion into the artery leading to the parathyroid gland of normal dogs. They followed the level of PTH in the vein draining the vascular bed of the parathyroid gland. The results show an intriguing relationship: administration of $1,25(OH)_2D_3$ and $24,25(OH)_2D_3$ results in each case in a perturbation of the circulating level of iPTH. These effects, however, appear to be obtained by distinctly different mechanisms for each steroid. Administration of $1,25(OH)_2D_3$ acutely stimulates the release of pre-existing PTH in the gland, followed by apparent inhibition of the biosynthesis of the additional hormone. Conversely, the administration of $24,25(OH)_2D_3$ results in an acute decrease in the secretion of (immuno-PTH), followed by an intermediate time period of increased secretion of iPTH and then by a chronic achievement of reduced PTH levels.

With the demonstration of the potentially stimulatory effects of PTH on the production of $1,25(OH)_2D_3$ and the associated feedback regulation of $1,25(OH)_2D_3$ and $24,25(OH)_2D_3$ in PTH secretion, the possibility of a classic endocrine regulatory mechanism exists, particularly when considered in concert with the well-documented feedback actions of elevated serum calcium levels on the parathyroid gland. As shown in Figure 8.12, the analogy between this calcium endocrine system and the neurohypophysis relay system is striking. There are "short-loop" and "long-loop" feedback relationships in both systems. It is well known that feedback and feedforward controls in biochemical and endocrine systems represent mechanisms for the transfer of information. Chemical messengers indicate to one part of the cell or organism the state of or activity in another part of the cell or organism; in order to ensure the proper flow of information throughout the biologic system, specific chemical messengers or transmitters must exist. In endocrine systems, this implies the existence of specific hormonal receptors on or within the relevant cells of the endocrine glands so that they can respond to incoming information.

The primary attribute of an endocrinologic system is that it exists and operates as a "closed-loop system" rather than as an "open-loop system." The distinction between the two systems, although simple, has profound implications for the mechanisms that are operative therein and the consequences of the operation. With a closed-loop system, the output influences the behavior of the system, which becomes, in terms of its responses, a "feedback input." That is, stimulus (input) leads to a response, but response (output) must ultimately influence the original stimulus. In this regard, the most important aspect of the closed-loop operation is one of "feedback control" and particularly "negative feedback control."

It has become increasingly apparent in recent years that one of the hallmarks in the regulation of integrated peptide hormone and steroid hormone endocrine systems is feedback loops. Thus, peptide hormones are known in several systems to have a trophic action on the production of steroid hormones, for example, ACTH on adrenal cortical hormones and leuteinizing hormone on estrogen or testosterone production. These steroid hormones then initiate specific biologic function, which produces defined biologic responses. These responses in some way feed back and diminish the secretion of both the steroid hormone and the trophic peptide hormone. Thus, as shown in Figure 8-12, as well as in Figure 8-3, one can identify the "long-loop" and "short-loop" feedback steps in both the calcium arena and the pituitary axis. It should be apparent that this is an area of investigation that is far from complete. At present, there are only the barest outlines in biochemical and molecular terms of the stimulatory actions of PTH on the renal production of $1,25(OH)_2D_3$ as well as the putative feedback action of renal vitamin D metabolites on the actions of the parathyroid gland. It is intriguing, however, to speculate as to the involvement of bone cells in this homeostatic mechanism. Certainly, given the complexity of cellular organization in bone and the dominant role of bone in calcium metabolism it would not be surprising to learn that it is intimately involved in feedback loops of this endocrine system.

Calcitonin

The present understanding of the relationship between vitamin D and its metabolism and its inter-relationship with calcitonin is even less well defined than that of PTH. Calcitonin is most noted for its hypocalcemic actions. In one study, within 1 hr after subcutaneous administration of calcitonin to rats, the plasma calcium concentration reached its lowest level; the same acute hypocalcemic effect was also observed in rats that had been given actinomycin D or that were parathyroidectomized. In this same study, the plasma calcium concentration returned to normal in the control rats within 1 to 3 hr, whereas in the actinomycin D–treated or parathyroidectomized rats, the plasma calcium concentration did not return to normal. This data demonstrated that in an actinomycin D–treated rat, the parathyroid glands cannot maintain a normal plasma calcium concentration and that the short duration of the hypocalcemic effect of calcitonin is due in large part to the actions of the parathyroid gland. In retrospect, it can be appreciated that the failure of the actinomycin D-treated animals, which also received calcitonin, to respond normally was caused by a blockage of the responses generated by the vitamin D metabolite $1,25(OH)_2D_3$.

Several workers have studied the relationship among vitamin D deficiency, calcitonin, and PTH. It has been reported that calcitonin is capable of lowering serum calcium levels in vitamin D–deficient animals, whereas PTH was incapable of acting in a hypercalcemic fashion. These results tend to support the view that calcitonin can act when vitamin D is lacking. These studies were followed by a report that calcitonin produced a hypocalcemic response in rats with hypercalcemia caused by hypervitaminosis D. Thus, calcitonin was capable of mediating hypocalcemic effects in the presence of excess vitamin D and when it was lacking.

Adrenal and cortical steroids

The relation of adrenal steroids to calcium and bone metabolism is well documented. Osteoporosis is often a prominent sign of Cushing's disease, which is, in essence, an overproduction of adrenal glucocorticoids. The bone disease osteoporosis also occurs frequently after prolonged adrenal corticoid therapy, which is often associated with rheumatoid arthritis. It is known that administration of cortisol or other adrenal steroids may cause a decrease in intestinal absorption of calcium and also in the renal tubular reabsorption of calcium. In addition, cortisol and related steroids are known to have effects on bone resorption and bone accretion. The mode of action of cortisol in any of these target tissues (intestine, kidney, and bone) remains to be elucidated; however, there is some evidence that cortisol or steroid treatment has antivitamin D–like activity.

Estrogens

The effect of estrogens on bone metabolism has been of interest for at least 30 yr, largely because of the therapeutic use of this sex steroid in the treatment of osteoporosis. It is well known that with the onset of menopause, the secretion of estradiol is limited and that many post-menopausal women develop osteoporosis.

Several laboratories have reported that estrogen and testosterone administration to Japanese quail and chicks, respectively, interferes with $25(OH)D_3$ conversion to $1,25(OH)_2D_3$. There is the possibility that sex steroids may indeed be intimately involved in the regulation of vitamin D metabolism and action; however, at the present time we do not have a detailed description of these relationships.

Thyroxine

The thyroid hormones thyroxine and triiodothyronine are known to influence mineral metabolism and bone calcium turnover. Thus, certain abnormalities of bone metabolism are noted in the disease states of hypothyroidism and hyperthyroidism. It has been shown that patients who suffer from hyperthyroidism also have an associated hypercalcemia. It is not clear whether the hypercalcemia is related to an associated hyperparathyroidism that occurs from nearest-neighbor endocrine gland perturbation or whether some long-range physiologic signals are generated to produce the hypercalcemia in another manner. Several research groups have reported that patients with thyrotoxicosis have significantly lowered levels of plasma $25(OH)D_3$.

Growth hormone-somatomedin

One of the major target organs for the action of growth hormone in the developing animal is the skeleton. When growth hormone is lacking, skeletal development is markedly slowed and in the extreme, dwarfism may result. It has been shown that most of the effects of growth hormone are in fact mediated by somatomedin. Thus, a critical need may develop for one of these hormones during the period of development, during which time there is a marked increase in calcium demand by the animal. However, it is known that in the adult human growth hormone is not necessary for normal mineral homeostasis.

It is to be anticipated that new relationships between growth and endocrine signals related to generation of growth may intervene in some aspect of calcium and phosphorus homeostasis. There are already several reports suggesting that growth hormone can stimulate the production of $1,25(OH)_2D_3$.

Insulin

It has been shown that individuals with either juvenile-onset or adult-onset diabetes have a reduced bone mass as compared with age-matched controls. Abnormalities of skeletal mass can also be produced by inducing diabetes in experimental animals. As yet, the pathogenesis of the reduced bone mass in humans with diabetes is not clearly known.

A series of experiments on diabetic rats implicated a defect in vitamin D metabolism in the production of calcium malabsorption in these animals. It was shown that in this experimental model there was intestinal malabsorption of calcium and a decreased quantity of a specific intestinal calcium-binding protein that is similar to the protein induced by the administration of vitamin D. The transport defect could be corrected by the administration of $1,25(OH)_2D_3$, but not by the administration of $25(OH)D_3$ or vitamin D_3 itself, suggesting that there was a defect in the production of $1,25(OH)_2D_3$. More recently, it has been reported that the serum level of $1,25(OH)_2D_3$ is significantly lowered in rats with streptozotocin-induced diabetes. Even more recently, the presence in the chick pancreas of a cytosol receptor for $1\alpha,25(OH)_2D_3$ as well as a vitamin D–dependent calcium binding protein has been demonstrated. No studies of vitamin D metabolism have been done as yet in human diabetics, but it can be anticipated that this will be a fertile field of investigation in the future.

Prolactin

An exciting new development concerns the possible involvement of the vitamin D endocrine system with changes in hormonal concentrations that occur during pregnancy and lactation. It has been reported that a single acute dose or chronic administration of ovine prolactin to the chick was effective in increasing the activity of the renal $25(OH)D_3$-1-hydroxylase as measured *in vitro*. Further support for this action was obtained by measuring changes in the plasma levels of $1,25(OH)_2D_3$ that occurred after prolactin administration; a significant elevation in plasma $1,25(OH)_2D_3$ levels was noted. Care must be taken in the interpretation of these results, since an action of ovine prolactin in chicks may not necessarily reflect an action of the hormone in mammals.

It should be clear from the foregoing remarks that although it is certain that the presence of vitamin D and its metabolites is essential to many aspects of bone morphology and metabolism, it is not at all apparent what the biochemical basis of many of these effects is. On the one hand, the development of our understanding of the vitamin D endocrine system permits the conceptualization of many new and complex relationships among the various endocrine regulators of calcium and phosphorus homeostasis; on the other hand, our appreciation of the existence of this new endocrine system and its relationship to and interaction on bone has made possible the formulation of ever-more-complex research projects. Certainly, research on bone biochemistry may be anticipated to have a productive and informative future.

References

Selected references are given here that can provide both a more detailed discussion of the major areas of focus on this chapter as well as access to the original literature.

General references on bone

 1. Avioli, L. V., and Krane, S. M. (eds.): Metabolic Bone Disease, Vol. 1, New York, Academic Press, 1977.
 2. Bourne, G. H. (ed.): The Biochemistry and Physiology of Bone, Vol. 2, New York, Academic Press, 1971.
 3. Bourne, G. H. (ed.): The Biochemistry and Physiology of Bone, Vol. 3, New York, Academic Press, 1977.
 4. Rasmussen, H., and Bordier, P.: The Physiological and Cellular Basis of Metabolic Bone Disease, Baltimore, Williams & Wilkins Co., 1974.
 5. Vaughn, J. M.: The Physiology of Bone, London and New York, Oxford University Press (Clarendon), 1970.

General references on vitamin D metabolism

 6. DeLuca, H. F., and Schnoes, H. K.: Metabolism and Mechanism of Action of Vitamin D, Ann. Rev. Biochem. 45:631–642, 1976.
 7. Lawson, D. E. M. (ed.): Vitamin D, pp. 1–433, London and New York, Academic Press, 1978.
 8. Marks, J.: A Guide to the Vitamins: Their Role in Health and Disease, University Park, 1976.
 9. Norman, A. W.: Vitamin D: The Calcium Homeostatic Steroid Hormone, pp. 1–490, New York, Academic Press, 1979.
10. Norman, A. W. (ed.): Clinical and Nutritional Aspects of Vitamin D, New York, Dekker Publishing Co., 1980.
11. Norman, A. W., and Henry, H. L.: 1,25-Dihydroxycholecalciferol—a hormonally active form of vitamin D$_3$, Greep, R. O. (ed.): Recent Progress in Hormone Research, pp. 431–480, New York, Academic Press, 30, 1974.
12. Norman, A. W., and Henry, H. L.: Vitamin D to 1,25-dihydroxycholecalciferol: Evolution of a steroid hormone, Trends in Biochem. Sci. 4:14, 1979.
13. Norman, A. W., Schaefer, K., v. Herrath, D., Grigoleit, H.-G., Coburn, J. W., DeLuca, H. F., Mawer, E. B., and Suda, T. (eds.): Vitamin D: Recent Advances and Their Clinical Implications, pp. 1–1251, New York, Walter de Gruyter Publishing Co., 1979.

Vitamin D and bone

EFFECTS ON COLLAGEN

14. Barnes, M. J., Constable, B. J., Morton, L. F., and Kodicek, E.: Bone collagen metabolism in vitamin D deficiency, Biochem. J. 132:113, 1973.
15. Baylink, D., Stauffer, M., Wergedal, J., and Rich, D.: Formation, mineralization and resorption of bone in vitamin D-deficient rats, J. Clin. Invest. 49:1122, 1970.
16. Canas, F., Brand, J. S., Neumann, W. F., and Terepka, A. R.: Some effects of vitamin D$_3$ on collagen synthesis in rachitic chick cortical bone, Am. J. Physiol. 216:1092, 1969.
17. Mechanic, G. L., Toverud, S. U., and Ramp, W. K.: Quantitative changes of bone collagen crosslinks and precursors in vitamin D deficiency, Biochem. Biophys. Res. Commun. 47:760, 1972.
18. Mechanic, G. L., Toverud, S. U., Ramp, W. K., and Gonnerman, W. A.: The effect of vitamin D on the structural crosslinks and maturation of chick bone collagen, Biochim. Biophys. Acta 393:419, 1975.

BONE ACCRETION

19. Crenshaw, M. A., Ramp, W. K., Gonnerman, W. A., and Toverud, S. U.: Effects of dietary vitamin D levels on the *in vitro* mineralization of chick metaphyses, Proc. Soc. Exp. Biol. Med. 146:488, 1974.
20. Haavaldsen, R., and Nicolaysen, R.: Studies in calcium metabolism in rats. I. A long term study in rats given an optimal diet with and without vitamin D, Acta Physiol. Scand. 36:103, 1956.
21. Kream, B. E., Jose, M., Yamada, S., and DeLuca, H. F.: A specific high affinity binding macromolecule for 1,25-dihydroxyvitamin D$_3$ in fetal bone, Science 197:1086, 1977.
22. Nicolaysen, R., and Jansen, J.: Vitamin D and

bone formation in rats, Acta Paediatr. (Stockholm) 23:405, 1939.

23. Nicolaysen, R., and Nordbo, R.: Calcium metabolism and citric acid, Acta Physiol. Scand. 5:212, 1943.

BONE RESORPTION

24. Carlsson, A., and Lindquist, B.: Comparison of intestinal and skeletal effects of vitamin D in relation to dosage, Acta Physiol. Scand. 35:53, 1955.
25. Carttar, M. S., McLean, F. C., and Urist, M. R.: The effect of the calcium and phosphorus content of the diet upon the formation and structure of bone, Am. J. Pathol. 26:307, 1950.
26. Reynolds, J. J., Holick, M. F., and DeLuca, H. F.: The role of vitamin D metabolites in bone resorption, Calcif. Tissue Res. 12:295, 1973.
27. Reynolds, J. J., Holick, M. F., and DeLuca, H. F.: Effects of vitamin D analogs on bone resorption, Calcif. Tissue Res. 15:333, 1974.
28. Wong, R. G., Myrtle, J. F., Tsai, H. C., and Norman, A. W.: Studies on calciferol metabolism V. The occurrence and biological activity of 1,25-dihydroxy-vitamin D_3 in bone, J. Biol. Chem. 247:5728, 1972.

Interactions of hormones with vitamin D

29. Arnaud, C., Rasmussen, H., and Anast, C.: Further studies on the interrelationship between parathyroid hormone and vitamin D, J. Clin. Invest. 45:1955, 1966.
30. Canterbury, J. M., Lerman, S., Claflin, A. J., Henry, H. L., Norman, A. W., and Reiss, E.: Effects of vitamin D metabolites on parathyroid hormone secretion, J. Clin. Invest. 61:1375, 1978.
31. Christakos, S., and Norman, A. W.: Interaction of the vitamin D endocrine system with other hormones, J. Mineral and Electrolyte Metab. 1:231, 1978.
32. Harrison, H. E., and Harrison, H. C.: The renal excretion of inorganic phosphate in relation to the action of vitamin D and parathyroid hormone, J. Clin. Invest. 20:47, 1941.
33. Harrison, H. E., and Harrison, H. C.: The interaction of vitamin D and parathyroid hormone on calcium phosphorus and magnesium homeostasis in the rat, Metab. Clin. Exp. 13:952, 1964.
34. Rasmussen, H., DeLuca, H. F., Arnaud, C., Hawker, C., and von Stedingk, M.: The relationship between vitamin D and parathyroid hormone, J. Clin. Invest. 42:1940, 1963.

Whereas biochemists have been interested in phosphate for a long time in view of its key function in a great many biochemical functions, this compound has been rather neglected by physiologists. Calcium homeostasis has been investigated in great detail; phosphate, however, has been given little more than benign neglect with the exception of its renal handling. One explanation of this situation is the difficulty in isotopically measuring *in vivo* phosphate fluxes, because of the distribution of the isotopes in a large number of different pools. Another explanation is the belief that plasma phosphate is not regulated or is regulated badly, and is thus uninteresting for the physiologist. It is only recently, with the realization that phosphate is implicated in the homeostasis of other ions—especially calcium—and is important in various diseases such as rickets, phosphate deficiency, renal failure, and renal stones, that interest in this compound has grown. The aim of this review is to sum up the knowledge available today.

H. FLEISCH

9

homeostasis of inorganic phosphate

Distribution of phosphate in the body

The adult human body contains between 15 and 20 mol of phosphate in the male and somewhat less in the female. This value decreases after the age of about 40 yr. Eighty to 90% is located in bone, more precisely in bone mineral as hydroxyapatite. The other 10 to 20% is in soft tissues, mainly muscle and internal organs, in extracellular fluid, and in erythrocytes. In soft tissues phosphate represents between 0.1 and 0.3% of the wet weight, and is contained nearly totally within the cells. It exists mainly in the form of phosphate in sugars, phospholipids, phosphoproteins, nucleic acids, and inorganic phosphate. In this text, total phosphate will be called P; inorganic phosphate will be called Pi.

Phosphate in blood

Phosphate is present both in erythrocytes and in plasma (Table 9-1). In erythrocytes, phosphate esters are the major fraction, followed by phospholipids, with Pi being the smallest fraction; in

TABLE 9-1 DISTRIBUTION OF PHOSPHATE IN ADULT HUMAN BLOOD IN MMOL/LITER

	ERYTHROCYTES	*PLASMA*
Ester-P	12.3–19.0	0.86–1.45
Lipid-P	4.13–4.81	2.23–3.13
Inorganic P	0.03–0.13	0.71–1.36

(From Wissenschaftliche Tabellen, Tielband Hämatologie und Humangenetik, 8 Auflage, Cibe-Geigy, Basel, 1979)

plasma, however, phospholipids are the main fraction followed by phosphate esters and Pi.

Plasma inorganic phosphate

The concentration in plasma of Pi varies largely according to the animal species. It is highest in certain fish and lowest in adult humans. In the fasting human, values of plasma Pi depend on age: whereas they vary between 0.71 and 1.36 mmol/liter in the adult, they lie between 1.28 and 2.0 mmol/liter in children, and between 1.39 and 2.67 mmol/liter in newborn babies.

The form of Pi in plasma is still somewhat controversial. When plasma is ultrafiltered *in vitro*, Pi concentration in the ultrafiltrate varies between 90 and 100% of that found in plasma. The same seems to be true *in vivo*. Thus, in the so-called Munich rats, which have glomerula at the surface, the concentrations of Pi in the glomerular ultrafiltrate is also comparable with those in plasma in females but are somewhat lower in males. This identity is, however, fortuitous, since a completely ultrafiltrable substance should have in the ultrafiltrate the concentration of plasma water, that is, 1.07 times that in plasma. Furthermore, if a correction for the Donnan equilibrium, which is about 1.09, is made, Pi in the ultrafiltrate should be about 1.17 times that in plasma. Thus, when the concentration in glomerular ultrafiltrate is similar to that in plasma, about 17% of the Pi is really nonfilterable, being bound to plasma proteins. In the case of the ultrafiltrability being below 100%, the phosphate binding is higher. In humans, values must be derived from data obtained by ultrafiltration *in vitro* through membranes, a technique that has various problems and results of which

should be interpreted with caution. The data suggest that protein binding is between 10 and 20% under normal conditions. Furthermore, the nonprotein-bound Pi is not all free, about 35% being in association with sodium, calcium, and magnesium. Thus, only a part of the Pi measurable in plasma, probably somewhat more than half, is available for chemical reactions.

It has been known for a long time that plasma Pi follows a circadian rhythm. It is at a minimum in the morning and at a maximum after 9 PM. Urinary excretion follows a very similar pattern. The cause of this rhythm is not yet known but is probably multifactorial. The intake of food plays a role, since fasting attenuates the variations. Food could act through the intake of P itself, or through various hormones, such as insulin, glucagon, and calcitonin, the secretion of which is influenced by intake of food. Furthermore, other yet badly defined mechanisms involving conditioned reflexes come into play. Part of the circadian variations, however, are independent of food intake. This rhythm is independent of other electrolytes and is not due only to changes in parathyroid hormone (PTH) or calcitonin. It is also independent of the recumbent position, of sleep, and until now has not been explained by hormonal variations. Whether the kidney plays a role in this rhythm, and if so to what extent, is not known.

Phosphate homeostasis

Two aspects of homeostasis have to be considered: the regulation of whole body phosphate and the regulation of the plasma level of Pi.

Homeostasis of whole body phosphate

As mentioned earlier, the greatest part of the body P lies within the mineral of bone, in which it helps to give this tissue its mechanical strength. Besides this structural role it could be envisaged that the bone Pi also plays the role of a Pi bank, allowing this ion to be released when it is needed by the organism. Bone mineral could then serve as an *ad interim* supply, to allow the maintenance of P in cells in which it plays a series of vital roles.

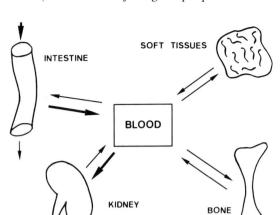

FIGURE 9-1 *Fluxes of Pi in and out of blood.*

The body takes up its P from the diet by absorption in the small intestine, and excretes it through the kidney. In the adult in steady state, the amount excreted in urine equals the net amount absorbed in the gut. It should be noted here that a change in renal reabsorption of Pi will lead to a change in plasma Pi, but not necessarily to an alteration of Pi balance. Indeed, as discussed later, the initial increase in urinary Pi induced by the change in tubular handling will rapidly disappear when plasma Pi has reached its new steady state value.

Homeostasis of plasma inorganic phosphate

The amount of Pi in plasma and extracellular fluid, about 15 mmol in the adult human, represents less than 0.1% of the total P present in the body. It is not yet known whether the concentration in the extracellular fluid is regulated by a feedback mechanism, sensitive to any change from the set value, as is the case for calcium. It has been claimed that if such a control does exist, it is not as tight as for calcium, since plasma levels vary a great deal more in percentage of the initial value when the steady state is disturbed, for example, by food intake. This argument is not necessarily correct, however, since the disturbing signal, that is, the change in flux reaching the extracellular fluid induced by food intake, is greater in relation to the extracellular pool for Pi than for calcium. Thus, it is by no means certain that the efficiency of the regulation of the plasma values is better for calcium than for Pi.

Plasma concentrations are the reflection of the various fluxes entering and leaving the extracellular pool. As shown in Figure 9-1, Pi enters this pool from the intestine, from the various soft tissues, and from bone. It leaves the extracellular fluid by way of the urine, through backflux into the gut lumen, and through passage back into both bone and soft tissues. The magnitude of these various fluxes for Pi are less well known than they are for calcium. Glomerular filtration and tubular reabsorption are among the most important if not the most important ones. With a plasma Pi of 1.2 mmol, the filtered load in an adult human will be about 200 mmol/d. If the urinary excretion is about 20 to 30 mmol, the tubular reabsorptive flux amounts to around 170 mmol, that is, nearly seven times the net flux from the gut. Extrapolation from work on the rat to humans would suggest that fluxes of this magnitude also exist into and out of the liver, muscles, and bone. From these data it would appear that all these tissues should be able to influence the plasma level of Pi, too. However, with the possible exception of bone, the amount of Pi present in these tissues is sufficient only for short-term influence, but is too small to be effective over a longer period. This is supported by the finding that if Pi is removed from blood by selective ion exchange, it is replenished rapidly from body stores only in the first period.

It is therefore likely that the main determinant of long-term plasma Pi is renal tubular reabsorption. Indeed, it is only the kidney that allows either elimination from the extracellular pool of large amounts of Pi over an unlimited time or its complete retention. Furthermore, it is to our present knowledge the only organ that has been shown to adapt its handling of Pi in a homeostatic way. There is no question, however, that besides tubular reabsorption the net inflow of Pi into the extracellular pool, which has been termed throughput, is also of importance. In the case of zero balance, that is, when Pi is neither retained nor lost by the organism, this throughput will obviously just correspond to the net amount absorbed in the gut.

Intestinal absorption of phosphate

The P source for noncarnivorous animals is plants. In the human diet, P is widespread. The largest concentration, 30 to 200 mmol, is found in fish, liver and other organs, eggs, meat, milk, and cheese, with the exception of human milk in which it is much lower. Furthermore, P is present in bread (30–60 mmol), vegetables (10–30 mmol) and fruit (3–10 mmol). Wine and beer (below 5 mmol) have a relatively low content, whereas, of course, all distilled products have no P at all. The presence of P in so many of our foodstuffs explains the rarity of its deficiency. Usually, a diet with enough calcium and enough protein is largely sufficient in P.

The average intake in humans lies between 30 and 50 mmol P/d. The minimum requirement is about 25 mmol/d for males and somewhat more for children and pregnant women.

Both inorganic and organic P can be absorbed. The absorption occurs in the whole small intestine, absorptive capacity being highest in the

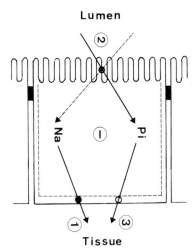

FIGURE 9-2. *Scheme of Pi absorption in the intestinal mucosa cell.* ① *Active Na-K-ATPase–dependent Na pump.* ② *Electroneutral Pi cotransport with Na⁺, driven by Na gradient.* ③ *Na-independent Pi efflux, perhaps carrier-mediated, driven by electrochemical gradient. (After Kinne, R., Berner, W., Hoffmann, N. and Murer, H.: In Massry, S. G. and Ritz, E. (eds.), Phosphate Metabolism. New York, Plenum Press, 1977)*

duodenum and lowest in the ileum. This does not mean that fluxes *in vivo* follow the same pattern, since food stays much longer in the latter segments. It is thought that P is absorbed actively at the luminal membrane against an electrochemical gradient (Fig. 9-2). The movement involves an energy-requiring sodium-dependent saturable process. $1,25(OH)_2D_3$ stimulates this process. Release from the cell through the basolateral membrane is probably through simple or facilitated diffusion. The transmural transport is, at least partly, independent of that of calcium. Besides this cellular mediated active component there is an important, probably paracellular, transmural Pi flux, which responds to the criteria of simple diffusion. This explains why in the whole animal, increasing Pi intake results in a proportional increment in net Pi absorption, with no indication of saturation. In contrast to calcium, in which the percentage of absorption decreases markedly when the intake goes up, this percentage for Pi, which is about 70% of the intake, changes to a relatively small extent. These small alterations in the intestinal Pi transport capacity in response to variations in the intake appear to be mainly mediated by the hormonal form of vitamin D_3, $1,25(OH)_2D_3$. The relative importance of this regulatory process is, however, small compared with that of Pi supply, which is thus the preponderant variable (Fig. 9-3). This explains why clinically inadequate Pi absorption results mainly from abnormal availability of absorbable Pi and not from changes in the intrinsic capacity of intestinal transport.

Such clinical syndromes are rare. Excessive absorption can occur when Pi is administered therapeutically in too large amounts. This leads to an increase in the blood level of Pi and ectopic precipitation of calcium phosphate in the soft tissues, especially in blood vessels, kidney, and heart. Lack of P is practically restricted to conditions when feeding is by infusion of P-free fluids. It can be seen occasionally in low-P diets, for example, in certain alcoholics, especially when antacids such as aluminum or magnesium salts, which strongly bind P in the intestine and render it unabsorbable, are used. This lack of P leads to a recently described syndrome of P de-

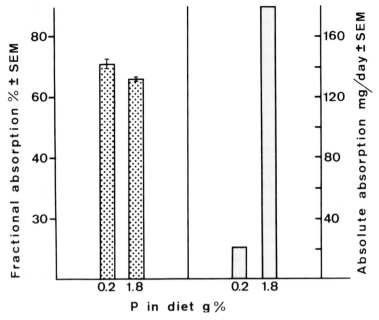

FIGURE 9-3 *Influence of various intakes of Pi during 18 d on fractional net absorption of Pi and on the actual amount absorbed. (Rizzoli, R., Fleisch, H., and Bonjóur, J.-P.: J. Clin. Invest. 60 639–647, 1977)*

pletion. In view of the importance of P in many biochemical processes in the body, it is not surprising that such a depletion leads to a widespread range of symptoms.

Extrarenal soft tissue handling of phosphate

Little is known yet about the regulation of the fluxes out of and into the soft tissues, other than the kidney, and their importance in setting of plasma Pi over the day. It is also barely known to what extent and for how long they can buffer any change induced by a change in P intake. There are, however, data suggesting that they do play a role in short-term regulation, which should not be neglected. Part of this regulation is likely to be through hormones, since several hormones have an effect on soft tissue P handling.

Calcitonin, PTH, and vitamin D

It has been known for a long time that calcitonin decreases plasma Pi. This was first attributed to a decrease in bone resorption. It has been shown, however, that the decrease in blood Pi is larger than the decrease in blood calcium, suggesting that the effect is not likely to be a result of diminished bone resorption only. Moreover, in various conditions the hypophosphatemic effect can be separated from the hypocalcemic one. Further, studies have shown that in nephrectomized animals calcitonin increases Pi exit from plasma, whereas it has no effect on the disappearance of calcium, again emphasizing the difference between the effect of calcium and Pi. The role of the various soft tissues and of the bone in this condition is still open.

Calcitonin also seems to be involved in the relationship between food intake and blood Pi levels, possibly through the secretion of gastrin. Thus, in the rat, plasma Pi levels as well as calcium levels are lowest before the onset and during the first hour of feeding, this fall being blunted by the removal of the thyroid gland. The finding that this fall can occur even 1 hr before feeding, suggests that a conditioned reflex is also involved, with the aim of attenuating the increase brought about by food intake. It appears that calcitonin will have to be investigated in more detail in the future with respect to its effect on P homeostasis. The suggestion that it is more a P hormone than a calcium hormone is a tempting one.

Similarly, in studies concerning the acute effect of PTH, it has been shown that phosphaturia induced by this hormone can only be accounted for by about half by loss from extracellular fluid and increased bone resorption. Furthermore, the hypophosphatemia occurring after PTH is less marked than what would be expected from urinary losses and bone resorption. Some Pi must therefore be liberated into the plasma from another source. The nature of this source is not yet clear. Some data suggest that both Pi and acid-soluble phosphate are decreased to some extent in erythrocytes, muscle, liver, lung, and brain. Another suggestion is that Pi comes from bone, but is not accompanied by a loss of calcium. Thus, it seems that PTH does play a role in regulating Pi fluxes from various organs. This is supported by various findings that PTH influences cellular transport of Pi. The extent and nature of this effect has, however, yet to be determined.

It has been suggested that vitamin D also plays a role in the transfer of Pi between extra- and intracellular compartments; $25(OH)D_3$ stimulates Pi uptake by muscles. The importance of such mechanisms has, however, yet to be assessed.

Fasting

Further circumstantial evidence of the participation of the soft tissues in plasma Pi homeostasis is derived from observations in patients and animals deprived of food. It has long been known that the rachitic lesions of vitamin D- and Pi-depletion could be healed by a period of starvation. This is possibly caused by the conspicuous rise of plasma Pi that occurs during fasting. Such a rise also occurs in normal animals, especially when previously fed a low-P diet. This explains the seemingly paradoxical behavior of phosphatemia in the rat, which rises during the day when the animal is fasting and falls during the night, when it is eating. Since there is no exogenous supply of Pi during fasting, this increased phosphatemia must be due to a mobilization of Pi from body stores. As renal Pi reabsorption is nearly complete with a low-Pi diet, the source of this Pi cannot be the kidney, but has to come from bone and/or the soft tissues. The latter are at least partially involved, since feeding increases both liver weight and acid-soluble phosphate, whereas fasting induces a loss in both. If such a mechanism is present for the liver, it could also be present for other soft tissues.

Carbohydrate metabolism

Part of the variation of Pi in relation to food intake could be due to carbohydrate metabolism and its regulatory hormones. Indeed, it has been known for quite some time that glucose induces a decrease in blood Pi levels. Since insulin has the same effect, and glucose has no action in pancreatectomized animals, the effect of glucose seems to be caused by an increase in the production of insulin. This hormone actually increases the uptake of Pi in heart and muscle and decreases the liberation of Pi by the liver.

Conversely, glucagon also decreases plasma Pi, an effect present in pancreatectomized animals as well as in nephrectomized animals. Since glucagon increases the Pi uptake by the liver, this hormone too appears to act through soft tissues. Finally, both epinephrine and cyclic-AMP also decrease plasma Pi and increase its uptake by the perfused liver.

The physiologic meaning of these various effects has yet to be defined.

Inorganic phosphate and bone

Little is known as to whether bone has a specific role in Pi homeostasis. Most studies have been directed toward assessing the role of bone mineral as a bank of calcium—the liberation of Pi, whenever there is a net destruction of bone, being regarded as a secondary event. It has been suggested, however, that bone may liberate Pi without calcium under such stimuli as calcitonin and PTH. Furthermore, the findings concerning $1,25(OH)_2D_3$, the active metabolite of vitamin D, point to the possibility of a feedback loop in Pi regulation. A low-Pi diet leads to an increase in bone resorption (Fig. 9-4). Since the production of $1,25(OH)_2D_3$ is increased in this situa-

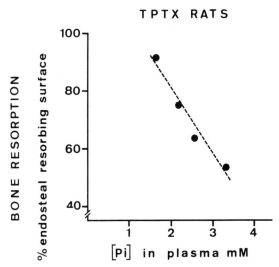

FIGURE 9-4 *Relationship between plasma Pi and endosteal bone resorption in TPTX rats fed various amounts of Pi. (After Baylink, D., Werdegal, J., and Stauffer, M.: J. Clin. Invest. 50 2519–2530, 1971)*

tion, and since this metabolite has the property of enhancing bone resorption, it is possible that the increase seen with a low-Pi diet is mediated by $1,25(OH)_2D_3$. In the future, bone should also perhaps be considered as a P reservoir.

Renal handling of phosphate

As discussed previously, the kidney plays a major role in setting and regulating the plasma level of Pi. In recent years, great progress has been made in the understanding of the renal handling of Pi and its regulation. The main aspects will be reviewed in this chapter.

Measurement of the renal handling

A series of approaches have been used to assess the renal handling of Pi. One of the oldest is simply to measure the urinary excretion. It must be stressed that in a steady state this variable reflects only the net input of Pi in the extracellular compartment, which in the nonfasting state is mainly the net amount absorbed by the gut. Urinary Pi will thus not give any indication about how this ion is handled in the kidney. Only in nonsteady state situations, such as after

acute administration of PTH, will the urinary Pi reflect to some extent what occurs in the kidney. This change rapidly subsides when a new steady state has been reached, urinary Pi going back to the original values and only plasma Pi remaining altered. Although this seems straightforward theoretically, many investigators still extrapolate changes in urinary Pi in some way or another to draw conclusions about the renal handling, or conclusions are made about urinary Pi from the renal handling. Thus, it is often claimed that in hyperparathyroidism, urinary Pi is increased. This is actually not the case in most instances, despite the fact that the renal handling of Pi is altered. In the few cases in which urinary excretion is increased, it is not due to the change in the renal handling but to a greater inflow of Pi into the extracellular compartment either from the gut and/or bone.

A better method, which better reflects the actual renal handling, is Pi clearance. This variable is, however, dependent on the glomerular filtration rate (GFR). This has been corrected by measuring the ratio of the clearance of Pi to that of inulin, which is the same as the fractional excretion of Pi. Unfortunately, both clearance and fractional excretion depend upon the level of plasma Pi. This dependence is due to the fact that the net tubular reabsorption of Pi is a saturable process. Therefore, a clearance or a fractional excretion determined at one plasma level cannot be compared with a clearance at another level in order to characterize the renal handling in terms of transport capacity. This fact has been disregarded in a great number of studies, which makes the interpretation of the literature on the actual renal handling of Pi very difficult and confused.

There is no advantage in using the fractional reabsorption of Pi, which is just the reciprocal of the fractional excretion. This is unfortunate, since a great proportion of the data in the literature, both in animals and in humans, report tubular reabsorption. Today, this method, if determined at one plasma Pi level only, should be abandoned for both investigative and clinical use.

The fractional excretion values have been corrected to some extent for the influence of plasma values, by introducing for diagnostic use an empirical formula, but without a physiologic meaning, called the Pi excretion index. This is calculated from a series of data under acute phosphate infusion. Unfortunately, the data on which the formula is based are somewhat questionable, since they were not obtained under steady state conditions. Furthermore, the formula is calculated from data under acute Pi infusion, but is then applied to conditions at steady state endogenous Pi, which are not necessarily identical, especially with respect to PTH concentration.

The tubular reabsorption of Pi in many animals as well as in humans is limited to a maximum value called the tubular maximum reabsorption, or TmPi (Fig. 9-5). This variable can be determined by infusing Pi and measuring its urinary excretion. In order to correct for kidney mass, TmPi is currently normalized by the ratio TmPi:GFR. This latter value actually corresponds to the theoretical renal threshold shown in Figure 9-5. The determination of Tm:GFR by means of Pi infusion is the method of choice for assessing tubular capacity to transport Pi. Clinically, the drawback of infusing Pi in each individual patient has been solved by the demonstration that in humans TmPi:GFR can be determined merely by measuring in the fasting state, urinary Pi, urinary creatinine, blood Pi, and blood creatinine and using a nomogram. Since this nomogram was derived from data obtained under Pi infusions, the intrinsic drawbacks of the latter are, however, not avoided. This procedure by itself changes the Tm both through an increased secretion of PTH induced by the decrease in ionized calcium and by a PTH-independent process. Unfortunately, there is today no way to avoid Pi infusion.

Despite this drawback the assessment of TmPi:GFR remains the best method available to evaluate the renal handling of Pi. It has also a physiologic basis, since it represents roughly the reabsorption capacity/individual nephron. In the light of the importance of the kidney in setting plasma Pi, it is interesting that TmPi:GFR is closely related to blood Pi at least in a population under the usual Pi intake. Moreover, a multiple regression analysis showed that 70% of the variation of plasma Pi in the fasting state in the individual without renal failure is determined by this parameter for the variables examined.

Localization of tubular reabsorption

Pi is filtered relatively freely through the glomerulum. As mentioned earlier, the filtered load can normally be calculated by using the plasma Pi, since the concentration in the glomerular filtrate happens to equal that of plasma Pi. However, this might not be true anymore, when plasma Pi or calcium is increased to high levels, because of nonfilterable calcium phosphate complexes.

Studies by free-flow micropuncture, microperfusion, stationary microperfusion, and *in vitro* microperfusion showed that a large part—in the view of some authors the totality of the Pi reabsorption—occurs in the proximal tubule. The reabsorption is maximum near the glomerulum, and then decreases to its lowest level, yet significant, in the pars recta. In the first part of the nephron the ratio of the concentration tubular fluid over plasma ultrafiltrate decreases from 1 to 0.6 to 0.8, showing that at this location Pi is absorbed faster than water. In the later part of the proximal tubule the ratio stays

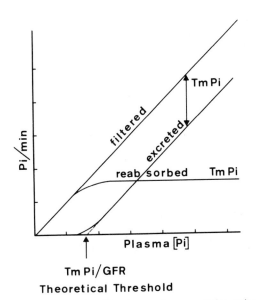

FIGURE 9-5 *Relationship among urinary excretion, tubular reabsorption, and plasma concentration of Pi.*

about the same, so that both water and Pi are absorbed at the same rate.

The question whether Pi is reabsorbed in the distal and the terminal nephron is still debated. From the data available it has to be concluded that distal reabsorption does exist, at least in some strains of rats. However, its relative importance in overall reabsorption has yet to be determined.

Tubular secretion

Secretion should be defined as unidirectional flux from peritubular space into the lumen. This has to be distinguished from the net addition of Pi within a segment, which requires that the secretory flux is greater than the reabsorptive flux. Some authors call only this latter situation secretion. Methodologically unidirectional flux can

only be assessed using radioactive isotopes. Clearance methods will only assess net addition. When present, this obviously implies unidirectional flux, but when lacking by no means excludes it.

Net addition has been shown to be present in various species such as aglomerular and glomerular fish, alligator, amphibians, and chicken. In humans and animals, clearances of Pi above that of inulin, that is, net addition of Pi, have been reported, but only in renal failure and in hypophosphatemic X-linked rickets. In experimental animals a unidirectional flux of Pi has been demonstrated in studies involving stop-flow techniques, microperfusion, stationary microperfusion, microperfusion *in vitro*, and transport of radioactive Pi. If one sums up all the data, it appears that under normal conditions, secretion of Pi does exist, but that in the seg-

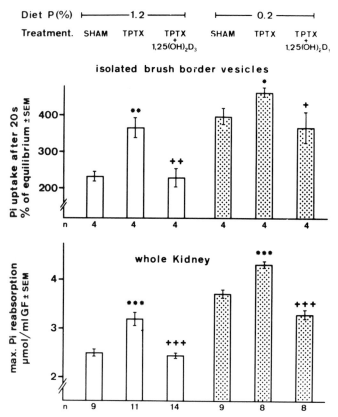

FIGURE 9-6 *Pi uptake* in vitro *by isolated brush border vesicles and maximum tubular Pi reabsorption* in vivo *in the rat under various experimental conditions.*

ments that have been investigated its magnitude is probably only minor. This could be different in pathologic conditions, especially in renal failure.

Mechanisms of tubular reabsorption

Although a ratio of tubular fluid over plasma ultrafiltrate of $0.6:0.8$ may be compatible with a passive diffusion and some small negative transtubular potential, this mechanism is probably not the one driving Pi reabsorption. Indeed, since the interior of the cell is negative with respect to the lumen, the passage from the lumen into the cell has to be against an electrochemical gradient and has to be driven by an active process. Conversely, the exit from the cell to the peritubular fluid could be passive. Various data support such a mechanism. The tubular absorption of Pi has been found to depend to a large extent on sodium transport, but not on water transport. No Pi is reabsorbed without sodium, and an inhibition of the sodium potassium ATPase diminishes the absorption.

Studies on isolated brush border membrane vesicles have also largely supported this view. These vesicles have been shown to take up Pi actively into their interior. This pumping is driven by sodium and decreased by arsenate. Kinetic studies have suggested that two sodiums are probably absorbed for one Pi, and that the divalent $HPO_4^=$ is likely to be the absorbed form. In contrast, the basolateral membranes have no concentrative uptake and are only influenced to a small extent by sodium. The more precise mechanisms by which Pi is pumped into the cell at the brush border membrane are still conjectural. It has been suggested that cyclic-AMP stimulates a protein kinase that would then phosphorylate a protein involved in Pi transport.

The relevance of the Pi uptake by the vesicles to the whole kidney Pi reabsorption is emphasized by the very close correlation found between the vesicle uptake *in vitro* and the renal Pi reabsorption *in vivo* in a large number of different situations, such as an excess and a lack of PTH, or a change in dietary P (Fig. 9-6). This shows that the measurement of Pi transport into the vesicles *in vitro* is a reliable tool that will allow us in the future to get closer to the mechanisms of transport and their regulation.

Factors influencing tubular Pi reabsorption

Tubular reabsorption is influenced by a number of factors, among them several hormones, the most important one being PTH.

PARATHYROID HORMONE (PTH)

It has been known for a long time that acute administration of PTH increases phosphaturia and that chronically PTH decreases plasma Pi levels. The effect of PTH is influenced by various factors, especially the Pi status of the animal or the individual, and the previous dietary Pi intake. In Pi depletion or after a period of low Pi intake, the phosphaturia is less or can be completely suppressed.

Renal artery infusions showed that the effect of PTH is due to a direct action on the kidney, altering the renal handling. Studies using stopflow techniques, free-flow micropuncture, microperfusion, and *in vitro* microperfusion showed that the main action of this hormone is on the proximal tubule, both in the middle convoluted part and in the pars recta. It has been claimed that PTH also has an effect on the reabsorption in the distal tubule.

PTH has been shown to alter specifically the Pi transport system within the brush border membrane of the proximal tubule. This effect is probably mediated by the increase in renal cyclic-AMP induced by PTH. It is thought that PTH reaches the renal tubule from the capillary blood at the basolateral membrane at which point it induces the production of the cyclic-AMP. The latter would then diffuse to the luminal membrane at which point it binds and produces its effect.

CALCITONIN

The role of calcitonin is less clear-cut than that of PTH. Although it has been found that pharmacologic amounts of calcitonin induce a phosphaturic effect, no data have shown that physiologic amounts produce a direct effect on the renal handling of Pi.

GROWTH HORMONE

Growth hormone increases TmPi in both dogs and humans. Furthermore, the TmPi : GFR is increased in acromegaly. It is probable that this effect is at least partly the cause of the higher plasma Pi levels in children compared with adults. Whether the effect on the renal handling is direct or indirect has not yet been ascertained.

THYROXIN

It is known that in thyroxicosis, blood Pi levels, TmPi and TmPi : GFR are increased and return to normal after treatment. Animal studies showed that thyroxin indeed increases the tubular reabsorption capacity of Pi both in normal and in thyroparathyroidectomized rats. However, whether this is due to a direct renal effect of thyroxin is again not yet known.

CORTICOSTEROIDS

The results on studies of these hormones are contradictory, so that no definitive statement can be made.

VITAMIN D AND ITS METABOLITES

The effect of these compounds is also still a subject of controversy. Results on the action of vitamin D are difficult to interpret, since they are contradictory and could often be due to other changes, especially PTH, calcemia, and Pi needs of the organism through an alteration in the mineralization rate.

When given acutely, $25(OH)D_3$ has been found by some authors and in some conditions to increase fractional Pi reabsorption. Other investigators have not been able to reproduce this effect. Even when present, there is as yet no strong evidence that this effect is really due to a change in the tubular capacity to reabsorb Pi when PTH is lacking. Some data in the literature show that $1,25(OH)_2D_3$ given acutely in pharmacologic amounts increases the fractional reab-

sorption of Pi. Again, this effect has been difficult to reproduce, and no evidence of an actual change in the renal capacity to reabsorb Pi has been provided when PTH is lacking. When given chronically in physiologic doses, however, $1,25(OH)_2D_3$ decrease the tubular reabsorbing capacity of Pi in both hypoparathyroid humans and animals. This effect is not present in normal animals and humans, suggesting that a state of $1,25(OH)_2D_3$ deficiency is required for the expression of the effect. Of special interest is the fact that this physiologic amount of $1,25(OH)_2D_3$ actually restores in thyroparathyroidectomized rats the Pi handling to normal, raising the question about the relative role of PTH and $1,25(OH)_2D_3$ in PTH deficiency. Whether the effect of $1,25(OH)_2D_3$ is direct or indirect, possibly partially through an increase in calcemia, is not yet known.

GLUCAGON

Glucagon increases the urinary excretion of Pi while decreasing the plasma level. Infusing glucose gives the same result, so that it is not clear whether the effect of the hormone is a direct one or mediated by glucose.

EXTRACELLULAR VOLUME EXPANSION

Various laboratories found that acute isotonic saline expansion of the extracellular volume promptly increases the fractional excretion of Pi and diminishes TmPi. This effect is only in part explained by a change in PTH and is not due to an increase in GFR. There is a linear relationship between the change in Pi clearance and that in sodium clearance, so that the changes in Pi are possibly secondary to the inhibition of sodium reabsorption in the proximal tubule. Although this mechanism is certainly relevant in acute experimental studies, it has not been proved yet to play a role in physiologic conditions.

ACID-BASE

The effects of acidosis and alkalosis are difficult to interpret, since it is not easy to distinguish between a direct and indirect action. Both chronic acidosis and alkalosis induce only small changes in the renal handling of phosphate. Conversely, an acute infusion of bicarbonate or alkalinization with acetazolamide decreases the tubular reabsorption. This effect is not due to changes in PTH and has been explained by competition between phosphate and bicarbonate or by a change in intracellular pH.

CALCIUM

The role of the calcium concentration in blood on the renal handling of Pi has been most controversial. The difficulty arises from the facts that calcium influences PTH secretion, calcium infusion produces a decrease in GFR, and if the calcium concentration in blood is raised too high, it makes nonfilterable complexes with Pi, rendering the interpretation of renal handling difficult. Nevertheless, taking into account all the data, the conclusion can be drawn that the chronic administration of calcium leads to a decrease in the tubular reabsorption of Pi, both in animals and in humans, independently of PTH. In contrast, the acute increase in calcemia or calcium concentration *in situ* seems to produce an increase in reabsorption.

Regulation of the tubular Pi reabsorption

As seen from the previous discussion, various factors can influence renal handling of Pi. They cannot, however, be claimed to regulate this function, since for regulation, a homeostatic feedback mechanism has to come into play. Even PTH cannot be considered as a regulator, since its production is not influenced directly by plasma Pi. The changes induced indirectly through an alteration of ionized calcium could be considered in some situations as part of a feedback loop. However, this loop can be of only minor importance, since PTH is above all a calcium regulating hormone (Fig. 9-7).

A new development in these past years has been the finding that the kidney possesses a very powerful mechanism over-riding all others, allowing it to adapt its Pi reabsorption to the need of the organism for this element. It has been known for many years that a restriction in the Pi supply leads to a sharp reduction in both the absolute and the fractional excretion of Pi. Until recently, this effect has been thought to be caused by a change in the filtered load of Pi and PTH secretion. Recently, it was found that this mechanism is independent of $\sqrt{PTH}$ the load, serum calcium, extracellular volume expansion, intratubular bicarbonate concentration, and urine pH (Fig. 9-8). Interestingly, it is also not linked to a change in cyclic-AMP excretion.

The question can be posed as to whether the effect is a result of some gastrointestinal information, for example a gastrointestinal hormone. This seems not to be the case, since similar changes in the renal Pi handling are brought about by changing the mineralization of bone in treating growing animals, in which about 80% of the phosphate absorbed in the intestine is taken up by the skeleton, with a calcification inhibitor. By changing the amount of Pi in the diet or altering its use by the organism leads, therefore, to a change in its renal handling. Thus, it seems that the kidney is able to adapt already within a day to the needs of the organism. This concept would explain why renal reabsorption, and thus plasma Pi concentration, is larger in young individuals than in adults, since the former has a greater need of P.

Free-flow micropuncture studies have shown that the adaptation takes place mainly in the first part of the proximal tubule, and possibly along the terminal nephron. In the proximal tubule, the adaptive response is expressed at the level of the Pi transport system within the brush border membrane.

Besides altering the basaline tubular Pi transport capacity, changes in the needs of the organism also modify the response of the kidney to PTH. Changing from a high- to a low-P diet blunts or even suppresses the phosphaturic effect of PTH. This effect is not caused by a change in filtered load as previously believed, but to a change in the response of the renal tubule itself. Conversely, reducing the Pi demand of bone by blocking its mineralization induces a greater response to PTH. Again, these effects are not mediated by a change in cyclic-AMP excretion.

The nature of the mechanisms underlying this

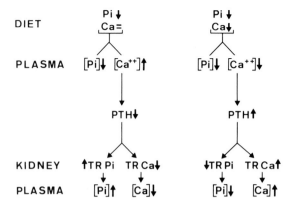

FIGURE 9-7 *Effect of changing Pi and calcium intake on the PTH-induced changes in the renal handling of this ion.*

renal adaptive response to the needs of the organism is still unknown. A humoral factor is of course a tempting possibility.

Diseases with alterations of the renal handling of Pi

Of the group of diseases with alterations of the renal handling of Pi, the main one is renal failure. In this disturbance, plasma Pi increases when GFR is below about 25 ml/min. The explanation that this increase occurs only at such low levels of GFR is severalfold. First, every increase in plasma Pi is compensated to some extent by an increase in its fractional excretion. Furthermore, an increase in Pi leads to a decrease in ionized calcium, and therefore to a stimulation of PTH secretion, which decreases tubular reabsorption. This secondary hyperparathyroidism is still thought by many to be the main correcting

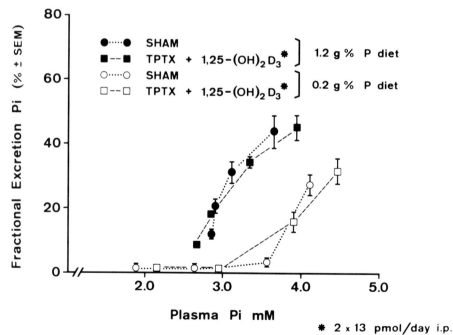

FIGURE 9-8 *Influence of dietary Pi on the fractional excretion of Pi in normal rats and TPTX animals given a physiologic dose of 1,25(OH)₂D₃.*

mechanism. It is, however, quite possible that mechanisms involving the adaptation of the kidney to the need of the organism also play a role. Indeed, reducing the number of functioning nephrons induces an elevation of the load/nephron, thus mimicking the situation of increased dietary Pi in the healthy individual.

In renal failure, the relative importance of the various fluxes for the setting of plasma Pi undergoes a drastic change. With progressive renal failure, the reabsorptive flux decreases, so that the importance of the flux coming from the intestine increases proportionately. This concept is currently made use of in clinical practice. Plasma Pi is decreased efficiently in renal failure by reducing P in the diet, or by inhibiting its intestinal absorption with Pi binders such as aluminum or magnesium salts. Besides the intestinal flux, the glomerular filtration also becomes a critical determinant of plasma Pi in renal failure. This is explained by the fact that the role of the filtered load increases with respect to the reabsorption flux.

Another disease of Pi metabolism involving the kidney is the hereditary X-linked hypophosphatemic rickets. A decrease in the tubular capacity for Pi reabsorption, which leads to low levels of plasma Pi, is one of the main features of this affliction. Whether this effect is the primary and unique cause of the bone mineralization defect has, however, as yet not been ascertained, either in the human disease or in its experimental model in the mouse.

A disturbance of tubular Pi reabsorption has also been suggested to occur in urinary stone patients with hyperabsorptive hypercalciuria. In this disease a decrease in TmPi:GFR and plasma Pi levels has been recorded. It has been proposed that this finding would represent a primary defect in the tubular Pi reabsorption, which would lead to an increased production of $1,25(OH)_2D_3$. Such an increase would then be responsible for the increase in the intestinal calcium absorption and urinary calcium excretion. More information is necessary before the existence of this pathophysiologic mechanism can be accepted as a reality.

Other diseases that affect the renal Pi handling, such as hyper- and hypoparathyroidism, thyrotoxicosis, and acromegaly, are charac-

terized only by a change in plasma Pi, but without pathophysiologic consequences.

CONCLUSIONS

Substantial progress has been made in these last years in the understanding of Pi homeostasis and its control by gut, kidney, bone and soft tissues. Our knowledge in this field is, however, still considerably behind that which we have for other minerals. Future research into the mechanisms controlling Pi handling by the various tissues, and into the influence of Pi on the functioning of the latter, especially bone, is likely to be very promising.

This work was supported by the Swiss National Science Foundation (3.725.76), and by the Ausbildungs- und Förderungsfonds der Arbeitsgemeinschaft für Osteosynthese (AO), Switzerland.

Suggested reading

Distribution of phosphate in the body

Marshall, R. W., and Nordin, B. E. C.: The state of inorganic phosphate in plasma and its relation to other ions. *In* Hioco, D. J. (ed.): Phosphate et Métabolisme Phosphocalcique, pp. 127–138, Paris, Laboratoires Sandoz, l'Expansion Scientifique Française, 1971.

Mills, J. N.: Human circadian rhythms, Physiol. Rev. 46:128–171, 1966.

Phosphate homeostasis

Robertson, W. G.: Plasma phosphate homeostasis. *In* Nordin, B. E. C. (ed.): Calcium, Phosphate and Magnesium Metabolism, pp. 217–229, Edinburgh, Churchill Livingstone, 1976.

Intestinal absorption of phosphate

Kinne, R., Berner, W., Hoffmann, N., and Murer, H.: Phosphate transport by isolated renal and intestinal plasma membranes. *In* Massry, S. G., and Ritz, E. (eds.): Phosphate Metabolism, pp. 265–277, New York and London, Plenum Press, 1977.

Massry, S. G.: The clinical syndrome of phosphate depletion. *In* Massry, S. G., Ritz, E., and

Rapado, A. (eds.): Homeostasis of Phosphate and Other Minerals, pp. 301–312, New York and London, Plenum Press, 1978.

Walling, M. W.: Intestinal inorganic phosphate transport. *In* Massry, S. G., Ritz, E., and Rapado, A. (eds.): Homeostasis of Phosphate and Other Minerals, pp. 131–147, New York and London, Plenum Press, 1978.

Extrarenal soft tissue handling of phosphate

Birge, S. J.: Vitamin D, muscle and phosphate homeostasis, Min. Electr. Metab. 1:57–64, 1978.

Talmage, R. V., Grubb, S. A., and Doppelt, S. H.: The physiology of calcium and phosphate homeostasis, *In* Proceedings of the Fifth International Congress of Endocrinology, Vol. 2, pp. 268–274, Amsterdam, Excerpta Medica Foundation, 1977.

Inorganic phosphate and bone

DeLuca, H. F.: Vitamin D metabolism and function. Springer-Verlag, New York, 1979.

Renal handling of phosphate

Bijvoet, O. L. M.: The importance of the kidneys in phosphate homeostasis. *In* Phosphate Metabolism, Kidney and Bone, pp. 421–474, Paris, Armour Montagu, 1976.

Coburn, J. W., Saltzman, R. L., and Massry, S. G.: Interactions between vitamin D and the kidney. *In* Martinez-Maldonado, M. (ed.): Methods in Pharmacology, Vol. 4A: Renal Pharmacology, pp. 227–267, New York, Plenum Press, 1976.

Dennis, V. W., Stead, W. W., and Myers, J. L.: Renal handling of phosphate and calcium, Ann. Rev. Physiol. 41:257–271, 1979.

Knox, F. G., Osswald, H., Marchand, G. R., Spielman, W. S., Haas, J. A., Berndt, T., and Youngberg, S. P.: Phosphate transport along the nephron, Am. J. Physiol. 233:F261–F268, 1977.

Massry, S. G., and Fleisch, H. (eds.): Renal Handling of Phosphate, New York, Plenum Press, in press.

Massry, S. G., Friedler, R. M., and Coburn, J. W.: Excretion of phosphate and calcium. Physiology of their renal handling and relation to clinical medicine, Arch. Intern. Med. 131:828–859, 1973.

Mudge, G. H., Berndt, W. O., and Valtin, H.: Tubular transport of urea, glucose, phosphate, uric acid, sulfate, and thiosulfate. *In* Orloff, J., Berliner, R. W., and Geiger, S. R. (eds.): Handbook of Physiology, Section 8: Renal Physiology, pp. 587–652, Washington, D. C., American Physiological Society, 1973.

Saltopolsky, E. and Rutherford, W. E.: The metabolism of phosphate in chronic renal disease. *In* Phosphate Metabolism, Kidney and Bone, pp. 35–45, Paris, Armour Montagu, 1976.

Ullrich, K. J.: Mechanisms of cellular phosphate transport in rat kidney proximal tubule. *In* Massry, S. G., Ritz, E., and Rapado, A. (eds.): Homeostasis of Phosphate and Other Minerals, pp. 21–35, New York and London, Plenum Press, 1978.

A fracture is technically an abrupt break of the calcified structure of a bone caused by an extrinsic or intrinsic mechanical force. It is a very common injury; perhaps 2 million fractures occur in the United States alone each year.[2] Many of these fractures are debilitative in the sense that they remove the individual from the work force for some period of time. The "economics" of bone fractures are aggravated by the knowledge that a significant number of fractures do not heal properly, even after skilled surgical intervention. The best data suggest that perhaps 5% (about 100,000 cases) of fractures go on to malunion or nonunion, thus adding to the personal and national economic burden.

In a gross sense, it is possible to erect several classes of fractures. A gross break, with and without shattering of the cortex of a long bone, is spoken of as a comminuted fracture. These **traumatic fractures** contrast with small breaks of a spur of bone, a segment of a thin cortex, or a few trabeculae, which are also common. Some of these can be **stress fractures** in the sense that they occur in an otherwise normal bone that has been subjected to repeated stresses, that is, in association with strenuous physical activity. Stress fractures occur most commonly in the bones of the foot (calcaneous, metatarsals), the proximal shaft (diaphysis) of the tibia, the distal shaft of the femur, the femoral neck, and the pubic ramus. The third category of fractures is the **pathologic fracture,** which is secondary to an underlying disease process. Some authors include osteoporosis in this category, but here one must distinguish between the osteoporosis that occurs as a normal part of the aging process (predominately in females), and the osteoporosis that occurs as a consequence of endocrine disturbances (Cushings Disease, hyperparathyroidism, osteomalacia). Pathologic fractures are associated with congenital or developmental disease entities such as fibrous dysplasia, cysts, endochondromas, and Paget's disease. Fractures are also very prevalent in individuals who suffer from osteogenesis imperfecta congenita. The cortical bone thinning attendant to osteosarcoma and metastatic disease (e.g., prostate and mammary carcinoma) will commonly produce fractures, and there is much evidence to suggest that local

DAVID J. SIMMONS

10

fracture healing

tumor-produced factors such as prostaglandins can exert local bone resorptive activity. In this way, the tumor can expand intraosseously.[35,46,47] Pathologic fractures can also occur if osteomyelitic lesions thin the cortex through endosteal resorption, and this can be a severe complication since it impairs the normal functioning of the bone cells that will participate in fracture repair. Osteomyelitic lesions either can be a primary reason why bone fractures occur or they can occur as a secondary process to surgical intervention or a wound in the skin over the fracture site. Thus, one speaks of an **open fracture** when the injury involves the skin or of a **closed fracture** when the skin is not broken or otherwise involved.

In this chapter, we will consider first the general way in which different fractures heal. I have chosen three models: (1) the comminuted but generally transverse fracture of a long bone, which has a periosteum, (2) the flat cranial bone fracture, which has a periosteum, and (3) the transcervical fracture of the femur—a site that lacks a periosteum. Within this context, the special problems of fracture healing can be appreciated, and delayed unions are one of these problems. We will then consider the natural histories of the cells that participate in fracture healing and the properties of the matrices they produce. We will also discuss some of the biophysical and biochemical characteristics of the tissue that plays a role in matrix-cell interactions. It is these matrix-cell interactions, in turn, that may provide the driving force or forces for the entire process of fracture repair. Here, we will consider factors such as oxygen tension and bioelectrical and osteoinductive phenomena.

General features of healing fractures

The histologic perspective

When a bone is fractured, the tissue responses are quite specific during all phases of the healing process. Under most circumstances, there is an orderly development of different tissue types. In classic descriptions of the process, there are three stages. The initial stage is represented by the formation of granulation tissue, and this is no different than that which occurs following a deep skin lesion. This first stage is gradually replaced by a fibrocartilaginous phase and finally by a bony phase. The nature of the process is such that each of the three phases is usually present to some degree when fracture sites are explored surgically. In fractures that fail to heal normally (e.g., infection), the early stages may even persist for unusually long periods of time. The sequence of histomorphological changes that occur at the fracture site from injury to healing are outlined in Table 10-1. This is basically a *précis* of Urist's classic descriptions.[131]

Although we have stated that this classic outline of fracture repair is consistent for *most* fractures, some qualifications are required. This scheme is not consistent with observations about

TABLE 10-1 SEQUENCE OF HISTOMORPHOLOGICAL CHANGES DURING REPAIR OF A LONG BONE FRACTURE

POSTFRACTURE TIME	HISTOLOGY	PHYSIOLOGY
Immediate	Extravasation of blood	
24 h	Aseptic inflammation → clot	
48 h	Organization of the clot	
4 d	Intramembranous bone formation	Resorption of dead bone
	Subperiosteal bone formation	
5–10 d	Subperiosteal bone formation ↓ Hyaline cartilage	
	↓	
	Fibrocartilage + calcification	Remodeling of callus
	↓	
30 d until time of healing	Trabecular bone formation	
	↓	
	Cortical bone formation	

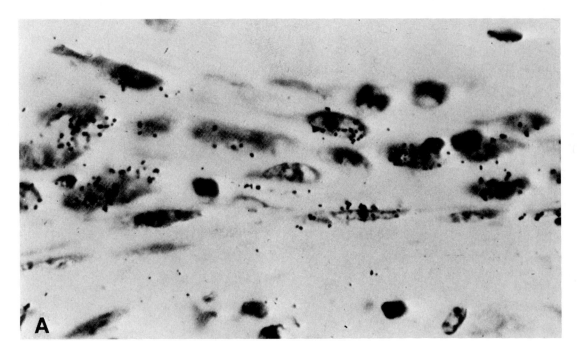

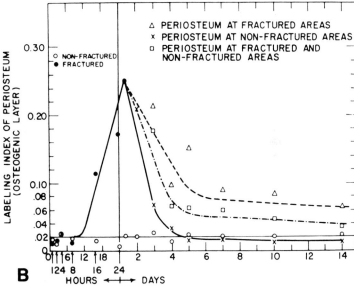

FIGURE 10-1 **(A)** *Autoradiograph of tritiated thymidine-labeled cells in the periosteum of a Swiss albino mouse following fracture. (Provided by E. A. Tonna, New York University College of Dentistry).* **(B)** *Graph of the labeling indices of cells in the periosteum of fractured and nonfractured femora of 5-wk-old Swiss albino mice (Brookhaven National Laboratory strain). Initially, increased labeling is observed throughout the periosteum, both at and proximodistal to the midshaft fracture site. Increased labeling is recorded up to 32 hr after fracture. During the ensuing time periods, there is subsidance of the periosteal reaction, but the labeling index at the fracture site remains higher than the nonfractured areas for several weeks. (Tonna, E. A., and Cronkite, E. P.: J. Bone Joint Surg. 43A:352–362, 1961)*

transcervical fractures of the femoral neck, nor is it entirely satisfactory for fractures of the long bones stabilized by compression plates or for fractures of the flat bones of the skull. The femoral neck, for example, lacks a periosteum. Fractures of the flat bones are not usually displaced, and the bone surfaces are in intimate contact. Compression plating results in the lack of an external callus. Finally, it should be appreciated that fractures of different bones and at different levels within a single bone may heal at significantly different rates. Najjar and Kahn[86] have published a brief chronicle of these events in the dog and rabbit, but it is a rather useful paper for the purposes of general orientation.

Repair in long bones with periosteum

Within the first few hours after an individual sustains a fracture of a long bone, the cells that make up the inner lining of the periosteum (cambium layer) begin to synthesize DNA and proliferate. Direct evidence of this process has been provided by Tonna[128] who followed the cell kinetics of the tissue in mice by labeling the cells with tritiated thymidine (^{3}HTdr). His studies showed, moreover, that proliferative activity occurred throughout the periosteum of the injured bone, not just at the site of injury (Fig. 10-1). Although the cells of the cambium layer are thought of as producers of osteoblasts, these cells are pluripotential, and early on they also produce fibroblasts and cells with chondrogenic capacities. The full potential of periosteal cells can be directly visualized *in vivo* and in special tissue culture systems. In collaboration with Dr. David Cohn's laboratory at the V.A. Hospital in Kansas City, this laboratory[116] loaded millipore diffusion chambers with osteoblast-like cells that had been isolated from murine calvaria, and we implanted these chambers in the peritoneal cavities of isologous mice. Within 3 wk, the cells had organized to form bone and fivrous connective tissue. When calvaria were also placed into millipore chambers with the cells, bone, fibrous tissue, *and* cartilage tissue developed (Fig. 10-2).

A hematoma also forms within the fracture site, owing to damage to the blood vessels in the marrow, periosteum, endosteum, and the capillaries contained within the haversian canals. We note here that the lining cells of the marrow cavity and the haversian canals are coextensive, and henceforth, we will simply refer to them as the endosteum. Periosteal healing by way of its pro-

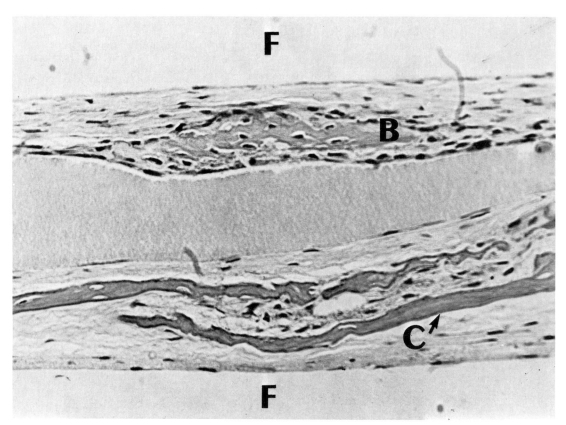

FIGURE 10-2 *Photomicrograph of bone* **(B)** *formed within a millipore* **(F)** *chamber that had been loaded with murine periosteal osteoblast populations and cryolytic calvarium* **(C)**. *The chamber had been implanted intraperitoneally in a CD-1 mouse for 3 wk.*

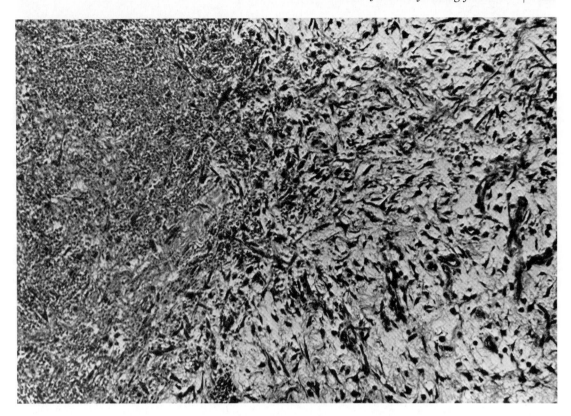

FIGURE 10-3 *Photomicrograph of fracture site showing the central portion of the hematoma at the left and granulation tissue at the right. Fibroblasts and capillary buds appear at the interface of the two tissues and invade the clot. (Aegerter, E., and Kirkpatrick, J. P.: Orthopedic Diseases, Philadelphia, W. B. Saunders Co., 1975)*

liferative activity and the restitution of vascular continuity with the overlying muscle are essential first steps in the healing process. In our laboratory at Washington University, Whiteside[148] has been intensively studying bone-blood flow in laboratory animals using the hydrogen washout technique, and he has reported convincingly that extraperiosteal dissection destroys periosteal vessels that would be so necessary to the healing of fractures. Dramatic changes occur within the bloodclot during the first 2 wk after fracture, and the older literature placed great stress on the importance of the hematoma to the successive stages of healing. Although the hematoma is invaded by a variety of blood-borne formed elements (Fig. 10-3) including macrophages that doubtless resorb fibrin, and a fibroblast-rich granulation tissue does form, this sequence occurs only when the clot is very large. It is evident from experimental animal studies that osteo-

blasts, not fibroblasts, invade clots when they are small.[51] Moreover, other investigators have demonstrated experimentally that fracture healing is not impaired after the early clot is removed by aspiration.

The early fracture site also contains devitalized muscle and bone fragments. The muscle fragments undergo autolysis within 5 to 10 d. When they occur as pedicled flaps with an initially intact blood supply, they tend to undergo fibrous degeneration, and the scar tissue does not generally offer a real impediment to healing—unless, of course, the fragments are very large and come to lie transversely across the fracture line. In fact, fibrous scars may ossify. Likewise, the bony fragments usually show some surface deposition of new bone, presumably stemming from migrating cells of periosteal origin. During this early time period, the medullary components that were deprived of their blood supply

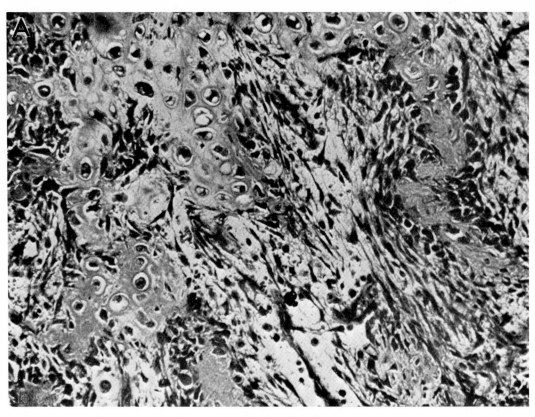

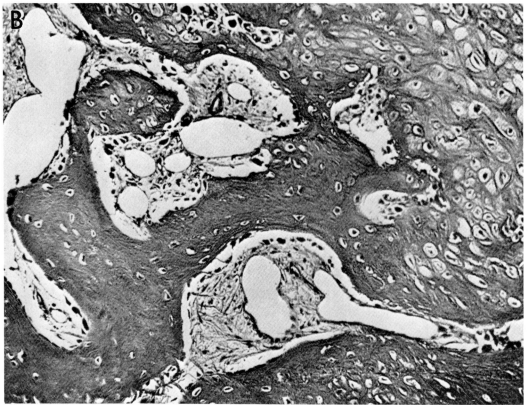

undergo fatty degeneration. However, in situations in which the medullary circulation has not been seriously compromised by injury, some endosteal new bone formation is possible. Although osteoblasts can form in the early callus, it is important to note that osteoclasts are not usually present.

The vascular compromise and the somewhat anaerobic conditions that prevail early after fracture appear to provide a microenvironment that favors the evolution of a callus that becomes more cartilaginous than osseous.

FIBROCARTILAGINOUS CALLUS STAGE

When mature, the fibrocartilaginous callus (Fig. 10-4) consists of a translucent mass of dense fibrous tissue, fibrocartilage, and cartilage. Unmineralized cartilage tissue predominates, however, during the formative stages. The cartilage occurs in nodules that are separated by irregular bands of fibrocartilage. By 3 wk postfracture, the callus is grossly wedge-shaped, with the fibrous septa converging at the middle of the fracture gap. These septa carry relatively large-caliber vessels that originate from the repaired periosteal and medullary circulation. The fracture gap itself consists of primitive marrow and spindle-shaped cells, and these elements are classified as osteoprogenitor cells capable of generating osteoblasts. The richer vascular supply of the fibrocartilaginous callus doubtless serves to increase the oxygen tension of the tissue, and this changed microenvironment seems to favor two additional changes that appear concomitantly. *First,* the fibrocartilaginous components calcify, and the chondrocytes at the periphery of the nodules appear to undergo a direct conversion to osteocytes. Possibly, other chondrocytes can be liberated from their lacunae and modulate to osteoblasts that begin to lay down bone in a manner identical to the sequence of changes that are typical of endochondral ossification. *Second,* osteoclasts appear for the first time. Thus, ossification

and resorption may proceed on different parts of the same trabeculae that begin to form in the callus. Moreover, the devitalized portions of cortical bone begin to be resorbed and remodel. Importantly, in terms of the increasing stability and strength of the fractured bone, the trabeculae closest to the fracture gap become thicker and take on the circumferential arrangement of bone lamellae typical of haversian systems. In this manner, the fibrocartilaginous callus is gradually converted to a bony callus.

BONY CALLUS STAGE

This stage culminates when the chondrosteoid tissue of the fibrocartilaginous callus is totally converted to bone, that is, when the fractured ends of the cortex have joined (Fig. 10-5).

Histologically (see Fig. 10-8), we know that cortical bone has a rich vascular supply and that because there are many collateral intracortical vessels, most of the endosteal cells and osteocytes survive following fracture. Some osteocyte death does occur locally after fracture—about 1 cm back from the break in cortical bone and about 1 mm back from a break in trabecular bone. During the formation of the osseous callus, osteoclastic resorption removes some dead bone from the periosteal and endosteal surfaces, and the cortex begins to become trabecularized even beyond the zone of osteoclastic activity. It appears from the increase in lacunar volume that some osteocytes are capable of resorbing their matrices—that they become uninuclear osteoclasts. This may be a real phenomenon; it was "codified" by Bélanger[10] at the University of Ottawa, and the process is known as **osteocytic osteolysis.** In the intact skeleton, only perhaps 1% of the osteocytes are normally in a resorptive phase. To a certain extent, resorption is matched in intensity by bone formation, so that radiologically one sees an apparent increase in the density of subperiosteal bone.

The ultimate consolidation of the bony shaft

◄ FIGURE 10-4 **(A)** *Island of cartilage cells surrounded by granulation tissue. The cartilage is coextensive with newly formed bony trabeculae, and on some aspects, it is undergoing endochondral ossification.* **(B)** *Chondro-osseous tissue indicating a more mature stage of callus than that seen in* **A.** *The cartilage appears to be undergoing direct conversion to bone (see Fig. 10-14). The intertrabecular spaces are filled with fibrous tissue. (Aegerter, E., and Kirkpatrick, J. P.: Orthopedic Diseases, Philadelphia, W. B. Saunders Co., 1975)*

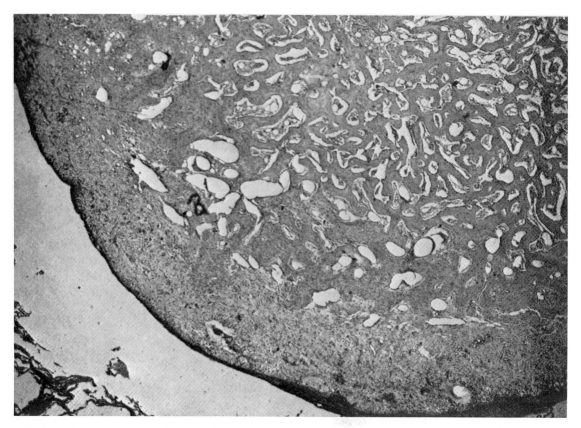

FIGURE 10-5 *A transverse section through the cortex of a fractured bone. The cartilage-fibrocartilage of the callus and the medullary tissue have been replaced by dense trabecular bone. The trabeculae closest to the endosteum are thickest. (Aegerter, E., and Kirkpatrick, J. P.: Orthopedic Diseases, Philadelphia, W. B. Saunders Co., 1975)*

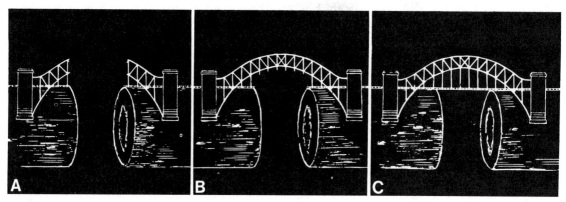

FIGURE 10-6 *Comparison of the union of a fracture of a long bone with the construction of a fixed arch bridge.* **(A)** *Stage 1: fracture—initial periosteal bone formation; bridge—a tower or elevated abutment is constructed on each embankment of the gap to be spanned.* **(B)** *Stage 2: fracture—new bone from both fragments grows over the fracture line but not between the main fragments; bridge—by the method of cantilevering out, an arch is constructed over the gap.* **(C)** *Stage 3: fracture—new bone, showing the formative structure of haversian systems of the compacta, appears between the arch of the periosteal trabecular bone callus; and formation continues to replace the remnants of the fibrocartilaginous callus until the fracture line is consolidated; bridge—the deck or roadway of the bridge is laid down between the ribs and spandrels are suspended from the arch. (Mclean, F. C., and Urist, M. R.: Bone, Chicago, University of Chicago Press, 1955)*

depends upon two events: (1) the continued formation and strengthening of the subperiosteal trabeculae that begin to bridge the fracture gap, and (2) continued remodeling of the cortex. This final structural phase of fracture repair has been likened to a fixed arch bridge. Figure 10-6 shows that the delicately formed subperiosteal trabeculae resemble the arch, whereas the consolidating compact bone of the cortex resembles the roadway. As the fibrocartilaginous callus recedes, the roadway extends to fill the gap. The rate of healing is, in a sense, dependent upon the length of the "span" and the surface area of the fracture line. Thus, a comminuted fracture may take a longer time to consolidate than a spiral fracture because the latter brings into play a proportionately larger number of potential osteoprogenitor cells (Table 10-2). Attempts to improve bone formation in difficult to heal fractures have included roughening of the ends of the stumps for this reason. The technique has been called "petalling."[58]

This description of fracture healing applies to the situation in which the broken ends are approximated or fixed without compression plating. We will deal with the effects of compression plating in a later section, since these fractures heal without the formation of an external stabilizing callus. Here the mechanism involves only intracortical remodeling.

REPAIR OF FLAT BONE FRACTURES

In experimental animal models, the evidence is that linear fractures of the skull heal without forming an intermediate cartilage-fibrocartilage tissue. Some elevation of the periosteum and proliferation of osteoblasts from its cambial layer occur on both sides of the fracture line. This rather direct mode of healing is related to the rich vascular supply of the cranial bones. The importance of maintaining a good vascular supply is recognized in an operational sense, and for this reason, craniotomies are done using bone flaps hinged on the temporalis musculature to preserve periosteal integrity. Scraping the periosteum will obviously ablate vessels, lower the oxygen tensions, and favor the formation of cartilage. This was, in fact, observed after Girgis and Pritchard[48] fractured an area of the skull of rats devoid of periosteum.

The problems presented by fracture of the flat bones are similar to those occurring after trauma to long bones. Provided that the lesion is not too large and brain or other tissues do not bulge into the gap, a periosteal callus will bridge the gap, and repair occurs directly. If the fracture line is wider than the area of heaped-up periosteal bone at the edge of the lesion, a fibrous nonunion will most likely occur. We would, as before, expect this tissue to have a cartilaginous component and the biochemical characteristics of a fibrous nonunion (see section on immobilization). For this reason, sizable cranial defects have been grafted with finely ground autogenous iliac crest bone molded to the contours of the skull. This type of graft (bone blend) will contain a rich supply of progenitor cells, both osseous and marrow-derived. Studies of this type have been pioneered by Boyne[17] as a natural extension of knowledge about the intrinsic osteogenic power of marrow cells (see sections on osteoclastic origins and osteogenic role of marrow).

It is realized, generally, that the time to healing in untended cranial defects is proportional to the size of the defect and the degree of vascular damage. Osteoblasts lay down bone at a rate of 1 to 2 μm/d, diminishing to less than 1 μm/d after

TABLE 10-2 TIME TO REPAIR IN LONG BONE FRACTURES

	UPPER EXTREMITY		LOWER EXTREMITY	
TYPE OF FRACTURE	*NO. WK. TO BRIDGE THE FRACTURE GAP*	*NO. WK. TO REPAIR THE CORTEX*	*NO. WK. TO BRIDGE THE FRACTURE GAP*	*NO. WK. TO REPAIR THE CORTEX*
Spiral or long oblique	3	6–12	6	12
Transverse	6	12–18	12	24

From Urist, M. R., and Johnson, R. W. Jr.: J. Bone Joint Surg. 25:375–426, 1943.

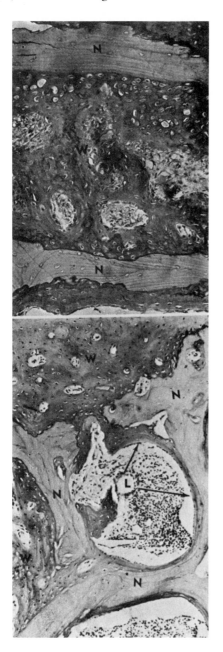

FIGURE 10-7 *Photomicrograph of the local biologic responses during healing of a necrotic femoral head in adult rabbits. The head was "killed" by transcervical osteotomy. The histologic appearance shows fiber bone (above) and lamellar bone (below) formed on the pre-existing but now "dead" bone trabeculae. This increase in bone mass is responsible for the radiologic density of the femoral head in aseptic necrosis. N-dead bone trabeculae. L-Lamellae of new bone.*

70 to 80 yr of age. The prospect for a satisfactory result will be better if, say, the fracture did not compromise the circulation to the inner vault of the skull. Kramer[67] followed healing of parietal bone trepans in rabbits, noting that healing from endosteal and periosteal proliferation took 8 to 16 wk and 20 wk, respectively. Osteotomies (0.5cm × 1.0cm) covered by periosteum heal more rapidly—within 6 to 8 wk.[86]

Bone repair when a periosteum is lacking

The importance of the periosteum to bone repair is everywhere evident, except when the femoral neck is involved. This is the only site in the skeleton not covered, externally at least, by osteogenic tissue. In fractures of the femoral neck, one of the fragments is almost invariably nonvital. The vascular supply to the head is particularly compromised, since the fracture line commonly occurs proximal to the major ring of nutrient vessels (medial femoral circumflex) that penetrate the bone and arborize toward the subchondral metaphyseal tissue. Cell death by aseptic necrosis is widespread in the head. Adequate reduction of the fractured ends accomplishes two purposes. First, it enables repair to proceed at the fracture line, and second, it permits the revascularization and internal remodeling of the subchondral trabecular bone within the head. In this instance, the endosteum and marrow stroma become the sole source of the osteogenic cells that are mobilized to form repair bone.

Once revascularization of the head begins, histologic sections show the construction of viable bone lamellae on the original (but now dead) trabeculae (Fig. 10-7). This is a gradual process, involving both the formation and resorption of old surfaces, "creeping" so to speak, from the site of injury up to the subchondral bony plate under the articular cartilage. Early on, the formation of new bone occurs in advance of osteoclastic resorption, so there is initially an increase in the volume of calcified bone tissue. Because dead bone does not demineralize, the femoral neck-head tends to become radiologically dense.

It is clear that some procedures such as grafting the head-neck do not usually improve the rate of healing. These procedures may provide some structural support and thereby contravene (to a degree) complications such as segmental or massive collapse of the femoral head and the onset of degenerative arthritis. Healing depends upon the rate of vascular penetration and the size of the population of osteogenic cells. As we will note subsequently, the census of osteogenic cells in the red marrow declines with age.

It would be clinically important to have some way to predict the vigor of the cell populations in fractures of this type, and at least one attempt to do this has been reported. Richters[95] cultured core biopsies of peritrabecular marrow cells from the femoral heads of patients with displaced (57) or undisplaced (14) subcapital fractures and intertrochanteric fractures (23). As one might have anticipated, the survival and proliferative capacity of the cell outgrowths from the devitalized heads was relatively poor compared with those from the neck, and the survival of cells from cases with undisplaced cervical fractures was better than that from cases with displaced fractures. Unfortunately, the report did not provide information about the clinical outcome in this patient population. Better-refined methodologies applied to this problem could happily "wed" the basic and clinical sciences. One must ask how many of the cells (fibroblasts, and so forth) that grew out of the explants had osteogenic potential, that is, could serve as the stem cells for osteoblasts.

Blood flow

Major trauma immediately reduces bone marrow pressure and bone-blood flow in the marrow. These effects have been measured directly using a variety of techniques such as ^{133}Xe and hydrogen washout.[34a,126] It is likely that the reduced marrow flow is due to vasoconstrictive effects. As early as 1922, Drinker[36] established that pressor amines decreased marrow blood flow, and many authors have since shown that blood flow to bone and bone marrow is sensitive to vasomotor substances such as acetylcholine and histamine. Sciatic nerve section or sympathectomy increases blood flow (see review by Brookes[21]).

As will be alluded to frequently in this chapter, surgeons must be cognizant that internal fixation by tight-fitting intramedullary rods or plates does interfere with bone-blood flow. Barron,[6] in Kelly's laboratory at the Mayo Clinic, compared the effects of these devices in 57 dogs with standard midulnar fractures. Here, ^{85}Sr clearance was used to measure blood flow, and tetracycline labeling was used to measure the appositional bone formation rates. Both types of fixation disturbed diaphyseal blood flow and the rate of bone formation, but the effect resulting from the plates was less severe. Despite this difference, most of the bones were healed after 90 d. Interestingly, the plated bones retained a well-developed and unremodeled periosteal callus that might have been a reaction to the plate *per se*. It was clear from this study that bone does compensate for widespread destruction of its medullary circulation. Most likely, the collateral circulation and associated perivascular osteogenic precursor cells were mobilized to effect healing. In several valuable reviews of the blood supply to bone, Brookes[21] and Rhinelander[93] emphasize that there are numerous active anastamoses between the medullary and metaphyseal arterial systems. Bone, therefore, has a back-up system that predisposes toward repair, unless there are physical obstructions such as interposing large masses of fibrocartilage and/or fragments of devitalized bone and soft tissue. In lieu of these complications, displaced fractures that have been satisfactorily reduced and maintained in a stable position without hardware show regeneration of the major medullary arteries within 3 wk. Figure 10-8 shows microangiograms taken from Rhinelander's monograph to demonstrate this point.

Compression plating

Ham and Harris[51] indicate that there are two terms adopted from wound healing studies that are frequently used to describe the repair of fracture—primary and secondary intention. In primary intention, the edge of a wound unites directly without the formation of granulation tissue. In secondary intention, the edge of a wound unites with the intervention of granulation tissue.

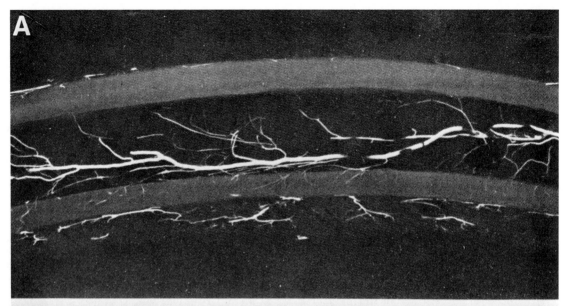

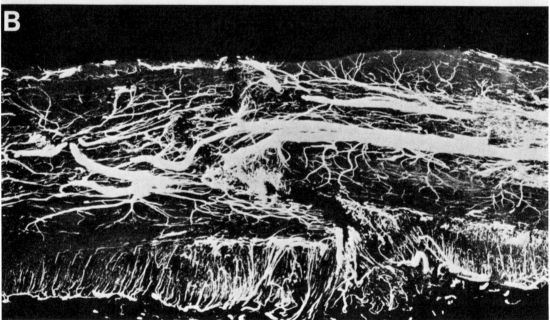

FIGURE 10.8 **(A)** *Microangiogram from the diaphysis of a normal canine radius with the circulation in a "resting" state.* **(B)** *Microangiogram from a 3 wk diaphyseal displaced fracture of a canine radius with the bone fragments in a "stable" position. Large medullary arteries have been reconstituted across the fracture line. Note the characteristic vascular pattern of early periosteal callus, with blood vessels perpendicular to the cortical surface. (Rhinelander, F. S.: Clin. Orthop. 105:34–81, 1974)*

Despite awareness that these terms do not accurately describe the processes of fracture repair, the classification has served as the basis of one modern clinical concept of fracture management—that of compression plating. The theory states that if bone ends can be closely apposed and compressed to a degree that pressure necrosis does not occur, bones will "knit" by a process that has been called autogenous welding. No external or internal callus will develop, but healing will occur by the growth of haversian systems across the fracture line. Presumably, the lack of callus reflects the lack of some stimulus that calls forth the expression of the osteogenic cells in the inner cambial layer of the periosteum. The classic tenant of Wolff's law is obeyed in the sense that it states that the degree of bone proliferation is proportional to the mechanical need for it to occur. The rigidity afforded by compression plates obviates, then, the need to form a stabilizing callus.

As noted previously, compression plating "forces" repair processes to procede in a unique way. The illustration in Figure 10-9 shows that new haversian systems originate by breakout resorption from endosteal channels that contain viable cells. The osteoclasts that are in the vanguard of the "cutting cones" migrate across the fracture gap at a rate of 50 to 80 μm/d.[108] In their wake, osteoblasts begin to generate new circumferential lamellae of haverian bone at a rate of perhaps 2 μm/d in younger individuals and at

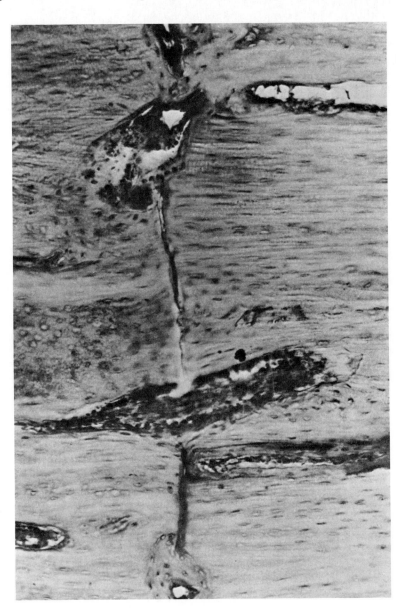

FIGURE 10-9 *Photomicrograph of an osteotomy site in one of the cortices of a canine radius 4 wk after fixation by a four-hole compression plate. On both sides of the cleft, cutter heads with osteoclasts are advancing to conduct additional osteons with new bone across the osteotomy. (Rhinelander, F. W.: In G. H. Bourne (ed.): New York, Academic Press, 1972)*

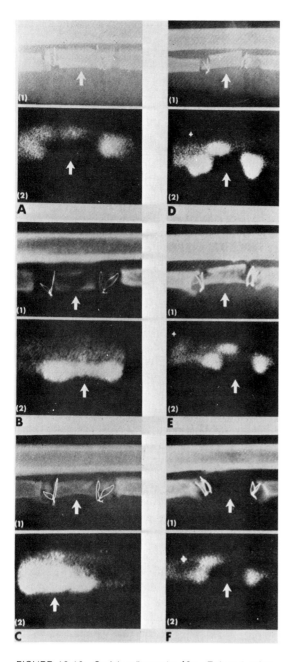

FIGURE 10-10 *Serial radiographs* (**A**1–**F**1) *and scinto-grams* (**A**2–**F**2) *comparing the healing in 2-cm defects in a dog ulna after packing with segments of autogenous* (**A** *to* **C**) *or allogeneic* (**D** *to* **F**) *bone. The scintograms show the failure of allogeneic bone to vascularize* (**E**) *and survive* (**F**) *long before the radiographs show that it has been re-sorbed.* (Stevenson J. S., Bright, R. W., and Dunson, G. L.: Radiology 110:391–394, 1974)

a rate of 0.5 to 1.0 μm/d in older individuals. It has been estimated from animal studies (dogs) that within a single developing haversian system, about 200 new osteoblasts are born from the perivascular osteogenic connective tissues each day. In the laboratory dog, the fracture line is crossed by cutting cones in 2 to 3 wk, and radiologic lucency between the bone fragments disappears in 5 to 8 wk. Of course, if compression is less complete, to the extent that there remains a 1-mm gap, it may take somewhat *less* time to heal the fracture. In this instance, new capillaries and osteogenic cells can migrate into the gap from the healed periosteum and endosteum, and a seal of lamellar bone forms within 2 to 3 wk.

Diagnostic techniques to predict bone repair

Clinical evaluation of fracture repair is based on three methods—radiology, sophisticated photon absorption techniques, and radionuclide imaging. Absorptiometry involves measurements of the attenuation of the emissions of a point source (e.g., [241]Am, ^{131}I) by bone, and therefore it measures bone mass.[87] Radionuclide imaging using [99m]Te or other short-lived isotopes that deliver only a very small dose to the healing tissues are especially useful in distinguishing delayed fracture union from nonunions. The technique is also capable of diagnosing stress fractures prior to radiologic change. The basis of imaging methodologies has recently been reviewed by Mattar and Friedman;[78] the visualization of the isotope depends upon its uptake on mineralized bone surfaces.

When grafting is used as an aid to fracture healing, those grafts that will fail to vascularize and go on to nonunion can be predicted by scanning 3 to 6 wk prior to the time when the situation can be diagnosed by x-ray. The power of the method is shown in Figure 10-10, which shows serial radionuclide imaging of healing in surgically created 2-cm defects in dog ulnae after packing with autogenous or allogeneic bone. Because the defects filled with allogeneic bone failed to vascularize, there was a progressively negative uptake image.[125] The early failure of the graft "to take" was not as obvious by normal x-ray evaluation of the fracture site. Radionuclide imaging will clearly visualize regions of ectopic bone formation as well.[83]

Sonic diagnosis—a three-needle excitation sensory system (electrical) may in the future provide a quantitative measure of the restoration of skeletal integrity following fracture. Preliminary dog and human studies reported by Sonstegard and Matthews[122] at the University of Michigan indicate that the method can differentiate between developing nonunions and the onset of the normal sequence of fracture repair.

Certain clinical problems in fracture repair

Delayed union

Fractures that require longer than the expected time to consolidate are not uncommon, but they can present special clinical problems. Poor healing can occur when a large volume of bone or soft tissue fragments interposes between the broken ends of bone. This problem is "relative," since the fracture site usually contains small fragments of bone, muscle, fascia, nerve, and tendon. Urist[131,132] indicates that most large soft tissue fragments will scar and ossify and be resorbed eventually. There are circumstances in which poor healing will occur without soft tissue interposition. Fractures in individuals with mineralization deficits caused by untreated rickets or osteomalacia are difficult to heal. Patients treated with anticonvulsants may also be difficult to heal because the drugs impair the conversion of vitamin D to its more active polar metabolites such as $1,25(OH)_2VD_3$.[50,73] Steroid therapy also delays fracture repair because these agents reduce both the proliferative potential of the osteoprogenitor cells in marrow and the functional capacities of the osteoblasts. They do not appear to have a consistent effect upon osteoclast numbers or function, although chronic treatment does impair leukopoiesis and therefore the production of monocytes, which are believed to be the precursor cells for osteoclasts.

Nonunion

There is no suitable animal model for the study of nonunions, and so the biologic basis for the problem remains unresolved. Somewhat heroic measures have to be taken to produce nonunions in animals, and these conditions are not always present in the clinical situation. The principle causes of nonunions are infections, but they can arise if the bone fragments are extensively displaced. Edwards[37] reviewed 492 fractures of the tibias and noted that nonunions were relatively common when there was an external wound or when the fractures were treated by open reduction. Ham and Harris[51] and Rhinelander[93] have reviewed the literature on cases of nonunions, and suggest a common etiology—that of damage to the periosteum. When the integrity of the periosteum is disrupted, there is opportunity for scarring fibrous tissue to invade the fracture gap. However, impaired periosteal circulation would interfere with callus formation and place at risk the survival of the intracortical cells with osteogenic potential. If, in addition, the medullary circulation were compromised or the bone was reamed for the insertion of rods, the survival of osteogenic cells in the marrow would also be at risk for a significant period of time after trauma.

We have essentially been talking about an adult problem, since nonunions are rare in children. In the younger patient group, the periosteum is thick and compliant, and better able to regenerate than the thinner periosteum of older adults.

There may be reason to delay open or closed internal fixation procedures in long bone fractures for 1 to 3 wk. Delayed internal fixation is apparently effective in reducing the incidence of nonunions from 30% to less than 1%. Table 10-3 summarizes these clinical findings. In effect, reinjury of the periosteum after it has undergone an initial period of healing causes a marked proliferation of cells in the cambial layer. The resultant callus is generally much larger, and the time to consolidation of the fracture is hastened. The exuberant callus produced as a result of a "second injury" to the periosteum has been duplicated in animal studies, and this emphasizes the importance of this form of healing. Figure 10-11

TABLE 10-3 THE COMPARATIVE EFFICACY OF EARLY AND DELAYED INTERNAL FIXATION OF FRACTURES IN ADULT MAN

		EARLY OPERATED GROUP				LATE OPERATED GROUP				RECOMM. TIME FOR SURGERY AFTER FX. (WEEKS)
AUTHOR	FRACTURE SITE	NO. OF FRACTURES	POST-FX. TIME OF FIXATION	% DELAYED OR NONUNION	TIME TO UNION	NO. OF FXS	POST-FX. TIME OF FIXATION (DAYS)	% DELAYED OR NONUNION	TIME TO UNION	
Smith & Sage (1957)	radius, ulna, radius/ulna	>253	1–6 days	19.7 / 80.0 / —	— / — / —	89 / 16 / 45	50–90 / 91–182 / >182	19.3 / — / —	— / — / —	— / —
Smith (1959)	radius/ulna radius/ulna	78	1–6 days	24.0	24.9% in 12 mo.	52	7	1.0	(100% in 12 mo.)	10–14 days
Emery (1965)	ulna	27 / 14	1–7 days / 1–7 days	53.0 / 44.0	— / —	36 / 22	8–30 / 8–30	11.0 / 9.0	— / —	1–4 / 1–4
Charnley & Guindy (1961)	femur	24	1–6 days	25.0	—	14	7–28	7.14	—	1
Smith (1964)	femur	85	1–6 days	23.0	—	126	7	0.8	—	2–3
Lam (1964)	femur, tibia	64 / 95	1–7 days / 1–7 days	9.4△ / 9.5	20.2 wks / 22.3 wks	66 / 79	14–42* / 14–42*	1.5 / 3.9	14.2 wks / 22 wks	2–4▽ / 2–4
Smith (1974)	tibia	180 / 219	1–6 wks / immediate	30.0 / 48.0	26.0 wks / 33.0 wks	78	7–21*	16.6	20 wks†	2–3

* Average time = 2.5 wks.
† Not later than 6 wks.
‡ Closed Fx = 18 wks; compound Fx = 27 wks.
△ Excluded when fractures
▽ Except for patients >60 yrs.

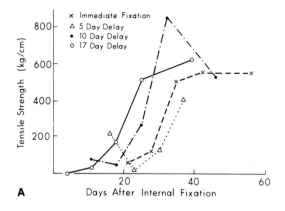

A

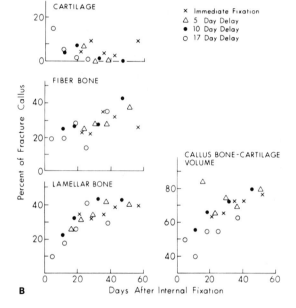

B

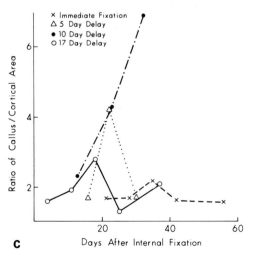

C

shows that in experimental animals, the tensile strength of the callus produced by a delayed operation is maximized early, but the components of the callus are normally distributed. The current recommendations of management of long bone fractures by cast bracing,[105,106] a procedure that also involves some manipulations and probable "movement" of the bone at the fracture line, suggest that a period of delay ensures a favorable result (see Table 10-6).

Origin of cells in fracture callus

We have described the changes in the histotypic characteristics of the fracture callus during healing as a continuum. There is little question that the periosteum contributes cells that, initially at least, modulate to the fibroblasts and chondroblasts of the early procallus and fibrocartilaginous callus. With the maturation of the callus vascular supply and the onset of bone formation, we continue to witness the pluripotency of the cells generated by the periosteum and by the undifferentiated cells of the marrow stroma. This scheme forms only a part of the story, which concerns the natural history of the cells that participate in fracture healing. Some of the original ideas about the cellular kinetics in the callus, for instance, were that (1) the chondrocytes could modulate directly to osteocytes and osteoblasts, (2) that the osteogenic cells were carried to bone from an extraosseous site, and (3) that the histotypic multinucleated osteoclasts were fusions of stem cells, osteoblasts, and/or fibroblasts and

FIGURE 10-11 **(A)** *Healing radial fractures in rabbits stabilized by intramedullary K-wires at various postfracture delay times versus time after initial fixation. Bones pinned 10 d after fracture attained maximum strength earlier than those pinned after 5 or 17 d.* **(B)** *Plots showing that the percentages of cartilage, fiber bone, and lamellar bone in the fracture callus were similar, but the greater strength of the 10-d callus (plots C) was due predominately to its larger size. (Ellsasser, J. C., Moyer, C. F., Losker, P. A., and Simmons, D. J.: J. Trauma 15:869–876, 1975).* **(C)** *Plots showing that the strength of callus which formed after fixation at different postfracture delay times was related to the size of the callus mass.*

that they could subsequently disaggregate to form osteoblasts. The over-riding concept was that both osteoblasts and osteoclasts were physiologic expressions of the same undifferentiated stem cells, and that in marrow, these stem cells were called reticular cells.

This view of the "world of bone cells" was based purely on our best interpretations of the size and shape of the cells as viewed in histologic sections. There were definitive cell types and cell types that seemed to form morphological intermediate types. Like anthropologists of old, bone physiologists searched for "missing links" in the line of morphological cell species. Our "type species," if we can so term it, were the apparent cellular transitions that took place in the medullary cavities of birds during the egg laying cycle, and in the long bones of mice treated with estrogen. For instance, in the laying hen[11] and pigeon[12] the preovulatory phase of the egg laying cycle was characterized by bone formation, and ultimately the marrow cavity filled up with trabecular bone. We saw a gradient of cell types in marrow around the bone surfaces; cells called preosteoblasts seemed to be differentiating into osteoblasts. After ovulation and at the time when the egg had reached the shell gland (and mineral was required to form the shell), we saw that much of the marrow bone was resorbed. The cell population in the marrow cavities then became markedly osteoclastic, and it was natural to believe that the mechanism involved fusions of osteoblasts and other fibroblastic cells in the vicinities of the bone trabeculae. Thus, the bird became the classic example for bone researchers interested in this problem of cell kinetics. As a matter of fact, this view of bone cell kinetics survived the initial years when, after 1962, more specific ways were found to "tag" the DNA of bone progenitor cells with radioactive nuclear markers such as ^{3}HTdr.[89,128,155,156] With high resolution autoradiographic techniques, we were able to follow the various ways in which bone cells could differentiate.

Animals systemically injected with ^{3}HTdr showed that the tracer was initially and permanently taken up by cells we once identified as preosteoblasts. Several hours later, we witnessed that these "tagged" preosteoblasts had

formed osteoblasts. Within 24 hr, some but not all of the tagged osteoblasts had formed sufficient bone around themselves (about one seventh) and had become osteocytes. There were other labeled cells in the marrow and on bone surfaces as well. Then, after 48 to 72 hr, we began to find the nuclear label in osteoclast nuclei. To make matters even more complex, and interesting, Young[155,156] at U.C.L.A. reported that with time, there was a continual gain and loss of nuclei within osteoclasts. Jaworski (personal communication) has since visualized this process in the osteoclasts that are responsible for tunneling through bone to form new Haversian systems. Young believed that there could be no reason why the nuclei lost to osteoclasts could not be "recycled" to form new osteoblasts. All that would be needed was for these nuclei to dedifferentiate to precursor cells and then to definitive osteoblasts. Subsequent research described a similar sequence of cell transformations in the origin of the cells that participated in fracture healing.[63,133]

There was only one problem with this scheme—the fact that in most studies, the tracer was administered *systemically*. Bone cell physiologists suffered from a rather myopic view of bone as a "closed cell system." It presumed that the cells labeled with ^{3}HTdr were bone-bound—that no cells left bone and, importantly, that no potential bone precursor cells ever entered bone from extraosseous sites. Several very imaginitive animal models have been developed within the last decade to test this proposition. They have revealed that osteoblasts and osteoclasts are derived from separate cell populations. Most of these new methodologies have involved a tissue regeneration model that is pertinent to fracture healing. Let us first consider the osteoclast.

Origin of osteoclasts

At Harvard, Fishman and Hayes[40] studied the origin and fate of bone cells in the regenerating amphibian limb. They injected ^{3}HTdr and waited until the only labeled cells in the circulation were monocytes and macrophages. Then they amputated a limb and sampled the site of regeneration at various times thereafter. During healing, they reported that some of the osteoclasts on bone surfaces had radioactively labeled nuclei. This was the first evidence that osteoclasts might be derived from cells in the circulation. This evidence was made more compelling when Gothlin and Ericsson[49] in Stockholm studied fracture healing in parabiosed pairs of rats and reported similar phenomena. In their model, the two animals share a common circulation by way of a skin flap. One of the animals was x-irradiated to kill its marrow and was subsequently fractured. The other animal was injected with ^{3}HTdr after the circulation between the rats was clamped off. When the circulation between the rats was restored and the fracture callus was biopsied, the only radioactively labeled nuclei in the blood were monocytes and macrophages, and the only radioactively labeled nuclei in the callus were in osteoclasts.

The migratory nature of the osteoclast precursor cell has since been affirmed in an experimental situation that involves the creation of chimeric bone rudiments in avian embryos that contain cells of both Japanese quail and domestic chickens. In our laboratory, Dr. Arnold Kahn and I[60] grafted embryonic quail limb bone rudiments onto the chorioallantoic membrane (CAM) of the developing chick. Subsequent to revascularization, the quail explants continued to grow and ossify. The species origin of the cells in these rudiments can be determined, since the interphase nuclei of quail cells typically contain one or more Feulgen-positive nucleoli, and the heterochromatin of chick nuclei is diffusely distributed (Fig. 10-12). Histologic analysis of the intact chimeric rudiments indicated that the osteoblasts and osteocytes were derived from progenitor cells originating *within* the graft; they contained the quail nucleolar marker. In contrast, most of the osteoclasts contained chick-like nuclei and must therefore have been derived from the host's circulation. These same results were achieved when embryonic quail rudiments were carefully fractured after they had revascularized on the chick egg CAM.[115]

Studies in animals with inherited disorders of osteoclast function have also contributed to this story. At Johns Hopkins University, Walker[144] was able to cure osteopetrotic mice by irradiating them and infusing spleen cells and/or bone marrow cells from normal litter mates. The excess bone was completely resorbed. The disease could be re-established in "cured" mice if the infused cells were derived from another mutant mouse. A cure was also achieved by parabiosing the osteopetrotic and normal litter mates. The same sequence of events was noted in osteopetrotic strains of rats.[77] The clinical relevance of these experimental animal models has been most powerfully demonstrates by Ballet and Griscelli in Paris[4] and by Coccia[28] at the University of Minnesota. Coccia confronted the problem of treating an infant girl with congenital osteopetrosis by transplanting marrow from a normal male sibling. Radiologic investigations have shown not only that the excessive bone was resorbed but also that the attendant visual and auditory deficits (through bone impaction on nerves) common to this disease improved. Histologically, serial iliac crest biopsies showed a progressive normalization of the peritrabecular bone. The important finding was that the nuclei in the patient's osteoclasts carried the male heterochromatin (sex chromatin) marker, and this patient is, in effect, a human chimera.

We do not know the precise nature of the osteoclast stem cell, although we are reasonably certain that it is a monocyte or a mononuclear phagocyte. This opinion is not based solely upon the results of the parabiotic studies described. It is an obvious conclusion from studies that follow the fate of human monocytes or murine peritoneal macrophages after they are placed into culture with radiocalcium-labeled bone chips.[62,84,85,127] The cells are seen to aggregate as multinucleated entities around the bone particles, and some of the radioactive label is released into the culture medium. Microcinematography shows that the cells are actively resorbing the bone (Fig. 10-13). Electron microscopy indicates, however, that the multinucleated cells do not appear exactly like osteoclasts; they have a rich supply of lysosomal bodies that are known to contain degradative acid hydrolases, but they lack the definitive ruffled membranes and clear

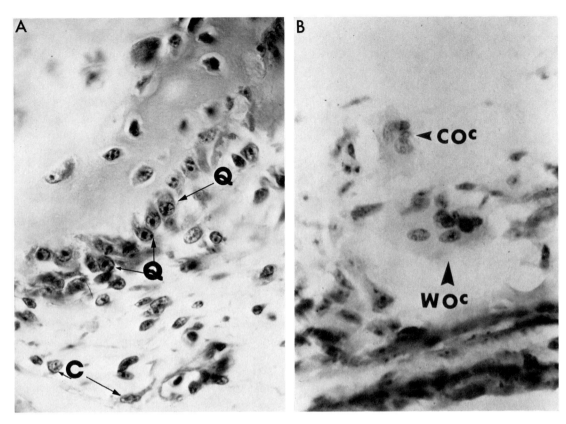

FIGURE 10-12 *Photomicrographs of developing bone from an embryonic quail limb bone grafted to the chorioallantoic membrane of a chick embryo. (A) A trabeculum of bone, showing surface osteoblasts with quail-type nuclei (Q). Other cells have nuclei with diffuse chromatin distribution typical of host chick cells (C). (B) Two osteoclasts in the graft. The nuclei of osteoclast COc are all of the host chick type, indicating a source from an extraosseous site. The nuclei of osteoclast WOc are mostly derived from the host chick circulation, but one nucleus (arrowhead) contains a quail-like nucleus. (Kahn, A. J., and Simmons, D. J.: Nature 258:325–327, 1975)*

zones typical of osteoclasts (see Chapter 2). Either we are trapped by our definitions of what certain cells ought to look like—differences that are not really physiologically meaningful—or the full differentiation of osteoclasts in this experimental system requires local factors that can only be supplied in the osseous environment *in vivo*. The *in vitro* culture systems do not, for instance, supply plasma components such as osteoclast activating factor (OAF)—a lymphokine in buffy coat cells that accelerates bone resorption *in vivo*.[56,66,74] Certain *in vitro* studies indicate that local factors in the bone environment must be important for the expression of resorption. For instance, peritoneal macrophages do not resorb [45]Ca-labeled bone particles from uremic animals in which the collagen is abnor-

mally cross-linked as readily as they resorb [45]Ca-labeled bone from normal animals.[75]

Origin of osteoblasts-osteocytes

With respect to the origin of osteoblasts and osteocytes, the quail-chick chimeric system has provided good evidence that they can be derived from chondrocytes as well as from the marrow stromal reticular cells.[61] Figure 10-14 shows that when periochondrial free pieces of quail cartilage are grafted to the CAM of the chick, some chondrocytes are liberated from their lacunae and these chondrocytes form an osteogenic tissue that resembles a periosteum. All of these cells and the osteoblasts that are laying down periosteal bone have the dense nucleolar chroma-

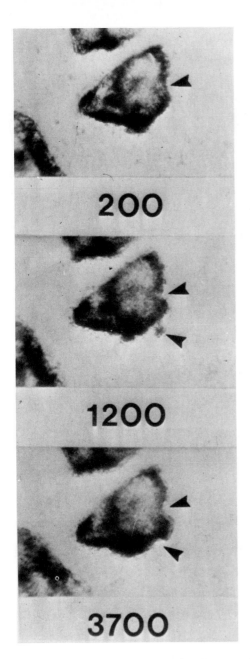

FIGURE 10-13 *Three frames from a time lapse motion picture showing the removal of matrix (arrowheads) from a particle of human adult bone by human monocytes in vitro. The cells are not seen in these reproductions. The time interval between frames 200 and 1200 was 33.3 h and that between frames 1200 and 3700 was 83.3 h. The cell concentration was 1 × 10⁵. (Kahn, A. J., Stewart, C. C., Teitebaum, S. L.: Science 199:988–990, 1978)*

tin marker typical of the donor quail cells. Other chondrocytes begin to form thick collagen fibers within their lacunae, and these fibers look like typical bone collagen. It is easy to see that there are obvious differences between the collagen in cartilage and bone. The cartilage collagen fibers are thin and irregularly dispersed in the intercellular matrix. The collagen fibers we think are bone-like[141,142] are much more massive and better oriented.

The osteogenic role of marrow

"Leads" to the conclusion that certain cells in marrow are capable of differentiating to osteoblasts are provided by several clinical and experimental observations. First, fractures of bone in the area of red marrow form consolidating bony trabeculae more rapidly than do fractures in areas of yellow fatty marrow. Second, new bone is formed when red marrow is grafted to an immunologically privileged site such as the anterior chamber of the eye. To reiterate a portion of our earlier discussion on the origin of intramedullary bone in avian species, it was early believed that marrow reticular cells were the osteogenic precursor cells. Nothing has shaken that conclusion, since surgeons have always favored the use of autologous bone marrow grafts to fill large osseous defects. Corroborating evidence has been gathered for over 40 yr. The more modern evidence about the osteogenic power of marrow cell populations begins with the experiments on composite bone grafts by Burwell and his collaborators in England.[24,25]

Autogenous cancellous bone grafting may be an important adjunct to the initial treatment of fractures when care is immediate. It can also be performed effectively 4 to 6 wk after injury if fractures are to be treated by open procedures after the danger of infection has passed. The experiences of Whiteside and colleagues[147] confirm the very extensive studies of Barth and Phemister (cited by Lance[70]), which showed that autogenous grafts do not serve a useful function if their purpose is to speed the pace of bone repair.

Burwell's[24,25] classic experiments (in rabbits) indicated that the osteogenic potential of bone bank material (allogeneic or xenogeneic grafts)

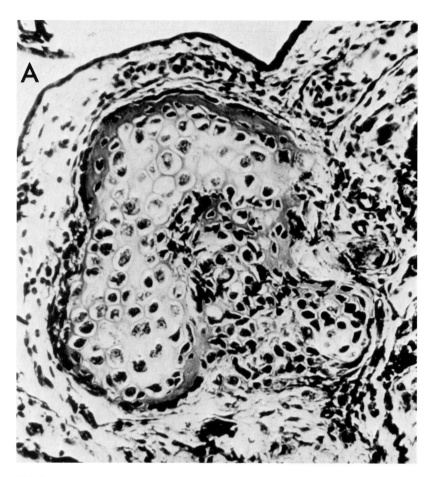

FIGURE 10-14 **(A)** *Photomicrograph of a quail embryonic cartilage grafted to the chorioallantoic membrane of an embryonic chick. The cells in the periosteum and bone were derived from the graft not from the host chick tissues (see Fig. 12A). (Kahn, A. J., and Simmons, D. J.: Nature 258:325–327, 1975)* **(B)** *An electron micrograph of a chondrocyte in a perichondrium-free graft of quail cartilage to the chorioallantoic membrane of the chick embryo. The chondrocyte is forming thick, banded bone-like collagen fibers in the lacunar space. Note the thinner and irregularly distributed collagen fibers in the original cartilage matrix.*

can be maximized if the bone is first impregnated with autologous marrow (Fig. 10-15). Such composite "alloautografts" are effective in producing bone in paravertebral muscle even though this site has competent mesenchymal cells that can be "induced" to become osteogenic elements.[134] Burwell suggested however, that it was the autologous undifferentiated reticuloendothelial cells in the marrow that were induced to form new bone—not the muscle elements. When the bony portion of the graft was impregnated with dead marrow cells, no new bone

was produced. Our own observations support this contention. When new bone formed around composite grafts in host rabbits that were prelabeled with [3]HTdr to "mark" the potential stem cells of the connective tissue, none of the new osteoblasts and osteocytes in the graft became labeled.[112] When the bone was impregnated with marrow cells from syngeneic rabbits that had been prelabeled with [3]HTdr, the newly formed osteoblasts and osteocytes did carry the nuclear marker. Related studies by Morris[81] and Cummine and Nade[30] have since shown that demin-

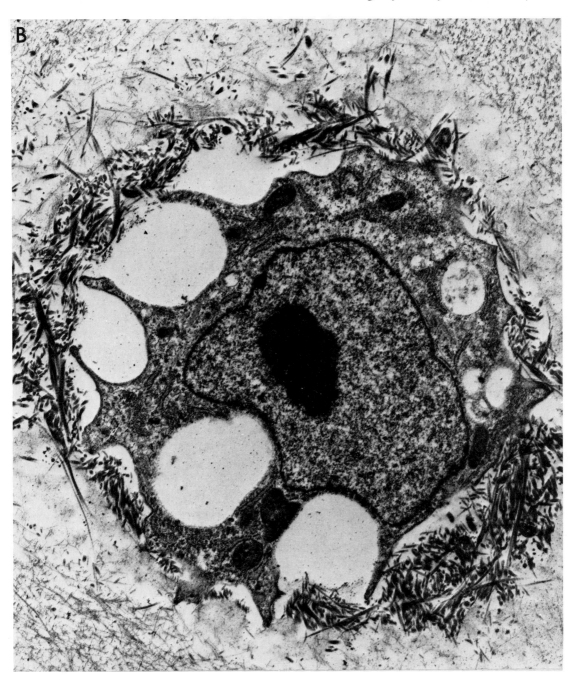

eralized grafts of allogeneic dentine and bone implanted in the subcutaneous tissues of rats and guinea pigs, respectively, had little or no osteogenic capacity unless they were packed with autologous marrow cells.

Optimizing the success of the composite graft appears to involve having the proper ratio of marrow cells : bone. Our studies in rabbits indicate that composite grafts, *equivalent in potency to autografts,* can be produced using as few as 2000

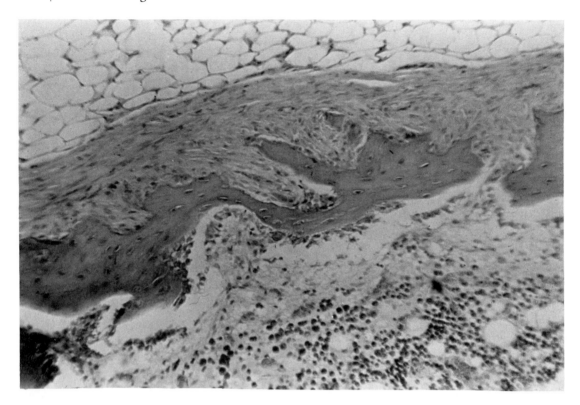

FIGURE 10-15 *Photomicrograph of an ossicle of bone formed from a composite graft of allogeneic bone and autologous marrow implanted in the rectus muscle of rabbits. The graft was harvested after 5 wk.*

autologous marrow cells/mg bone. Furthermore, such cells retained their osteogenic potential even after they were grown in tissue culture for 4 d prior to use. Interestingly, composite grafts with initially suboptimal numbers of autologous marrow cells could be made fully effective if the host rabbits were treated postoperatively with multiple injections of the lectin phytohemagglutinin (PHA). PHA's functions include an immunologic component and a mitogenic component.

The results of these experiments demonstrate the clinical potential of composite grafts. Autologous marrow cells could even be obtained by sternal or trochanteric biopsy and, if necessary, grown in tissue culture with PHA until sufficient numbers have been produced for grafting. We have cited all of these studies, however, simply as a prelude to describing the actual clinical application of the methodology. Salama and Weissman[102,103] have effectively treated 28 patients, some of whom were casualties of the 1973 Arab-Israeli conflict (Yom Kippur War), with composite grafts. In the majority of cases, the bony portion was sterilized deproteinized ox bone (Kiel bone), but cancellous autogenous bone was used adjunctively in a few operations. They reported good results after excision of benign bone lesions for athrodeses, pseudarthroses, and traumatic bone defects. They state: "Preliminary immunological studies of our patients, including agglutination, complement fixation, lymphocytotoxicity tests and hematologic studies suggested that Kiel bone is very weakly antigenic in the human host, if at all. It is therefore not very surprising that such satisfactory results have been obtained."

We can conclude our discussion about the osteogenic capabilities of some cells in marrow by alluding to the valuable insights of Friedenstein and his collaborators.[44,45] By use of *in vitro* culture methods, these workers have shown that bone marrow contains a resident population of cells with both clonogenic (i.e., stem cells) and osteogenic potential. Some of these cells are capable of giving rise to progeny that can become osteoblastic without any inductive substances, and they are called determined osteogenic–precursor cells (DOPC). Other marrow cells also appear to become osteogenic, but require an inducer (e.g., urinary bladder epithelium or decalcified bone matrix) to express this potential. These cells are called inducible osteogenic precursor cells (IOPC). Osteogenic precursor cells thus occur as a fixed fraction of the marrow population, and as might be expected, the size of the population seems to decline with age. They are also relatively sensitive to insults such as ionizing radiation.

While DOPCs have been observed only in bone marrow, IOPCs have been reported in spleen, thymus, peripheral blood, and peritoneal fluid. The blood vascular IOPCs are strong candidates for a role in heterotopic bone formation. Danis[31] and Urist[134] have also detected IOPC-like components of the mesenchyme in tendon, dermis, subcutaneous tissue, and muscle, and these cells are virtually as responsive to an osteoinductive stimulus as are bone marrow cells. All of these experiences are likely to be widely applied to orthopedics in the future when certain "conditions" of the graft *per se* and the transplant bed are inherently unfavorable. As noted previously, the host bed or graft has to contain cells capable of sustaining an osteogenic response. Host-cell-deficient states may occur in aging, in some kinds of infection, following irradiation, or in the presence of abundant scar tissue produced by surgery. Composite grafts contain the ingredients essential for surgical success in the sense that they provide their own complement of osteogenic precursor cells.

One further remark about marrow cells and their competency to produce new bone is warranted at this time. Everything we have said to this point indicates that marrow-bone graft success probably depends more upon the complement of marrow cells than the influence of the bone and whatever osteoinductive effects it might have (see Chapter 11). We say this because composite grafts fashioned from classically potent osteoinductive substrates such as surface-demineralized bone or freeze-dried bone do not

[in our hands] express an unusually powerful osteogenic response (in an intramuscular site in rabbits) (Table 10-4). If this is so, there might be some advantage to procuring marrow samples from patients (scheduled for grafting) at a "time of day" when their proliferative potential is maximal. From the work of Mauer,[79] we know that the population of human bone marrow reticulocytes exhibits a mitotic peak in the early evening—at a time when there are other signs of peak production and turnover of connective tissues such as collagen (urinary hydroxyproline)[92] and glycosaminoglycans.[109] There is some experimental evidence that suggests, further, that there may be a "best time" for grafting, but this type of investigation has only been carried out in rats.[113,114] We produced standardized midshaft fibular defects in rats at different times of day, and these defects were immediately overlayed with autograft bone *or* fresh, demineralized or freeze-dried allogeneic bone. Clinical and histologic healing was evaluated 3 wk later. The grafts performed at night were more firmly united than those performed during the day (Fig. 10-16). These data were, not surprisingly, consonant with a suite of diurnal metabolic profiles of cortical bone growth in rats.[116a] Tetracycline labeling studies[100] have detected significantly greater cortical appositional bone growth rates at night in rats, both at the periosteum and the endosteum (Fig. 10-17). The rate of endosteal growth is, of course, dependent in part upon the rate at which osteogenic precursor cells are supplied from the marrow.

It is now clear that marrow cells with osteogenic potential are not the fixed elements of marrow—they are stem cells distinct from the stem cells that give rise to the granulocytes and the erythroid series. When red bone marrow of femurs and tibias of laboratory animals is ablated by either flushing (saline) or irradiation, it is the endosteal cells in the vascular channels that migrate into the empty marrow cavity and begin to lay down masses of trabecular bone.[90] It is data of this type that contributes to our understanding of the basic biologic mechanisms of how fractures heal following modern compression plating techniques (see subsequent discussion).

The potential applications of composite grafts

TABLE 10-4 PERCENT BONE GRAFT SURFACES COVERED WITH NEWLY INDUCED BONE (5 WK)

GRAFT CLASS	GRAFT TYPE	NO. OF MARROW CELLS/MG BONE	RECONSTITUTED*		
			BONE-MARROW GRAFT	INTACT BONE-MARROW GRAFT	WASHED BONE GRAFT†
Autologous Bone + autologous marrow	Fresh bone	500	40.0 ± 12.7 (3)	71.3 ± 2.8 (36)	61.3 ± 5.9 (6)
		1000	64.7 ± 16.7 (4)		
		2000	81.9 ± 9.1 (7)		
Allogeneic bone ± allogeneic marrow	Fresh bone		0 (11)	0 (11)	0 (24)
	Decalcified bone				0 (3)
	Decalcified ± IAA bone‡				0 (3)
	Freeze-dried bone				0 (7)
Composite Grafts: Allogeneic bone + Autologous Marrow	Fresh bone	1000	39.5 ± 9.9 (6)		
	Decalcified bone	1000	76.9 ± 17.5 (3)		
	Freeze-dried bone	1000	40.8 ± 18.5 (4)		
	Fresh bone	2200	67.5 ± 4.8 (21)		
	Fresh bone + dead marrow cells	2500	2.9 ± 1.9 (11)		
		Ratio of autologous marrow to allogeneic spleen cells (%)			
Composite Grafts: Allogeneic bone + Autologous marrow + Allogeneic spleen	Fresh Bone	100M/0S	81.9 ± 9.1 (7)		
		50M/50S	29.5 ± 3.7 (6)		
		37M/66S	38.7 ± 4.8 (21)		
		0M/100S	5.1 ± 3.8 (11)		

* Grafts in which the marrow is flushed out and then replaced.
† Grafts in which the marrow is flushed out and is not replaced.
‡ Bone incubated in iodoacetic acid.

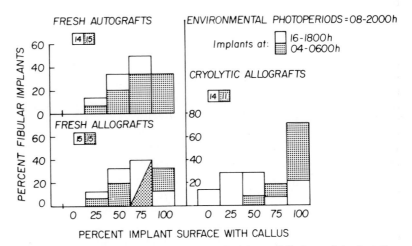

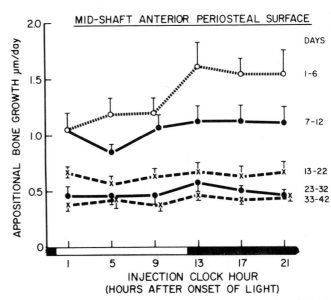

FIGURE 10-16 *Relationship between the clock hour of fibular graft implantation and callus formation in rats 4 wk postoperatively. The grafts of various matrices into fibular defects were better healed when the operations were performed at night (0400–0600 h) rather than during the day (1600–1800 h). (Simmons, D. J., Bratberg, J. J., Lesker, P. A., and Aab, L.: Clin. Orthop. 116:227–239, 1976)*

FIGURE 10-17 *Appositional bone formation rates on the midshaft anterior periosteal surface of femurs from rats weighing 250 g at different times in a 24-h day.* **DAYS,** *at the right of the figure, represents the segments of time when bone formation rates were estimated by administering tetracycline time markers. Each point in the charts represents a different group of 15 rats that always received saline and/or tetracycline injections at either 1, 5, 9, 13, or 17 h after the onset of the environmental photoperiod. The daytime groups received injections at 1, 5, and 9 h; nighttime groups received injections at 13, 17, and 21 h. Note that the younger rats displayed the most pronounced growth rhythms and that here, bone formation rates were highest at night. The loss of rhythmicity in "older" rats from the 13th to the 42nd d of the study might have been due to age per se or to disturbance of the animals by the daily injection schedule.*

309

for orthopedics are many. Children, for instance, may have insufficient bone to "donate" in the event they suffer a substantial loss of skeletal mass. Similarly, adult patients requiring repeated grafts for chronic nonunions may ultimately have too little suitable bone from which to fashion additional grafts. In older individuals, there is the further problem that the osteogenic potential of the cambial layer of the periosteum may have become so diminished that inclusion of this tissue might not be expected to produce a favorable outcome when defects must be filled to achieve a functional result. Finally, in patients with bone tumors that have been treated both surgically and with large doses of ionizing radiation, the lesion site is usually rendered fibrotic and necrotic. The prognosis of treating such lesions is poor, even with the best autogenous grafts currently available.

There are few alternatives to the autograft and composite graft. Allografts and xenografts have proved to be poor substitutes for autogenous tissue. There is the obvious problem of potential graft rejection resulting from their antigenicity, however weak. Despite the fact that allogeneic bone grafts may survive for extended periods of time and initially, at least, support some new bone formation, the osteogenic response is usually not of long duration. Various measures have been taken to extend the survival periods for allografts, but techniques such as immunosuppression of the recipient by steroids or by agents such as mercaptopurine may compromise the overall health of the patient and diminish the osteogenic capacity of the cells at the graft site. Alternatively, graft antigenicity can be reduced by chemically and physically modifying the matrix, and there is a large amount of literature about these effects. Allogeneic and xenogeneic bone grafts have been boiled, frozen, freeze-dried, sterilized by x-rays, or deproteinized in attempts to rid them of their antigenicity—all with less than satisfactory results. Lance[70] and Burchardt and Enneking[22] have reviewed these studies comprehensively. It is now realized that bone matrix contains an as-yet-undefined "principle" that is osteoinductive, but this is so labile that it is destroyed by all the measures that have been used heretofore to prepare a biocompatible graft.

Total body response to injury

Blood changes

When sustained, a fracture elicits a stress response due to hemorrhage and traumatic shock. This is a generalized stimulus in the sense that there are fairly immediate changes in the concentrations of protein fractions, hormones, and enzymes in blood. Rokkanen[98] used the pig, which has a mineral metabolism picture much like that of humans. He reported that fracture induces a short-term (3–6 h) metabolic acidosis and increased lactate concentrations in blood, changes that may be due to impaired tissue perfusion. Serum phospholipids, triglycerides, and cholesterol levels remained within normal limits. Arterial pressure falls, causing an associated decline in bone marrow pressure. These changes precede the onset of the skeletal responses, but may persist long enough so that there is some overlap. However, much laboratory energy has been expended to find correlates that could be used to predict the progress of fracture healing.

Hertzberg[54] followed the changes in blood protein in 143 patients with tibial fracture. In over 50% of cases, their serum glycoproteins were within normal limits. However, they did detect an increase in the α_1 and α_2 globulins in another 50% of this population from days 2 to 10 after trauma. On the average, the changes occurred within the first 4 d, and normalized by 30 d. The α_2 globulins may act to detoxify products (kallikreins, leukotaxine, bradykinin) that are released from the injured tissues and wound debris into the fracture site, and they may be chemotactic for the monocytic precursors of osteoclasts.

The blood protein patterns are doubtless related to the general increase in circulating corticosteroids and the subsequent impairment of growth hormone levels. There are usually no post-traumatic changes in plasma and serum alkaline phosphatase, calcium, and phosphorus levels comparable to those that occur in bone—

except, perhaps, in geriatric patients who have values of 30 King-Armstrong units alkaline phosphatase after experiencing fractures of the femoral neck. Even patients immobilized in plaster casts fail to show untoward changes in serum alkaline phosphatase levels. It is of some interest, in this regard, that laboratory animals such as rats do show some elevated titers of enzyme following fracture, but here as well, most of the enzyme is of intestinal origin and not from bone. Thus, the serum alkaline phosphatase values do not reflect the stages of healing in callus tissue. They can, of course, be somewhat lower than normal in certain disease states of collagen or mineral metabolism (e.g., rickets, osteomalacia, lathyrism, corticosteroid or anticonvulsant therapy), but no evidence exists that these populations show elevated alkaline phosphatase values after fracture. One also recalls that the serum titers of alkaline phosphatase are normal in individuals with certain inherited disorders such as hypophosphatemia and osteogenesis imperfecta, in which fractures are common.

In terms of a local reaction in bone, some species such as the rat do show a transient but marked osteoclasia within 3 hr after bleeding or femoral fracture.[59] This is accompanied by a fall in the serum albumin level in the face of increasing blood calcium values, indicating a shift toward higher ionized calcium levels resulting from hypersecretion of parathyroid hormone (PTH). These responses are probably peculiar to the rat, since patient populations generally fail to develop post-traumatic hypercalcemia unless at bedrest.[99]

Postfracture linear bone growth

The anoxia at the site of fracture that occurs immediately after trauma due to the disruption of the local blood supply does not fully describe the consequences of trauma on the blood vascular supply of bone. It is here that we see that the sequelae of injury are not simply confined to the area of trauma. Shortly after trauma, the entire skeleton becomes hyperemic,[21,87,152] and there are bursts of periosteal proliferative activity even in the intact bones.[128] It has also been shown that the vascular supply of long bones is shunted away from the fracture site toward its epiphyseal growth cartilages. This oxygen-enriching event has been associated with stimulated linear bone growth, particularly in the injured element.[23,29,33,124,129,151] The length differential between a broken bone and the intact contralateral member at the end of healing may be as much as 2 cm in growing children less than 10 to 12 yr of age. Surgeons may attempt to compensate for this expected overgrowth by stabilizing a fracture with the bone ends overlapping, rather than setting them end to end. However, it is perhaps significant that postfracture linear bone growth does not always occur. These exceptions can signal the influence of an as-yet-undefined interface between the metabolic state of bone and cartilage cells and some systemic factor present at the time of injury.

Studies from our laboratory[114] suggest that the degree of postfracture growth in rats is dependent, at least in part, upon the relative level of growth hormone in the circulation at the time of injury (Fig. 10-18). Bone growth and metaphyseal bone alkaline phosphatase values were stimulated only when the time of fracture coincided with the phase in the body rhythm when pituitary growth hormone concentrations peaked (midday). The differential growth response was not present in hypophysectomized rats. We do not know if there is such an association clinically, since the times of injury are never reported in the literature. But the rat data suggest that the propensity for overgrowth of limb length will be greatest if trauma occurs at night when human plasma growth hormone levels are at their highest.

Biochemistry of fracture healing

Normal healing

The sequential development of different tissue types during the healing of a fracture means that the biochemical characterization of the callus is complex. We can predict certain obvious events. The process of callus formation and maturation

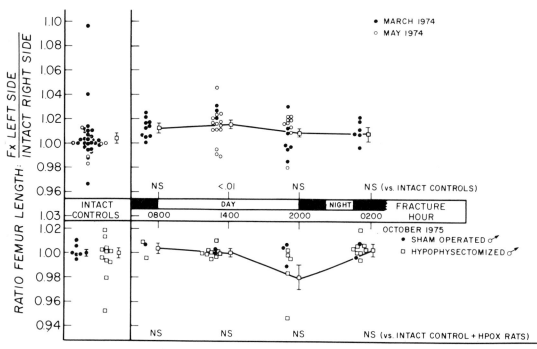

FIGURE 10-18 *Plots showing the relationship between the clock hour of tibial fracture and linear bone growth of femurs 1 mo after trauma in intact and hypophysectomized rats. The P values compare the ratios of femur length (fractured-controls) in the traumatized rats versus the ratios of bone lengths in intact control rats. Note that significant differences in intact rats were observed only after fracture at mid-day (1400 h), and hypophysectomy abolished this differential response to trauma.*

calls into play elements that resemble the mechanism of endochondral ossification in the epiphyseal plates of the long bones during the growth years. The glycosaminoglycan-rich ground substance and collagen framework of the cartilaginous components will be expected to form first, but its intensity will wane as the callus becomes better ossified and calcified. Bone normally has a lower concentration of glycosaminoglycan and a richer supply of collagen than cartilage. Moreover, cartilage and bone have distinctly different collagen types.[91] The collagen of cartilage consists of three identical α_1 chains of amino acids, and its notation is type II—that is, $(\alpha_1[II])_3$. The collagen of bone consists of 2 identical α_1 chains and one α_2 chain, having the shorthand notation $(\alpha_1[I])_2\alpha_2$. The fibrous tissue component of the intermediate fibrocartilaginous callus consists of both type I and type III collagens. These shifts in the appearance of the different collagens have been identified in the avian embryonic epiphyseal cartilage by immunofluorescence tech-

niques.[141,142] Thus, type I bone collagen is formed by maturing chondrocytes in the zone of provisional calcification prior to the time when most of the cartilage matrix will be partly resorbed. The unresorbed calcified matrix is destined to form the cores of the early bony trabeculae that develop in the callus, thus preserving the tissue "mix" until the callus is totally converted to bone.

Because the different tissue types have vastly different biochemical characteristics, it has been possible to time the stages of callus formation with good accuracy. Radioactively labeled precursors such as ^{35}S-sulfate have been used to quantitate the formation of the sulfated glycosaminoglycans of the early cartilaginous callus. Tritiated or ^{14}C-labeled glycine or proline are markers for collagen formation, since glycine forms every third residue, and proline content is about 12% by weight of collagen. Proline is also converted by prolyl hydroxylase (within osteoblasts) to form hydroxyproline. The incorporation of alkaline earth elements such as isotopes of strontium (^{85}Sr) or calcium (^{45}Ca or ^{47}Ca) following pulse injections have been used as markers for mineralization. Typically, the processes by which callus forms have been visualized in tissue sections by autoradiography following radiotracer injection, or they have been quantitated (specific activity measurements) by scintillation counting of chemically extracted labeled matrical components. Alternatively, the rate of incorporation and duration of retention of ^{85}Sr and ^{45}Ca in the calcifying new bone have been quantitated by external counting above the fracture site. The latter was a relatively common clinical technique to evaluate the pace of fracture healing in humans during the middle 1950s and 1960s. Wendenberg[146] injected ^{85}Sr intravenously in patients with tibial fractures and followed the retention of the isotope by external counting above the fracture site. There was an initial peak in retention (i.e., new mineralization) shortly after administration, but the count rate in the fractured bone was still higher than that in the uninjured areas as long as 6 to 9 yr after fracture. This showed that the reorganization of the bone tissue occurred long after healing was clinically and radiologically complete.

Laboratory investigations in small animals have been the only means to establish the general sequence of tissue development in and around fractures. The radiologic series of a healing fibular fracture in rats shown in Figure 10-19 is rather typical for most models. Babicky and Kolar[3] describe a similar sequence in the rat femur as follows: During the early period of post-traumatic hyperemia, there is an initial increase in the content of (sulfated) proteoglycans such as hexosamine and uronic acid. The volume and ash weight of callus increases during the first 2 to 3 wk, and ^{45}Ca accretion maximizes from the 10th to 16th d. Union is radiologically complete at the end of this time. From 20 to 60 d, the callus volume and ash weights decrease about 50% and 20%, respectively, whereas the rate of ^{45}Ca uptake decreases about 65% (following pulse injections). Radiocalcium uptake will not, of course, be expected to exceed the amount normally incorporated at newly mineralizing sites in uninjured bone after tissue repair has been completed.

Immobilization

The effects of immobilization (by roding) on the biochemistry of the healing fractured tibiae of rats were tested by Lane[71] and Li[72] at the Hospi-

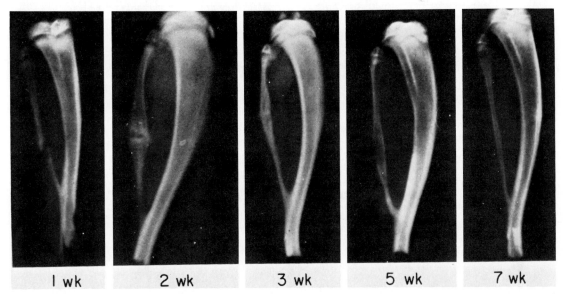

FIGURE 10-19 *Radiographs showing healing of standardized midshaft fibular fractures in rats. The callus size is maximum at 2 wk, and the lucency of the fracture line disappears at 3 wk. Note that repair is generally complete at 7 wk.*

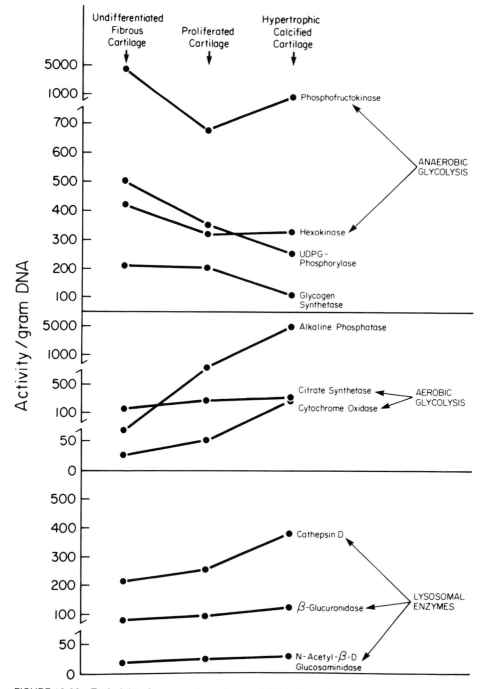

FIGURE 10-20   *Typical data from a study on fractured tibial of rats. (Ketenjian, A. Y., and Arsenis, C.: Clin. Orthop. 107:266–273, 1975)*

tal for Special Surgery in New York. Compared with the femur, the maximum callus size in mobilized tibias was achieved at 4 wk, somewhat later than the femur. The fracture line itself looses its radiolucency by 7 wk. In this model, the firmly fixed and immobilized limbs developed a very sparse external callus with negligible amounts of cartilage. Moreover, the bone healed by direct membranous bone formation. These differences were reflected biochemically by the early, more active synthesis of proteoglycan (hexosamine) and collagen (hydroxyproline and hydroxylysine) in the mobilized limb callus. What is important is that the rate of healing was roughly equal in the mobilized and immobilized bones even though the mechanism was different. And, after this occurred, there were no biochemical differences between them with respect to the soft tissue components. Nevertheless, the formation of mineralized tissue in the immobilized callus was somewhat slower.

The matrix constituents of experimentally produced fibrous nonunions can be expected to vary significantly from the normal situation during repair. Moreover, the biochemical profiles will depend upon whether the nonunion site is sampled from the middle of the lesion or from areas closest to the broken ends of the bone. Typical data from a fractured rat study are shown in Figure 10-20. Here, we compare the pattern of healing in an immobilized tibia versus that in a nonunion maintained by inserting an Ω-shaped pin into the marrow cavities exposed at the time of fracture. As noted previously, the immobilized bone healed by intramembranous bone formation without forming substantial callus. In the case of the distracted tibia with the nonunion, an early gradient of proteoglycan and collagen (types I and II) concentration was established. A small callus formed at the fracture edge; it was even less extensive than that which formed in the immobilized limb, and it never mineralized. Throughout the study, the center of the nonunion showed collagen formation only. As evidenced by the presence of a disproportionately high proteoglycan content and the mixed collagen types, the tissue formed in the nonunion had never matured beyond the mesenchymal cartilaginous stage.

There is every reason to consider that the rat nonunion model mimicks the way nonunions develop in humans.[132] In human long bone fractures that fail to form bridges of rigid bone, the area of repeated motion frequently forms a pseudarthrosis. Fibrous tissue (type I and type II collagen) persist and frequently transform into (proteoglycan-rich) cartilage.

Enzymic profiles in fractured bones

When developing callus tissue is dissected into its component parts and analyzed by sensitive microchemical techniques, it has been possible to further resolve the role of cartilage and bone cells in the repair process. This work, of course, can only be performed in laboratory animals, but the results of these endeavors have provided much detailed information about the biologic requirements for repair. Chapter 6 deals with these processes in some detail, so we will report only certain of the data that are needed to complete our understanding of repair.

There are sequential temporal alterations in enzymic and ultrastructural processes leading or accompanying cartilage calcification and conversion to bone. Different enzymes active in anaerobic and aerobic glycolysis predominate at different stages of callus maturation, and carbohydrate metabolism provides the structural intermediates and energy for repair. A portion of Ketenjian and Arsenis's work[64] is illustrated in Figure 10-21, because it provides a useful overview of the metabolic inter-relationships within the callus. Although glycolytic pathways dominate the early undifferentiated fibrocartilage and proliferative cartilage, there is a shift to an aerobic pattern as the callus matures. The change seems to be associated with the increasing richness of the blood supply. This observation has, in fact, contributed one (untested) theoretical clinical rationale for fracture management, that is, hyperbaric oxygen therapy (see subsequent discussion). For the moment, however, the plots also demonstrate two further phenomena. In the ossifying callus, there are coordinated increases in the concentrations of (1) degradative lysosomal enzymes, which probably contribute to chondrocyte hypertrophy, and (2)

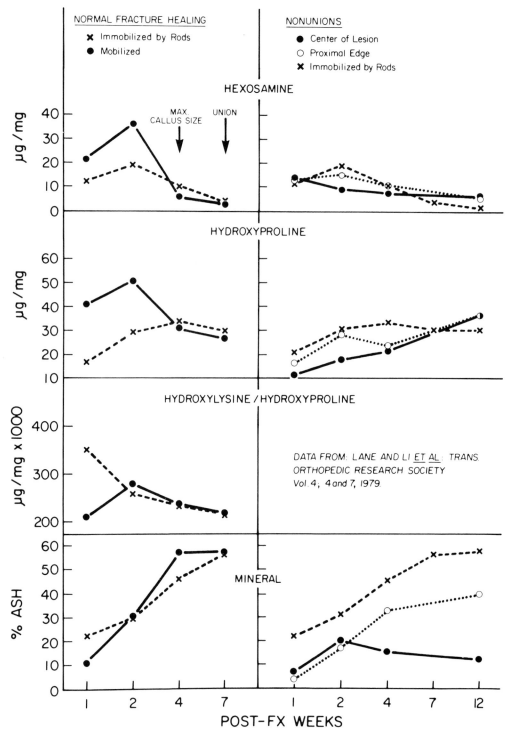

FIGURE 10-21 *An overview of the metabolic inter-relationships within the callus. (Ketenjian, A. Y., and Arsenis, C.: Clin. Orthop. 107:266–273, 1975)*

TABLE 10-5 COMPARISONS OF ENZYMATIC REACTIONS IN FIBROCYTES CHONDROCYTES, OSTEOCYTES AND OSTEOCLASTS

	FIBROCYTES	*CHONDROCYTES*	*OSTEOCYTES*	*OSTEOCLASTS*
Aminopeptidase	+3	+3	+3	0
Alkaline phosphatase	+4	+3–+4	+3–+4	0
Acid phosphatase	+2–+4	+2–+4	+2–+4	+4
Succinate dehydrogenase	+1–+2	+1–+2	+1–+2	+4
Lactate dehydrogenase	+4	+4	+4	+4

From Mori, M., Ohta, T., Okada, Y., Makino, M., and Murakami, M.: Acta Histochem. Cytochem. 8:8–17, 1975.

alkaline phosphatase, which has long been thought to play an active role in mineralization. The biochemical correlates described by Kuhlman[68] also show that the calcified regions of fracture callus are rich in the inorganic pyrophosphatases that "destroy" a pyrophosphate calcification inhibitor. The precise localization of a wide suite of oxidative enzymes in fracture callus has also been achieved by histochemical methods,[80] and we present certain of these semiquantitative data in Table 10-5.

Oxygen tensions

From early *in vitro* studies of Bassett and Herrmann,[7] we learned that 20-d embryonic chick tibial cortex formed bone when subjected to high oxygen tensions and mechanical compac-

tion. The same preparations were chondrogenic in low oxygen tensions and compaction. Fibroblasts were a major product when they were subjected to high oxygen tensions and tensile forces. Based upon these experiences, Brighton and Krebs[18] correlated the histologic differentiation within the callus tissue of fractured rabbit fibulas with direct measurements of oxygen tensions. These findings are summarized in Figure 10-22. The data indicates that hematoma has the lowest oxygen tensions (6.25 mm Hg), whereas diaphyseal bone has the highest values. A gradient during healing was thus discerned. The callus composed predominately of cartilage continued to show low oxygen tensions, even through the fibrocartilaginous and fiber bone stages. However, with increasing maturity, the oxygen tensions gradually increased until they were essen-

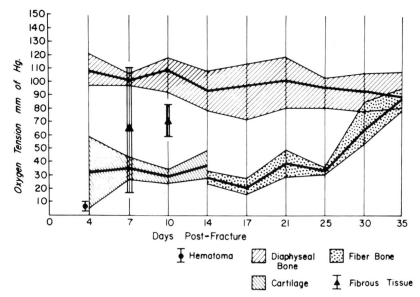

FIGURE 10-22 *Plots of oxygen tensions in the various tissues of the fracture calluses of rabbits at different postfracture days. (Brighton, C. T., and Krebs, A. G.: J. Bone Joint Surg. 54A:323–332, 1977)*

tially identical with that of diaphyseal bone. These patterns would appear to be consonant with the biochemical evolution of the healing callus glycolytic enzyme patterns. The data may also reflect increased oxygen consumption by the cells (in the anaerobic enzyme phase) in the early callus, and some corroborative *in vitro* data have been developed in Brighton's laboratory.[18]

The overall message is that direct measurements of oxygen tensions, in rabbit fractures at least, do reflect the increasing vascularization of the fracture site. These observations do not correlate with the biomechanical test results of tensile strength of fractured bone, since radiologically, the fractures are consolidated by the 17th day when oxygen tensions in the fiber bone callus are still much lower than normal. Moreover, Brighton's laboratory[19] has indicated that oxygen tensions may not be as precise an indicator of tissue differentiation as might be hoped. In experimentally produced nonunions of rabbit femurs in which there is motion at the fracture site, the nonunion fibrous tissue callus (cartilage and fiber bone) showed consistently higher oxygen tensions than a healing fracture. He concluded that although cartilage formation and bone formation have optima that are both low, these tissues can be formed at higher than optimum oxygen tensions. The persistence of fibrous tissue and cartilage could, however, be due to their higher oxygen tensions.

Heppenstall and his coworkers[53] conducted a particularly instructive series of studies on the effects of oxygen in bone repair at the University of Pennsylvania. They induced chronic systemic hypoxia in dogs by a right-to-left cardiac shunt and noted a significant delay in the healing of transverse fibular fractures. In the shunted dogs whose arterial oxygen levels had decreased from a normal 76 mm Hg to 42.8 mm Hg, their bone histologic appearance showed abundant, persistent cartilage in the callus. Impaired healing was also noted by radiology and biophysical bending tests. Conversely, hyperbaric oxygenation does favor fracture repair in rats (callus size, collagen content and mineralization),[52,153] and it enhances the survival of transplanted cartilages in rabbit long bones.[26] To the author's knowledge, the effects of chronic hypoxia and environmentally induced hyperoxia on fracture repair in humans have not been evaluated.

Mineralization

Mineralization of the callus begins · concomitantly with the formation of fibrocartilage and lamellar bone. These matrices become calcifiable by virtue of their complement of a calcium-phospholipid-phosphate complex.[14] Two acid phospholipids—phosphatydyl serine and phosphatydyl inositol—are throught to be the most important components, but there is as yet no concensus about how this complex functions in mineralization. It may serve *in situ* as a nucleation site, as a calcium reservoir, or as a means of transporting calcium to nucleation sites. These complexes seem to be exported to extracellular matrices in small vesicles that pinch off from cell membranes (see Chapter 2). In the nonimmobilized rat tibia fracture model already noted (see Fig. 10-19), the calcium-phospholipid-phosphate complexes are most concentrated in the 2-wk callus, and this time correlates with the initial increase in the ash content.[15]

The healing stimulus

Motion at the fracture site

A variety of internal fixation devices are used in orthopedic practice to stabilize a fracture. The purpose of internal fixation is, overall, to maintain correct alignment of bone fragments, to prevent muscle wasting, to bring about early weight-bearing and early discharge from hospitals. King writes[65] that within the last 20 yr, the techniques "have become more refined, technically stronger and physiologically less destructive."

In terms of being physiologically destructive, it is clear that implantation of intramedullary pins requires the sacrifice of medullary vessels by reaming.[32] Plates require prior subperiosteal dissection and stripping, which compromises the periosteal circulation. Screws destroy intracortical and medullary vessels, and they create stress-risers that weaken bone. There is a balance to be struck, and one must make choices based upon the knowledge of the alternate responses of bone at the tissue level. From our discussions on compression plating, surgeons can choose to decrease the period of bed rest and morbidity at the expense of the rate of fracture healing.

Motion at the fracture ends to some degree is definitely advantageous from the standpoint of stimulating a stabilizing callus. Rhinelander[93] points out that "bones vary in their requirements for stabilization. Ribs heal well with persistent motion; long bones do not." The callus tissue response is perhaps a function of bioelectrical potentials that are generated within bone and stimulate osteoblast production and activity. The application of rigid plates (and screws) with compression induces porotic changes through osteoclastic resorption in cortical bone, even at some distance from the fractured area, and the cortex is thinned. Here, rigidity is achieved at the expense of maintaining skeletal integrity. In rabbits, the phase of bone destruction can occur for as long as 18 wk and can persist for as long as 36 wk. The tissue obeys Wolff's Law, since the stresses are carried by the rigid plates, not the bone.

Recently, Woo[150] and Akeson[1] have begun to experiment with less rigid plates composed of graphite fiber and methylmethacrylate. These "resin composite plates" (GFMM) have not as yet been made biocompatible for use in humans, but they would be of theoretical and practical value; their lower modulus of elasticity forces the bone to share the responsibility for carrying stress. In an experiment designed to compare the effects of graphite composite plates with stainless steel plates, these investigators[1] reported that the GFMM plates induced osteoporosis in canine radii 4 wk after osteotomy by 50%—both at the fracture site and proximal to the osteotomy. Tetracycline labeling patterns were interpreted to signify that composite plate fixation resulted in a higher rate of bone formation. Despite these favorable signs, biomechanical tests indicated that the composite plates and the stainless steel plates promoted the same quality of healing; the maximum shear stresses, the torque and angular deformity, and the energy absorbed before fracture were identical, despite the greater tendency

for the GFMM plates to promote osteogenesis. Subsequently, Moyen and his collaborators[82] at the Massachusetts General Hospital have tested the effect of thinner, more flexible (and biocompatible) plates composed of titanium, 6-aluminum, and 4-vanadium on intact dog femora. The results after 6 and 9 mo indicated that the flexible plates had significantly reduced the degree of osteoporosis that developed at the endosteum below the devices (15 vs 26% at 6 mo, and 20 vs 31% at 9 mo). In these intact bones, they reported increased rates of bone formation, particularly during the first two mo after plate application.

These observations have an impact on various theories of fracture management. One school of thought believes that fractures of the long bones should be treated by immobilization of the injured element and adjacent joints. Another school denies that this assumption should be rigidly followed in certain of these fractures, and they point to the abundant callus formed around fractures of active patients. The latter observations confirm that some motion of the fracture fragments benefits fracture repair. They also justify the assertions of advocates of treatment of fractures of the femur and tibia by early weight-bearing. In the 1976 Instructional Course Lectures and elsewhere, Sarmiento[104–106] stresses the importance of "functional bracing" in the treatment of all long bone fractures. The techniques assure that after alignment, the fractured fragments would continue to receive normal deforming forces, assuring stimulation of bone formation. Table 10-6 summarizes these results.

In the laboratory, Sarmiento[107] has worked to develop experimental models that could confirm this concept. We have reproduced one of his illustrations (Fig. 10-23), which compares a femur from a rat that was permitted to walk as soon as it would following femoral fracture, with a bone from an immobilized limb. The femur from the functional limb had the better-consolidated fracture. Somewhat related are observations that athletes have the greatest bone mass in their exercised limbs. Avioli[2] has stressed, however, that bone mass is related to the duration of exercise and that, accordingly, an

TABLE 10-6 MEDIAN TIME TO HEALING WITH FUNCTIONAL CAST BRACING OF ACUTE FRACTURES OF LONG BONES

| BONE | N | FRACTURE | | | | LOCATION | | | TYPE | | RECOM-MENDED TIME TO CAST BRACING |
		TRANS-VERSE	COM-MIN-UTED	OBLIQUE	SEG-MEN-TAL	PROX-IMAL 1/3	MID-SHAFT	DIST 1/3	OPEN	CLOSED	
Tibia*	532	16 wk	14.5 wk	15 wk	17.5 wk	14.5 wk	14.5 wk	15 wk	17.5 wk	14.5 wk	4 wk
Femur*	191								17.5 wk	14.5 wk	5+ wk
Forearm*	117										
Ulna	70								10 wk (5–26 wk)		First 2 wks
Radius	25								9.6 wk (5–26 wk)		First 2 wks
Ulna/Radius	22								16.4 wk (9–33 wk)		
Humerus†	51								8.5 wk		

* Data from Sarmiento, A., Latta, L., and Sinclair, W. F.: Instructional Course Lectures, XXV: 184–239, 1976.
† Data from Sarmiento, A., Kinman, P. B., Galvin, E. G., Schmitt, R. H., and Phillips, J. G.: J. Bone Joint Surg. 59A: 596–601, 1977.

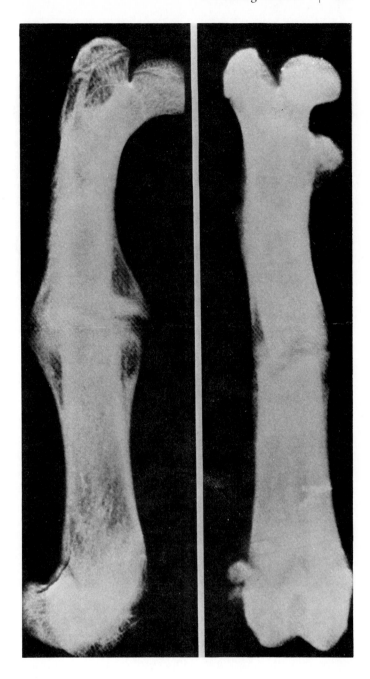

FIGURE 10-23 *Comparison of roentgenograms of 3-wk-old femoral fractures from rats permitted to bear weight after trauma (left) versus rats immobilized in a cast (right). The well-developed callus of the better-healed bone (left) contrasts with the lesser degree of change seen around the fracture site from the immobilized bone (right) (Sarmiento, A., Schaeffer, J. F., Beckerman, L., Latta, L. L., and Enis, J. E.: J. Bone Joint Surg. 59A:369–375, 1977)*

exercise regimen would probably not be immediately helpful to sedentary individuals whose risk of fracture increases with age.

The literature does suggest that prior physical conditioning could benefit the course of fracture healing. When mice subjected to a graded program of exercise on a treadmill sustained a (tibial) fracture, they were better able to repair their bone than unexercised mice. On biochemical evaluation, the rates of callus collagen formation and mineralization were markedly improved after exercise. On the basis of these studies, Heikkinen[52] suggested that physical training increased the oxygen tension in muscle and the periosteal blood supply, and, as we have seen, this would favor the rapid conversion of repair tissue into bone. Some caution is warranted in transcribing these effects to humans, since on a relative scale, the role of periosteal bone formation in the repair of fractures in small animals is perhaps more important than it is in humans.

Bioelectrical events

We have noted that stresses generated in bone by "relative motion" of the bone ends could provide a stimulus for bone repair. The stimulus is currently believed to be electrical in nature. Bassett and Becker[8] and others[76] found that slabs of cortical bone could generate small piezoelectrical currents on the order of 1 to 2 mv when subjected to compressive or tensile forces. The response was present only when bone was mineralized. Bone that had been decalcified before testing did not generate potential differences. Further investigations indicated that the concave surfaces tended to be electronegative, whereas convex surfaces were electropositive.[41] Clinical experience showing that bones develop a more robust callus on concave surfaces following reduction of fractures also seems to suggest that electrical phenomena might play an important role in the healing mechanism. In rabbits, fracture increases the electronegativity of bone.[42] This was a proposition that could be readily tested in the laboratory. It was soon realized that when active electrodes were inserted through the bony cortex, new bone formed around the cathode and bone resorption occurred around the anode, especially when the applied voltages were large.[94] In the laboratory[42] and clinic[20] direct currents have accelerated fracture healing and the results in treatment of nonunions appear promising. Much of the research has been collected in a series of papers published in Clinical Orthopedics and Related Research, No. 124, 1978, and in a recent symposium volume (*Electrical Properties of Bone and Cartilage*, eds. Brighton *et al.*, Grune and Stratton, N.Y., 1979).

The biochemical basis for the osteogenic response to applied currents has been advanced by a group of scientists at the University of Connecticut led by Rodan.[16,96,97] He believes that the useful small electrical currents provide a "trigger stimulus" or threshold that initiates a sequence of cellular events. These involve the dedifferentiation or proliferation of uncommitted (stem) cells and their subsequent differentiation into an osteogenic cell line. This concept is supported by observations that direct currents (1) stimulate DNA synthesis in chick cartilage cells and in the calvaria of 19-d-old rat embryos, (2) increase the ultrastructural features of bone cells associated with collagen formation (ribosomes, rough endoplasmic reticulum, microsomes, and so forth), (3) alter the morphologies of the cells at the light microscope level, and (4) increase the accumulation of alkaline phosphatase on osteogenic cell surfaces. These effects are specific to bone cells. Fibroblasts and lymphocytes from rat spleens do not respond to electrical (direct) currents. This evidence is made even more compelling by the knowledge that osteogenic cell lines respond to direct currents with increased production of $3',5'$-GMP and Ca^{++}, and by decreased $3',5'$-cyclic-AMP. The growth phase of most cells is always associated with low cyclic-AMP production. Davidovich[34] recorded a similar pattern of change in bone cells, that is, toward low cyclic-AMP levels when cells were mobilized to remodel the jaws of cats in response to an applied orthodontic stress-producing device. Thus, the trigger stimulus provided by bioelectrical currents may involve an initial depolarization of cell membranes.

There is currently much clinical interest in the applicability of electrical currents to patients with difficult to heal fractures. The clinical experiences with nonunions has been summarized by Spadaro,[123] who suggests that currents of 5 to 25 Hz, 2 uA/mm^2 and 52 Hz, 6 uA/mm^2 can best benefit the pace of bone formation at fracture sites. He calculated that when this treatment produced healing, the energy dissipated in bone was on the order of 7 joules. In all of these cases, the field strength appears to be the very critical limiting factor that determines whether the sequence of cellular events responsible for producing bone healing will proceed in a normal fashion. It is not inconceivable that the optimal field strength differs at each stage of fracture callus maturity, since different cells are involved at different times. Several commercially available intramedullary cathodes are now available to surgeons, and less invasive techniques are under development. In this respect, reasonable experimental outcomes have been achieved using coils that can be wrapped around a fracture site (ELECTRET).[154] One must keep in mind that the implantable internal and external devices are in a sense both nonspecific, since there is no way that the field strengths they produce can be directed to a selected line of osteogenic cells. Imposed field strengths are attractive, since there is less chance of developing an infection at the fracture site.

The osteoinductive stimulus

Heretofore, we have primarily stressed the cellular control of bone repair. We have noted that there are proliferative elements in periosteum, endosteum, and marrow, and we have considered some of the microenvironmental condition (bioelectrical potentials, oxygen tensions, and so forth) that provide a stimulus to activate these populations. The bone graft, which has been an important clinical tool, has not been emphasized as an active participant in the repair process.

The old concept that an autologous bone graft may contribute a *significant* number of actively osteogenic cells to the repair process probably exaggerates this function of an implant. If the site is favorable, many osteocytes probably do survive.[55] However, there is little hard evidence that these osteocytes can form an important reserve population of osteogenic cells once their circumlacunar matrix has been resorbed. Deprived of their nutritive supply, it is also unlikely that most osteoblasts on the bone surfaces of an autologous graft will survive long. Bone allograft osteocytes may survive 24 hr.[22] Intralesional grafts of periosteal tissues have not always produced a successful clinical outcome, even when microsurgical procedures have been able to initially restore vascular continuity with the host tissues.[70] The best guess was that a bone graft's main function was to survive long enough to provide a structural mass upon which the host's tissues could grow. For the most part, the bone implants—autologous, allogeneic, or xenogeneic—played a passive role. A great deal of effort and research has been directed toward making the graft—any graft—survive, and it was noted that freezing, irradiation, sterilization, or deproteinization did tend to make allogeneic or xenogeneic bone more biocompatible by reducing its (already weak) antigenic potential.

Over the past decade, work that has principally been performed at Urist's laboratory at U.C.L.A. has done much to avert and change the opinion that bone grafts were passive participants in repair mechanisms. Urist has amassed much evidence that the graft contains a biologically active substance that causes resident cells at the site of injury to become active in healing processes. It is not yet known if this property of the graft elicits an angiogenic or chemotactic phenomena. The biologically active substance is called BMP—an acronym for bone morphogenetic protein. Chapters 11 and 12 deal with the properties of BMP in substantial detail. Here, we note that there is now reason to suspect that a BMP is released from the fractured ends of bone at the site of injury, and that this will cause primitive or undifferentiated cells in the area to differentiate into competent osteogenic cells. The efficacy of a matrix rich in BMP has not been rigorously tested in a large animal model system, but there are some observations in rats and rabbits that we will summarize at the end of this section. The bulk of the evidence that bone contains such an osteogenic promoting substance is provided by systems which utilize intramuscular implants of BMP-rich matrix either placed directly in muscle or implanted within millipore diffusion chambers. In the former, the cells that migrate into the revascularizing graft first form a cartilage that is later transformed to bone. New bone lamellae also form around the periphery of the matrix. In the latter, new bone forms from the mesenchymal cells in the muscle bed around the millipore chamber.

The osteoinductive substance released from bone is probably associated with the collagenous fraction. The evidence to this point is based in part upon information that BMP activity can be destroyed by endogenous proteases found only in dentin and bone, by trypsin digestion under conditions that do not release hydroxyproline, and by dinitrophenylation. BMP is also alkali-labile and its activity is suppressed by scission of tyrosine and phenylalanine residues, or abolished by deamination and mercaptoethanol reduction. Again, its presence in bone (and dentin) is most powerfully demonstrated when the implanted matrices are first demineralized and sequentially extracted to remove small strongly antigenic glycoprotein moieties.[135–137,139]

Although we have noted that this concept has not been critically tested in a fracture healing model in large animals, our laboratory[113] has tested the osteogenic properties of surface demineralized and freeze-dried grafts of allogeneic bone in a fibular defect model in rats. The work was done within a circadian context—different animals were grafted at different times in their body rhythm. A substantial difference was found in the ability of the host to provide osteogenic cell populations at different clock hours. After a 3-wk postoperative period, we found that the firmest unions occurred in those groups of rats grafted at night, e.g. when the normal diurnal peak of marrow reticular (osteoprogenitor) cell mitoses occurred. This rather unconventional approach to the problem of fracture healing may be evidence that some biologically active substance, presumably a BMP, was released from the graft and stimulated progenitor cell proliferation.

More recently, Oikarinen and Korhonen[88] have also compared the osteoinductive property of fresh autologous calcified and surface demineralized allogeneic matrices (BIM) in a fibular defect model in rats. Three months after these matrices were packed into 2-mm defects, all but 1 of 16 BIM-treated fibulas showed abundant callus, and 11 were firmly united with bone. Conversely, only 4 of 16 fibulas treated with autogenous bone showed bony union, and 12 sites were not healed; 5 of these showed pseudarthroses. The same principles should be applicable to clinical situations. In addition, it would be valuable to know if electrically induced field strengths operate to promote repair of fractures by an influence on the osteogenic potential of bone cells *per se*, or whether this effect is due to accelerated diffusion of a BMP from bone (i.e., cell-matrix interactions). Given the reality of BMP, it would be safe to anticipate that both mechanisms are operative at a fracture site.

References

1. Akeson, W. H., Woo, S. L.-Y., Coutts, R. D., Matthews, J. V., Gonslaves, M., and Amiel, D.: Quantitative histological evaluation of early fracture healing of cortical bone immobilized by stainless steel and composite plates, Calcif. Tissue Res. 19:27–37, 1975.
2. Avioli, L. V.: Osteoporosis: pathogenesis and therapy. *In* Avioli, L. V., and Krane, S. M. (eds.): Metabolic Bone Disease, Vol. 1, pp. 307–385, New York, Academic Press, 1977.
3. Babicky, A., Kolar, J., and Vyhnanek, L.: Generalized skeletal response to local injuries—a part of wide mesenchymal reaction, Nature 212:410–411, 1966.
4. Ballet, J. J., and Griscelli, C.: Lymphoid cell transplantation in human osteopetrosis. *In* Horton, J. E., Tarpley, T. M., and Davis, W. H. (eds.): Mechanisms of Localized Bone Loss, pp. 399–414, Calcif. Tissue Abstracts (Suppl.) 1978.
5. Balogh, K., Jr., and Hajek, J. V.: Oxidative enzymes in intermediary metabolism in healing bone fractures, Am. J. Anat. 116:429–448, 1965.
6. Barron, S. E., Robb, R. A., Taylor, W. F., and Kelly, P. J.: The effect of fixation with intramedullary rods and plates on fracture-site blood flow and bone remodeling in dogs, J. Bone Joint Surg. 59A:376–385, 1977.
7. Bassett, C. A. L., and Herrmann, I.: Influence of oxygen concentration and mechanical factors in differentiation of connective tissues in vivo, Nature 190:460–461, 1961.
8. Bassett, C. A. L., and Becker, R. O.: Generation of electrical potentials by bone in response to mechanical stress, Science 137:1063, 1962.
9. Bauer, G. C. H., Carlsson, A., and Lindquist, B.: Metabolism and homeostatic functions of bone. *In* Comar, C. L., and Bronner, F. (eds.): Mineral Metabolism, Vol. IB, pp. 609–676, New York, Academic Press, 1961.
10. Belanger, L. F.: Osteocyte resorption. *In* Bourne, G. H. (ed.): Biochemistry and Physiology of Bone, Vol. III, pp. 240–270, New York, Academic Press, 1971.
11. Bloom, M. A., Bloom, W., Domm, L. V., and McLean, F. C.: Changes in avian bone due to

injected estrogen and during the reproductive cycle, Anat. Rec. 78(Suppl.):1–43, 1941.

12. Bloom, W., Bloom, M. A., and McLean, F. C.: Calcification and ossification. Medullary bone changes in the reproductive cycle of female pigeons, Anat. Rec. 81:443–475, 1941.

13. Borden, J., and Smith, W. S.: Refracture of the shaft of the femur, South. Med. J. 45:874–876, 1952.

14. Boskey, A. L., and Posner, A. S.: Extraction of a calcium-phospholipid-phosphate complex from bone, Calcif. Tissue Res. 19:273–283, 1976.

15. Boskey, A. L., Lane, J. M., Li, W. K., and Cordella, D. M.: Lipid and phospholipid content and metabolism in early fracture repair, Trans. Orthop. Res. Soc. 4:5, 1979.

16. Bourret, L. A., and Rodan, G. A.: The role of calcium in the inhibition of cAMP accumulation in epiphyseal cartilage exposed to physiological pressure, J. Cell. Physiol. 88:358–361, 1976.

17. Boyne, P.: Use of marrow-cancellous bone grafts in maxillary alveolar and palatal clefts, J. Dent. Res. 53:821–824, 1974.

18. Brighton, C. T., and Krebs, A. G.: Oxygen tension of healing fractures in the rabbit, J. Bone Joint Surg. 54A:323–332, 1972.

19. Brighton, C. T., and Krebs, A. G.: Oxygen tensions of nonunion of fractured femurs in the rabbit, Surgery 135:379–385, 1972.

20. Brighton, C. T., Friedenberg, Z. B., Mitchell, E. I., and Booth, R. E.: Treatment of nonunion with constant direct current, Clin. Orthop. 124:106–123, 1977.

21. Brookes, M. The Blood Supply to Bone, London, Butterworths, 1971.

22. Burchardt, H., and Enneking, W. F.: Transplantation of bone, Surg. Clin. N. Am. 58:403–427, 1978.

23. Burdick, C. G., and Siris, I. E.: Fractures of the femur in children. Treatment and end results in 268 cases, Ann. Surg. 77:736–753, 1923.

24. Burwell, R. G.: Studies in the transplantation of bone. VII. The fresh composite homograft-autograft of cancellous bone. An analysis of factors leading to osteogenesis in marrow transplants and in marrow-containing bone grafts, J. Bone Joint Surg. 46B:110–140, 1964.

25. Burwell, R. G.: Studies in the transplantation of bone. VIII. Treated composite homograft-autograft of cancellous bone. An analysis of inductive mechanisms in bone transplantation, J. Bone Joint Surg. 48B:532, 1966.

26. Calderwood, J. W.: The effect of hyperbaris oxygen on the transplantation of epiphyseal growth cartilage in the rabbit, J. Bone Joint Surg. 56B:753–759, 1974.

27. Charnley, J., and Guindy, A.: Delayed operation in the open reduction of fractures of long bones, J. Bone Joint Surg. 43B:664–671, 1961.

28. Coccia, P. F., Cervenka, J., Teitelbaum, S. L., Kahn, A. J., Clawson, C. C., and Brown, D. M.: Reversal of human osteopetrosis by bone marrow transplantation: etiologic implications, Am. Soc. Clin. Invest. in press.

29. Cole, W. H.: Compensatory lengthening of the femur in children after fracture, Ann. Surg. 82:609–616, 1925.

30. Cummine, J., and Nade, S.: Osteogenesis after bone and bone marrow transplantation. 1. Studies with combined myeloosseous grafts in the guinea pig, Acta Orthop. Scand. 48:15–24, 1977.

31. Danis, A.: Etude de l'ossification dans les greffes de moelle osseuse, Bruxelles, Les Editions "Acta Medica Belgica," 1–120, 1957.

32. Dankwardt-Lilliestrom, G.: Reaming of the medullary cavity and its effect on diaphyseal bone, Acta Orthop. Scand. (Suppl.) 128:1–153, 1969.

33. David, V. C.: Shortening and compensatory overgrowth following fractures of the femur in children, Arch. Surg. 9:438–449, 1924.

34. Davidovich, Z., and Shanfeld, J. L.: Cyclic AMP levels in alveolar bone of orthodontically treated cats, Arch. Oral. Biol. 20:567, 1975.

34a. Davies, D. R., Bassingthwaighte, J. B., and Kelly, P. J.: Blood flow and ion exchange in bone. *In* Simmons, D. J., and Kunin, A. S. (eds.): Skeletal Research—An Experimental Approach, pp. 397–419, New York, Academic Press, 1979.

35. Dowsett, M., Easty, G. C., Powles, T. J., Easty, D. M., and Neville, A. M.: Human breast tumor—induced osteolysis and prostaglandins, Prostaglandins 11:447, 1976.

36. Drinker, C. K., Drinker, K. R., and Lund, C. C.: Circulation in mammalian bone marrow, Am. J. Physiol. 62:1–92, 1922.

37. Edwards, P.: Fracture of the shaft of the tibia: 492 consecutive cases in adults. Importance of soft tissue injury, Acta Orthop. Scand. (Suppl.) 76:1–82, 1965.

38. Ellsasser, J. C., Moyer, C. F., Lesker, P. A., and Simmons, D. J.: Improved healing of experimental long bone fractures in rabbits by de-

layed internal fixation, J. Trauma 15:869–876, 1975.

39. Emery, M. A.: The incidence of delayed union and non-union following fractures of both bones of the forearm in adults, Can. J. Surg. 8:285–287, 1965.

40. Fischman, D. A., and Hayes, E. D.: Origin of osteoclasts from mononuclear leucocytes in regenerating newt limbs, Anat. Rec. 143:329–338, 1962.

41. Friedenberg, Z. B.: Bioelectrical potentials in bone, J. Bone Joint Surg. 48A:915–923, 1966.

42. Friedenberg, Z. B., and Smith, H. G.: Electrical potentials in intact and fractured tibia, Clin. Orthop. 63:222–225, 1969.

43. Friedenberg, Z. B., Roberts, P. G., Jr., Didizian, N. H., and Brighton, C. T.: Stimulation of fracture healing by direct current in the rabbit fibula, J. Bone Joint Surg. 53A:1400–1408, 1971.

44. Friedenstein, A. J., Chailakhjan, R. K., and Lalykina, K. S.: The development of fibroblast colonies in monolayer cultures of guinea pig bone marrow and spleen cells, Cell Tissue Kinet. 3:393–403, 1970.

45. Friedenstein, A. J.: Determined and inducible osteogenic precursor cells. *In* Hard Tissue Growth and Repair, Ciba Foundation Symposium 11:169–185, 1973.

46. Galasko, C. S. B., and Bennett, A.: Relationship of bone destruction in skeletal metastases to osteoclast activation and prostaglandins, Nature 263:508–510, 1976.

47. Galasko, C. S. B.: Mechanisms of bone destruction in the development of skeletal metastases, Nature 263:507–508, 1976.

48. Girgis, F. G., and Pritchard, J. J.: Experimental production of cartilage during the repair of fractures of the skull vault in rats, J. Bone Joint Surg. 40B:274, 1958.

49. Gothlin, G., and Ericsson, J. L. E.: Electron microscopic studies on the uptake and storage of thorium dioxide molecules in different cell types of fracture callus, Acta Pathol. Microbiol. Scand. 81A:523–542, 1973.

50. Hahn, T. J.: Bone complications of anticonvulsants, Drugs 12:201–211, 1976.

51. Ham, A. W., and Harris, W. R.: Repair and transplantation. *In* Bourne, G. H. (ed.): Biochemistry and Physiology of Bone, Vol. I, pp. 338–399, New York, Academic Press, 1971.

52. Heikkinen, E., Vihersaari, T., and Penttinen, R.: Effect of previous exercise on fracture healing: a biochemical study with mice, Acta Orthop. Scand. 45:481–489, 1974.

53. Heppenstall, R. B., Goodwin, C. W., and Brighton, C. T.: Fracture healing in the presence of chronic hypoxia. J. Bone Joint Surg. 58A:1153–1156, 1976.

54. Hertzberg, M., Oberman, Z., Weissman, S. L., and Herold, H. Z.: Serum glycoproteins and proteins after fracture, Clin. Chem. 11:920–924, 1965.

55. Heslop, B. F., Zeiss, I. M., and Nisbet, N. W.: Studies on transference of bone. I. A comparison of autologous and homologous bone implants with reference to osteocyte survival, osteogenesis and host reaction, Br. J. Exp. Pathol. 41:269–297, 1960.

56. Horton, J. E., Raisz, L. G., Simmons, H. A., Oppenheim, J. J., and Mergenhagen, S. F.: Bone resorbing activity in supernatant fluid from cultured human peripheral blood leucocytes, Science 177:793–795, 1972.

57. Hyldebrandt, N., Damholt, W., and Nordentoft, E. L.: Investigation of the cellular response to fracture assessed by autoradiography of the periosteum, Acta Orthop. Scand. 45:175–181, 1974.

58. Jarry, L., and Uhthoff, H. K.: Activation of osteogenesis by the "Petal" technique. An experimental study, J. Bone Joint Surg. 42B:126–136, 1960.

59. Johnell, O., and Hulth, A.: Proliferation of osteoclasts in rat bone following bleeding and femoral fractures, Calcif. Tissue Res. 23:241–244, 1977.

60. Kahn, A. J., and Simmons, D. J.: Investigation of cell lineage in bone using chimera of chick and quail embryonic tissue, Nature 258:325–327, 1975.

61. Kahn, A. J., and Simmons, D. J.: Chondrocyte-to-osteocyte transformation in grafts of perichondrium-free epiphyseal cartilage, Clin. Orthop. 129:299–304, 1977.

62. Kahn, A. J., Stewart, C. C., and Teitelbaum, S. L.: Contact mediated bone resorption by human monocytes in vitro, Science 199:988–990, 1978.

63. Kernek, C. B., and Wray, J. B.: Cellular proliferation in the formation of fracture callus in the rat tibia, Clin. Orthop. 91:197–209, 1973.

64. Ketenjian, A. Y., and Arsenis, C.: Morphological and biochemical studies during differentiation and calcification of fracture callus cartilage, Clin. Orthop. 107:266–273, 1975.

65. King, K. F.: Recent advances in the treatment of long bone fractures of the lower limb, Med. J. Aust. 1:548–551, 1978.

66. Koeffler, H. P., Mundy, G. R., Golde, D. W., and Cline, J.: Production of bone resorbing activity in poorly differentiated monocyte malignancy, Cancer 41:2438–2443, 1978.

67. Kramer, I. R. H., Killey, H. C., and Wright, H. C.: A histological and radiological comparison of the healing of defects in the rabbit calvaria with and without implanted heterogenous anorganic bone, Arch. Oral Biol. 13:1095–1106, 1968.

68. Kuhlman, R. E., and Bakowski, M. J.: The biochemical activity of fracture callus in relation to bone production, Clin. Orthop. 107:258–265, 1975.

69. Lam, S. J.: The place of delayed internal fixation in the treatment of fractures of long bones, J. Bone Joint Surg. 46B:393–397, 1964.

70. Lance, E. M.: Bone and cartilage. In Najarian, J. S., and Simmons, R. L. (eds.): Transplantation, pp. 655–697, Philadelphia, Lea & Febiger, 1972.

71. Lane, J. M., Li, W. K. P., Eaton, B., Dick, B. L., and Blaine, G.: Effect of immobilization on the fracture callus matrix: collagen, proteoglycan and mineral metabolism, Trans. Orthop. Res. Soc. 4:4, 1979.

72. Li, W. K., Lane, J. M., Siegal, T., Horowitz, D., Eaton, B., and Dick, B. L.: Matrix constituent alterations in fracture non-union, Trans. Orthop. Res. Soc. 4:7, 1979.

73. Lindgren, L., and Walloe, A.: Incidence of fracture in epileptics, Acta Orthop. Scand. 48:356–361, 1977.

74. Luben, R. A.: Purification of a lymphokine osteoclast activating factor from human tonsil lymphocytes, Biochem. Biophys. Res. Commun. 84:15–32, 1978.

75. Malone, D., Kahn, A. J., and Teitelbaum, S. L.: An in vitro analysis of uremic bone, Abstract submitted to American Society of Nephrology, 1979.

76. Marino, A. A., and Becker, R. O.: Piezoelectricity in bone as a function of age, Calcif. Tissue Res. 14:327–331, 1974.

77. Marks, S. C., Jr. and Schneider, G. B.: Evidence for a relationship between lymphoid cells and osteoclasts: bone resorption restored in *ia* (osteopetrotic) rats by lymphocytes, monocytes and macrophages from a normal littermate, Am. J. Anat. 152:331–342, 1978.

78. Mattar, A. G., and Friedman, B. A.: Bone tracers: radionuclide imaging and related techniques. In Simmons, D. J., and Kunin, A. S. (eds.): Skeletal Research—An Experimental Approach, pp. 458–486, New York, Academic Press, 1979.

79. Mauer, A. M.: Diurnal variations of proliferative activity in the human bone marrow, Blood 26:1–7, 1965.

80. Mori, M., Ohta, T., Okada, Y., Makino, M., and Murakami, M.: Aminopeptidase histochemistry in healing bone fractures, Acta Histochem. Cytochem. 8:8–17, 1975.

81. Morris, M. L.: The effects of freezing human dentin and cementum before implantation in the subcutaneous tissues of the rat, J. Periodont. Res. 46:286–291, 1969.

82. Moyen, B. J.-L., Lahey, P. J., Weinberg, E. H., and Harris, W. H.: Effects of intact femora of dogs on the application and removal of metal plates, J. Bone Joint Surg. 60A:940–947, 1978.

83. Muheim, G., Donath, A., and Rossier, A. B.: Serial scintograms in the course of ectopic bone formation in paraplegic patients, Am. J. Roentgenol. Rad. Therap. Nucl. Med. 118:865–869, 1973.

84. Mundy, G. R., Altman, A. J., Gondek, M. D., and Bandelin, J. G.: Direct resorption of bone by human monocytes, Science 196:1109–1111, 1977.

85. Mundy, G. R., Varani, J., Orr, W., Gondek W., and Ward, P. A.: Resorbing bone is chemotactic for monocytes, Nature 275:132–135, 1978.

86. Najjar, T. A., and Kahn, D.: Comparative study of healing and remodeling in various bones, J. Oral Surg. 35:375–379, 1977.

87. Nilsson, B. E. R.: Posttraumatic osteopenia. A quantitative study of bone mineral mass in the femur following fracture of the tibia in man using Americium-241 as a photon source, Acta Orthop. Scand. (Suppl.) 37:1–55, 1966.

88. Oikarinen, J., and Korhonen, K.: Repair of bone defects by bone inductive material, Acta Orthop. Scand. 50:21–26, 1979.

89. Owen, M. R.: Cellular dynamics of bone. In Bourne, G. H. (ed.): Biochemistry and Physiology of Bone, Vol. III, pp. 271–298, New York, Academic Press, 1971.

90. Patt, H. M., and Moloney, M. A.: Bone formation and resorption as a requirement for marrow development, Proc. Soc. Exp. Biol. Med. 140:205–207, 1972.

91. Prockop, D. J., Kivirikko, K. I., Tuderman, L.,

and Guzman, N. A.: The biosynthesis of collagen and its disorders, New Engl. J. Med. 301:13–23, 1979.

92. Radom, S., Zulawski, M., and Dahlig, E.: Circadian rhythm of total urinary hydroxyproline excretion and ³H-hydroxyproline test, Clin. Chim. Acta 39:277–278, 1972.

93. Rhinelander, F. W.: Tibial blood supply in relation to fracture healing, Clin. Orthop. 105:34–81, 1974.

94. Richez, J., Chamay, A., and Bieler, L.: Bone changes due to pulses of direct electric microcurrent, Virchows Arch. (Pathol. Anat.) 357:11–18, 1972.

95. Richters, V., Meyers, M. H., and Sherwin, R. P.: Tissue culture studies of bone from the fractured hip, Clin. Orthop. 101:268–277, 1974.

96. Rodan, G. A., Bourret, L. A., and Norton, I. A.: DNA synthesis in cartilage cells in stimulated by oscillating electric fields, Science 199:690–692, 1978.

97. Rodan, G. A., Bourret, L. A., Harvey, A., and Mensi, G.: 3′,5′ cyclic AMP and 3′,5′ cyclic GMP: mediators of the mechanical effects on bone remodelling, Science 189:467–469, 1975.

98. Rokkanen, P., Jussila, J., Paatsama, S., Lahdensuu, M., Makela, V., Ehnholm, C., and Myllyla, G.: Traumatic shock after severe limb tissue damage in pigs, Acta Chir. Scand. 140:85–90, 1974.

99. Rosen, J. F., Wolin, D. A., and Finberg, L.: Immobilization hypercalcemia after single limb fractures in children and adolescents, Am. J. Dis. Child. 132:560–564, 1978.

100. Rosenberg, G. D., Simmons, D. J., Halberg, F., Nelson, W., and Burstein, A.: Skeletal effects of methylprednisolone sodium succinate administration on an every day or alternate day chronopharmacologic dose schedule. Hayes, D., Scheving, L. E., and Halberg, F. (eds.): Proceedings of XII International Congress on Chronobiology, Science Press, New York, in press.

101. Ruthersford, R. E., and Bell, J. P.: Delayed open reduction of isolated fractures of the femoral shaft, South. Med. J. 68:1243–1244, 1975.

102. Salama, R.: Experimental appraisal and clinical applications of recombined xenografts of bone and autologous red marrow, Isr. J. Med. Sci. 12:14–15, 1976.

103. Salama, R., and Wiseman, S. L.: The clinical use of combined xenografts of bone and autologous red marrow. A preliminary report, J. Bone Joint Surg. 60B:111–115, 1978.

104. Sarmiento, A., Cooper, J. S., and Sinclair, W. F.: Forearm fractures. Early functional bracing—a preliminary report. J. Bone Joint Surg. 57A:297–304, 1975.

105. Sarmiento, A., Latta, L., and Sinclair, W. F.: Functional bracing of fractures. Instructional Course Lectures, XXV: 184–239, 1976.

106. Sarmiento, A., Kinman, P. B., Galvin, E. G., Schmitt, R. H., and Phillips, J. G.: Functional bracing of fractures of the shaft of the humerus, J. Bone Joint Surg. 59A:596–601, 1977.

107. Sarmiento, A., Schaeffer, J. F., Beckerman, L., Latta, L. L., and Enis, J. E.: Fracture healing in rat femora as affected by functional weight-bearing, J. Bone Joint Surg. 59A:369–375, 1977.

108. Schenk, R., and Willenengger, H.: Fluroreszenmikrosckopische Untersuchungen zur Heilung von Schaftfrakturen nach Stabiler Osteosynthese am Hund. *In* Richelle, L. J., and Dallemagne, M. J. (eds.): Calcified Tissues, pp. 125–133, Liege, Belgium, University of Liege Press, 1965.

109. Scott, J. E., and Newton, D. J.: The recovery and characterization of acid glycosaminoglycans in normal human urine. Influence of a circadian rhythm, Connect. Tissue Res. 3:157–164, 1975.

110. Simmons, D. J., Ellsasser, J. C., Cummins, H., and Lesker, P.: The bone inductive potential of a composite bone allograft-marrow autograft in rabbits, Clin. Orthop. 97:237–247, 1973.

111. Simmons, D. J., Sherman, N. E., and Lesker, P. A.: Allograft induced osteoinduction in rats. A circadian rhythm, Clin. Orthop. 103:252–261, 1974.

112. Simmons, D. J., Lesker, P. A., and Ellsasser, J. C.: Survival of osteocompetent cells in vitro and the effect of PHA-stimulation on osteoinduction in composite bone grafts, Proc. Soc. Exp. Biol. Med. 143:986–989, 1975.

113. Simmons, D. J., Bratberg, J. J., Lesker, P. A., and Aab, L.: What is the best time of day to schedule a bone graft operation? Clin. Orthop. 116:227–239, 1976.

114. Simmons, D. J., Lesker, P. A., Cohen, M., and McDonald, D.: Chronobiology of fracture healing. *In* Lassmann, G., and Seitelberger, F. (eds.): Rhythmische Funktionen in Biologischen Systemen, Teil II, pp. 140–150, Facultas-Verlag, Wien, 1977.

115. Simmons, D. J., and Kahn, A. J.: Cell lineage in fracture healing in chimeric bone grafts, Calcif. Tissue Int. 27:247–253, 1979.

116. Simmons, D. J., Cohn D. V., Jilka, R. L., Kent, G. N., and Whiteside, L. A.: Isolated PT cells grown in vitro are osteogenic, Trans. Orthop. Res. Soc. 5:343, 1980.

116a. Simmons, D. J., Whiteside, L. A., and Whitson, S. W.: Biorhythmic profiles in the rat skeleton, Metab. Bone Dis. 2:49–64, 1979.

117. Slatis, P., Karaharju, E., Holmstrom, T. Ahomen, J., and Paavolainen, P.: Structural changes in intact tubular bone after application of rigid plates with and without compression, J. Bone Joint Surg. 60A:516–522, 1978.

118. Smith, J. E. M.: Internal fixation in the treatment of fractures of the shaft of the radius and ulna in adults. The value of delayed operation in the prevention of non-union, J. Bone Joint Surg. 41B:28–31, 1959.

119. Smith, J. E. M.: The results of early and delayed internal fixation of fractures of the shaft of the femur, J. Bone Joint Surg. 46B:28–31, 1964.

120. Smith, J. E. M., and Sage, F. P.: Medullary fixation of forearm fractures, J. Bone Joint Surg. 39A:91–98, 1957.

121. Smith, J. E. M.: Results of early and delayed internal fixation for tibial shaft fractures, J. Bone Joint Surg. 56B:469–477, 1974.

122. Sonstegard, D. A., and Matthews, L. S.: Sonic diagnosis of bone fracture healing—a preliminary study, J. Biomechanics 9:689–694, 1976.

123. Spadaro, J. A.: Electrically stimulated bone growth in animals and man, Clin. Orthop. 122:325–332, 1977.

124. Staheli, L. T.: Femoral and tibial growth following femoral shaft fracture in childhood, Clin. Orthop. 55L:159–163, 1967.

125. Stevenson, J. S., Bright, R. W., and Dunson, G. L.: Technicium-99m phosphate bone imaging: a method for assessing bone graft healing. Radiology 110:391–394, 1974.

126. Szabo, Z., and Szabo, G.: The effect of hemorrhage and bone fracture on bone marrow circulation, Res. Exp. Med. 172:7–17, 1978.

127. Teitelbaum, S. L., Stewart, C. C., and Kahn, A. J.: Rodent peritoneal macrophages as bone resorbing cells, Calcif. Tissue Int. 27:255–261, 1979.

128. Tonna, E. A., and Cronkite, E. P.: Cellular response to fracture studied with tritiated thymidine. J. Bone Joint Surg. 43A:352–362, 1961.

129. Truesdale, E. D.: Inequality of the lower extremities following fracture of the shaft of the femur in children, Ann. Surg. 74:498–500, 1921.

130. Tull, S. M., and Singh, A. D.: The osteoinductive property of decalcified bone matrix, J. Bone Joint Surg. 60B:116–123, 1978.

131. Urist, M. R., and Johnson, R. W., Jr.: Calcification and ossification. IV. Healing of fractures in man under clinical conditions, J. Bone Joint Surg. 25:375–426, 1943.

132. Urist, M. R., Matzet, R., Jr., and McLean, F. C.: The pathogenesis and treatment of delayed union and non-union. A survey of eighty-five ununited fractures of the shaft of the tibia and one hundred control cases with similar injuries, J. Bone Joint Surg. 34A:931–967, 1954.

133. Urist, M. R., Wallace, T. H., and Adams, T.: The function of fibrocartilaginous fracture callus. Observations on transplants labelled with tritiated thymidine, J. Bone Joint Surg. 47B:304–318, 1965.

134. Urist, M. R., Silverman, B. F., Buring, K., Dubuc, F. L., and Rosenberg, J. M.: The bone induction principle, Clin. Orthop. 59:59–96, 1968.

135. Urist, M. R., Iwata, H., and Strates, B. S.: Bone morphogenetic protein and proteinase in the guinea pig, Clin. Orthop. 85:275–290, 1972.

136. Urist, M. R., and Hisashi, I.: Preservation and biodegradation of the morphogenetic property of bone matrix, J. Theoret. Biol. 38:155–167, 1973.

137. Urist, M. R., Iwata, H., Ceccotti, P. L., Dorfman, R. L., Boyd, S. D., McDowell, R. M., and Chien, C.: Bone morphogenesis in implants of insoluble bone gelatin, Proc. Natl. Acad. Sci, (U.S.A.) 70:3511–3515, 1973.

138. Urist, M. R., and Hernandez, A.: Excitation transfer in bone. Deleterious effects of cobalt-60 radiation-sterilization of bank bone, Arch. Surg. 109:436–493, 1974.

139. Urist, M. R., Mikulski, A., and Conteas, C. N.: Reversible extinction of the morphogen in bone matrix by reduction and oxidation of disulfide bonds, Calcif. Tissues Res. 19:73–83, 1975.

140. Veldhuijzen, J. P., Bourret, L. A., and Rodan, G. A.: In vitro studies of the effect of intermittant compressive forces on cartilage cell proliferation, J. Cell. Physiol. 98:299–306, 1979.

141. von der Mark, H., von der Mark, K. and Gay, S.: Study of differential collagen synthesis during development of the chick embryo by im-

munofluorescence. II. Localization of Type I and Type II collagen during long bone development, Dev. Biol. 55:153–170, 1976.

142. von der Mark, K., and von der Mark, H.: The role of three genetically distinct collagen types in endochondral ossification and calcification of cartilage, J. Bone Joint Surg. 59B:458–463, 1977.

143. Wahner, H. W.: Radionuclides in the diagnosis of fracture healing. J. Nucl. Med. 19:1356–1357, 1978.

144. Walker, D. G.: Control of bone resorption by hematopoietic tissue. The induction and reversal of congenital osteopetrosis in mice through use of bone marrow and splenic transplants, J. Exp. Med. 142:651–663, 1975.

145. Weinberg, E. D., and Ward, G. E.: Diathermy and regeneration of bone, Arch. Surg. 28:1121–1129, 1934.

146. Wendenberg, B.: Mineral metabolism of fractures of the tibia in man studied with external counting of Sr⁸⁵. Acta Orthop. Scand. (Suppl.) 52:1–79, 1961.

147. Whiteside, L. A., Reynolds, F. C., Lesker, P. A., and Ogata, K.: Effect of acute bone autograft on early fracture healing. Surg. Forum XXVIII: 488–490, 1977.

148. Whiteside, L. A., and Lesker, P. A.: The effects of extraperiosteal and subperiosteal dissection. II. On fracture healing, J. Bone Joint Surg. 60A:26–30, 1978.

149. Wilber, M. C., and Evans, E. B.: Fractures of the femoral shaft treated surgically. Comparative results of early and delayed operative stabilization, J. Bone Joint Surg. 60A:489–491, 1978.

150. Woo, S. L.-Y., Akeson, W. H., Levenetz, B., Coutts, R. D., Matthews, J. V., and Amiel, D.: Potential application of graphite fiber and methylmethacrylate resin composites as internal fixation plates, J. Biomed. Mater. Res. 8:321–338, 1974.

151. Wood, S. K.: Growth disturbance following femoral fracture in children, J. Bone Joint Surg. 54B:201, 1972.

152. Wray, J. B., and Goodman, H.: Post-fracture vascular phenomena and long-bone overgrowth in the immature skeleton of the rat, J. Bone Joint Surg. 43A:1047–1055, 1961.

153. Yablon, I. G., and Cruess, R. L.: The effect of hyperbaric oxygenation on fracture healing in rats, J. Trauma 8:162–202, 1968.

154. Yasuda, I.: Electrical callus and callus formation by ELECTRET, Clin. Orthop. 124:53–56, 1977.

155. Young, R. W.: Cell proliferation and specialization during endochondral osteogenesis in young rats, J. Cell Biol. 14:357, 1962.

156. Young, R. W.: Specialization of bone cells. In Frost, H. M. (ed.): Bone Biodynamics, Boston, Little Brown & Co., 1964.

Bone is one of the most frequently transplanted tissues in the body, and it is routinely used for the repair of defects from injury, neoplasms, congenital malformations, and infections. Tissue banks also issue far more units of bone than skin, fascia, tendons, dura, arteries, veins, or any other part of the body. The reason is that bone performs an allostructural function and its encorporation does not depend upon tissue survival. Bone, particularly cortical bone, as free of marrow as possible, is very slowly resorbed and incites a relatively low immune response. Bone also induces an embryonic type of bone morphogenetic response even in postfetal life. This unique response is the basis of the high regenerative capacity of the skeleton of higher vertebrates and has been the object of laboratory and clinical investigations for over a century. The subject is only just beginning to be explored with the aid of the incisive methods of modern molecular biochemistry.

Bone grafts, implants, and their derivatives

Present knowledge of bone graft surgery encompasses the field of bone cell differentiation, the mechanism of osteoinduction, and the immunology of allogeneic transplants and implants. The international terminology relating to the principles and practice of bone graft surgery conforms to the general field of transplantation surgery. The terminology, presented in Table 11-1, is based on the genome of the donor and the recipient's immunosurveillance not only of viable bone grafts but also of biochemical components of nonviable alloimplants. The term implant applies to nonviable bone that has been frozen, freeze-dried, or sterilized by irradiation. The term also applies to bone exposed to chemical solutions for extraction of antigenic substances or for chemosterilization. Implants of chemically extracted chemosterilized bone, in the strict sense, are not bone but are derivatives of bone.

MARSHALL R. URIST

bone transplants and implants *

* Supported by a grant in aid from the USPHS, NIH, NIDR #DE02103, Kroc Foundation, Solo Cup Foundation, and the Harcourt Fund.

TABLE 11-1 OLD AND NEW TERMINOLOGY FOR BONE GRAFT OPERATIONS*

OLD NOUN	OLD ADJECTIVE	NEW NOUN	NEW ADJECTIVE	DONOR
Autograft	Autologous	Autograft	Autogeneic	Same individual
Isograft	Isogenous	Isograft	Isogeneic	Identical twin or inbred strain
Homograft	Homogenous	Allograft	Allogeneic	Same species, living
Homoimplant	Homogenous	Alloimplant†	Allogeneic	Same species, dead
Heterograft	Heterogenous	Xenograft	Xenogeneic	Another species
Heteroimplant	Heterogenous	Xenoimplant	Xenogeneic	Another species

* Modified from Russe., P. S., and Monaco, A. P.: The Biology of Tissue Transplantation, Boston, Little Brown & Co., 1965.
† An alloimplant is nonviable bone prepared by chemical agents, irradiation sterilization, freezing or freeze-drying, and so forth. The term lyophilization means "promotion of lysis" and is not applicable to bone because vacuum drying does not facilitate solubilization of bone matrix, as occurs with vacuum drying of purified soluble substances.

Survival of donor cells

A relatively small number of the donor's cells in compact bone and a large number of these cells in cancellous bone survive autologous transplantation. The proliferation of histocompatible cells accounts for the obvious superiority of autologous over allogeneic bone for transplantation. Autologous osteoprogenitor cells, or preosteoblasts proliferate and bridge the gap between the surfaces of donor and recipient. The earliest deposits, identifiable either by sex chromatin[1] or by ^{3}H-thymidine-labeling techniques,[55] develop from the preosteoblasts. Transplanted osteocytes generally die in response to anoxia and injury of surgery. The dead cells disintegrate by autolysis and leave empty lacunae.

Preosteoclasts, preosteoblasts, and osteoclasts may survive transplantation. Transplanted osteoclasts may initiate resorption of the donor tissue but the process of resorption depends upon revascularization.

Osteoclasts

Observations on parabiosed rats by Buring[7] affirm the theory that preosteoclasts and osteoclasts are derived from the monocyte-macrophage cell lines. The preosteoclast precursor cells originate from blood-borne bone marrow–derived cells that migrate into areas of bone formation generally concurrent with the remodeling of woven bone into lamellar bone. Consequently, the generation of preosteoclasts and osteoclasts first requires transport of precursor cells through the blood stream and then requires

such microenvironmental factors as found in remodeling bone. Too few of the donor tissue osteoclasts survive transplantation to be identified either in an allograft or in a composite bone graft. It is possible that multinucleation and osteoclast formation occur only on mineralized living bone surfaces. Transplantation of demineralized allogeneic bone powders induce aggregation of foreign body–type multinucleated cells called matrix-clasts. These possibly develop by fusion of macrophages and may or may not be entirely comparable to osteoclasts. Osteoclasts are activated by parathyroid hormone, osteoclast-activating factor, and other agents unrelated to foreign body giant cell phagocytic functions. The ultimate fate of osteoclasts is not known. Fission and recycling along a preosteoblast line of development seems not to have been ruled out.

Revascularization

In autografts of embryonic bone rudiments onto chorionic allantoic membrane and in transplants of postfetal cancellous bone, the tissue circulation is restored by formation of microanastomoses.[25,55,29] Microanastomoses restore circulation, supply nutrients for synthesis of cell products, support proliferation of osteoprogenitor cells and sustain differentiation of new osteoblasts as well as formation of new osteoclasts. Proliferation occurs in a layer of only about 1 mm of the bone tissue of the surface of an autograft that is in direct contact with the recipient bone bed. Alloimplants revascularize—not by microanastomosis but by invasion of capillary sprouts from the host bed during the process of resorption of the old matrix.

Vascularized bone grafts

Bone defects caused by resection of tumors are sometimes too large to successfully bridge even with autologous bone. Two- or three-stage supplementary operations may be necessary to restore the continuity of the bone. Two new surgical approaches are used in an effort to perform a massive autologous bone graft operation in one stage. The first is a muscle pedicle bone graft. The second is a vascularized pedicle graft. The muscle pedicle graft is limited in applicability to a few anatomical sites, that is, fibula to tibia, and so forth. Vascular pedicle and free vascularized grafts, stemming from recent advances in microvascular surgery, have almost unlimited applicability. The transplant is constructured of bone and soft tissue. The donor tissue blood vessels are joined by end-to-end anastomosis to host blood vessels inside the recipient bed. The diameter of donor and host bed vessels must approximate each other as closely as possible. The operation is long, tedious, and difficult. The donor sites are generally rib, iliac crest, clavicle, and fibula. Angiographic studies and rehearsal of the procedure on a cadaver are absolutely essential. When the operation is successful, the process of bone repair is more like a segmental fracture than a free bone graft, and the healing time is correspondingly reduced. The indications for free vascular pedicle bone grafts are bone loss from extensive injury, bone tumor defects, irradiated recipient fields, and congenital pseudoarthrosis.

Autologous bone graft incorporation

The process of envelopment and interdigitation of the donor bone tissue with new bone deposited by the recipient is termed incorporation. Interdigitation occurs during resorption of variable quantities of the old dead bone and by remodeling of the new living bone structure. In the course of remodeling, all surfaces of contact between new and old bone are covered with a film of metachromatic-staining cement substance. The zone of interdigitation and the quantity of resorbed donor bone is greater in cancellous than in cortical bone autografts and greater in autografts than in alloimplants. In every case, the end point of incorporation falls short of complete replacement by entirely living bone. The bulk of the unresorbed structure of the donor may be as much as 90% of the volume of a cortical bone graft in an adult recipient. The donor tissue may be unresorbed for as long as 20 yr after the operation. In growing bones in children, bone resorption and new tissue remodeling is so much more rapid than in adults that only microscopic quantities of the structure of the donor may be recognizable by the second year after the operation.

Enneking[24] quantitatively analyzed the rate at which cortical bone autografts are incorporated and the relationship between the stage of incorporation and the physical properties of the transplanted bone by measuring resorption, apposition, porosity, and cumulative new bone formation within the transplant. In dogs, a 4-cm diaphyseal cortical autograft is substantially weakened by porosity at 6 wk to 6 mo and does not completely recover after 1 yr. Resorption produces porosity rapidly over a period of 6 wk, whereas apposition reduces porosity, occurs relatively slowly and increases gradually in the interval from 8 to 12 wk after the operation.

Whereas appositional bone formation in the skeleton as a whole is regulated by the metabolic rate, the progress of resorption of the transplanted bone process procedes independent of systemic skeletal metabolism. The spatial pattern of repair is also ordered rather than random. Torsional stress failure is correlated more with porosity than with microanastomic features. Most remarkable, the interstitial lamellae are unreplaced and are retained as islands of necrotic matrix. Thus, the strength of the transplant is inversely proportional to the porosity rather than to the completeness of incorporation. After 48 wk of incorporation when the physical resistance to torsional stress is nearly normal, only about 60% of the structure of the transplant has been resorbed and replaced by new bone. A large part of the nearly 40% unreplaced bone consists of unresorbed interstitial lamallae (densely calcified old dead bone filling spaces between osteons).

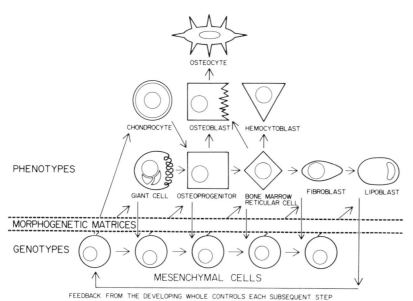

FIGURE 11-1 *Diagrammatic representation of the spectrum of phenotypic differentiation in a bone morphogenetic response to an implant of bone matrix. The process is morphogenetic because it leads to the development of an ossicle composed of a cortex and a marrow cavity filled with hematopoietic tissue.*

Osteoconduction

The three-dimensional process of ingrowth of sprouting capillaries, perivascular tissue, and osteoprogenitor cells from the recipient bed into the structure of an implant or bone graft is called osteoconduction. Osteoconduction occurs within a framework of nonbiologic materials such as glass tubes, ceramics, and plastics, as well as within nonviable biologic materials such as autoclaved bone, deproteinized bone, chemosterilized, demineralized-trypsinized bone and frozen or freeze-dried allogeneic bone. In nonbiologic frameworks, osteoconduction may occur without resorption of the implanted material. In the incorporation of a bone graft, osteoconduction

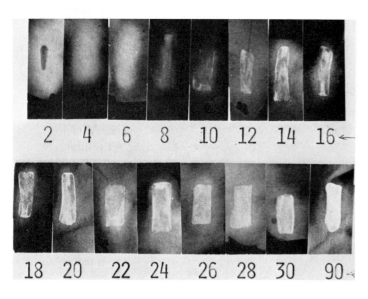

FIGURE 11-2 Roentgenograms of alloimplants of demineralized bone, illustrating the time sequences in matrix-induced heterotopic bone formation in muscle in rats. An air bubble occupies the center of the implant at 2 d, and areas of increased soft tissue density delineate the implant at the 4 and 6 d intervals. By the 8th d, the outlines of the implanted matrix are radiopaque and by the 10th to the 18th d, deposits of calcified new woven bone appear. In the intervals from the 20th to the 90th d, the new woven bone is remodeled into lamellar bone and there is a corresponding progressive increase in radiopacity.

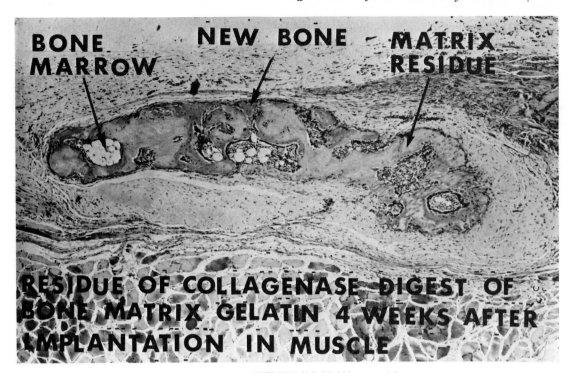

BONE MARROW **NEW BONE** **MATRIX RESIDUE**

RESIDUE OF COLLAGENASE DIGEST OF BONE MATRIX GELATIN 4 WEEKS AFTER IMPLANTATION IN MUSCLE

FIGURE 11-3 *Photomicrograph of the undigested remnant of rat bone matrix gelatin that had been incubated in a solution of bacterial collagenase for 24 hr and then implanted in a muscle. The formation of new bone and bone marrow in and upon the surfaces of the implant in volumes equal to the matrix residue suggest that BMP is collagenase-resistant. The same experiment performed with trypsin produces no bone and is evidence that BMP is trypsin-labile.*

and osteoinduction are inter-related processes; as a consequence, the donor tissue is more rapidly and more completely incorporated than is any kind of nonbiologic material.

Differentiation of new bone cells by induction

The process of recruitment of mesenchymal-type cells into cartilage and bone under the influence of a diffusible bone morphogenetic protein (BMP) is termed osteoinduction. Present evidence for a diffusible BMP[81] is derived from observations on transplants, implants, and soluble hydrophobic glycoproteins in muscle pouches.[80,81] The mode of action of BMP is not known. Hypothetically, a BMP would diffuse from the organic matrix of the donor to cell surface receptors of mesenchymal type cells of the recipient (Figs. 11-1–11-3). Tangible evidence in support of this hypothesis is lacking because

immunochemical localization on cell surfaces will be possible only when a well-purified BMP becomes available.

Historically, there are two unresolved diametrically opposed theories about the origin of bone cells in postfetal life. The first and longest-held theory is that in postfetal life, new bone develops from pre-existing bone, particularly a population of osteoprogenitor cells (preosteoblasts) in periosteum endosteum, marrow reticulum.[4,29,55] The second and newest theory is that new osteoprogenitor cells are recruited by induction of residual mesenchymal-type cells in marrow reticulum, endosteum, periosteum, and even in the connective tissue framework of the surrounding muscle.[10–12,19,31,33,44,47,48,56,68,69] Both theories are correct because in an autologous graft new bone originates in early stages from surviving osteoprogenitor cells, and in later stages from the inductive response of the host.

Conceptually, the inductive process is regulated by a diffusion gradient of BMP.[76] The arguments against the osteoinduction concept is the supposition that nonspecific injury[92] can incite proliferation of osteoprogenitor cells and generation of bone. A further supposition is that cells of regenerating injured muscle may grow into nonbiologic or nonviable bone implants by osteoconduction alone. Even though pre-existing preosteoblasts are sufficient to account for the superiority of autografts over alloimplants of bone, the evidence for the osteoinduction concept is firmly supported by experimental research. In rats, bone cells differentiate in postfetal life in implants of either nonviable demineralized bone matrix or soluble BMP in a diffusion chamber in muscle pouch with no possible contact with pre-existing bone or significant damage to muscle. Moreover, the quantity of new bone is proportional to the mass of the matrix implant or the dose of the BMP.[78]

The literature on the biochemistry of BMP[81] and the physiology of the mesenchymal cell response is extensive in laboratory rodents but relatively limited in dogs, monkeys, human beings, and other long-lived animals.[56,68-86] Mesenchymal-type cells with a high level of competence to respond to BMP are present in the connective tissue framework of muscle, tendon, fascia, subcutis, and other somatic structures. The same structures exhibit a significantly lower level of competence in long-lived animals. In human beings, a mesenchymal cell population with a level of competence to respond to BMP comparable to that in rodent muscle is found in bone marrow stroma. That muscle and other somatic connective tissue mesenchymal cells are competent to respond to BMP and produce heterotopic bone is easy to observe in animals. That heterotopic bone formation is induced by injury to muscle attachments to bone[92] and by other regional or local disorders is also commonly observed in patients. In fact, the propensity of the muscle connective tissues to produce bone is hardly realized and is as yet unexpressed for useful purposes of reconstructive surgery. This propensity is strikingly demonstrated by an extraordinarily wide, but highly specific, variety of experimental models. For example, transplants of urinary bladder, HeLa cells, placenta, and vaccinia-transformed fibroblasts induce muscle

mesenchymal-type cells to differentiate into bone.[49,90] The biochemical mechanism is unknown but clearly develops through epithelial mesenchymal cell interaction. Clinically, as will be outlined in detail in Chapter 11, mesenchymal cells differentiate into bone in response to trauma, paraplegia, total hip arthroplasties, and urinary bladder operations. With allowances for species-specific differences in competence, bone matrix–induced bone formation is the most consistently reproducible of any of these heterotopic systems.

BMP is a hydrophobic glycoprotein and evokes a cross-species bone morphogenetic response.[81] Speculation about net positive or negative surface alterations, streaming potentials, and prizoelectric effects as possible mechanisms of bone induction are now under intensive investigation by research workers all over the world. Whatever the net surface charge on an osteoinductive alloimplant may prove to have, the matrix of bone transplants have a BMP component that distinguishes bone-inducing from noninducing systems. This component also might be proved by further research to account for the capacity of bone to remodel in postfetal life and to regenerate following transplantation.

Immune response to allogeneic bone

Bone transplantation antigens

The term antigen means that which generates antagonism in the form of antibodies. Antigens derived from a bone transplant or implant are termed transplantation antigens. The immune response to bone transplantation alloantigens is chiefly cell mediated. There are three methods of isolating transplantation antigens from bone: extraction with detergents, extraction with fat solvents, and autodigestion.[43,57] Lipid extraction with chloroform-methanol and autodigestion constitute an efficient combination of methods of removal of transplantation antigens from the organic matrix of bone. A hydrophobic glycopeptide (HGP), extractable from allogeneic cortical bone as well as from other tissues by chloroform-methanol, has the essential properties of a transplantation antigen and is designated a haptenic antimorphogen. When combined with HGP, bone matrix induces differentiation not of osteoprogenitor cells but of mononuclear leukocytes and fibrous connective tissue cells that block the bone morphogenetic response of the recipient.[45]

Rejection by sequestration

An immune reaction, either cell mediated or humoral in nature, against a graft is termed rejection. The rejection of a skin graft is grossly visible by discoloration, separation, and shedding of the donor tissue from the host bed. Other organ grafts are buried in the body and sequestered by the host, but the immune reactions are the same. An immune reaction may be hyperacute, acute, or chronic. The hyperacute rejection is immediate and is the product of preformed antibodies initiating deposition of fibrin, platlet aggregation, neutrophil aggregation, and failure of the graft to survive. The acute rejection is delayed in onset but eventually has the same destructive end result. The chronic rejection is slowly progressive and gradually leads to isolation of the graft in a cocoon of fibrous tissue. The second set phenomenon is the antibody production and cell-mediated immunity induced by a previous first graft in the same host with the result that the rejection reaction is intensified.

The reaction to a free bone transplant differs from the reaction to skin and other organ transplants in that over 90% of the donor tissue does not survive the loss of blood supply. A rejected bone graft may be indistinguishable from the host bone for months. Only after a period of tissue development is the rejected donor tissue sequestered in a fibrous connective envelope formed by the host plasma cell, macrophage, and reticulocyte phase of the host immune response. This response blockades the transfer of BMP from the donor to the recipient bed and the osteoinductive response of the host.

In either autografts or allografts, osteocytes autolyse and disappear within the first day after the transplantation. Relatively few osteocytes are situated on surfaces in which survival by perfusion with the recipient bed tissue fluid is possible. In a cancellous bone autograft, osteo-cytes conceivably may survive for a few days, but eventually nucleases and other intracellular proteases autolyse osteocytes and release nucleoproteins. At the same time, extracellular proteases solubilize extracellular proteins of bone matrix.[67,71,74,75] The solubilized proteins and antigenic tissue degradation products are absorbed by the lymphatic system of the recipient.[3,4,10–12,14,15]

The infiltration of perivascular tissues and the blockage of capillaries in the zone of interdigitation of donor and recipient structures (about 14 d after an allograft or about 21 to 28 d after an alloimplant) are called a delayed hypersensitivity reaction. The reaction is more intense in xenoimplants and allografts than in alloimplants. Morphologically, the delayed hypersensitivity reaction resembles a tuberculin reaction. It is intense and prolonged in xenoimplants. It is weak and subsides in freeze-dried whole bone alloimplants in 6 to 8 wk. With the subsidence of the delayed hypersensitivity reaction, leukocytes are replaced by an envelope of fibrous scar tissue between the structure of the recipient and the donor. The thickness of the scar is proportional to the intensity of the delayed hypersensitivity reaction. Formation of microanastomoses between the blood vessels of the recipient and the donor tissue is obstructed by the delayed hypersensitivity reaction (Fig. 11-4).[3,29]

Antigenicity of freeze-dried bone implants

Indirect measurements of antigenicity by established immunologic techniques,[21,23] such as rejection time of skin grafts, lymph node localized enlargements, lymphocyte microtoxicity, and migration inhibition of leukocytes, are placed in a realistic perspective for the field of bone graft surgery by an important study by Burchardt and Ennecking.[5] Until Burchardt and coworkers made direct controlled quantitative histometric and biophysical observations on bone, freeze-drying was claimed to reduce antigenicity of allogeneic bone. This claim was based on indirect measurements and is now known to be unfounded. Freeze-dried allogeneic bone does not unite with the host bed as does either freeze-dried nonviable autologous bone or fresh viable

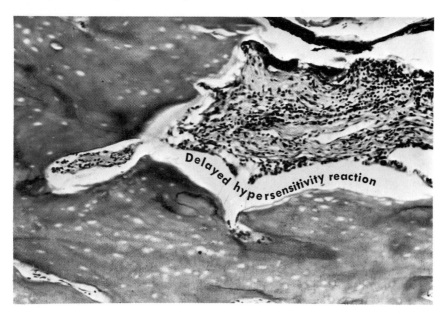

FIGURE 11-4 *Photomicrograph of an implant of aseptically collected whole freeze-dried rat allogeneic cortical bone in a muscle pouch, 4 wk after the operation. Note the acellular graft and collection of small, round cells surrounding the donor tissue, characteristic of an immune response of the recipient.*

autologous bone. Freeze-drying preserves enough donor cell antigen in allogeneic cancellous to incite a lymphocyte, plasma cell, and macrophage response at the interface between donor and host bed. This response blockades and transfer of BMP from the bone matrix of the donor to the responding mesenchymal cells of the host (see subsequent discussion).[45]

Alloimplant

A substitute for a bone graft derived from bone tissue of an individual of the same species that contains no viable cells is an alloimplant. An alloimplant prepared by freezing, freeze-drying, irradiation sterilization, or chemosterilization contains a full compliment of dead cells. When prepared by autolytic digestion and chemo-sterilization, an alloimplant contains few or no donor cells.[72,74,75] The components of the donor that are transferred to the recipient by an alloimplant are minerals, cell debris, enzymes, noncollagenous proteins, and collagen. All of the components of an alloimplant constitute alloantigen, but the least antigenic component is colla-

gen. Cortical bone is preferred for preparation of alloimplants because of the relatively large quantity of collagen and low antigenic activity. Because of its relatively high antigenic activity, cancellous bone is rapidly disappearing from use for alloimplantation.

Morphological and immunologic evaluations of a bone graft

Morphological incorporation or restoration of skeletal continuity is the only acceptable end point for evaluation of a bone graft operation. This end point is most likely to be reached with autologous bone and is unlikely to be reached with xenogeneic bone or irradiation-sterilized allogeneic bone. The order of probability that other allogeneic bone will be incorporated is as follows: autolysed antigen-extracted allogeneic (AAA) bone > freeze-dried bone > whole frozen bone.[73] Immunologic data indicate that cytotoxic serum (humoral) antibodies are produced by transplanted allogeneic bone and bone marrow grafts but not by the isologous bone grafts or grafts killed by low-dose irradiation, freezing, or freeze-drying.[22] The correlation of serum antibodies with the destruction of donor cells is positive in grafts with living cells that secrete transplantation antigens. The correlation is negative in grafts of nonviable allogeneic bone. The correlation is also negative with high-dose (3.5 mrad) irradiation-sterilized bone[8,9,77] but not with low-dose (3–5000 rad) irradiation devitalized bone.[22] The denaturation of BMP by high-dose irradiation is so complete as to advise against any further use of irradiation-sterilized bone in patients.[77]

Allografts

Autografts are routine for all kinds of orthopedic operations. Bone allografts are hardly even recommended. Soluble proteins, both intracellular (particularly nucleoproteins and ribonucleoproteins) and some extracellular proteins absorbed by the recipient of an allograft, are chemotactic for blood-borne mononuclear cells and initiate a cell-mediated immune response.[3,4,10–12,14,15] An allograft may survive if the donor is a parent or sibling, and tissue types of the donor and recipient match or if immunosuppression[25] is achieved in the recipient. Although documented cases suggest that living bone allografts are better than nonviable alloimplants, there is a significant amount of information only in recent literature on joint surface replacements with osteochondral allografts in patients with arthritis or tumors. The rationale in this line of research is that the host response to joint cartilage is different from the host response to bone.

Humoral immune response

Elves[21] reviewed the literature on the humoral antibodies produced by allografts and observed that marrow-containing cancellous bone elicited a typical pattern of antibody production. The humoral response was not as rapid as the response to allogeneic spleen cells injected intradermally, but it was nevertheless measurable. Marrow-free cortical and washed cancellous bone also gave rise to a humoral antibody response, but it was delayed in onset. Cytotoxic antibodies were identified in serum using donor

blood lymphocytes, and fluorochromatic microcytotoxicity plates were incubated at 20° C for 1 hr before the reactions were read. Serum samples, in which at least 25% of the lymphocytes were killed, were regarded as positive, but in most instances, 75% to 100% of lymphocytes were killed. Combined with the first and second set skin graft rejection time, these methods demonstrate the levels of the host humoral response to allografts of bone. Control grafts that are identical with the host for major Ag-B antigen systems fail to elicit a humoral immune response. Irradiation sterilization, freezing, or freeze-drying reduced the capacity of donor cells to secrete antigen and elicit a measurable humoral antibody response in short-term experiments in some strains of rats. However, in children exposed to large doses of antigen released by large doses of irradiated freeze-dried allogeneic bone, antibodies are measurable in the circulating blood for several years after the operation.[32,88]

Efforts to eliminate antigenicity

Graft rejection times in mice cannot be extrapolated to support claims that freeze-dried bone is less antigenic than frozen bone for bone graft operations.[6] Indeed, in preference to immediate freeze-drying or deep-freezing, which preserves undesirable antigenic material, Parrish[51] recommends first refrigeration for at least 3 wk, then chemical sterilization and extraction for at least 3 wk, and treatment in antibiotic solutions before implantation. Clinically, the product appears better tolerated than aseptically collected freeze-dried bone for large bone defects created by resection of tumors, and it is relatively slowly resorbed. Similar empirical observations have been reported by Cloward[17] and others.[12,14,89]

Enhancement

Langer and colleagues[47] demonstrated by three different methods that frozen allogeneic implants are immunogenic. By means of leukocyte migration, donor skin graft rejection time, and humoral cytotoxic antibody titer determinations, inbred strains of rats can be observed to produce an immune response to frozen allogeneic bone implants. However, recipients of both allografts and frozen allogeneic implants eventually develop enhancing factors that block detectable immunity and seem to protect the graft from rejection. The evidence for the phenomenon of blocking (enhancement) is defined as inhibition of transplantation immunity by the formation of serum blocking factors, which are believed to affix to the cells that are responsible for rejection, thus neutralizing their activity.

The levels of humoral cytoxic antibodies are sustained until 4 wk after transplantation of living allografts. In rats, humoral cytotoxic antibodies were not detectable in recipients of deep-frozen allogeneic implants. Both living and nonliving allogeneic bone accelerated the time of rejection of the skin grafts and prolonged the local inflammatory cell reaction to the donor tissue. In fact, the intensity of the inflammatory reaction was the same in both living and nonliving allogeneic bone for the first 8 wk after the operation. After 8 wk, blocking (enhancement) may have occurred and produced acceptance, the same being true in a frozen nonviable alloimplant as in an allograft. Blocking is attributable to substances present in the sera of bone graft recipients that can act to abrogate the normally observed transplantation immunity to allografts. Langer and coworkers[38] also conclude that because fresh viable allografts are acceptable, tissue matching for HL-A transplantation antigens should not be necessary. The facts that cytotoxic antibodies were only detectable in recipients of fresh allografts during the first 4 wk after grafting and that a similar pattern of toxic antibody levels has been described in animals with enhanced renal allografts would not have any bearing on bone grafts in which the donor tissue does not survive. A fact not sufficiently taken into consideration is that the immune response to either allografts or frozen bone alloimplants destroys the osteoinductive property, which is the critical difference between autologous and allogeneic donor tissues and accounts for the superiority of an autograft. Moreover, to validate the conclusions of Langer and colleagues[38] from experiments on small transplants in rats, it would be necessary to duplicate the data in patients with massive, slowly resorbing allografts and alloimplants.

Relevance of measurements of the alloantibody response in animal inbred strains

Total diaphyseal grafts in eight different strains of allogeneic mice by Halloran and colleagues[28] demonstrated that healing is impaired and skin graft rejection is accelerated by H-2 and H-7 antigens. Living immunogenic cells of the donor survived in the recipient for at least 4 wk. Comparable grafts that were frozen and thawed before transplantation were non immunogenic. These results in mice are contrary to observations in dogs and humans that indicate that frozen, freeze-dried, and irradiation-sterilized bone is not incorporated as early or as completely as either similarly devitalized autologous or chemosterilized antigen-extraced allogenic bone.[6,67] The explanation may be that quantities of alloantigen too small to be detected by skin graft rejection, microtoxicity, or cell migration inhibition tests are sufficient to produce enough cell-mediated immunity to blockade the transfer of BMP including the osteoinductive response of the recipient bed. Whether the enhancement factors are sufficient to permit the host osteoinductive response is not known.

Joint cartilage and subchondral bone allografts

Even though the underlying subchondral bone cells die, articular cartilage cells obtained from an autopsy subject within a very few hours after death may survive transplantation. Tissue typing, blood grouping, and leukocyte migration inhibition tests on donor cartilage show the expected evidence of histoincompatibility. However, there is no correlation of 2-yr successful transplants with immunocapability of the donor and host. Mankin and coworkers[42] preserved human allografts in 10% glycerol putatively to retain viability of cartilage during the process of freezing down to −70° C, and reported successes in 3-yr follow-up examinations. These observations on patients are supported by experimental operations. Allografts preserved by such methods are successfully incorporated and sustain joint function for several years in cats.[62] Thus the contentions are that (1) the immune response does not interfere with incorporation of a joint allograft that is placed in broad tight contact with the host subchondral bone bed, and (2) enhancement factors may promote survival of osteochondral allografts.

Xenogeneic implants

Efforts to prepare xenogeneic bone for implantation in human beings, comparable to xenogeneic collagen that is used for suture material and hemostatic sponges, have failed to produce a histocompatible implant. Within a few days, instead of weeks as occurs with freeze-dried al-loimplants, xenogeneic implants are enveloped in a pool of acute and chronic inflammatory tissue. The envelope around a xenoimplant consists of plasma cells, lymphocytes, macrophages, and even polymorphonuclear leukocytes. Xenoimplants of massive, dense cortical bone having a small surface area or low porosity produce a quantitatively low inflammatory tissue reaction, whereas xenoimplants of particulate or cancellous grafts having a large surface area produce a massive, quantitatively high inflammatory response. The final disposition of calf or sheep bone xenoimplants is sequestration or envelopment in a fibrous envelope (Fig. 11-5). Ramani and coworkers[54] investigated xenogeneic

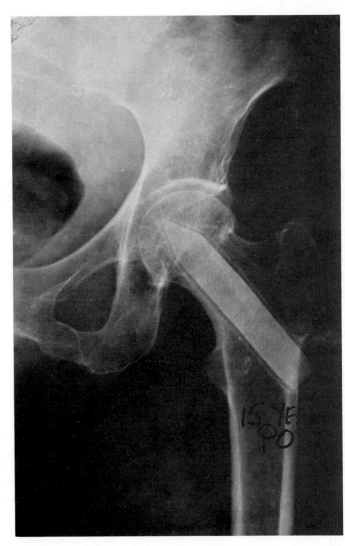

FIGURE 11-5 *Roentgenogram of a healed subcapital fracture of the hip joint 15 yr after internal fixation with a processed bovine xenoimplant (Boplant) in a 70-yr-old woman. Note the sequestration of the implant by radiolucent tissue more than 1 mm in thickness and the surrounding layer of sclerotic bone deposited by the host. (McLean, F. C., and Urist, M. R.: Bone, 3rd edition, Chicago, University of Chicago Press, 1968)*

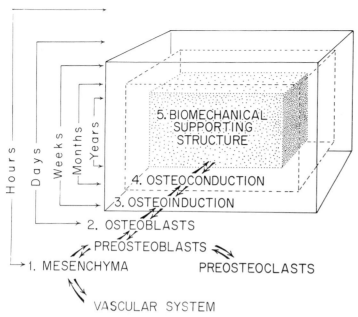

FIGURE 11-6 *Diagrammatic representation of the five phases of the incorporation of a bone graft, illustrating the three-dimensional relationships and time sequences. The end point is reached when the inert biomechanical structure of donor tissue is completely encased in remodeled lamellar bone deposits of the recipient.*

bone for anterior vertebral body fusions and observed the sequestration of the donor tissue even when arthodesis ensued. The quantity of xenogeneic protein that is sufficient to produce circulating cytotoxic antibodies in addition to a local hypersensitivity reaction is relatively small. Not even hydrogen peroxide maceration, alkali hydrolysis or detergent extraction, which either solubilizes or denatures bone collagenous as well as noncollagenous proteins, extracts enough cytotoxic antigen to produce an acceptable xenoimplant. Marrow and bone cell membranes resist degradation or digestion, persist longer than other parts of the tissue, and are believed to contain the most potent of all tissue xenoantigens.[43]

Phases of bone graft incorporation

The incorporation of autografts and properly prepared, biologically active alloimplants of bone occurs in five stages, which are illustrated diagrammatically in Fig. 11-6.

Phase 1 occurs within minutes to hours after a surgical wound and consists of inflammation, and proliferation of preosteoblasts and preosteoclasts in the recipient bed. BMP, along with various degradation products of transplanted tissue, initiates chemotactic-directional migration of cells toward all exposed surfaces outside and inside the structure of the graft. Phase 1 occurs in response to a bone graft; the same is true in autologous and allogeneic bone, irrespective of whether the donor tissue is living or dead.

Phases 2 and 3 are contiguous with phase 1; they occur from d 1 to d 7, and develop after inflammation of the surgical injury subsides. Phases 2 and 3 are characterized by the response of the recipient bed fibroblast-like mesenchymal cells to donor tissue BMP. In an autograft, BMP transfer and the osteoinductive response are also produced by secretions of osteoblasts. In an alloimplant, it is supplemented by transfer of BMP from the organic matrix to mesenchymal cell surfaces. The BMP is destroyed by autoclaving or irradiation sterilization. The osteoinductive response to BMP is *blockaded* by a hypersensitivity-like reaction, and a histoincompatibility immune response is observed by infiltration of blood-borne small, round cells, plasma cells, and reticulocytes. The blockade appears by the third week after a living allograft and by the fourth week after implantation of freeze-dried allogeneic raw bone. The blockade is further delayed and the osteoinductive response is relatively unimpeded in implants of antigen-extracted, antolysed allogeneic AAA bone.[82]

Phase 4 consists of osteoconduction and occurs over periods of months to years. Osteoconduction depends on growth of new bone *by extension* from a recipient bed. Osteoconduction is characterized by ingrowth of sprouting capillaries and new bone into nonbiologic structures such as methylmethacrylate, ceramics, and calcium sulfate or *denatured* biologic structures such as irradiation-sterilized bone or autoclaved bone. Osteoconduction is prevented by formation of a membrane of fibrous tissue between the host and donor, but it is promoted by contact compression or interdigitation of the interstices of the donor and host bone structure. In osteoconduction, the structure of the donor plays a passive role. The process is important and rapid in young, growing bones. Osteoconduction is more closely linked with osteoinductive processes in the incorporation of biologic undenatured resorbable grafts and implants than in nonbiologic nonabsorbable substances.

In phase 5, both autografts and alloimplants gradually (for periods as long as 2 to 20 yr depending on the quantity and shape of the donor tissue) perform a purely mechanical function. Successful autografts, alloimplants, and nonbiologic implants eventually become enmeshed in the structure of the recipient bone. Phase 5 is as important as the preceding four phases, because by the time the repair processes subside, only about 10% of the volume of the donor tissue may be remodeled or otherwise altered. Hence, nonviable bone (with osteocyte lacunae devoid of cells) constitutes 90% of the total mass of a successful cortical bone autograft of alloimplant. A small volume (possibly 20%) of bone with empty lacunae similarly fills cortical bone of some parts of the skeleton in aged normal individuals.

The rate of incorporation is optimum when information about the cellular activity of each phase is fed back to the preceding phase and transferred to the succeeding phase of development. Osteoinduction may occur without osteoconduction—as in osteogenesis in response to secretions of uroepithelium—but not in a bone autograft. Osteoinduction without donor-derived living osteoprogenitor cells occurs in alloimplants of demineralized freeze-dried or thimerosal (Merthiolate)-fixed bone matrix in a muscle pouch.[95] Provided that contact compression is applied to a fresh allograft, osteoinduction and osteoconduction may occur in sequence even in the presence of a delayed hypersensitivity reaction. Normally, the osteoinductive and osteoconductive phases are in a dynamic equilibrium or are closely associated processes steadily progressing toward donor tissue incorporation. The incorporation of allogeneic bone at a slower rate than autologous bone may be attributable to disassociation of osteoinductive from osteoconductive phases by delayed hypersensitivity reactions. Elimination of the osteoinductive stage, as in autoclave-sterilized, irradiation-sterilized, and β-propiolactone-sterilized, or benzalkonium-sterilized bone,[84,88] reduces the rate of incorporation. Thimersol and polyvinylpyrrolidone-iodine (Betadine) sterilization (unpublished experiments) do not extinguish the osteoinductive response in rats, but other methods of chemosterilization outlined in Table 3, are more applicable to human bone banks.

Although the experimental evidence for osteoinduction is now well established,[12,46] knowledge of the biophysical chemistry of substrata for expression of bone morphogenetic potential[90,93] is only beginning to materialize. Important information is also emerging from observations on histoincompatibility reactions that may blockade the inductive response more completely in human beings than in rats, rabbits, and other experimental animals.

Composite bone grafts

The combination of autologous iliac cancellous bone marrow and frozen or lyophilized cortical allogeneic bank bone is called a composite bone graft.[10–12,63] Burwell[12] demonstrates that either viable or nonviable frozen cortical bone serves as an osteoinductive substrate for the growth of new bone from transplants of cancellous bone or red bone marrow. Composite grafts of frozen bone and bone marrow are relatively well tolerated because almost all of the new bone is derived from the transplanted bone marrow reticulum.[52] The resorption and replacement rates as well as the quantity of bone are comparable to those of massive autologous cortical bone grafts. Composites of marrow and AAA bone or surface-demineralized allogeneic cortical bone is as effective as frozen whole bone.[52] The matrix provides the substratum for growth of transplanted iliac autologous osteogenetic cells. Salama and coworkers[60] claim that composite grafts of autologous marrow and xenogeneic calf or sheep cortical bone produces new bone in rats. No osteoinductive effect is ascribed to bovine or sheep cortical bone because the xenogeneic tissue is intensely immunogenic.

Quantitative correlated roentgenographic, histometric, and biochemical data on composite grafts of bone marrow and demineralized bone matrix or bone matrix gelatin demonstrate that a composite graft produces new bone by differentiation of marrow reticular or mesenchymal cells in the early stages and by induction of host mesenchymal cells in the later stages. By a combination of both mechanisms, the yield of new bone is always more than the sum of the yield obtained by either one alone. Of special interest is the fact that the transplantation of disaggregated marrow cells suspended in a minimum essential culture medium produces more bone than the original marrow tissue. These observations suggest that myelogenous elements and clotted blood in whole marrow may disassociate from reticular cells and when dissociation is complete, the induction is enhanced. More experimental research is required to determine how mesenchymal and reticular cells of bone marrow interact in relation to BMP.

The use of the composite graft of allogeneic bone and autologous cancellous bone marrow is necessary for treatment of patients with large bone defects, too large to fill with autologous bone alone. The composite graft is often mandatory in small children in which iliac crest and tibia combined are insufficient for a reconstructive operation. The success of a composite bone graft depends upon absolute, uninterrupted internal fixation to the host bed. Xenogeneic bone is not recommended for patients, even as a composite graft, because in human beings it incites a deleterious chronic inflammatory reaction at the interface between the donor and the recipient bone tissue. Neither chemical extraction of soluble proteins, nor freeze-drying, nor irradiation sterilization can make xenogeneic bone as well tolerated as allogeneic bone.

Conservation of viable cells

If the contributions of surviving cells of the endosteum and bone marrow stroma are important for successful incorporation of an autograft, more attention should be given to details of surgical procedure. Ideally, the recipient bed should first be thoroughly decorticated and carefully prepared. Then the graft should be excised, trimmed, and transferred from the donor site without delay or exposure to artifactual solutions. Saline solution reduces or eliminates the viability of the donor's osteoprogenitor cells.[2,53]

Bone banks

Frozen or freeze-dried aseptically excised allogeneic bone is obtained from cadavers, amputation specimens, and excised ribs and other parts of the skeleton for bone banks. The procedures for operation of a bone bank have not changed in over 40 yr of clinical investigation. The bone is cleaned of soft parts under aseptic operating room conditions, wrapped in a plastic bag, and transferred to a deep-freeze unit at a temperature of $-70°$ C. The tissue is cultured for contamination with bacterial organisms before it is encased in the plastic bag. The bone is tagged with the donors name, age, blood type, Rh factor, clinical diagnosis, date of surgical collection, serologic report, and confirmation of a negative history of tuberculosis, syphilis, hepatitis, malignancy, malaria, and gas gangrene. There is no age limitation, but young adults are preferable donors.

For many years, the bone was collected unsterile from autopsy specimens, placed in plastic containers equipped with glass dosimeter beads, and shipped out for sterilization by cathode irradiation by air express in containers of dry ice. The bone was returned in dry ice containers and stored in a deep freeze at −70° C. If the postirradiation bacteriologic culture was negative, the bone was used to fill bone cyst cavities and other small defects but was considered unreliable for arthrodesis or ununited fractures. Irradiation sterilization is much less accepted now than in previous years because recent research has shown that it destroys BMP of the organic matrix.[77]

Cobey[18] polled 160 surgeons in the United States to determine how many surgeons currently use "bank bone" for bone graft operations on bone cysts, nonunion of fractures, and ankylosed joints or congenital defects. Of 112 respondents, 44% used bone from the bone banks. Of the 56% of nonusers, 30% would use bank bone in selected cases if it were available to them and 26% had no use for bank bone even if it were available. If it were readily available, 480 patients a year would have had bank bone grafts. An undetermined number of surgeons now operate institutional bone banks. These are nonprofit organizations that sell allogeneic bone for patients of other orthopedic surgeons. Recently, an Association of Tissue Banks has been organized to improve and standardize tissue banking procedures.

Table 11-2 summarizes the literature on procedures observed to reduce the biologic or morphogenetic potential of the organic matrix of allogeneic bone. To retain BMP activity, the method of preparation should make allowances for (1) biodegradation time—the time elapsed between death of the donor and collection of the bone, (2) bacterial, fungal, and viral contamination during the process of collection, (3) preservation by freezing at −70° C with subsequent vacuum drying, (4) avoidance of irradiation sterilization, and (5) requirements for chemical inhibition of degradative enzymes.

Biodegradation time

Observations on alloimplants of bone matrix in muscle of rats demonstrate that about half of the BMP activity, as measured by the yield of new bone, is lost within 24 hr postmortem.[71,74,75] Consequently, the time between death and excision, termed the biodegradation time, determines how much BMP activity is retained in a preparation of autopsy bone. Bone collected in the minimal biodegradation time and treated to retain BMP requires a multidisciplinary pathology, tissue collection, pharmacology, and orthopedic laboratory group. The bone must be excised from the donor within 4 to 8 hr after death. Although the importance of early collection of bone from carefully selected donors cannot be overemphasized, chemosterilization by specific enzyme-inhibiting chemical reagents is necessary to preserve BMP. Only by community efforts and medical-legal procedures for securing bone with minimal delay in cases of accidental death can bone with optimum BMP activity be made available in unlimited quantities for allogeneic implantation.

TABLE 11-2 PROCEDURES WITH DETRIMENTAL EFFECTS ON BONE MORPHOGENETIC (OSTEOINDUCTIVE) PROPERTY

PROCEDURE	EFFECT	REFERENCE
Delayed collection time (more than 12 hr)	Activates endogeneous proteases	Urist and Iwata[74]
Prolonged storage, 0° C to 30° C	Digestion of bone morphogenetic property	Wilson[89]
Immediate freeze-drying	Preserves BMPase as well as antigenic substances	Urist, et al[75,80]
Irradiation sterilization (more than 2.0 mrad)	Denatures bone morphogenetic property	Buring and Urist[9] Buring[8] Urist and Hernandez[77]

Bacterial, fungal, and viral contamination—controlling measures

Although aseptically collected freeze-dried whole bone had been implanted in more than 4000 patients in the United States from 1941 to 1962[26] and has been reported to be satisfactory for bone cysts,[64] in other nations the procedure is regarded as bacteriologically unsafe when compared with irradiation-sterilized freeze-dried bone.[8,16,49,61] Several chemical methods of sterilization[27] have been abandoned after investigation by empirical random clinical trials. Statistically, however, the results with chemosterilization were not significantly different from the end results with either freeze-dried bone or bone prepared by physical methods of sterilization, such as irradiation[65,66,91] or even autoclaving.[59]

Preservation measures and antigenicity

Freezing and storage at −70° C has both adverse and beneficial effects. Freeze-drying may preserve enzymes that degrade constituents of bone matrix essential for the bone morphogenetic response[71–74] and, equally important, preserve soluble intra- and extracellular proteins responsible for a delayed hypersensitivity reaction.[4,6,23] Although not as intense as the hypersensitivity (histoincompatibility) reaction to viable allografts, it is not eliminated by irradiation, freezing, vacuum drying, or even autoclaving the donor tissue. Antibodies to allogeneic bone *accumulate* in the blood of children more than a year after transplantation of freeze-dried, irradiation-sterilized massive bone implants.[88]

Adverse effects of ionizing radiation sterilization

Ionizing radiation for sterilization preservation, for example, 3.5 mrad,[61] destroys the capacity of bone matrix to elicit a morphogenetic response[9,77] and is no longer recommended for bone banks. Owing to the high ionizing potential of the inorganic compared with the organic components, irradiation of undemineralized bone with only 2.0 mrad is sufficient to destroy the property of the matrix essential for bone

morphogenesis.[77] Retention of enzymic activity in bone tissue is not, as recently assumed,[88] an indication of the survival of biologic properties of bone tissue. The only constituents of bone not denatured by irradiation sterilization are undesirable degradative enzymes.[77,88] Inadequate incorporation of bone treated by irradiation sterilization was first noted in 1956[66] and again in 1963[30] but was either disregarded or considered unimportant for practical clinical purposes.[91] Statistics indicating good results in 70% to 85% of thousands of clinical operations with irradiation-sterilized bone are cited[65,88,91] but do not invalidate experimental evidence against irradiation sterilization for two reasons. The first is that equally good results are reported with autoclaved bone.[34–36,39,41,59] The second is that bone denatured by either irradiation sterilization or autoclaving can be incorporated in the skeleton in growing normal children by osteoconduction alone. The process is almost as rapid in an autograft, but only if the donor tissue is in tight contact with the recipient bed on all sides.

Specific effects of chemical agents for bone tissue preservation

A wide variety of bactericidal and fungicidal chemical reagents have been used for preservation of bone for bone banks. A remarkable coincidence is that a chemical agent, thimerosal, used by Reynolds and colleagues more than 20 years ago inhibits BMPase without denaturation of bone morphogenetic protein.[58,79] Polyvinylpyrrolidone-iodine neither denatures BMP nor inhibits BMPase degradation of BMP activity. Sterilization with other chemical agents, for example, beta-propiolactone and hydrogen peroxide, destroys BMP. Thimerosal (2.5 Mm/l) and Cialit (a similar organic mercurial compound) are both bactericidal and fungicidal and are capable of sterilizing dense cortical bone.[27]

The incorporation of thimerosal-preserved alloimplants is not as rapid as with autografts even in relatively normal host beds with benign tumors and fractures. The overall results are about the same as obtained with frozen or freeze-dried bone. In a random selection of cases, including pathologic host recipient beds, the results with autografts in large bone defects are only slightly better than those with frozen bone.[12,51] A statistical consideration that apparently has not been taken into account is the time interval between death of the donor and collection, preparation, or preservation of the bone in allogenic bone grafts. In this time interval, alterations would occur in the BMP and in BMPase activity of the donor bone.[71,72,73,74,75]

Resorption

The rate of resorption of an alloimplant is proportional to the surface area. The quantity of antigen in a bone alloimplant is also proportional to the mass of the preimplanted tissue. Autodigestion of dead cells leaves empty osteocyte lacunae. The process is catalyzed by intracellular endogenous proteolytic enzymes. Autolytic digestion is comparable to *in vitro* digestion of a bone by an exogenous neutral protease such as trypsin. Bone autografts and alloimplants, regardless of the method of preparation (frozen, freeze-dried, irradiated, thimersol-fixed, autoclaved, or even decalcified), transfer significant quantities of intracellular and extracellular proteins from the donor to the recipient through the lymphatic system. The donor's intracellular proteins are derived from remnants of bone marrow cells, fibrocytes, osteoprogenitor cells, and osteocytes. The osteocytes constitute only about 10% of the volume of marrow-free cortical bone.

Chemosterilized, autolysed antigen-extracted allogeneic (AAA) bone

To sterilize cortical bone without loss of BMP activity and at the same time lower the antigenicity of raw frozen cadaver tissue, the osteocytes should be removed by autolytic digestion in the presence of sulfhydral enzyme inhibitors; transplantation antigens can be extracted by chloroform methanol and resorption by the recipient may be facilitated by partial demineralization in 0.6N HCl at 2° C. When the cortical bone is sequentially processed by these reagents, the end product is AAA bone.

AAA bone is a substitute for autologous bone and is recommended for operations in which transfer of a massive graft is disadvantageous or detrimental to the welfare of the patient.[67] AAA bone evolved from research on bone morphogenesis and experimental bone graft operations on mice, rats, guinea pigs, rabbits, dogs, and monkeys.[49,68-86] In experimental defects in rabbits, AAA bone is more rapidly resorbed and replaced by new bone that frozen raw whole bone, and is almost as effective as autologous cancellous bone.[49] Clinical investigations on AAA bone are concerned with the rationale for autolytic digestion and chemical extraction of the matrix of cortical bone, informed consent procedures, and tissue typing.

Autolytic digestion of cells in vitro *for preparation of AAA bone*

Autodigestion of bone in neutral buffer solutions *in vitro* removes from the tissue soluble proteins that are capable of producing an alloimmune (delayed hypersensitivity) response. Specific enzyme inhibitors are added to the buffer solution to retain the BMP activity essential for osteoinductive function of a bone alloimplant during the process of extraction of transplantation antigens (Figs. 11-7–11-9). Figures 11-10 and 11-11 illustrate the AAA bone–induced osteogenetic response in a muscle pouch in an allogeneic recipient. Figures 11-12 and 11-13 demonstrate the same response in an athymic mouse and a cortisone-treated rat. Figures 11-14 and 11-15 show biopsy specimens of AAA human bone in allogeneic recipients.

Informed Consent Procedures

AAA bone is prepared from bone obtained at autopsy on persons who legally donate their bodies to the institution for organ transplantation and research. Guidelines for medical research adopted by the National Institutes of Health require that Informed Consent Statements should be signed by recipients of AAA bone in orthopedic operations.

Tissue Typing

When donors of kidneys for organ transplantation are also used as donors for AAA bone, typing information may be available for retrospec-

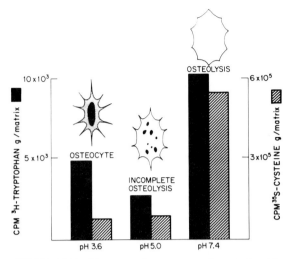

FIGURE 11-7 *Diagrammatic representation of the histochemistry of autolytic digestion of osteocytes and other bone cells to reduce the antigenicity of allogeneic cortical bone. Weanling rats were injected daily for 4 wk with ^{3}H-tryptophan and ^{35}S-cysteine to labile noncollagenous proteins of bone matrix. Freshly collected labeled bone was incubated in buffer solutions at the three levels of pH shown in the horizontal axis. The height of the bar graphs and drawings of the contents of osteocyte lacunae show the simultaneous disintegration of the osteocytes and the release of radioactivity into the incubation fluid. At pH 3.6, under conditions of inactivity of neutral proteases, DNAases, and RNAases, cell remain intact and there is minimal release of radioactivity. At pH 5.0, acid proteases degrade cells, but relatively little radioactivity is released from the bone matrix. At pH 7.4, under conditions of maximum activity of neutral proteases, the osteocyte lacunae become empty and the release of radioactivity from the matrix reaches maximum levels.*

tive observations on patients with AAA bone grafts. Tissue typing is based on isoantigens of leukocytes that have been identified and demonstrated by means of skin grafts to be transplantation antigens.[20,87] For this purpose the leukocyte groups are determined either on blood of living potential donors or on lymph nodes of autopsy subjects as soon as permissible after death. The serum of the recipient is tested for leukocyte agglutinins against the donor and compared with leukocytes of 100 persons chosen at random. In the laboratory of Terasaki the tests are performed using the method of Mittal and colleagues,[46] in which the readings are fed into a computer to establish whether the serum of the recipient, when compared with sera of other persons, recognizes the same antigens, and, if so,

whether some of the antigens are allelic to each other.

If transplantation antigens have been extracted by chloroform methanol, tissue typing is unnecessary in recipients of AAA bone. Theoretically, matched donors and recipients of unprocessed freeze-dried bone should produce incorporation as complete as observed with freeze-dried autologous bone by Burchardt and colleagues.[6] Records are available on the serologic reactions of HL-A antigens to cells obtained from (1) lymph nodes at autopsy of AAA bone donors, and (2) blood of recipients of AAA bone implants in selected patients before the operation and 3 wk to 3 mo after. Sera have been collected at 6-mo and 1-yr intervals from patients who have failed bone graft operations, but the level of circulating antibodies has been too low to measure. For further investigations, the lymphocytes of the donor have been isolated and typed by the microcytotoxicity test and the antisera of the recipient were then tested against known serotypes.

Preparation of AAA bone

Table 11-3 summarizes five steps in the preparation of AAA bone. Allogeneic cortical bone is aseptically collected as soon as possible at autopsy in a special operating room and cut into cylinders 15 cm long or in strips 10 cm × 2 cm. Old blood and marrow are washed out by vigorous stirring in a sterile cold water solution of sodium azide, 10 mmol/liter three times. The bone segments are sterilized, defatted, and extracted in 1:1 chloroform methanol for 24 hr and are then surface demineralized at 2° C in 0.6N HCl for 24 hr to increase the permeability of the matrix to solutions of enzyme inhibitors. The surface demineralized bone is then transferred to a phosphate buffer containing N-ethyl maleimide and sodium azide (10 mM/liter each) for 72 hr at 37° C to autolyse and further extract transplantation antigens. These enzyme inhibitors prevent degradation of BMP without inhibiting enzymes that digest bone cells of the donor and at the same time serve as antimicrobial agents.[80] Phosphate buffer, pH 7.4, activates intra- and extracellular enzymes for autolytic digestion of nearly all of the intralacunar stainable osteocytes. The evidence for this view is that acetate buffers at pH 5.5 remove only a small part of the stainable cellular material. After autolytic digestion of cells, the bone segments are finally washed in fresh buffer and frozen in liquid nitrogen at $-70°$ C over a period of 24 hr. The AAA bone segments are stored in sterile double plastic envelopes and sealed, labeled glass containers. AAA bone is white and is about 75% of the weight of freeze-dried whole cortical bone.

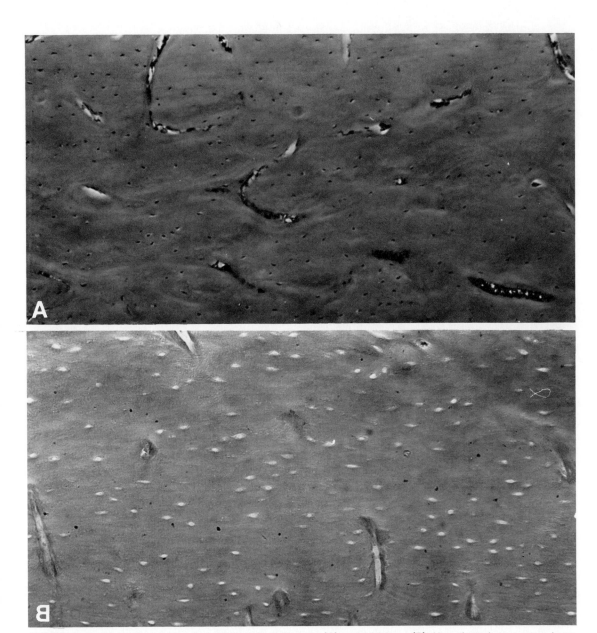

FIGURE 11-8 *Photomicrographs of preimplanted whole bone* **(A)** *and AAA bone* **(B)***. Note the enlargement and complete evacuation of the osteocyte lacunae by incubation of bone in buffer solutions containing sulfhydryl enzyme inhibitors used in the preparation of AAA bone. Hematoxylin eosin and azure II stain.*

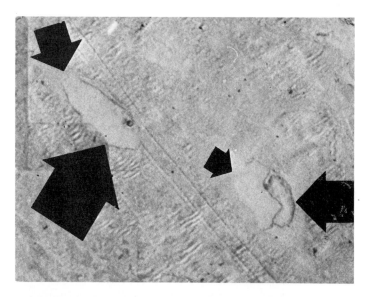

FIGURE 11-9 *Electron micrograph of plasma membranes retained in osteocyte lacunae following autolytic digestion of bone cells by activation of neutral proteases, DNAases, and RNAases in buffer solution containing sulfhydryl enzyme inhibitors.*

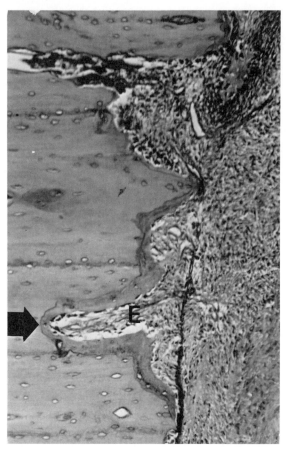

FIGURE 11-10 *Photomicrograph of an intramuscular implant of AAA bone in posterior cervical muscles of adult mongrel dog tested for osteoinductive activity 6 wk after the operation. The new bone (arrow) deposited on the walls of a resorption tunnel (E) is metachromatic-staining.*

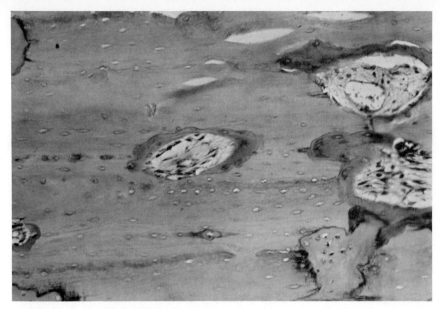

FIGURE 11-11   *Photomicrograph of the same test block shown in Figure 11-7, cut in cross-section to demonstrate cement lines between old and acellular bone of donor and appositional deposits of deeply stained cellular new bone of recipient.*

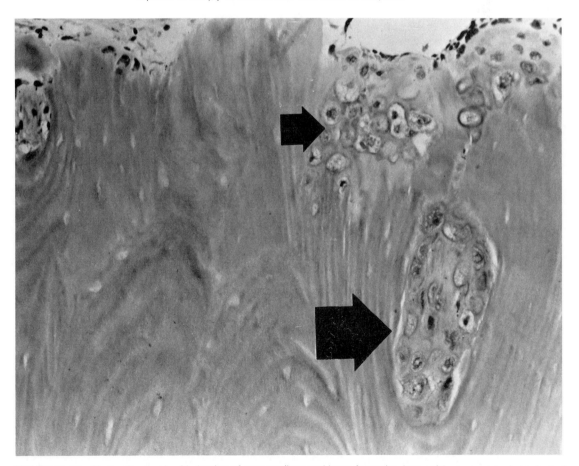

FIGURE 11-12   *Photomicrograph of induction of new cartilage and bone formation (arrows) by a xenogeneic implant of human AAA bone in an athymic nude mouse, 3 wk after the operation.*

351

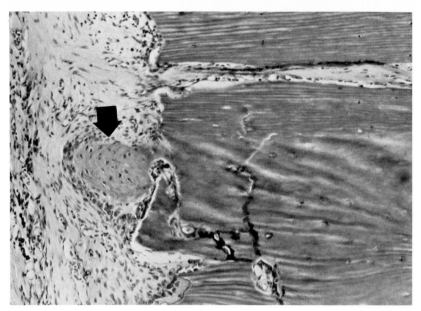

FIGURE 11-13   *Photomicrograph of an intramuscular implant of human AAA bone in an adult rat treated with daily injections of cortisone acetate for immunosuppression, 21 d after the operation. Note the deposits of new rat bone (arrow) induced by the AAA bone in the recipient muscle bed.*

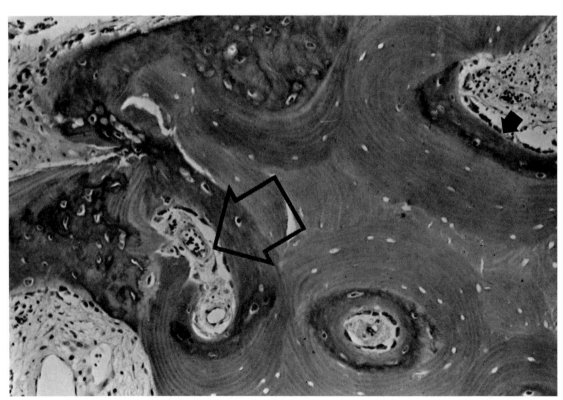

FIGURE 11-14   *Photomicrograph of AAA cortical bone implanted to fill excision biopsy defect in 24-yr-old man who died of synovial sarcoma. Note acellular AAA bone (right) and resorption cavities lined with osteoblasts and metachromatic, deeply stained layers of new bone (arrows).*

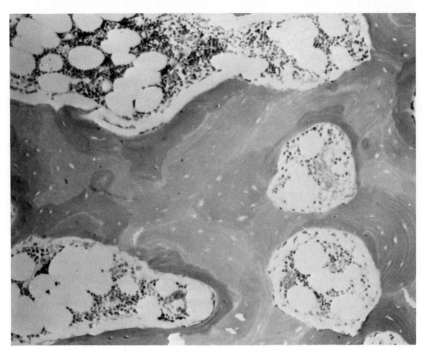

FIGURE 11-15 *Photomicrograph of a biopsy of an AAA human bone alloimplant after 6 mo in a two-stage laminectomy and spinal fusion for spinal stenosis in a 55-yr-old man. Note the cellular metachromatic-stained new bone and bone marrow deposits of the recipient surrounding the acellular pale-stained AAA bone of the donor.*

The breaking strength is only about one half that of whole undemineralized wet bone (Figs. 11-16 and 11-17).

Table 11-4 summarizes the surgical technical requirements for the use of AAA bone. Success-ful incorporation of AAA in the recipient bed of skeletal tissue is possible when there is strict adherence to the principle of autologous bone graft operations. Provided that these technical requirements are met, chemosterilized antigen-

TABLE 11-3 FIVE STEPS IN THE PREPARATION OF CHEMOSTERILIZED, ANTIGEN EXTRACTED, AUTOLYSED, ALLOGENEIC (AAA) BONE

STEP	SOLUTIONS AND PRESERVATION MEASURES	TEM-PERA-TURE °C	HOURS	PURPOSE
1	1 : 1 Chloroform-methanol	25	4	Extracts lipids and cell membrane lipoproteins, including antimorphogenetic hydrophobic glycopeptides (AHG)
2	0.6 N Hydrochloric acid	2	24	Extracts acid-soluble proteins and surface, demineralizes matrix
3	0.1 M Phosphate buffer, pH 7.4, containing 10 mM/liter iodoacetic acid and 10 mM/liter sodium azide	37	72	Endogenous intra- and extracellular enzymic autodigestion of transplantation antigens with preservation of BMP by sulfhydryl group enzyme inhibitors
4	Freeze-drying	−72	24	Dehydrates and preserves residual proteins, including BMP
5	Double plastic envelope in vacuum-sealed glass containers	25		Prevents rehydration and chemical deterioration

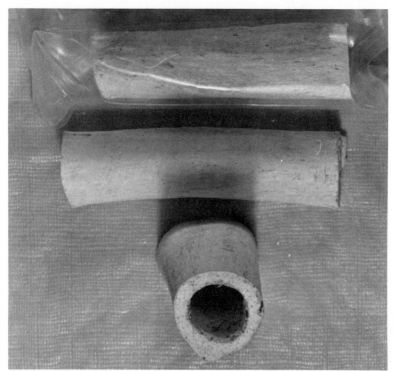

FIGURE 11-16 *Photographs of segments of freeze-dried AAA cortical bone on the operating table after removal from sterile glass containers. The bone at the top is dispensed in sterile double thickness plastic wrappers. The unwrapped cylinder in the middle is reconstituted in an antibiotic solution. The porosity of the AAA bone is shown in the surface cut in cross-section at the bottom.*

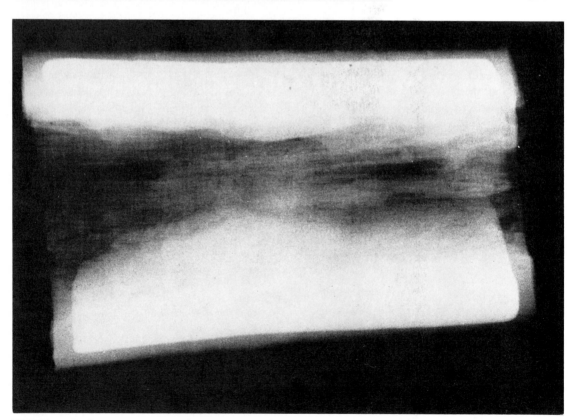

FIGURE 11-17 *Roentgenogram showing 1.0-mm surface layers of radiolucent matrix of a specimen of AAA tibial cortical bone, × 2.5.*

TABLE 11-4 AAA BONE GRAFT TECHNIQUE

DO:	DO NOT:
Mortice implants tightly in place in the host bone	Do not place AAA bone loosely on moving parts of the host bed
Use internal fixation and contact compression or plaster immobilization or both to obtain rigid immobilization of the recipient bone	Do not use AAA bone to bridge gaps between moving bone ends
Use continuous suction drainage	Do not allow AAA bone implants to float in a blood clot in a large bone defect
Preserve surface area of viable host bed by the principle of onlay instead of inlay	Do not slide massive segments of the recipient bed, which reduces the surface area of viable host
Encourage ambulation and exercises, even partial weightbearing, to increase bloodflow through segments of the limb above and below the recipient bone	Do not enforce absolute bed rest, nonweight-bearing, or abstinence from exercises
Surround the alloimplant with cancellous bone and bone marrow as completely as possible to apply the principle of a composite bone graft	

extracted bone should be incorporated more rapidly than either lyophilized (freeze-dried) or irradiation-sterilized bone.

Evaluation of clinical results of bone grafts and alloimplants

Although an autograft is superior to alloimplants for some orthopedic operations, it is not justified for all operations. It is not superior to an alloimplant for large bone defects caused by bone cysts, intraosseous ganglia, aneurysmal bone cysts, villonodular synovitis, giant cell tumors, and so forth. Autografts are either not available in sufficient quantities for operations on large bone defects in small patients or are accompanied by high morbidity attributable to the donor site, that is, sacroiliac pain, heterotopic bone infection, iliac hernia, neuroma, and deformity. When the surface area of the host bed is small and the volume of the bone defects is very large, the incorporation of the donor tissue may be enhanced by the addition of autologous cancellous bone (including bone marrow) to an AAA implant to produce a composite bone graft.

A prospective clinical investigation of a large number of cases is necessary to ascertain the indications and compare the results of operations with AAA bone implants with operations using frozen and freeze-dried whole bone in one group, autografts in another, and composite grafts in still another. Matched cases are absolutely essential for proper conclusive evaluation of the permutations and combinations of clinical factors.

High failure rates are observed from operations on infected or old fractures with missing substance, bone ends devitalized by metallic devices, or very large bone defects in middle-age adults. The lowest failure rates come from operations on young normal children with a high proliferative capacity of growing bones. However, even in children, autografts are unsuccessful in congenital pseudarthrosis, neurofibromatosis, and other disorders of the neurovascular supply of the bone. More successful results may come from combined operations using electrical stimulation devices and bone grafts. But not enough case reports are available at this time to warrant conclusive statements. In children, unicameral bone cysts will heal with almost any kind of implant, for example, freeze-dried, irradiated, wholly autoclaved, denatured allogeneic bone, ceramics, or even implants of plaster of Paris.[41,50] Bone repair around denatured bone and nonbiologic implants can occur by the process of osteoconduction. The process of repair with AAA bone depends upon the retention of BMP and is enhanced by the extraction of undesirable soluble tissue antigens from bone *in vitro*. The results are that AAA bone: is more rapidly resorbed and replaced by new bone than either frozen or freeze-dried whole bone, incites a relatively slight delayed hypersensitivity reaction, and possesses both osteoinductive and osteoconductive properties (see Figs. 11-14 and 11-15).

Donor sites

The three areas of the skeleton generally selected for donor sites for autologous bone grafts are the iliac crest, the anterior medial aspect of the tibia, and the midshaft of the fibula.

Iliac crest

The outer table including the cancellous bone of the iliac crest is the most frequently selected donor site for an autologous bone graft. After a graft of the desired dimensions is removed *en bloc* with an osteotome, the cancellous bone is removed from the margins of the donor site with a large curette. In the average adult, as much as 50 cm³ of cancellous bone can be removed. When a large graft is excised for a two-level spinal fusion, special care is necessary to retain the inner wall of the pelvis. If the curettage is too vigorous and the inner table is perforated, a number of complications are possible. Bone bleeding may be extensive, and precautions must be taken against hematoma formation and wound infection. Careful hemostasis and provisions for continuous suction drainage are absolutely essential. Challis and coworkers[13] recently reviewed the literature on lumbar hernia in iliac crest donor sites and reported a case of volvulus. Ramani and coworkers[54] noted a high morbidity; even fractures have been reported from removal of small quantities of bone from the ilium.

Tibia

The favorite donor site for full-thickness cortical grafts is the anterior medial aspect of the tibia. The graft is moved from the host bed with a parallel-bladed power saw. The upper end of the donor site may be curetted to remove additional cancellous bone. The typical complication of a cortical tibial bone graft is fatigue fracture across the donor site. The best precautionary measure is substitution of the autologous graft with an allogeneic cortical bank bone implant of exactly the same dimensions. The tibia as a donor site necessitates plaster cast immobilization for 2 or 3 mo and/or crutches to protect the leg against fatigue fracture.

Fibula

The midshaft of the fibula is an excellent donor site of cylindrical cortical bone grafts for repair of large defects in long bones (especially in the forearm) and for intramedullary bone grafts for ununited fractures of the neck of the femur in young adults. Except for the obvious need to protect the peroneal nerve against surgical injury, there are few instances of complications from removal of the adult fibula. Valgus deformities of the ankle may occur in children when the graft is taken too close to the lower third of the fibula, but this complication can be avoided by removing only the middle third of the fibula and by carefully preserving the periosteal tube. Because it is lacking in cancellous bone and bone marrow, the fibula is used less frequently than other bones. Lipscomb[40] reported that fibular grafts threaded over Kirschner wires are excellent for replacement for long bone defects in children. Cortical grafts in children are incorporated more rapidly than in adults. Stress fractures, sequestration, and resorption do not occur as frequently in children as they do in adults.

Choice of donor site

Lipschomb[40] observes that severe pain or morbidity that accompanies the removal of grafts from the ilium can and should be avoided and that, particularly in children, cortical bone grafts are superior to iliac grafts. In ununited fractures of the upper end of the tibia a sliding bone graft heals more slowly than an onlay graft and may be no more effective than an AAA cortical bone strip.

The recipient bone

Every bone and every part of the bone of the human skeleton responds to injury in its individual way and incorporates a bone graft at its own rate of repair. The factors intrinsic to the repair process are age, anatomical pattern of vascularity, immobilization, contact compression, and pathologic condition. The transplant should be dovetailed in place to secure maximum contact between the donor and the host bones. In sclerotic or otherwise pathologic recipient beds, sustained contact and even contact-compression by means of internal fixation devices can prevent undesirable motion along bone surfaces and increase the incidence of successful incorporation of the graft. The circulation and anatomical characteristics of each bone are so different from every other bone that bone graft operations on the individual parts of the skeleton must be considered separately. In general, the rate of failure of autologous bone grafts ranges from 13 to 30%, a percentage far too high to be acceptable. The overall failure rate of operations with raw allogeneic frozen or freeze-dried bone is even higher. The overall failure rate with AAA bone in a prospective study in progress on spinal fusion operations is about 14%.

Clavicle

When comminuted displaced fractures of the midshaft of the clavicle in adults are inadequately treated by closed methods, they heal slowly and may fail to unite. Comparable fractures in children almost invariably heal. Ununited fractures in adults may require an open operation with rigid internal fixation and an onlay or intermedullary peg for fixation. In these cases, the choice of a bone graft may be either an autologous only graft from the crest of the ilium or an intermedullary cortical bone peg from an allogeneic donor. In either case the adult clavicle may not unite without rigid internal fixation or external immobilization of the shoulder joint, or both, for periods of 8 to 12 wk.

Humerus

Nearly all bone graft operations on the humerus are performed on the diaphyseal portion of the bone. One of the most common conditions requiring a bone graft is an ununited fracture of the midshaft of the humerus in an adult. The surgical approach requires a careful dissection and retraction of the radial nerve. Pseudarthrosis should be excised and the bone ends trimmed to produce perfectly matching flat surfaces for a transfixion screw if the fracture is oblique or contact compression with a bone plate if the fracture is transverse. Because of the distracting force of gravity on the distal fragment, the efficiency of internal or external fixation of the humerus may mean the difference between success and failure.

One or two autologous onlay cancellous bone grafts at 90° angles to the plate should be placed in the closest possible contact with the recipient bone and well covered with muscle. In a normal nondiseased bone bed, cortical bone bank allogeneic implants may be substituted for autologous bone. Suction drainage for 24 hr is important, even in cases in which hemostasis seems adequate, particularly in fractures in which blocks of AAA bone are used to fill large defects. When there is any doubt about the efficiency of the internal fixation, the fracture should be immobilized in a shoulder spica for at least 3 mo. Only absolute, total restriction of rotation and distraction forces will prevent recurrence of a nonunion of the midshaft of the humerus in middle-aged persons.

Radius and ulna

Fractures of both bones of the forearm in adults are frequently difficult to reduce and immobilize, and in instances of interposition of a muscle may heal very slowly or fail to unite. Surgical management requires open reduction and internal fixation with an intermedullary pin for the ulna and a bone plate for the radius. Onlay autologous bone grafts or allogeneic cortical implants are placed at 90° angles to the plate on the volar aspect of the radium. A graft should never be placed in the interosseous space, in which a synostosis might ensue. A perfect anatomical fit of the fracture surfaces is essential for rapid healing. Even slight rotation forces are detrimental to union. A long arm plaster cast with the elbow at an angle of 100°, the wrist in slight dorsiflexion, and the hand in functional position is important for the first 3 mo of healing.

Carpal scaphoid

Although nearly all fractures of the carpal scaphoid unite if immobilized long enough, nonunion may occur in neglected cases and require a cancellous inlay or cortical bone peg graft. The technique is extremely exacting and requires a volar approach. The failure rate is 30%. Autologous bone is used almost exclusively.

Cervical spine

Anterior cervical body fusion and posterior interlaminar arthrodesis are best accomplished with iliac autologous bone. The compressive forces on the anterior vertebral body acting on a dovetailed autograft or AAA bone implant produces union in a high percentage of cases. Posterior interlaminar spinal fusion is subject to strain and a high failure rate; in adult patients, internal fixation with interspinous process wires is necessary to achieve an acceptable fusion rate. The quantity of bone required for cervical spinal fusion is relatively small and easily satisfied by an iliac half-thickness autologous bone graft.

Scoliotic spine

Spinal fusion with correction and internal fixation by means of Harrington instrumentation can be carried out with success using autologous bone alone or by supplementing autologous bone of the recipient bed with AAA bone. The apophyseal joints should be erased and packed with autologous bone. The alloimplant should be placed on the concave side of the curves in long, thin cortical bone strips. On the convex side of the curves, even autologous bone is generally resorbed. In most cases, enough is retained on the concave side to be remodeled and incorporated for fusion of the primary curves.

Lumbar spine

The highest rates of failure of autologous as well as of allogeneic bone grafts are reported in operations on the lumbosacral area of the spinal column. The success rate is improved by combining intertransverse process arthrodesis with posterior interlaminar fish-scaled bone grafts. The operation is called posterolateral fusion and is generally supplemented by cortical interspinous process H blocks for internal fixation. In a well-performed spinal fusion operation the laminae are decorticated, the apophyseal subchondral bone is also exposed for transfixion with cortical bone pegs. All the recipient bed bone surfaces should consist of bleeding spongiosa and red bone marrow. When a tibial cortical bone alloimplant in the form of an H block is dovetailed in place between the notches cut in spinous processes, the end product is a composite bone graft of viable autologous bone marrow and nonviable allogeneic cortical bone. Autologous iliac bone is mechanically inferior to allogeneic cortical bone for purposes of internal fixation. AAA cortical bone is ideal for multiple-level intertransverse process fusions in which large strips of cortical bone are advantageous. When dovetailed in slots cut in the sacrum and placed on the dunuded transverse processes, alloimplants can be as effective as cortical autografts. (Figs. 11-18–11-21).

Femur

For nonunion of the neck of the femur, either autologous fibula or AAA bone are effective (Fig. 11-22). For nonunion of the shaft of the femur, AAA bone grafts are very satisfactory. The success of the operation depends on absolute internal fixation with a physiologic degree of contact compression. Compression plates are helpful if the bone ends are in close contact and onlay grafts are placed across the fracture site on the medial cortex of the femur. For acceptable internal fixation, intramedullary rods must be tightly fit without any telescoping or rotary motion at fracture site.

Tibia

The shaft of the tibia is a common site of failure of autologous bone grafts. Bone grafts are advisable in patients with nonunion but not in fresh fractures with avascular bone ends, inadequate skin covering, and poor resistance to infection.

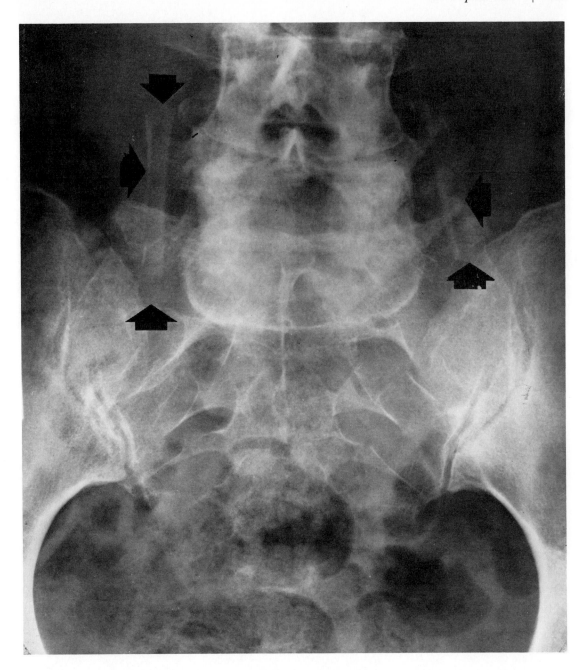

FIGURE 11-18   *Postoperative roentgenogram of intertransverse process AAA bone implant in a 45-yr-old woman treated by bilateral laminectomy for fifth lumbar degenerative disc and joint disease. Note the radiolucent AAA fibular bone overlapping the transverse processes of the fifth lumbar and first sacral vertebrae (arrows).*

The surgical approach in patients selected for bone alloimplants should include the minimum amount of dissection of soft tissue around the bone ends. Excision of the pseudarthrosis is not necessary. Continuous suction drainage for the first 3 d after the operation is absolutely essential. Bone alloimplants or grafts should be tightly in contact with fresh bleeding subperiosteal decorticated bone. Bone plates should not be applied to poorly vascularized sclerotic bone ends.

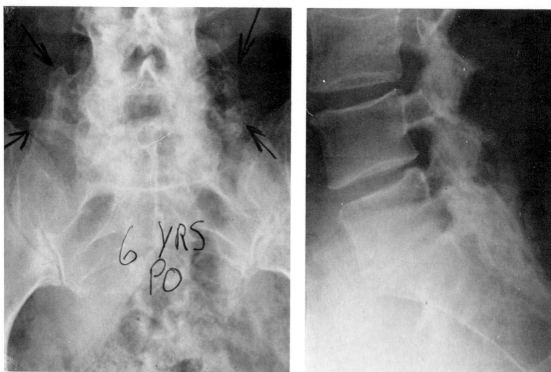

FIGURE 11-19   *Anterior and lateral view roentgenograms of the low back of the same patient as shown in Figure 11-18, 6 yr after the operation. Note the resorption of the overlapping ends and the incorporation of AAA bone between the transverse processes to produce a solid, permanent arthrodesis.*

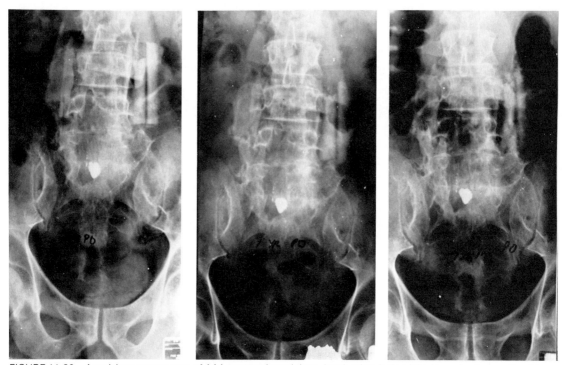

FIGURE 11-20   *A serial roentgenogram of AAA posterorlateral three-level arthrodesis of the lower lumbar and lumbosacral spine at 3, 12, and 21 mo (left to right) after bilateral laminectomy operations for spinal stenosis in a 50-yr-old man. Note the resorption, remodeling, and replacement of the cortical bone strips across the transverse process.*

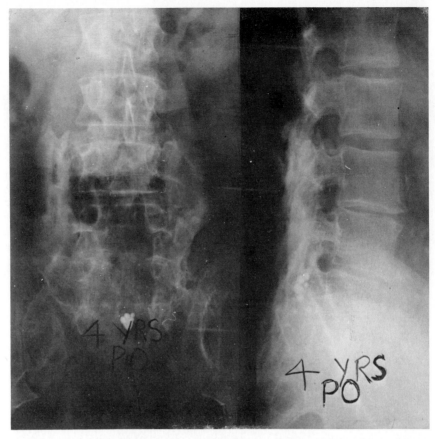

FIGURE 11-21   *Roentgenograms in the anteroposterior and lateral views of the same patient as shown in Figure 11-20, 4 yr after the operation. Note the continuous fusion mass across the transverse process from the fourth lumbar to the first sacral vertebrae.*

Onlay bone alloimplants in the *posterior* compartment or fibulotibial cross pegs above and below the fracture site will produce union in a high percentage of patients if the leg is immobilized in a hinged cast brace to encourage early weight-bearing exercises. AAA bone is an excellent supplement for autologous bone for arthrodesis of the ankle and other joints (Fig. 11-23).

Bone tumors

Bone cysts, giant cell tumors, aneurysmal bone cysts, and other benign tumors are excised or curetted as thoroughly as possible and filled with allogeneic bank bone (Figs. 11-24–11-26). After a course of chemotherapy, low-grade chon-drosarcomas may be removed by *en bloc* excision and repaired with a total diaphyseal replacement with allogeneic or composite allogeneic and autologous bone grafts held rigidly in place by internal fixation supplemented with an external plaster encasement. As autologous iliac bone is most readily available, it is most frequently used when the tumor is small in volume. If the graft is not replaced by new bone, it is resorbed and replaced by tumor or fibrous tissue. Roentgenographically, this is observed as a decrease in size and density and eventual dissolution of the graft. The causes of the dissolution of the graft are recurrence of a cyst or tumor, insufficient area of contact between the donor tissue and recipient bed, insufficient internal fixation or immobilization of the part, and infection.

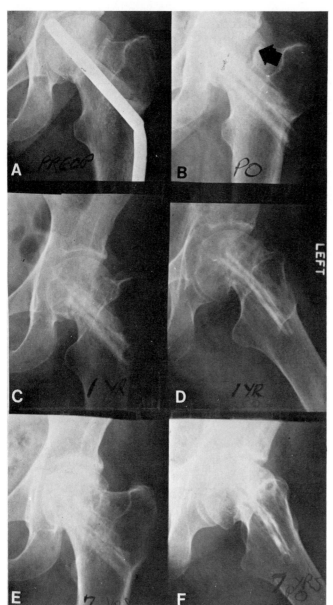

FIGURE 11-22 *Roentgenograms of ununited fracture of the neck of the femur, showing fracture line (arrow) and protrusion of the nail (Neufeld type) into the acetabulum* **(A)** *in a 68-yr-old woman. The nail was removed 2 mo after the fracture and the nail tract was filled with two AAA cortical bone pegs* **(B).** *Note the union at 1 yr after the operation* **(C** *and* **D)** *and the normal structure of the hip joint* **(E** *and* **F)** *7 yr after the operation.*

Summary

The terminology of bone graft surgery is based on the genome of the donor and the immunochemical reactions of the recipient. It is applicable to nonviable alloimplants as well as viable transplants. The process of imcorporation is a function of the recipient bed and depends on close contact with the conor tissue, time sequences, and synchronization of five biologic processes: (1) differentiation of osteoprogenitor cells, (2) deposition of woven bone by osteoblasts, (3) osteoinduction, (4) osteoconduction, and (5) biomechanical function of the unresorbed structure of the donor. Frozen and freeze-dried bone incite a delayed hypersensitivity response that eliminates the *osteoinductive bone morphogenetic phase* of incorporation of a bone graft.

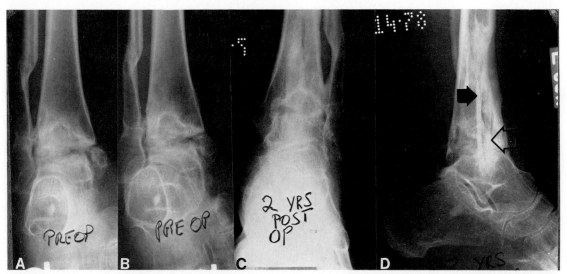

FIGURE 11-23 (**A** and **B**) Anterior and oblique view roentgenograms of the tibiotalar joint of a 20-yr-old student nurse, showing ununited septic compound fracture of the medial malleolus and destruction of the subchondral bone, 3 yr after injury. (**C** and **D**).Roentgenograms of the same ankle joint 2 yr after arthrodesis by a sliding inlay of autologous (black arrow) and AAA bone grafts. Note the union of the medial malleolus, fusion of the tibiotalar joint, and replacement of the anterior AAA graft with new bone (clear arrow).

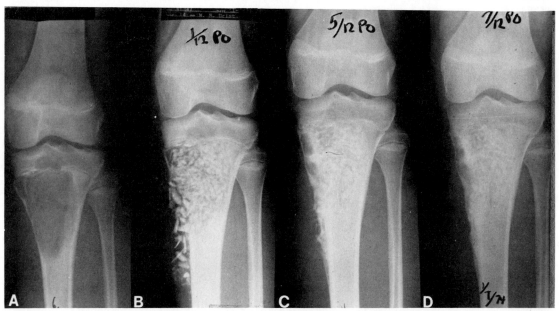

FIGURE 11-24 Roentgenograms of a unicameral bone cyst in a 14-yr-old girl treated by curettage and repair with AAA bone chips at intervals. (**A**) preoperative, (**B**) 1 mo postoperative, (**C**) 5 mo postoperative, (**D**) 7 mo postoperative. Note the rapid resorption and incorporation of the bone chips into the structure of the recipient bed.

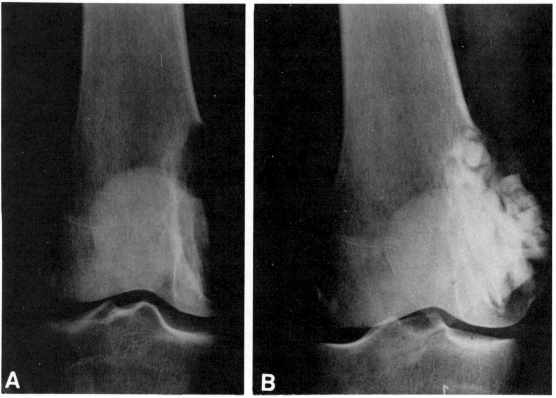

FIGURE 11-25   Roentgenogram of aneurysmal bone cyst destroying the medial femoral condyle of a 45-yr-old woman. **(A)** preoperative, **(B)** 1 mo postoperative. Excision and repair with AAA bone chips.

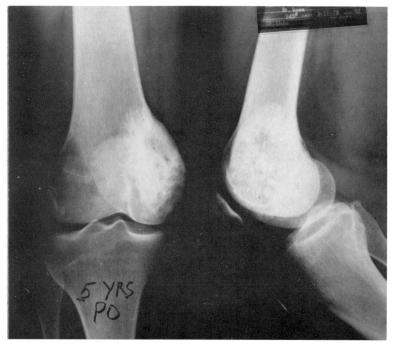

FIGURE 11-26   Roentgenogram of the same knee as shown in Figure 11-20, in anteroposterior (left) and lateral (right) views 5 yr after the operation. Note incorporation of the AAA bone and complete regeneration of the medial femoral condyle.

Freeze-dried new bone contains undesirable enzymes that degrade the matrix bone morphogenetic protein (BMP). These enzymes are extractable along with deleterious transplantation antigens. Irradiation sterilization destroys, by means of electron transfer, the BMP that is responsible for the osteoinductive process. Chemosterilization in buffer solutions containing enzyme inhibitors extract soluble antigeneic proteins without reduction in the bone morphogenetic glycoproteins in the organic matrix. Autolysed antigen-extracted allogeneic (AAA) bone differs from frozen or freeze-dried bone in that osteocyte lacunae are emptied of cell membranes, cytoplasmic proteins, and nucleoproteins. AAA bone consists chiefly of collagen, structural glycoproteins, and BMP. The structure of AAA bone is stabilized by dehydration and defatting in chloroform-methanol followed by freeze-drying and vacuum packing.

Osteoinduction is the process of recruitment of mesenchymal cells of the host bed by BMP to switch further development from a fibromorphogenetic (scar tissue) to an osteogenetic pathway of development. Bioassay of AAA bone for osteoinductive potential in extraskeletal sites in mice, rats, guinea pigs, and rabbits suggests that the osteoinduction plays an important part in the physiology of a bone graft. Present experience with AAA bone demonstrates that the organic matrix is readily resorbed with relatively little cell-mediated local immune reaction and with rapid incorporation of the donor tissue in the recipient bed. When the BMP in human bone matrix is isolated, sequenced, and synthesized, it could be complexed with various nonbiologic, relatively inert substances and become as available on the operating room shelf as suture material.

The individual bones of the human skeleton differ so much in anatomical features, circulation, and regenerative capacity that each bone has its own requirements for immobilization and type of bone graft. There is no all-purpose bone graft. No one type of bone graft can transfer viable osteogenetic cells in significant numbers and also provide the mechanical advantages of compact cortical bone. Composite bone grafts consisting of autologous iliac cancellous bone

and cortical allogeneic bank bone may provide living cells and structural support for repair of very large defects in long bones of adults with low regenerative capability.

References

1. Arora, B. K., and Laskin, D. M.: Sex chromatin as a cellular label of osteogenesis by bone grafts, J. Bone Joint Surg. 46A:1269, 1964.
2. Bohr, H., Ravn, H. O., and Werner, H.: The osteogenic effect of bone transplants in rabbits, J. Bone Joint Surg. 50B:866, 1968.
3. Bonfiglio, M., Jeter, W. S., and Smith, C. L.: The immune concept: its relation to bone transplantation, Ann. N.Y. Acad. Sci. 59:417, 1955.
4. Bonfiglio, M., and Jeter, W. S.: Immunological responses to bone, Clin. Orthop. 87:19, 1972.
5. Burchardt, H., and Enneking, W. F.: Transplantation of bone, Surg. Clin. North Am. 58:403, 1978.
6. Burchardt, H., Jones, H., Glowczewskie, B. S., Rudner, C., and Enneking, W. F.: Freeze-dried allogeneic segmental cortical bone grafts in dogs, J. Bone Joint Surg. 60A:1082–1090, 1978.
7. Buring, K.: The origin of cells in heterotopic bone formation, Clin. Orthop. 110:293, 1975.
8. Buring, K.: Ionizing radiation for sterilization of bone, Intern. Atomic Energy Agency, 1:70–75, 1970.
9. Buring, K., and Urist, M. R.: Effects of ionizing radiation of the bone induction principle in matrix of bone implants, Clin. Orthop. 55:225, 1967.
10. Burwell, R. G.: Studies on transplantation of bone, J. Bone Joint Surg. 48B:552, 1966.
11. Burwell, R. G.: Biological mechanisms in foreign bone transplantation. *In* J. P. H. Clark, (ed.): Modern Trends in Orthopedics, p. 138, Washington, Buttersworth, 1964.
12. Burwell, R. G.: The fate of bone grafts. *In* Apley, A. G. (ed.): Recent Advances in Orthopedics, p. 115, Baltimore, Williams & Wilkins Co., 1969.
13. Challis, J. H., Lyttle, J. A., and Stuart, A. E.: Strangulated lumbar hernia and volvulus following removal of iliac crest bone graft, Acta Orthop. Scand. 46:230, 1975.
14. Chalmers, J.: Bone transplantation. *In* Symposium on Tissue Organ Transplant, J. Clin. Pathol. 20:540, 1967.

15. Chalmers, J.: Transplantation immunity in bone homografting, J. Bone Joint Surg. 41B:160, 1959.

16. Christensen, E. A.: Bacterial evaluation of sterilization procedures, Ann. Pharm. 5:3, 1966.

17. Cloward, R. B.: Treatment of lumbar intervertebral disk by vertebral body fusion. III. Method of use of banked bone, Ann. Surg. 136:987, 1952.

18. Cobey, M. C.: A national bone bank survey, Clin. Orthop., in press.

19. Debruyn, P. H., and Kabisch, W. T.: Bone formations by fresh and frozen autogenous and homogenous transplants of bone, bone marrow, and periosteum, Am. J. Anat. 96:375, 1955.

20. Dick, H. N., and Crichton, W. B.: Tissue Typing Techniques, Baltimore, Williams & Wilkins Co., 1972.

21. Elves, M. W.: Humoral immune response to allografts of bone, Int. Arch. Allergy 47:708, 1974.

22. Elves, M. W., and Pratt, L. M.: The pattern of new bone formation in isografts of bone, Acta Orthop. Scand. 46:549, 1975.

23. Enneking, W. F.: Immunologic aspects of bone grafting, South Med. J. 55:894, 1962.

24. Enneking, W. F.: Physical and biological aspects of repair in dog cortical bone transplants, J. Bone Joint Surg. 57A:237, 1975.

25. Goldberg, V. M., and Lance, E. M.: Revascularization and accretion in transplantation, J. Bone Joint Surg. 54A:807, 1972.

26. Grishaw, R. B., Perry, V. P., and Wheeler, T. E.: U. S. Navy tissue bank, JAMA 183:99, 1963.

27. Guntz, E. W. H.: Experiences with the use of bone grafts preserved in cialit in over 800 operations, J. Bone Joint Surg. 43:290, 1961.

28. Halloran, P. F., Lee, E. H., Isreal, Z. F., Langer, F., and Gross, A. E.: Orthotopic bone transplantation in mice, Transplantation 27:420, 1979.

29. Hancox, M.: Survival of transplanted embryo bone grafted to chorvallantoic membrane; subsequent osteogenesis, J. Physiol. 106(3):279, 1947.

30. Heiple, K. G., Chase, S. N., and Herndon, C. H.: A comparative study of the healing process following different types of bone transplantation, J. Bone Joint Surg. 45A:1593, 1963.

31. Huggins, C., Wiseman, S., and Reddi, A. H.: Transformation of fibroblasts by allogeneic and xenogeneic transplants of demineralized tooth and bone, J. Exp. Med. 132:1250, 1970.

32. Imamaliev, A. S.: The preparation, preservation, and transplantation of articular bone ends. *In* Apley, A. G., (ed.): Advances in Orthopedics, Baltimore, Williams & Wilkins Co., 1969.

33. Iwata, H., and Urist, M. R.: Protein polysaccharide of bone morphogenetic matrix, Clin. Orthop. 87:257, 1972.

34. Kausch, W.: Ueber Knochenimplantation, Verh Deutsch Ges. Chir. 35:179, 1906.

35. Kausch, W.: Zur frage der freien transplantation toten knochens, Zbl. Chir. 36:1379, 1909.

36. Kausch, W.: Ueber knochenersatz. Beitrage zur transplantation toten knochens, Beitr. Klin. Chir. 68:670, 1910.

37. Lance, E. M.: Bone and cartilage in transplantation, *In* Transplantation, edited by J. S. Najarian, and R. L. Simmons, (eds.): P. 665, Philadelphia, Lea & Febiger, 1972.

38. Langer, F., Czitrom, A., Pritzker, K. P., and Gross, A. E.: The immunogenicity of fresh and frozen allogeneic bone, J. Bone Joint Surg. 57A:216, 1975.

39. Leriche, R.: Sur les graffes d'os mort et sur les greffes onoplastiques et heteroplastiques, Mem. Acad. Chir. 76:389, 1950.

40. Lipscomb, P. R.: When to use cortical bone grafts, Tex. Med. 70:76, 1974.

41. Lloyd-Roberts, G. C.: Experiences with boiled cadaveric bone, J. Bone Joint Surg. 34B:428, 1952.

42. Mankin, H. J., Fogelson, F., and Thrasher, A. J.: Massive allograft transplantation for bone tumors. J. Bone Joint Surg. 57A:1171–1172, 1952.

43. Manson, L. A.: Membrane associated histoincompatability antigens. *In* Nowatuy, A. (ed.): Cellular Antigens, New York, Springer-Verlag, 1972.

44. McLean, F. C., and Urist, M. R.: Bone, 3rd edition, Chicago, University of Chicago Press, 1968.

45. Mikulski, A. J., and Urist, M. R.: An antigenic antimorphogenetic bone hydrophobic glycopeptide, Prep. Biochem. 5:21, 1975.

46. Mittal, K. K., Mickey, M. R., and Terasaki, P. I.: Serotyping for homotransplantation XXI. A 45-minute microtoxicity test, Transplantation 8:801, 1969.

47. Nogami, H., and Urist, M. R.: A substratum of bone matrix for differentiation of mesenchymal cells into chondro-osseious tissues *in vitro*, Exp. Cell Res. 63:404, 1970.

48. Nogami, H., and Urist, M. R.: Transmembrane bone matrix gelatin-induced differentiation of bone, Calcif. Tissue Res., in press.

49. Oikarinen, J., and Korhonen, L.: The bone inductive capacity of various bone transplanting materials used for treatment of experimental bone defects, Clin. Orthop. 140:208, 1979.

50. Peltier, L. P.: The use of plaster of Paris to fill large defects in bone, Am. J. Surg. 97:311, 1959.

51. Parrish, F. F.: Allograft replacement of all or a part of the end of a long bone following excision of a tumor, J. Bone Joint Surg. 55A:1, 1973.

52. Pike, R. L., and Boyne, P. J.: Composite autogenous marrow and surface decalcified implants in mandibular defects, J. Oral Surg. 31:905, 1973.

53. Puranen, J.: Reorganization of fresh and preserved bone transplants, Acta Orthop. Scand. (Suppl.) 92:1, 1966.

54. Ramani, P. S., Kalbag, R. M., and Sengupeta, R. P.: Cervical spinal interbody fusion with Kiel bone, Br. J. Surg. 62:147, 1975.

55. Ray, R. D.: Vascularization of bone grafts and implants, Clin. Orthop. 87:43, 1972.

56. Reddi, A. H., and Huggins, C. B.: Biochemical sequences in the transformation of normal fibroblasts in adolescent rats, Proc. Nat. Acad. Sci. 69:1601, 1972.

57. Reisfeld, R. A., and Kahan, B. D.: Transplantation antigens, Adv. Immunol. 12:117, 1970.

58. Reynolds, F. C., Oliver, D. R., and Ramsey, R. R.: Clinical evaluation of merthiolate bone bank and homogenous bone, J. Bone Joint Surg. 33A:873, 1951.

59. Rocher, H. L.: Correspondence. Dead bone grafts in orthopaedic surgery, J. Bone Joint Surg. 35:328, 1953.

60. Salama, R., Burwell, R. G., and Dickson, I. R.: Recombined grafts of bone and marrow, J. Bone Joint Surg. 55B:402, 1973.

61. Santin, L. N.: Sterilization of bone tissues with gamma rays of cobalt 60, Radiobiologica 3:621, 1963.

62. Schachar, N. S., Fuller, T. C., Wadsworth, P. L., Henry, W. B., and Mankin, H. J.: A feline model for study of frozen osteoarticular allografts. II. Development of lymphotoxic antibodies in allograft recipients, Orthop. Transact. 2:150–151, 1978.

63. Simmons, D. J., Ellsasser, J. C., Cummins, J., and Lesker, P.: The bone inductive potential of a composite bone allograft marrow autograft in rabbits, Clin. Orthop. 97:237, 1973.

64. Spence, K. F., Sell, K. W., and Browen, R. H.: Solitary bone cysts: treatment with freeze-dried cancellous bone allograft, J. Bone Joint Surg. 51A:87, 1969.

65. Swanson, A. B., Glessner, J. R., Burdick, H. W., and Mahaney, R. C.: Seven years experience with irradiated bone graft material, Surg. Gynecol. Obstet. 117:573, 1963.

66. Turner, T. C., Basset, C. B., and Sawyer, P. N.: Sterilization of preserved bone grafts by high voltage cathode-irradiation, J. Bone Joint Surg. 38:862, 1956.

67. Urist, M. R.: Bone: transplants, implants, derivatives, and substitutes—a survey of research of the past decade, Am. Acad. Orthop. Surg. 17:184, 1960.

68. Urist, M. R.: Bone: formation by autoinduction, Science 150:893, 1965.

69. Urist, M. R.: The substratum for bone morphogenesis, 29th Symposium Society of Dev. Biol. (Suppl.) 4:125, 1970.

70. Urist, M. R.: Bone histogenesis and morphogenesis in implants of demineralized enamel and dentin, J. Oral Surg. 29:88, 1971.

71. Urist, M. R.: Osteoinduction in undemineralized bone implants modified by chemical inhibitors of endogenous matrix enzymes, Clin. Orthop. 87:132, 1972.

72. Urist, M. R.: Enzymes in bone morphogenesis: endogenous enzymic degradation of the bone morphogenetic property in bone in solutions buffered by ethylenediaminetetraacetic acid (EDTA). Hard Tissue Growth, Repair and Remineralization, p. 143, CIBA Symposium II. Amsterdam, Associated Scientific Publications, 1973.

73. Urist, M. R.: Practical applications of basic research on bone graft physiology. *In* Evans, B. (ed.): Instructional Course Lectures, Am. Acad. Orthoped. Surg. 25:1, St. Louis, The C. V. Mosby Co., 1976.

74. Urist, M. R., and Iwata, H.: Preservation and biodegradation of the morphogenetic property of bone matrix. J. Theor. Biol. 38:155, 1973.

75. Urist, M. R., Iwata, H., Boyd, S. D., and Ceccottik, P. L.: Observations implicating an extracellular enzymic mechanism of control of bone morphogenesis, J. Histochem. Cytochem. 22:88, 1974.

76. Urist, M. R., Iwata, H., Ceccotti, P. L., Dorfman, R. L., Boyd, S. D., McDowell, R. M., and Chien, C.: Bone morphogenesis in implants of insoluble bone gelatin, Proc. Nat. Acad. Sci. 70(12):3511, 1973.

77. Urist, M. R., and Hernandez, A.: Excitation transfer in bone-deleterious effects of cobalt 60 radiation-sterilization of bank bone, Arch. Surg. 109:486, 1974.

78. Urist, M. R., Jurist, J. M., Dubuc, F. L., and

Strates, B. S.: Quantitation of new bone formation in intramuscular implants of bone matrix in rabbits, Clin. Orthop. 68:279, 1970.

79. Urist, M. R., Mazet, R., Jr., and McLean, F. C.: The pathogenesis and treatment of delayed union and non-unions, J. Bone Joint Surg. 36A:931, 1954.

80. Urist, M. R., Mikulski, A. J., and Boyd, S. D.: A chemosterilized antigen extracted bone morphogenetic alloimplant, Arch. Surg. 110:416, 1975.

81. Urist, M. R., Mikulski, A. J., and Lietze, A.: Solubilized and unsolubilized bone morphogenetic protein. Proc. Nat. Acad. Sci. 76:1828, 1979.

82. Urist, M. R., Nogami, H., and Terashima, Y.: A substratum of bone gelatin for chondrogenesis in tissue culture and in vivo. *In* Slavkin, H. C., and Gruelich, R.: Extracellular Matrix Influences in Gene Expression, pp. 609–618, New York, Academic Press, 1975.

83. Urist, M. R., Silverman, B. G., Buring, K., Dubuc, F. L., and Rosenberg, J. M.: The bone induction principle, Clin. Orthop. 53:243, 1967.

84. Urist, M. R., and Strates, B. S.: Bone morphogenetic protein, J. Dent. Res. 50 (6) (Suppl.):1392–1406, 1971.

85. Urist, M. R., Earnest, F., Kimball, K. M., Di-Julio, T. P., and Iwata, H.: Bone morphogenesis in implants of residues of radioisotope labelled bone matrix, Calcif. Tissue Res. 15(4):269, 1974.

86. Van De Putte, K. A., and Urist, M. R.: Osteogenesis in the interior of intra-muscular implants of decalcified bone matrix, Clin. Orthop. 43:1966, 1966.

87. VanRood, J. J., Van L'Eeuwen, A., and Bruning, J. W.: The relevance of leucocyte antigens for allogeneic renal transplantation, J. Clin. Pathol. 20:504, 1967.

88. Volkov, M., and Bizer, V.: Homeotransplantation of bone tissue in children, Moscow, MIR Publ., pp. 232, 1972.

89. Wilson, P. D.: Follow-up study of the use of refrigerated homogenous bone transplants in orthopedic operations, J. Bone Joint Surg. 33A:307, 1951.

90. Wodarski, K., Hancox, N. M., and Brooks, B.: The influence of cortisone on the implantation site on bone and cartilage induction in various animals, J. Bone Joint Surg. 55B:595, 1973.

91. Wright, K. A., and Trump, J. G.: Cooperative studies in the use of ionizing radiation for sterilization and preservation of biological tissues. *In* Sterilization and Preservation of Biological Tissues by Ionizing Radiation. Vienna, International Atomics Energy Agency, 1970.

92. Zaccalini, P. S., and Urist, M. R.: Traumatic periosteal proliferations in rabbits, the enigma of myositis ossificans traumatica, J. Trauma 4:344, 1964.

The process of development of bone in extra-skeletal sites and musculotendinous parts that normally do not ossify is termed heterotopic or ectopic bone formation. Heterotopic bone formation is not difficult to distinguish from pathologic calcification. Roentgenographically, foci of pathologic calcification in soft parts are chalk white and considerably more radiopaque than in heterotopic bone. Pathologic calcification occurs in a matrix of a decomposed, caseous, or necrotic tissue. Pathologic heterotopic bone mineralization occurs in an organized matrix of living cells. Roentgenographically, living bone deposits are relatively gray and cast the shadow of an irregularly woven pattern. Microscopically, bone tissue is lamellated or trabecular in structure with an eosinophilic collagenous matrix and branching cells (osteocytes) and normally always includes hematopoietic bone marrow. In fact, the presence of bone marrow is indicative of benign or non-neoplastic heterotopic bone.

Heterotopic bone formation begins with a morphogenetic phase of development and ends with a cytodifferentiation phase of development. The morphogenetic phase is characterized by mesenchymal cell disaggregation and migration. The cytodifferentiation phase is characterized by cell reaggregation and specialization.[74] This sequence of events may be observed around hip joint muscle attachments to bone in paralyzed limbs in which tissue is damaged by prolonged stasis and edema. The damage incites a morphogenetic movement of cells. The local conditions associated with the morphogenetic movement of mesenchymal-type cells initiate cytodifferentiation of cartilage, woven bone, lamellar bone, and bone marrow. The biochemistry of the combination of systemic and physiochemical factors leading to the bone morphogenetic response is an unexplored and fascinating field of biomedical science.

MARSHALL R. URIST

12

heterotopic bone formation*

* Supported by a grant in aid from the USPHS, NIH, NIDR #DE02103, Kroc Foundation, Solo Cup Foundation, and the Harcourt Fund.

369

Species-characteristic extraskeletal ossification

The genetic program of nearly all vertebrate species includes some sites of extraskeletal ossification. This ossification occurs in ligaments and tendons in the form of accessory ossicles and should not be confused with heterotopic bone formation. A few examples are sufficient to illustrate the nature of extraskeletal bone in otherwise normal soft parts. The leg tendons of the domestic turkey, *Meleagrio gallapaveo*, ossify as a genetically determined time-dependent development. Ossicles normally form in the semilunar cartilages of the knee of the rat and many other mammals. In the domestic dog and other wild animals, ossicles develop in the penis in the fibrous septum between the corpus cavernosa and form the baculum. Some species develop ossicles in the sclera of the eyeball and some develop ossicles even in the base of the heart valves. The sesamoid bones of the great toe perform a weight bearing function and are thus associated with the upright posture of human beings.

Mechanical injury of muscle

To investigate mechanical trauma as a primary etiologic factor, Zaccalini and Urist[72] demonstrated the results of focal injury to the quadriceps of rabbits, a species previously considered to be especially susceptible to heterotopic bone formation in muscle. Calibrated blunt forces were applied to muscle alone or simultaneously to bone and muscle. Depending upon the level of the force and the selection of tissue, the reaction to injury was simply periosteal proliferation of bone. Isolated foci of heterotopic bone did not develop in muscle. The proliferation of new bone was correlated not so much with injury of muscle as with injury and resorption of juxtaposed previously existing bone structure. Comparable experiments were performed in sheep with identical results.[69]

Anderson and Coulter[3] reported that injury does not produce heterotopic ossification in thigh muscles of the mouse because surgical lacerations, implants of empty diffusion chambers, infusions of latex spheres, injections either of alcohol or acid alcohol, or inoculations of the sea-

weed polygalactose polymer causing carrageen granuloma, do not produce cartilage or bone in hybrid mice. Such observations emphasize the point that heterotopic bone develops as a response to conditions other than mechanical injury. Some of the conditions would include resorption of adjacent bone, deposition of calcium salts in injured muscle, and inclusions of mesenchymal cell remnants with predetermination or gene activation for bone cell differentiation. For example, in AKR mice, thin plates of bone develop from the following combination of local and genetic conditions: surgical injury of implantation of lucite rings in the thigh muscles, inflammation, calcification of muscle fibers, and resorption of calcified muscle (Fig. 12-1). The incidence of bone development is 30% and this form of heterotopic bone does not develop under identical conditions in other strains of mice (Syftestad and Urist, unpublished observations).

Unaware of the predifferentiated osteogenetic foci in some parts of the skeletal system, some investigators have erroneously observed heterotopic bone formation as a spontaneous reaction of muscle to injury. For example, transplantation of autologous minced gastrocnemius muscle to the anterior abdominal wall of the rat produces bone. In the rat, but not in the rabbit, guinea pig, or dog, the insertion of the gastrocnemius muscle contains a nest of fibrocartilaginous tissue that calcifies and is resorbed and replaced by bone following injury. The replacement by bone consistently occurs following tenotomy[5] and in the rat would be expected to occur following the injury of transplantation.[6] This reaction does not occur following tenotomy or transplantation of minced abdominal or other muscle tissue even in the rat. Species-determined focal areas of extraskeletal cartilaginous tissue can mislead the unwary and cause observers to dismiss ossification as a simple reaction to injury, thereby discouraging further research on the local biochemical conditions responsible for heterotopic ossification.

Chemical injury of skeletal muscle

Experiments on rabbit quadriceps muscles demonstrate that chemical injury alone is not sufficient to produce heterotopic ossification of mus-

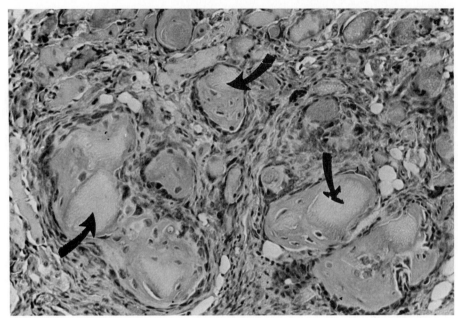

FIGURE 12-1 *Photomicrograph of heterotopic deposits of bone enveloping calcified muscle fibers (arrows) in response to the injury of an implant of an acrylic ring in the gluteus maximus of an AKR strain mouse.*

cle. Selle and Urist[44] injected 365 muscles with various necrotizing or calcifying inorganic and organic substances in graduated concentrations and volumes. Contrary to expectations, non-specific chemical injury and inflammation only infrequently produced heterotopic bone in rabbits. Injections of alcohol produced bone in 31% of the animals. The bone deposits always appeared on the periphery of focal areas of necrosis and in the adventitia of calcified blood vessels. The new bone was associated as well as unassociated with nodules of calcifying cartilage. Surprisingly, large volumes (5 to 21 ml) injected into the quadriceps by Heinen and colleagues[14] and Martin-Lagos and others[26] precludes the fact that, as contended by Levander,[23] the solutions of alcohol dissected along fascial planes produced cartilage and bone deposits derived from muscle attachments to the skeleton. Injections of alcoholic extracts of cartilage and bone produced bone in only slightly greater percentages than did alcohol alone.

Injections of 5 ml of calcium chloride ($CaCl_2$) produced pathologic calcification but not heterotopic cartilage or bone.[44] The reaction to 0.5 to 2.0% $CaCl_2$ was formation of calcified plaques in (1) elastic fibers in the walls of small arteries and veins, (2) an amorphous coagulum, possibly mucoprotein, between atrophied muscle cells, and (3) bundles of calcified collagen fibers and hyalinized connective tissue. There was no new bone or cartilage. Thus, although areas of osteogenesis are frequently seen in close relationship to areas of pathologic calcification, the two processes may be either associated or disassociated from one another.

Cardiac muscle

In rats, ligation of the apical parts of the ventricles initiates in succession, mural thrombi, interstitial granules positively stained for iron and with periodic acid-Schiff reagent (PAS), calcium deposits, foreign body giant cells, new cartilage, new woven bone, new lamellar bone, and bone marrow.[47] The deposits of new bone are comparable in every way to the ossified plaques within the heart and the large blood vessels found in patients with chronic heart disease. Selye[45] claims that calciphylactic deposits may evoke heterotopic bone formation. His observations are reminiscent of the descriptions of heterotopic bone formation in sites of experimental and clinical pathologic calcification observed

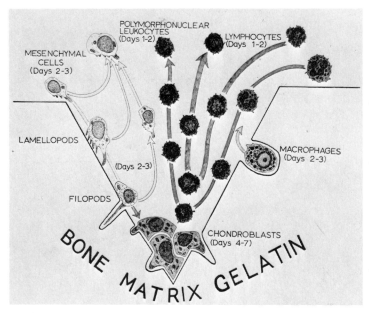

FIGURE 12-2 *Time and cell sequences in the development of heterotopic bone in an implant of bone matrix gelatin in a muscle pouch. Within 48 to 72 hr the mesenchymal-type cells migrate out of the host muscle connective tissue. Migration occurs by lamellopod locomotion. The migratory cells probe crevices in the matrix with filopodia. Contact migration-contact is followed in 4 to 7 d by cell aggregation and phenotypic differentiation in chondroblasts. In this time interval, other cells derived from the inflammatory reaction to surgical injury of implantation, that is, polymorphonuclear leucocytes, lymphocytes and macrophages, secrete proteolytic, collagenolytic, and other BMP-releasing enzymes and later migrate out of the area. Chondroblasts secrete intercellular matrix, and the formation of the cartilage follows.*

by Leriche and Policard[22] more than a half century ago.

Matrix-induced heterotopic bone formation

The most consistently reproducible method known to induce heterotopic bone formation is implantation of demineralized allogeneic bone matrix in muscle. Although it had been implanted for repair of bone defects for nearly a century, it was not until 1965 that the organic matrix of bone was observed to produce new bone in a heterotopic site.[52] The pathogenesis, local conditions, and species specificity are as follows. In all species, the matrix incites only a brief and mild inflammatory reaction to surgical

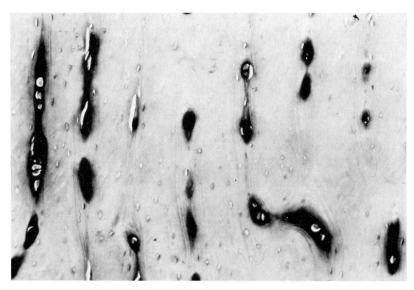

FIGURE 12-3 *Deposits of metachromatic-staining new cartilage differentiation from migratory mesenchymal cells in old vascular channels in the interior of the implanted matrix, 10 d after implantation in a muscle pouch.*

injury of implantation. In rats, the implant transfers a bone morphogenetic protein (BMP) from the matrix to perivascular connective tissue cells as early as 24 hr.[64-66] Within 48 hr after implantation, the matrix surfaces are covered with mesenchymal-type cells. By the end of 72 hr, the mesenchymal cells hypertrophy and become aligned perpendicular to the matrix surfaces. By the end of 1 wk, the hypertrophied cells differentiate into cartilage and by the end of the 2 wk they differentiate into bone.[54] In humans, monkeys, dogs, cats, and other long-lived animals, the morphogenetic response is delayed. Cartilage and bone may not develop on matrix surfaces until 6 to 12 wk after the implantation.

The cell sequences and movements in heterotopic bone formation rats are shown diagrammatically in Figure 12-2. As a general rule, the cartilage develops from cells in deep recesses of nonvascularized parts, and bone develops in vascularized parts of the implanted matrix (Fig.

12-3). Rat bone matrix-induced morphogenesis occurs in nonvascularized systems *in vitro* in the same time intervals as *in vivo*, but the end product is cartilage. Figure 12-4 is a diagrammatic summary of experimental systems designed for research work on BMP. Bone develops by chondroidal ossification when the matrix-induced cartilage is transplanted back into an isologous rat. All of the common strains of laboratory rats produce the response of muscle mesenchyma to bone matrix. Even myoblasts appear to respond.[29] Muscle satellite cell proliferation that is activated by injury may provide a new cell population capable of an osteogenetic response to BMP.

Osteoblasts differentiate on and beneath matrix surfaces penetrated by sprouting capillaries on or about the tenth day. Characteristically, osteoblasts have a deeply basophilic cytoplasm, extrude matrix vesicles, secrete calcifiable metachromatic-staining matrix, and thus deposit

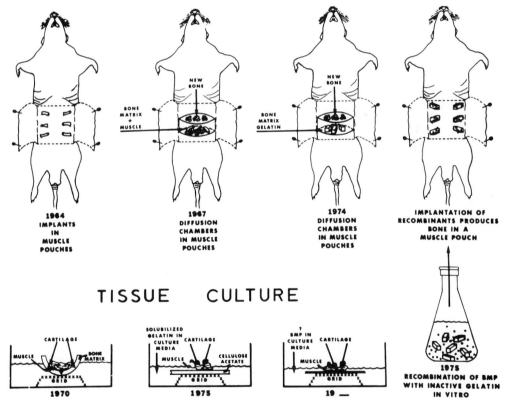

FIGURE 12-4 *Diagrammatic representation of experimental methods, along with the year they were first employed, for the induction of heterotopic bone formation in* in vivo *and* in vitro *muscle systems.*

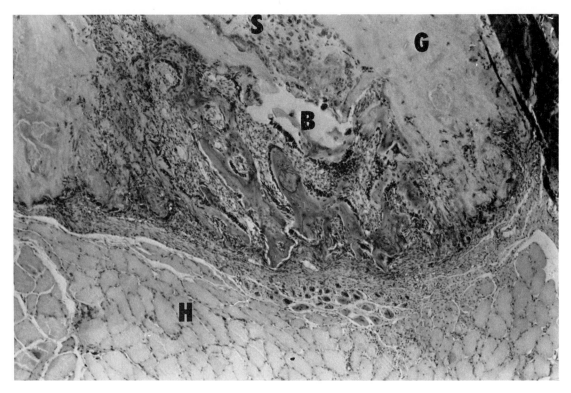

FIGURE 12-5 *Deposits of new bone* **(B)** *on and beneath resorbing surfaces of an implant of bone matrix gelatin* **(G)** *in a muscle pouch 14 d after the operation. Host muscle bed =* **H,** *hypertrophied mesenchymal cells =* **S.**

new woven bone (Figs. 12-5 and 12-6). The explanted matrix recalcifies but only on or near surfaces covered with deposits of new bone. The new bone deposits are resorbed and remodeled over a period of 14 to 28 d into lamellar bone and bone marrow (Fig. 12-7). The end product is an intramuscular heterotopic ossicle comparable to an ossicle formed in a patient with myositis ossificans. The volume of the heterotopic bone is proportional to the matrix mass, and the three-dimensional form is determined by the location or shape of the implant.[63]

Biochemical indicators of matrix-induced heterotopic bone formation appear as early as d 1 and 2. Hyaluronate accumulates in and around the implant on d 1, and is removed by hyaluronidase by d 2.[18,64] Proteoglycans secreted by cartilage cells is tissue-specific insofar as the chondroitin sulfate chains are larger than in proteoglycans synthesized by other tissues. Reddi and coworkers[40] observed that this cartilage-specific molecule, which appeared on d 7,

gradually disappeared and was replaced by smaller proteoglycans by d 11 to 14, coincidental with resorption of cartilage and endochondral ossification. A similar small molecular mass proteoglycan was synthesized prior to d 4 in the precartilagenous preosseous phase of heterotopic bone formation in muscle.

Rathe and Reddi[37] also demonstrated that levels of activity of ornithine decarboxylase (one of the key enzymes regulating polyamine synthesis and cell proliferation) can be correlated with two intervals of time in matrix induced bone formation. The first is the time of contact of cells with the inductive matrix on d 3. The second is the time of intense mitotic activity of newly differentiated preosteoblasts on d 8. The time of colonization of the heterotopic bone by marrow on d 18 to 21 was not associated with a rise in the activity of this enzyme. Reddi and colleagues[39] noted that tissue-specific collagen types change with the course of events preceding and during heterotopic ossification. On d 3 when

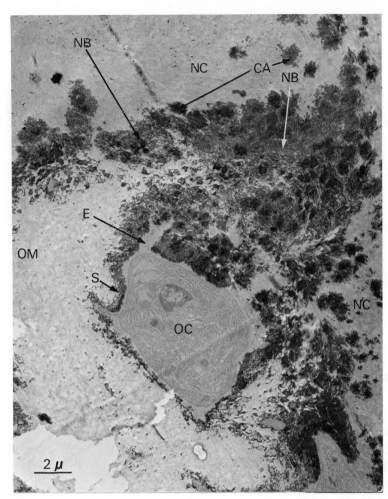

FIGURE 12-6 *Electron micrograph of interface between deposits of heterotopic bone cell* **(OC)** *and the implanted matrix* **(OM)***. The newly formed matrix* **(NC)** *includes matrix vesicles laden with calcium* **(CA)***. Coalescence of the matrix vesicles and clusters of mineral constitutes the calcified new bone matrix* **(NB)***. The calcified new bone also surrounds osteocyte cell extensions* **(E)***.*

fibroblasts proliferate on matrix surfaces, collagen type III predominates, whereas on d 4 to 6 type I again predominates when cartilage is replaced by bone, and type III returns coincidental with the colonization of the deposits of bone marrow, including the development of its reticular cell stroma. Reddi and Huggins[41] observed that incorporation of ^{59}Fe into heme provided a sensitive indicator of the formation of the first colonies of bone marrow cells on d 12. Complete occupation of the heterotopic bone by hematopoietic tissue occurs by d 23 to 28.

Autoradiographs of implants of rats injected either systematically or locally with ^{3}H-thymidine, show labeling of nuclei of perivascular mesenchymal-type cells and preosteoblasts at 72 hr. The label also appeared in the nuclei of osteoblasts at 96 hr.[67] By correlation of ^{3}H-thymidine uptake in DNA with ornithine decarboxylase activity, Rath and Reddi[38] found that bone matrix is mitogenic.[38] Although many developmental biologists observe that collagen is an important substratum for cell differentiation, it is misleading to extrapolate this view to bone matrix-induced heterotopic bone formation. Bone matrix is about 88% collagen but it also contains important tissue-specific noncollagenous proteins. Tendon shares with bone matrix the same collagen type III, but tendon matrix lacks these important proteins, and implants of tendon in muscle induce differentiation only of fibrous connective tissue. In this connection, it is interesting to note that even reconstituted collagens used for experiments in developmental biology

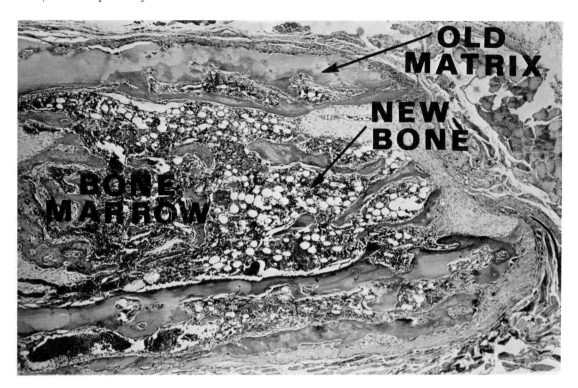

FIGURE 12-7 *Photomicrograph of bone formation induced in a muscle by an implant of an alloimplant of bone matrix in an adult rat, 28 d after the operation. Note: the central cavity of resorbed bone matrix is occupied by colonies of bone marrow; remnants of pale-staining unabsorbed old matrix is a substratum for the deposits of new bone.*

are impure because tightly bound glycoproteins are difficult to remove without digestion of the matrix with collagenase. The noncollagenous BMP fractions account for the high level of bone matrix mitogenic activity, as will be discussed further on.

In a systematic series of experiments on preparations of bone matrix modified by a wide selection of physical, nonenzymic, and enzymic chemical agents, the following evidence was gathered by our research group to support the concept of heterotopic bone formation induced by a matrix, noncollagenous BMP.[52-68] Physical absorption of energy of bone matrix by pulverization to particle sizes less than 200 μm^3, prolonged ultrasonification at 28° C) and doses of ^{60}Co irradiation in excess of 2.0 M rad or heat > 70° C to 100° C denatured BMP irreversibly and prevented formation of heterotopic bone. Chemical denaturation of bone matrix by nitrous acid deamination, dinitrophenylation of ϵ amino and other groups, Cu^{2+} complex formation

across amino and carboxyl groups, disruption of disulfide bonds by mercapthoethanol, cleavage of methionine residues by cyanogen bromide, simultaneous rupture of hydrophobic and hydrophilic bonds in acidic solutions of nonaqueous solvents (i.e., acid alcohol, acid ether, acid acetone, and so forth) prevent matrix-induced heterotopic bone formation. Limited digestion of bone noncollagenous proteins with dilute solutions of trypsin, chymotrypsin, or pronase degrade BMP, whereas collagenase does not. Endogenous sulfhydryl group neutral proteases in bone matrix, including a BMPase, similarly degrade BMP and extinguish matrix-induced heterotopic bone formation. BMP is protected by BMPase inhibitors such as iodoacetic acid, iodoacetamide, N-ethyl maleinide, and para-amino mercuribenzoic acid.[58,61] Incubated in solutions of these BMPase inhibitors even at pH 7.4, body temperature, and ionic strength of body fluids, matrix retains BMP activity. These observations constitute lines of indirect evidence for a BMP and are based on solid state properties of bone matrix. More direct evidence comes from the following experiments with implants of preparation of soluble BMP.

Bone matrix-induced heterotopic bone under the influence of a diffusible component of bone matrix

Two systems employing cellulose acetate diffusion chambers in a muscle pouch reveal that bone matrix releases a diffusible BMP and thereby induces heterotopic bone formation.[59,66] A third system employs tissue culture.[28] In the first system, autologous muscle transplants and bone matrix gelatin implants are placed in paired diffusion chambers; in response to components of the bone matrix gelatin diffusing from one chamber to the other, the host bed muscle mesenchymal-type connective tissue cells differentiate into cartilage (Fig. 12-8). In the second system, cartilage differentiates in the interior of transplants of muscle in diffusion chambers containing a soluble BMP released from bone matrix gelatin by the action of collagenase. In the third system, cartilage develops in an explant of muscle in a tissue culture medium containing bone

matrix gelatin. When transferred from the chambers or from tissue culture into an autologous or isologous muscle pouch, the cartilage is resorbed and replaced by new bone that is later colonized by bone marrow.

The character of a diffusible bone morphogenetic protein (BMP) in experimental heterotopic bone formation

The entire sequence of events in heterotopic bone formation can be produced by implantation of a soluble BMP that has been isolated from bone matrix. BMP also coprecipitates with calcium phosphate with some enhancement of biologic activity (Fig. 12-9). BMP is collagenase-resistant under specified conditions and is separated from solutions of collagenase-digested bone matrix gelatin by concanavalin A chromatography. The combination of carbohydrate recognition and hydrophobic interaction and a high content of hexosamines are presumptive evidence that BMP is a hydrophobic glycoprotein.[65] BMP is isolated without digestion of the matrix by chemical extraction with 50% ethylene glycol (EG) in phosphate buffered saline solutions.[64] In this nonaqueous solvent mixture, BMP retains

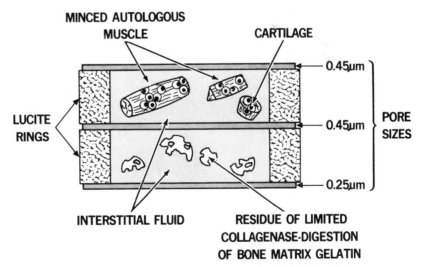

FIGURE 12-8 *Construction of a paired chamber of three cellulose acetate membranes with a pore size of 0.45 μ and a thickness of 150 μ cemented to two hard plastic rings. The upper compartment is filled with strips of muscle tissue. The lower compartment is filled with residue of limited collagenase digest of bone matrix gelatin. After implantation in muscle, the avascular conditions inside of the paired chamber promote induction of cartilage cell differentiation inside of an autograft of adult muscle.*

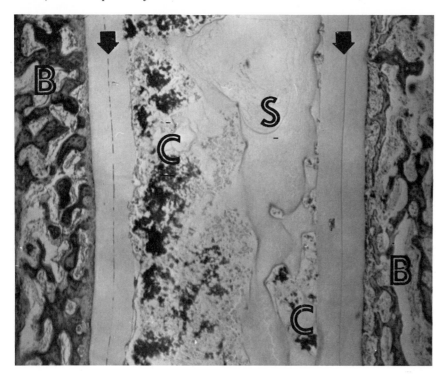

FIGURE 12-9 *Photomicrograph of transmembrane bone formation* **(B)** *on both sides of a double-walled diffusion chamber* (arrows). *The pore size is 0.45 μ and the thickness of each membrane is 150 μ. The chamber was loaded with a coprecipitate of calcium phosphate and BMP, that is dark-staining with hematoxylin and azure* **(C)**. *The intermediate material is eosin-stained precipitated serum* **(S)** *that percolates through the chamber, solubilizes, and transfers BMP. Undecalcified section.*

biologic activity but is difficult to dissociate from EG. Present preparations of soluble BMP are impure and contaminated with several other noncollagenous proteins. Much work lies ahead before the smallest unit of protein structure with BMP activity is known and defined in terms of amino acid composition, sequence, and precise molecular weight.

For the present, it is clear that the mesenchymal-type connective tissue cells in mammalian muscle are genetically coded for a bone morphogenetic pathway of development. These cells are the BMP-responding cells which enter into heterotopic bone formation.

Cartilage tissue differentiation in sites of heterotopic bone

Why differentiation is restricted to the chondrogenetic pathway of development in tissue culture but is permitted to extend to osteogenesis in a muscle pouch is not known. One possibility is that avascular hypoxic conditions are conducive to development of cartilage. In tissue culture, hypoxia promotes the synthesis of N-acetyl-glucosamine-1-t-UDP, a limiting step in the formation of chondroitin.[21] Anoxia may favor synthesis of collagen type II. In a muscle pouch, mesenchymal cells differentiate near sprouting capillaries in which the well oxygenated microenvironment may be conducive to synthesis of the highly cross-linked type I bone matrix collagen. High oxygen saturation and low carbon dioxide tension may be essential requirements for bone tissue development, but respiratory conditions like other general nutritional requirements are ubiquitous and hardly sufficient explanation for heterotopic bone formation. Considering that respiratory and nutritional requirements are also fulfilled, other conditions not yet clearly defined are provided, and BMP is present in the local environment, differentiation of mesenchymal type cells becomes switched from a fibrous connective tissue to a chondrogenic pathway of development.

Under the influence of BMP in bone matrix, cartilage cells differentiate from mature muscle-derived mesenchymal-type cells labeled with ^{3}H-thymidine in tissue culture. Transplants of the labeled cartilage cells differentiate into labeled osteocytes. Development of osteocytes from chondrocytes occurs by a process of chondroidal ossification and suggests that cartilage and bone are allelic expressions of the same gene function.[28,31–32]

The role of blood clot in matrix-induced bone formation

Fibrinous clot covers matrix surfaces immediately after implantation. The clot is resorbed and replaced by granulation tissue. The time required for replacement of all fibrinous material is determined by the volume of the clot. This time may vary from 1 d in the matrix implants in young rats to years in patients with damage to a large muscle. Fresh hematoma does not provide conditions for ossification, but the fibrous envelope around old, unabsorbed fibrin may necrose, calcify, revascularize, and then induce heterotopic bone formation.[23]

Austin[4] constructed a unique silicone tube system (12 × 4 mm in volume) to prolong the time interval of resorption of blood clot on matrix surfaces. By perforating the tube with 0.75-mm holes and filling the perforated tube with bone matrix embedded in clotted blood, Austin observed ingrowth of streams of granulation tissue cells and the progress of dissolution of hematoma. Matrix-induced heterotopic bone developed within 2 to 3 wk inside the tube. These experiments demonstrate that a specified volume of clotted blood and prolongation of the interval of resorption of old fibrin does not blockade the transfer of BMP to mesenchymal cell components of granulation tissue. The biochemical mechanism of heterotopic bone formation in the walls of an old hematoma is not known, but the association of bone deposits with old sites of pathologic calcification warrants investigation by biochemical methods. BMP coprecipitates with calcium phosphate *in vitro*[65] and conceivably might accumulate from some as yet undefined source in areas of pathologic calcification by a similar mechanism.

Marrow transplant–induced heterotopic bone

Within 7 d after transplantation of bone marrow into a muscle pouch, deposits of woven bone develop. The myelogenous cells migrate, regress, or degenerate, whereas the stromal cells proliferate and differentiate into bone. It is reasonable to suppose that bone marrow stroma includes resting osteoblasts (descended directly from osteoprogenitor cells), that a redistribution of this cell population occurs in the course of remodeling of woven bone into lamellar bone, and that in response to the injury of transplantation, stroma osteoblasts differentiate into bone cells. As bone marrow stroma cells include preosteoblasts or already differentiated cells, the classification of osteogenetic precursor cells into determined and inducible osteogenetic precursor cells by Friedenstein[11] serves no useful purpose. As there are no connective tissues that are not induced either by bone matrix or uroepithelium to form bone in a diffusion chamber, the classification of inducible is also redundant. Furthermore, bone marrow stroma includes both mesenchymal cells with unexpressed osteogenetic competence and endosteum-derived preosteoblasts.[24]

Mature marrow stroma consists chiefly of a branching, sponge-like network of reticular cells. By definition, a reticular cell elaborates argyophilic reticular fibers, constitues a large part of the sinusoidal perivascular connective tissue, and only infrequently undergoes mitotic division. However, in response to injury either *in situ* or in a transplant into a muscle pouch, reticular cells proliferate and become undistinguishable from mesenchymal cells, fibroblasts, or osteoprogenitor cells (preosteoblasts). Following injections of carbon particles and various colloidal materials, reticular cells differentiate into fixed macrophages. In this respect, bone marrow reticular cells perform the same function as reticular cells of the liver, spleen and lymph nodes (organs of the reticuloendothelial system), and are fixed macrophages as distinguished from monocyte-derived mobile macrophages.[7]

Unlike bone marrow reticulocytes, spleen and liver reticulocytes do not differentiate into osteoblasts following injury or exposure to bone matrix. Outside of the spleen and under the influence of bone matrix, reticulocytes of spleen may be able to differentiate into bone.[7] Having a lower level of DNA synthesis than hematopoietic cells, mesenchymal and reticular cells recover from irradiation damage more completely than do stem cells, and they will respond to an inductive substratum. The same is true of stromal reticular cell differentiation into bone in response to injury of irradiation.[8] Osteogenetic competence of the cell population is demonstrated simply by implantation of an inductive matrix in various organs of the body. The levels of competence of somatic mesenchyme cells *in situ* are: marrow > muscle > subcutaneous tissue > spleen > or liver or kidney parenchyma.

Speculation on the possibility that blood-borne bone marrow derived cells may lodge in extraskeletal sites and produce heterotopic bone appears in the literature,[9,11] but thus far lacks objective experimental evidence. In direct contrast, bone resorbing cells have been demonstrated to be derived from blood-borne precursor. For example, in parabiost animals, labeled monocytes may pass from the circulating blood into the bone, become pre-osteoclasts, proliferate, fuse and differentiate into osteoclasts. Macrophages in bone may originate either from local or circulating blood cell precursors. Working in tandem, osteoclasts resorb bone while macrophages phagocytose and remove insolubilized bone debris. A conclusive experiment on the fate of osteoclasts has not yet been devised. Until one is, it is impossible to discard the old concept of a cycle of bone cells or the concept that osteoclasts undergo fission[55] and generate either functional osteoblasts or reticular cells depending upon local conditions, i.e., a microenvironment conducive to recycling of bone cells.

Mesenchymal cell and myoblast determination for differentiation in tissue culture

Connective tissue of muscle (endomysium), including myoblasts, satellite cells, endothelial, and mesenchymal-type cells differentiates into cartilage in response to bone matrix in tissue culture.[31,32,50,68] Present evidence is that the mesenchymal-type cells are the responding cell population but other cell types are difficult to exclude.

Nathanson and coworkers[29] contend that the myoblast may not be a stable cell form and along with mesenchymal-type cells may differentiate into cartilage in response to bone matrix *in vitro*. Rat fibroblasts derived from endomysium clonal cultures were induced by matrix to differentiate into cartilage after 14 d in culture. Chick (but not rat) myoblasts differentiated into cartilage. These results are interpreted to suggest that phenotypic differentiation is dependent not simply upon rigidly predetermined genetic patterns but also upon bone matrix–derived environmental stimuli. Since in response to bone matrix, osteoblast differentiation from somatic mesenchymal-type cells in tendon, subcutaneous spaces, brain, and many organ systems[60] other than muscle may occur, unstable myoblasts could not be more than an auxillary group of complemented cells.

Nathanson and coworkers[29] observed that *in vitro* mesenchymal cells from the capsules of visceral organs differentiated into cartilage in response to bone matrix. *In situ*, visceral organ cells (e.g., spleen cells) inhibit matrix-induced cartilage and bone formation.[7] Further experiments are necessary to ascertain the existence of such epithelial mesenchymal cell inter-relationships as may inhibit differentiation of cells in one organ system and induce differentiation in another.

Aorta

Old calcified arteriosclerotic plaques are sometimes resorbed by new blood vessels and perivascular connective tissue, including mesenchymal-type cells and macrophages. In the process of resorption of the calcium salts, heterotopic ossification of arterial walls occurs spontaneously in both human beings and other mammals in the course of either aging or disease, and has been produced experimentally in animals. In rodents, chemical injury of the aorta with heavy metals initiates uptake of calcium ions by the tunica elastica, and calcification follows. In rats, the calcium deposits remain unabsorbed for months. In rabbits, the calcium deposits are rapidly resorbed, and bone formation appears in areas of revascularized calcified elastin and elastoid. Biochemical investigations on calcified blood vessels seem not to have been performed to elucidate the local biochemical conditions leading to intravascular heterotopic bone formation. The purpose would be to determine whether a blood-borne BMP may accumulate in old arterial wall calcium deposits by adsorption or coprecipitation, as has been observed *in vitro* with calcium phosphates.[64,65]

Tendon

Heterotopic ossification may occur in tendon, especially in tendon attachments to bone. In some instances, such as the rat achilles tendon, tenotomy is sufficient to produce bone in spaces between regenerating tendon fibers and scar tissue. The histopathologic process is described in detail by Buck[5] who discovered that following tenotomy, fibrocartilage in the interior of the rat achilles tendon undergoes endochondral ossification and accounts for heterotopic ossification in this location in this species. Injury of this part of the tendon initiates migration, proliferation, and differentiation of paratenon mesenchymal cells into bone. Ossification of a regenerating achilles tendon does not occur in the rabbit or other rodents and is a genetic characteristic of the rat. In this species, ossification may stem from an embryonic axial mesenchymal cell nest that is activated by injury to differentiate into bone. A similar genetic trait characterized by ossification in tendon, but not associated with mechanical injury, occurs in the leg muscle of the domestic turkey.

The mechanism of ossification in the tendon can be observed in intramuscular transplants of viable and nonviable autologous tendon implants in muscle.[56] Viable autologous tendon is simply resorbed and replaced by fibrous tissue. Tendon pretreated in calcium chloride to initiate calcification *in vivo*, then excised and reimplanted in a second site in muscle produces differentiation of new bone on surfaces of previously calcified tendon. Why calcified but not uncalcified rabbit tendon initiates differentiation of mesenchymal cells into cartilage and bone cells requires investigation with the use of biochemical methods for extraction of BMP.[64,65]

Glass tubes in subcutaneous spaces

Glass chambers, 20 mm in height and 30 mm in diameter, subcutaneously implanted on the back muscles of a rat for 60 d are found to contain columns of connective tissue surrounded by exudates of interstitial fluid.[46] The columns measure 3 to 4 mm in diameter and contain calcified granules within histocytes, calcified necrotic connective tissue containing foci of cartilage, bone, bone marrow, and adipose tissue. The bone includes cords of bone marrow. Adipose tissue surrounds the deposits of bone. Injections of carbon particles into the glass chamber produce carbon-laden histocytes or macrophages, which blockade induction of heterotopic bone formation. A similar diversion with charcoal particles, thorium dioxide, or trypan blue occurs in implants of bone matrix[6] (Fig. 12-10). Heterotopic bone formation in glass chambers is relatively low in incidence, in fact so low that other research groups have not confirmed the observation. Nevertheless, the possible association of the bone deposits with foci of pathologic calcification inside of glass chambers warrants further pursuit of this line of investigation.

Implants of plastics

Observations on inbred strains of mice suggest that a combination of local and systematic factors are involved in heterotopic bone formation around plastic implants. Syftestad and Urist[49] implanted bone matrix and various nonbiologic materials, such as cellulose acetate, acrylic, or hydron sponge, inside of hip muscles and observed heterotopic bone formation in over 90% of AKR strain mice. DBA, C_3H and hybrid strains rarely developed bone. However, both the incidence and quantity of bone in AKR mice were far greater with implants of bone matrix.

Winter and colleagues[70] described heterotopic bone in subcutaneous implants of hydron sponge in pigs. The fibrous tissue and necrotic debris

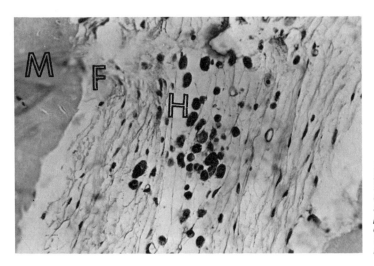

FIGURE 12-10 *Retardation of matrix-induced heterotopic bone formation by intravenous injections of a solution of charcoal particles on the seventh day and accumulation of histocytes (macrophages* **H***) by the 21st day after the operation. Note the paucity of fibroblasts* **(F)** *on the surfaces of the implanted matrix* **(M)**.

calcified in and around the sponge and scanty deposits of bone appeared in adjacent sites after an interval of time in a small percentage of implants. Other species failed to similarly produce heterotopic bone.

Ceramic calcium phosphate and other solid support systems

An affinity for solid state surfaces, particularly surfaces composed of physiochemically inert structure, is characteristic of growing bone. The process of inextension of bone growth onto and into inert substances is known as osteoconduction. For example, the pores of ceramics of β-calcium phosphate and other compounds conduct the ingrowth of preosteoblasts or bone marrow reticular cells and formation of new bone.[27] Regenerating bone tissue similarly grows on surfaces of metallic carbon, methylmethacrylate, cellulose acetate films, and other plastics that are osteoconductive when implanted in bone defects.

Epithelium-induced heterotopic bone formation

In postfetal life, bone can be produced experimentally in heterotopic sites by transplantation of uroepithelium (Fig. 12-11), gall bladder epithelium, gastric epithelium, skin, and stable cell lines derived from either placenta or cervix.[2,71] The circumstances are reminiscent of the mechanism of embryonic development of cranial bones from a condensation of mesenchymal cells in response to the pressure of the growing brain. The mechanism is more complex than a reaction to purely mechanical pressure because only a particular selection of epithelial tissues induces the osteogenetic response.[12] Moreover, some epithelial cells (e.g., urinary bladder, gall bladder, and gastric epithelium) induce bone formation only whereas others, (e.g., HeLa and amnion Fl cell lines) first induce development of cartilage then induce development of bone. Whatever the inducing epithelium may be, the induced cell population is perivascular mesenchymal-like connective tissue.

Attention has been given to the problem of exclusion of endothelium as the responsive cell population. The evidence against this point of view is that cartilage cell induction occurs in systems *in vitro* and in areas of a bone matrix implant (see Fig. 12-3), in which there is no endothelium or capillary ingrowth.[54] Moreover, neither cartilage nor bone forms in endothelium-rich tissues of liver, spleen, or kidney parenchyma.[60] There is some speculation on blood-borne bone marrow–derived stem cells as a source of preosteoblasts.[9,11] Evidence against this possibility is the failure of heterotopic bone to form in liver, spleen, and kidney parenchyma, in which stem cells statistically may lodge as frequently as in muscle.[60] Even when composite

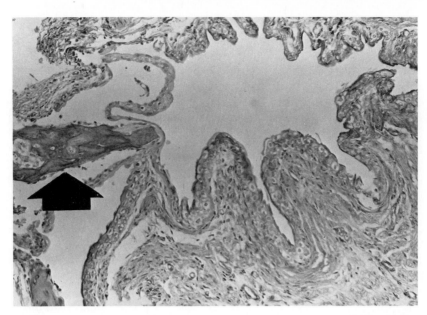

FIGURE 12-11 *Photomicrograph of a cyst produced by an autologous transplant of guinea pig urinary bladder. Note the convolutions of proliferating transitional epithelium, the encysted space previously occupied by fluid (center), and a deposit of heterotopic bone in the wall of the cyst (arrow).*

grafts of inflammatory connective tissues and inductive matrix are implanted in these organs, neither cartilage nor bone differentiates, but when the same composites are first implanted in muscle and then transferred to liver, spleen, and kidney, bone formation ensues.[7] Bone matrix induces bone formation in a larger variety of tissues than does any epithelial cell type. Subcutaneous perivascular connective tissue cells do not interact with epithelial osteoinductive cell lines but are consistently induced by bone matrix to produce new bone.[60]

Włodarski and Jakobisiak[71] irradiated inbred mice with sublethal doses (700 rad) and lethal doses (850 rad). The mice treated with sublethal doses did *not* produce heterotopic bone in response to an established human cell line (HEp-2) or dog transitional (bladder) epithelium transplants in muscle. The mice treated with lethal doses and protected with an infusion of syngeneic bone marrow cells did produce heterotopic bone. Although the experimental design does not discriminate between recovery of muscle mesenchymal cells from irradiation damage and the activity of blood-borne bone marrow–derived cell population, the develop-

ment of large deposits of heterotopic bone in lethally irradiated bone marrow–infused mice renews speculation on the view that circulating blood cells might be induced to differentiate into bone cells. However, the experiment that is necessary to submit unequivocal evidence for the blood cell origin of preosteoblasts has not yet been designed.

The permutations and combinations of transplants and donor site factors leading to induction of bone by epithelium are discussed in detail in review articles by Anderson[2] and by Ostrowski and Włodarski.[34] The difficulties inherent in research on osteogenetic epithelial mesenchymal cell interactions are exemplified by the present state of research on uroepithelium-induced bone formation. After more than a half century of research on Huggins'[17] key observation on bone deposits in transplants of uroepithelium, the literature is a collection of merely empirical or negative information. Uroepithelium induces bone formation in muscle or fascia consistently in human beings, dogs, cats, and guinea pigs (but seldom in rabbits, rats, or mice). Nothing is known about the biochemical mechanism. Transitional uroepithelial transplants proliferate and secrete a hyaloid substance and become encysted. Although patches of bone differentiate in the *walls* of the cyst, there is no objective evidence of any association of the new bone with either the epithelial cells or the cyst contents.

Malignant mucosal cells of gastrointestinal cancers, particularly cancer of the distal segment of the large bowel, generate calcifying metastases. The host bed connective tissue cells surrounding the calcified cancer cells differentiate into bone. The association of secretory byproducts of transplants of all of these normal epithelial tissue and neoplastic cell lines, calcifying or noncalcifying, is more than circumstantial. Only a select group of epithelial cells are osteoinductive. Investigations on BMP in epithelial mesenchymal interactions should be pursued by means of immunofluorescent antibody techniques.

Clinical pathologic conditions

Myositis ossificans traumatica

Heterotopic bone formed in muscle in response to trauma is commonly termed myositis ossificans traumatica (MOT). The term has gained the permanence of common usage because the earliest or preroentgenographic symptoms and signs are pain, local heat, and swelling—the classic clinical symptoms of inflammation. The term is constantly criticized yet almost impossible to extricate from the literature. The objections are that inflammation is not the characteristic feature and muscle fibers are not the focal points of the pathologic lesion. The characteristic feature is reaction of mesenchymal-like fibroblasts that migrate, proliferate, and differentiate into cartilage and bone. The focal point of the lesion is the connective tissue septa between, not in, muscle fibers.

There are no recorded statistics on the incidence of MOT. The clinical impression is that MOT appears more frequently in sports injuries in growing high school athletes (aged 14 to 17 yr) than in college athletes (aged 18 to 24 yr) and more frequently in college athletes than in professional athletes (aged 25 to 35).

In experimental muscle contusions in laboratory animals and in sports injuries in young people, myositis ossificans occurs in or near hemorrhagic muscle attachments to bone. In abdominal scars heterotopic bone is generally not attached to the xiphisternum, but attachments may eventually develop. The low incidence of ossification either in abdominal scars (only 21 case reports up to 1974) or in myositis ossificans in hermorrhagic muscle after all kinds of orthopedic operations indicates that muscle is not normally predisposed to ossification. In MOT, either the traumatic or idiopathic form, roentgenographically demonstrable bone formation may begin at some distance from bone, but eventually the deposits grow toward and become attached to the nearest skeletal part. The earliest deposits also contain cartilage that later undergoes endochondral ossification.

Ossification of muscle in cerebral injury, paraplegia, and burns

Normal muscle is refractory to ossification. Paralyzed muscle, by some unknown mechanism, becomes susceptible to ossification. A combination of local, regional, and presently undefined systemic factors induce proliferation and differentiation of the muscle connective tissue cells into cartilage and bone. Systemic factors are suspect, because only about 30% of paraplegics are disposed to heterotopic bone formation. The local factors are stasis, edema, swelling, inflammation, and prolonged immobility of the limb. The deposits are always periarticular and are generally in the shoulder, elbow, and hip muscles. Resorption and atrophy invariable occur in the adjacent bone tissue. The process is enhanced by injuries to ligamentous attachments from overzealous passive exercises which may accelerate heterotopic ossification in patients with spinal cord injuries.

Heterotopic bone formation typically occurs below the level of damage to the spinal cord lesion.[19] The bone develops in muscle and tendon attachments to bone, and not in joint capsules or articular structures. When the growing bone deposits are extensive, or if surgical excision is performed before the deposits are mature, the levels of the serum alkaline phosphatase and urinary hydroxyproline may rise. Either a high uptake of technetium-99 diphosphonate in bone scintograms or elevated levels of alkaline phosphatase (as long as 1.5 yr after the first appearance of heterotopic bone in roentgenograms) are contraindications to surgical excision. The elbow joint is most commonly involved. The deposits occur in the first 6 mo after the injury, and may appear either in posterior or anterior musculature. The brachialis anticus is especially susceptible (Fig. 12-12). The articular surfaces and capsular ligaments are surprisingly uninvolved or resistant.

Myositis ossificans circumscripta

Extraosseous non-neoplastic localized development of bone without a history of trauma is termed myositis ossificans circumscripta (MOC). Although localized heterotopic bone develops in paraplegic, poliomyelitis, and bedridden patients with extensive burns or chronic infections, MOC occurs in otherwise normal patients. In four cases reported in the thigh or buttock of young adults by Paterson,[35] the blood chemistry studies were entirely normal. The differential diagnosis of osteosarcoma is important and can be worrisome. Osteosarcoma usually occurs near the ends of the bones, continues to increase in size, and erodes cortical bone. MOC diminishes in size, does not erode cortical bone, or invade muscle may be successfully excised and is even known to spontaneously regress under conservative management. Recurrences may follow excision but are as benign as the original tumor. Microscopically, MOC is isolated from the host muscle by a fibrous connective tissue capsule, and is organized in three zones: an inner zone of proliferating spindle shaped cells, a central zone of osteoblasts and osteoid, and an outer zone of lamellar bone including bone marrow (Figs. 12-13 to 12-15). The etiology is not known, but the clinical picture points to a local biochemical

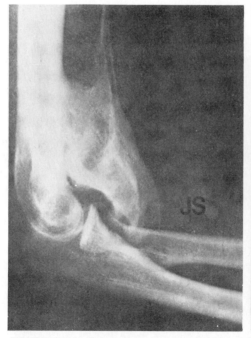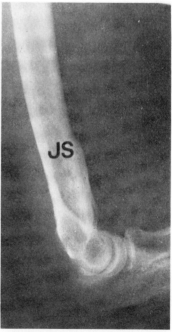

FIGURE 12-12 *Roentgenograms of ankylosis of the elbow (left) caused by heterotopic ossification associated with brain injury and long-term coma. The patient was a 27-yr-old woman who also developed heterotopic bone in both hip joints. The elbow heterotopic bone mass was extra-articular and was excised 15 mo after the injury. There was no recurrence 11 mo later at the time of the last x-ray film (right). (Roberts, J. B., and Pankratz, D. G.: J. Bone and Joint Surg. 61A:760–763, 1979)*

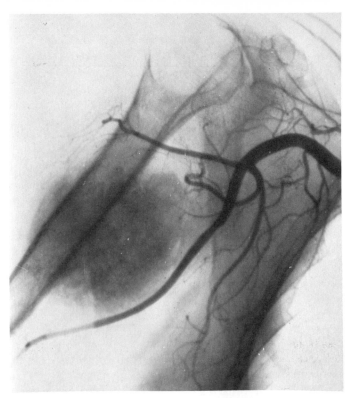

FIGURE 12-13 *Angiogram of a 55-yr-old woman with myositis ossificans circumscripta. Note the lack of tumor blood vessels. For relief of radial nerve paresis and pain, the tumor was excised. There was no recurrence, but the recovery of the radial nerve was incomplete.*

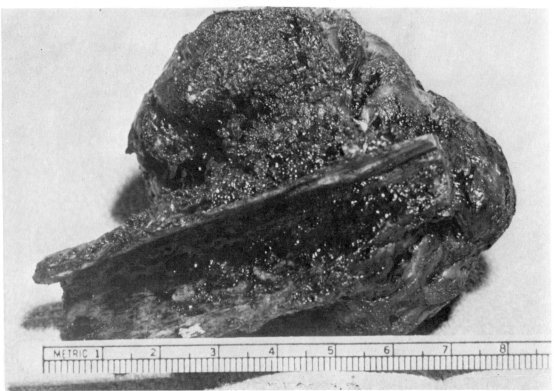

FIGURE 12-14 *Photograph of a specimen of myositis ossificans circumscripta shown in Figure 12-13, removed by excision, including the en bloc site of attachment to the medial aspect of the shaft of the humerus. The host bone bed defect was repaired with an allogeneic bone graft.*

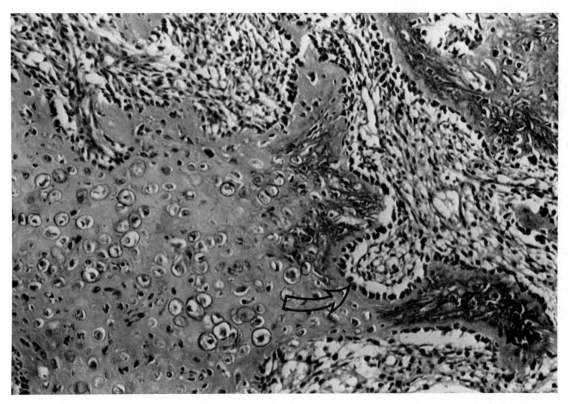

FIGURE 12-15 *Photomicrograph of cartilage and bone in the tumor shown in Figure 12-14. The layers of osteoblasts aligned at right angles to the bone surfaces (arrow) are evidence of the benign character of myositis ossificans circumscripta.*

abnormality of the muscle tissue cortical bone interface in combination with a metabolic factor of undetermined nature. A search for metabolic abnormalities related to blood or tissue BMP activity is compelling in the patient with MOC and disseminated pulmonary deposits of typical heterotopic bone and bone marrow.

Myositis (fibrodysplasia) ossificans progressiva

A generalized progressive disease characterized by ossification in the paravertebral, shoulder, pelvic girdle, jaw, and head musculature is known as myositis ossificans progressiva (MOP; Fig. 12-16). Neither smooth nor cardiac muscle is involved. The condition develops from an autosomal dominant mutation and does not appear in siblings. The diagnosis can be established at birth by the abnormalities of the hands and feet. Microdactyly of the thumbs and great toes oc-

curs in nearly every case. Reproductive fitness is low because the patients frequently die of respiratory failure before childbearing age.

The most significant feature of MOP is the genetic predisposition of the connective tissue cells to differentiation into cartilage and bone at the site of injections, injuries, and surgical operations. The bone develops without the influence of any obvious exogenous agent. The possibility of a blood-borne or systemic BMP has not yet been investigated. Microscopically, muscle fibers degenerate, calcify, and are replaced by connective tissue, bone, and bone marrow. The serum levels of alkaline phosphatase may be slightly elevated, but otherwise the blood chemistry is generally normal. The etiology is congenital, but the local pathologic changes are remarkably similar to myositis ossificans associated with injuries in young athletes. Muscle fibers degenerate and calcify, and in the after-

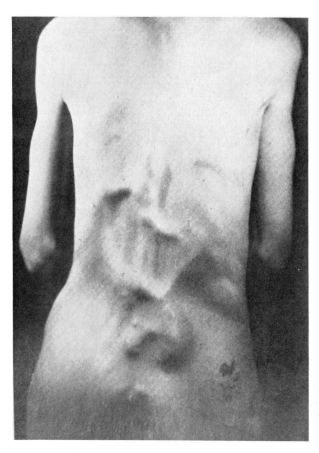

FIGURE 12-16 *Photograph of the plaques, plates, bars, and irregular masses of heterotopic bone in the trunk muscles of a patient with myositis ossificans progressiva (fibroplasia ossificans progressiva). (Fairbanks, Atlas of General Affections of the Skeleton, London, Churchill Livingston, 1976)*

math of resorption and revascularization of degenerated calcified tissue, endomyseal perivascular connective tissue mesenchymal-type cells differentiate into bone. The literature has been reviewed by Smith and coworkers[48] and Lutwak,[25] who performed detailed metabolic studies and reported unsuccessful results of treatment with a variety of systemic hormonal and biochemical agents. As has been demonstrated both in experimental animals[36,49] and in patients[15,16] diphosphonate EHDP therapy of MOP inhibits calcification but not heterotopic bone matrix formation.

Surgical trauma and joint implant operations

Heterotopic bone formation occurs in response to implantation of metallic devices for fixation and plastic devices for artificial joints. The movement of tissues around an intramedullary nail protruding from the greater trochanter of the hip produces injury, inflammation, and calcification of muscle fibers. Over a period of months, the injured tissues are resorbed or enveloped in deposits of heterotopic bone. Fracture of the humerus at the attachment of the brachialis anticus muscles may induce heterotopic bone formation in children and young adults.

Heterotopic bone is frequently encountered in patients with total hip arthroplasties. Some surgical approaches may produce a slightly higher incidence than others. The average occurrence is 8 to 12% but it may be as high as 21% with the anterior approaches. The average quantity of heterotopic bone generally does not limit flexion and other functions of the hip. The incidence of above-average obstructive quantities of heterotopic bone varies from 5 to 8% and is three times more common in men than in women. DeLee and colleagues[10] reviewed the literature and reported an overall incidence of 14.6% in a series of 2311 cases. Unexpectedly, the occurrence of obstructive heterotopic bone formation was not greater in revision than in initial operations and was not greater in cases with trochanteric osteotomy or osteophytectomy, but was higher (16.9%) in osteoarthritis or ankylosing spondylitis than in other forms of joint disease. Because patients with heterotopic bone in one total hip arthroplasty develop heterotopic bone in the contralateral hip, constitutional factors of unknown character have been assumed to play a role in the etiology. Individuals who are predisposed to periarticular heterotopic ossification warrant investigation of biopsy specimens for levels of tissue BMP activity by xenografts in athymic mice.

Heterotopic ossification in fibrous capsules of old hematomas

Extra vasated blood normally does not induce bone formation, but areas of the fibrous connective tissue envelope around an old unabsorbed hematoma may necrotize and calcify. Such areas of focal calcification are slowly resorbed and in the process produce deposits of marrow. Zadek[73] described a 22-yr-old unabsorbed massive hematoma surrounded by lamellar bone and bone marrow. On the basis of circumstantial evidence alone, the patient was diagnosed as having an ossifying hematoma. The condition is distinguished from MOT by the lack of any attachments to an adjacent bone and by the failure of the heterotopic bone to mature, remodel, regress, and disappear with time. Since the heterotopic bone develops in sites of calcified necrotic fibrous tissue and not in clotted blood, the term ossifying hematoma is misleading.

Laparotomy scars, abdominal incisions for suprapubic prostatectomy, and uroepithelial-induced heterotopic bone formation

Heterotopic bone formation may be discovered by palpation in patients with midline laparotomy incisional scars. The deposits may or may not be attached to the xiphoid segment of the sternum. The condition is more common in males than in females and generally occurs in middle-aged individuals. The time sequence of events and the pathologic features are the same as in MOT.[30]

Heterotopic bone formation sometimes occurs in suprapubic abdominal scars. Bladder mucosal grafts for repair of experimental hypospadias in dogs generally form bone. Either fascia or muscle tissue grafts for repair of fluid-filled bladder cysts frequently ossify. Bone deposits also develop in bladder transplants in humans. Heterotopic bone may occur in the aftermath of healing of surgical defects in the ureter. All parts of the urinary tract that are lined with transitional epithelium are similarly predisposed to heterotopic bone formation. Although knowledge of the biochemical mechanism is lacking, the pathologic process is identical to that observed in epithelial mesenchymal cell–induced bone formation in animals.

Ossification of spinal ligaments

One of the characteristic signs of anklyosing spondylitis, spondylosis, and other seronegative arthropathies is ossification of the longitudinal ligaments of the spine. A similar condition is typically localized in the cervical spine, sometimes causing cervical myelopathy, but may present no signs or symptoms. The condition appears to be endemic in Japanese, and is named diffuse idiopathic skeletal hyperostosis (DISH).[33] The symptoms in patients with cervical myelopathy are parathesias, numbness and tingling in upper and lower extremities, anesthesia of areas of the trunk, motor weakness, instability, incoordination, head pain and neck stiffness, urinary and rectal incontinence, and loss of libido. The physical findings include muscle atrophy, fasciculations, hyper-reflexia, and sensory loss.

Resnick, and colleagues[42] reviewed the literature on DISH and reported four cases in a non-Japanese population. Autopsy examinations revealed calcification of a thickened deep layer and ossification of the superficial layers of the posterior longitudinal ligaments. Hyperplasia of connective tissue and differentiation of cartilage cells occurred at the interface between deep and superficial layers. The pathogenesis of DISH and other ossifying diseases of the spinal column ligaments is unknown and presents unusual opportunities for laboratory investigation of blood and tissue levels of BMP activity.

Treatment of heterotopic bone formation

The treatment of heterotopic ossification is surgical excision, but it is recommended only in patients who have interference with function of an essential joint, and then only after an interval of 18 mo after the onset of the condition. Early excision is almost invariably followed by reformation of the heterotopic bone. The following measures have been reported with uncertain success to prevent heterotopic bone formation: immobilization, aspiration of hematomas, local injections of hydrocortisone, diphosphonate therapy, and irradiation. No one measure or combination of measures is known to be effective. Until more research is done on both systemic and regional as well as local biochemical mechanisms, the treatment of heterotopic bone formation is bound to be unsatisfactory.

Research retrospect and prospects

The extraordinary diversity of systems of bone induction systems in both experimental animals and patients suggests that a further understanding of the biochemistry of heterotopic bone will bring fundamental knowledge of the mechanisms of formation of normal bone. Heterotopic bone formation is a benign, self-limiting growth with no obvious function. Heterotopic bone formation is an abnormality of interacting systemic, regional, and local biochemical factors that induce differentiation of postfetal mesenchymal-type cells into cartilage, bone, and bone marrow. Neither individually nor in combinations are the effects of presently known factors on cell development known, except possibly one. A bone morphogenetic protein (BMP) has been isolated from bone matrix in solubilized form and as a coprecipitate with calcium phosphate.[64,65] The purification of BMP is incomplete. Whether a BMP also initiates epithelial-mesenchymal (i.e., uroepithelium and fascia connective tissue) cell systems in heterotopic bone formation is not known. One engaging prospect to heterotopic bone deposits is that BMP may be chemotactic for mesenchymal type cells which in turn differentiate and induce interaction with blood-borne cells. Heterotopic bone initiates a homing response by blood-borne bone marrow precursor cells. In fact, the presence of bone marrow in a BMP-induced bone deposit distinguishes host normal bone from neoplastic bone.

References

1. Ackerman, I. V.: Extraosseous localized non-neoplastic bone and cartilage formation (so called myositis ossificans), J. Bone Joint Surg. 40A:279–289, 1958.
2. Anderson, H. C.: Osteogenetic epithelial-mesenchymal cell interactions, Clin. Orthop. 119: 211–224, 1976.
3. Anderson, H. C., and Coulter, P. R.: Bone-inducing capability of cultured human cells (Fl and HeLa) compared to that of various types of injury, Fed. Proc. 27:475, 1968.
4. Austin, J. C.: The induction of bone in organizing haematomata in rats, South Afr. J. Med. 38:95, 1973.
5. Buck, R. C.: Regeneration of tendon, Pathol. Bact. 67:1, 1953.
6. Carlson, B. M.: The Regeneration of Minced Muscles, New York, S. Karger, 1972.
7. Chalmers, J., Gray, D. H., and Rush, J.: Observations on the induction of bone in soft tissues, J. Bone Joint Surg. 57B:36–45, 1975.
8. Craven, P. L., and Urist, M. R.: Osteogenesis by radioisotope labelled cell populations in implants of bone matrix under the influence of ionizing irradiation, Clin. Orthop. 76:231–243, 1971.
9. Danis, A.: Etude de l'ossification de les greffes de moelle osseuse, Acta Med. Belg. (Suppl.) 56(3):1–120, 1957.
10. DeLee, J., Ferrari, A., and Charnley, J.: Ectopic bone formation following low friction arthroplasty of the hip, Clin. Orthop. 121:53–60, 1976.
11. Friedenstein, A. J.: Determined and inducible osteogenic precursor cells, *In* R. F. Sognnaes and J. Vaughan: Hard Tissue, Ciba Symposium II (new series), p. 169, Amsterdam, Associated Scientific Publications, 1973.

12. Hall, B. K.: Developmental and Cellular Skeletal Biology, New York, Academic Press, 1979.

13. Harvey, W. H.: Experimental bone formation in arteries, J. Med. Res. 17:25–36, 1907.

14. Heinen, J. H., Jr., Dabbs, G. H., and Mason, H. A.: The experimental production of ectopic cartilage and bone in the muscles of rabbits, J. Bone Joint Surg. 31A:765, 1949.

15. Hentzer, B., Jacobsen, H. H., and Asboe-Hansen, G.: Fibrodysplasia (myositis) ossificans progressiva treated with disodium etidronate, Clin. Radiol. 29(1):69–75, 1978.

16. Holmsen, H., Ljunghall, S., and Hierton, T.: Myosificans ossificans progressiva, Acta Orthop. Scand. 50:33, 1979.

17. Huggins, C. B.: The formation of bone under the influence of epithelium of the urinary tract, Arch. Surg. 22:377, 1931.

18. Iwata, H., and Urist, M. R.: Hyaluronic acid production and removal during bone morphogenesis in implants of bone matrix in rats, Clin. Orthop. 90:236–245, 1973.

19. Kewalramani, L. S.: Ectopic ossification, Am. J. Phys. Med. 56:99, 1977.

20. Kubacek, V., Fait, M., and Poul, J.: A case of heterotopic ossification in the hip joint area following skin burn, Acta Chir. Plast. 19(3–4):209–214, 1977.

21. Lash, J. W.: Chondrogenesis: genotypic and phenotypic expression, J. Cell Physiol. 72:35, 1968.

22. Leriche, R., and Policard, A.: The Normal and Pathological Physiology of Bone: Its Problems, translated from the French by Sherwood Moore and J. A. Key, St. Louis, the C. V. Mosby Co., 1928.

23. Levander, G.: Induction phenomena in tissue regeneration, Baltimore, Williams & Wilkins Co., 1964.

24. Lindholm, T. S., and Urist, M. R.: A quantitative analysis of new bone formation by induction in composite grafts of bone marrow and bone matrix, Clin. Orthop. (in press).

25. Lutwak, L.: Myositis ossificans progressiva, Am. J. Med. 37:269–293, 1964.

26. Martin-Lagos, F., and Zarapico Romero, M.: Obtension experimental de hueso metaplasico, Trab. Inst. Nac. Cien. Med. 6:173–215, 1946.

27. McDavid, P. T., Boone, M. E., Kafrawy, A. H., and Mitchell, D. F.: Effect of autogenous marrow and calcitonin on reactions to a ceramic, J. Dent. Res. 58:1478–1483, 1979.

28. Nakagawa, M., and Urist, M. R.: Chon-drogenesis in tissue cultures of muscle under the influence of a diffusible component of bone matrix, Proc. Soc. Exp. Biol. Med. 154:568–572, 1977.

29. Nathanson, M. A., Hilfer, S. R., and Searle, R. L.: Formation of cartilage by non-chondrogenetic cell types, Dev. Biol. 64:99, 1978.

30. Nilsson, F., and Simonsson, N.: Heterotopic bone formation in upper midline abdominal incisions, Acta Chir. Scand. 143(7–8):435–437, 1977.

31. Nogami, H., and Urist, M. R.: Substrata prepared from bone matrix for chondrogenesis in tissue culture, J. Cell Biol. 62:510–519, 1974.

32. Nogami, H., and Urist, M. R.: Explants, transplants and implants of a cartilage and bone morphogenetic matrix, Clin. Orthop. 103:235, 1974.

33. Ono, K., Ota, H., Toda, K., Hamoda, H., and Takoaka, K.: Ossified posterior longitudinal ligament, Spine 2:126, 1977.

34. Ostrowski, K., and Włodarski, K.: Induction of heterotopic bone formation. *In* Bourne, G. H. (ed.): The Biochemistry and Physiology of Bone, 2nd edition, New York, Academic Press.

35. Paterson, D. C.: Myositis ossificans circumscripta, J. Bone Joint Surg. 52B:296–301, 1970.

36. Plasmans, C.: The influence of diphosphonates on induced heterotopic bone, Ph.D. thesis, Catholic University, Nijmegen, The Netherlands, Van Mameran, Publishers, 1977.

37. Rath, N. C., and Reddi, A. H.: Changes in ornithine decarboxylase activity during matrix induced cartilage, bone, and bone marrow differentiation, Biochem. Biophys. Res. Commun. 81:106–113, 1978.

38. Rath, N. C., and Reddi, A. H.: Collagenous matrix is a local mitogen, Nature 278:855, 1979.

39. Reddi, A. H., Gay, R., Gay, S., and Miller, E. J.: Transitions in collagen types during matrix induced cartilage, bone and bone marrow formation, Proc. Nat. Acad. Sci. 74:5589, 1977.

40. Reddi, A. H., Hascall, V. C., and Hascall, G. K.: Changes in proteoglycan types during matrix induced cartilage and bone development, J. Biol. Chem. 253:2429, 1978.

41. Reddi, A. H., and Huggins, C. B.: Formation of bone marrow in fibroblast transformation ossicles, Proc. Nat. Acad. Sci. 72:2212, 1975.

42. Resnick, D., Guerra, J., Robinson, C. A., and Vinton, C. V.: Association of diffuse idiopathic skeletal hyperostosis (DISH) and calcification and ossification of the posterior longitudinal ligament, Am. J. Roentgenol. 131:1049–1053, 1978.

43. Roberts, J. B., and Pankrotz, D. G.: The surgical treatment of heterotopic ossification at the elbow following long term coma, J. Bone Joint Surg. 61A:760–763, 1979.

44. Selle, R., and Urist, M. R.: Calcium deposits and new bone formation in muscle in rabbits, J. Surg. Res. 1:132–142, 1961.

45. Selye, H.: Calciphylaxis, Chicago, University of Chicago Press, 1962.

46. Selye, H., Lemire, Y., and Bajusz, E.: Induction of bone, cartilage and hemopoietic tissue by subcutaneously implanted tissue diaphragms, Roux' Archiv für Entwicklungsmechanik 151:572–585, 1960.

47. Selye, H., Mahajan, S., and Mahajan, R. S.: Histogenesis of experimentally induced myositis ossificans in the heart, Am. Heart J. 73(2):195–201, 1967.

48. Smith, R., Russell, R. G. G., and Woods, C. G.: Myositis ossificans circumscripta, J. Bone Joint Surg. 58B:48, 1976.

49. Strates, B. S., and Urist, M. R.: The origin of the inductive signal in implants of normal and lathyritic bone matrix, Clin. Orthop. 66:226–240, 1969.

50. Terashima, Y., and Urist, M. R.: BrdU-inhibition of substratum-controlled chondrogenesis, Proc. Soc. Exp. Biol. Med. 146:855–858, 1974.

51. Tibone, J., Sakimura, I., Niekel, V. L., and Hsu, J. D.: Heterotopic ossification around the hip in spinal cord injured patients, J. Bone Joint Surg. 60A:769, 1978.

52. Urist, M. R.: Bone: Formation by autoinduction, Science 150:893, 1965.

53. Urist, M. R.: Bone morphodifferentiation and tumorigenesis, Persp. Biol. Med. 22:589, 1979.

54. Urist, M. R.: The substratum for bone morphogenesis, 29th Symposium Soc. for Develop. Biol. (Suppl.) 4:125, 1970.

55. Urist, M. R., and Craven, P. L.: Bone cell differentiation in avian species: with comments on multinucleation and morphogenesis, Fed. Proc. 29:1680–1693, 1970.

56. Urist, M. R., de la Sierra, J., and Strates, B. S.: The substratum for new bone formation in tendon, Clin. Orthop. 63:210–221, 1969.

57. Urist, M. R., Dowell, T. A., Hay, P. H., and Strates, B. S.: Inductive substrates for bone formation, Clin. Orthop. 59:59, 1968.

58. Urist, M. R., Earnest, F., Kimball, K. M., DiJulio, T. P., and Iwata, H.: Bone morphogenesis in implants of residues of radioisotope labelled bone matrix, Calcif. Tissue Res. 15:269–286, 1974.

59. Urist, M. R., Granstein, R., Nogami, H., Svenson, L., and Murphy, R.: Transmembrane bone morphogenesis across multiple-walled chambers: new evidence of a diffusible bone morphogenetic property, Arch. Surg. 112:612–619, 1977.

60. Urist, M. R., Hay, P. H., Dubuc, F., and Buring, K.: Osteogenetic competence, Clin. Orthop. 64:194, 1969.

61. Urist, M. R., Iwata, H., Boyd, S. D., and Ceccotti, P. L.: Observations implicating an extracellular enzymic mechanism of control of bone morphogenesis, J. Histochem. Cytochem. 22:88–103, 1974.

62. Urist, M. R., Iwata, H., Ceccotti, P. W. L., Dorfman, R. L., Boyd, S. D., McDowell, R. M., and Chien, C.: Bone morphogenesis in implants of insoluble bone gelatin, Proc. Nat. Acad. Sci. 70:3511–3515, 1973.

63. Urist, M. R., Jurist, J. M., Dubec, F. L., and Strates, B. S.: Quantitation of new bone formation in intramuscular implants of bone matrix in rabbits, Clin. Orthop. 68:279–293, 1970.

64. Urist, M. R., and Mikulski, A. J.: A soluble bone morphogenetic protein extracted from bone matrix with a mixed aqueous non-aqueous solvent, Proc. Soc. Exp. Biol. Med., 162:48–53, 1979.

65. Urist, M. R., Mikulski, A. J. and Lietze, A.: Solubilized and insolubilized bone morphogenetic protein, Proc. Nat. Acad. Sci. 76:1828–1832, 1979.

66. Urist, M. R., Nakagawa, M., Nakata, N., and Nogami, H.: Experimental myositis ossificans: cartilage and bone formation in muscle in response to a diffusible bone matrix-derived morphogen, Arch. Pathol. Lab. Med. 102(6):312, 1978.

67. Urist, M. R., Silverman, B. F., Buring, K., Dubec, F. L., and Rosenberg, J. M.: The bone induction principle, Clin. Orthop. 53:243–283, 1967.

68. Urist, M. R., Terashima, Y., Nakagawa, M., and Stamos, C.: Cartilage tissue differentiation from mesenchymal cells derived from mature muscle in tissue culture, *in vitro* 14(8):697, 1978.

69. Walton, M., and Rothwell, A. G.: An animal model for the study of ossifying quadriceps hematoma, Proceedings of University of Otago Medical School 56:1–2, 1978.

70. Winter, G. D.: Heterotopic bone induced by synthetic sponge implants, Biochem. Biophys. Aspects 7:433, 1971.

71. Włodarski, K., and Jakobisiak, M.: Attempts of bone induction by xenogeneic epithelial cells in sublethally and lethally irradiated mice. Preliminary report, Arch. Immunol. Ther. Exp. (Warsz) 26:1047–1051, 1978.

72. Zaccalini, P. S., and Urist, M. R.: Traumatic periosteal proliferations in rabbits: The enigma of experimental myositis ossificans traumatica, J. Trauma 4:344–357, 1964.

73. Zadek, I.: Ossifying hematoma in the thigh, J. Bone Joint Surg. 51A:386–390, 1969.

74. Zwilling, E.: Morphogenetic phases in development, Dev. Biol. (Suppl.) 2:184–207, 1968.

This chapter will cover the essentials of the present knowledge of osteoporosis, osteomalacia and rickets, hyperparathyroid and hypoparathyroid bone disease, and Paget's disease of bone—the most common of systemic diseases of bone.

Osteoporosis

Definition

Osteoporosis may be defined as a decrease in the amount of bone below the level required to maintain skeletal integrity. The bone that remains is histologically normal. This clearly separates osteoporosis from osteomalacia, in which there is an excessive amount of unmineralized or poorly mineralized osteoid tissue.

Osteoporosis is a heterogeneous disorder that is associated with numerous diseases (Table 13-1). Several conditions superficially resemble primary osteoporosis and must be clearly differentiated from it because the prognosis and mode of therapy are different. Examples of such conditions are osteomalacia and rickets, hyperparathyroid bone disease, multiple myeloma, carcinomatosis, and osteogenesis imperfecta. A radiologic term, osteopenia, must not be regarded as synonymous with osteoporosis. Osteoporotic bones are osteopenic but so are hyperparathyroid and osteomalacic bones in some instances.

Morphology and histology

Both trabecular bone and cortical bone are decreased. Trabecular bone has the greatest area of resorbing surface[21,22] (endosteal surface) per unit of bone volume; thus, trabecular bone loss exceeds cortical bone loss. Therefore, bones with the most trabecular bone are more severely affected by osteoporosis. This accounts for the principal features of the disease—fractures of the vertebrae (90% trabecular bone), proximal femur (50% trabecular bone), and distal radius (30% trabecular bone). The branching or secondary trabeculae are lost, and the primary trabeculae appear more prominent. In the vertebrae,

RAJIV KUMAR AND
B. LAWRENCE RIGGS

13

pathologic bone physiology

trabecular bone loss may be so severe that only the upper and lower plates of the individual vertebrae are visible on roentgenologic examination of the spine. The intervertebral disks may be invaginated into the body of the vertebra. Cortical bone also is lost; this occurs almost exclusively on the endosteal surface. The haversian canals are normal or enlarged and also may be plugged in places. Inasmuch as similar changes are found with normal aging, some investigators have interpreted these findings as an indication that osteoporosis represents premature senescence.

Bone cell dynamics also are altered. There is increased resorptive surface,[21] attributed by some to increased osteoclastic activity. The resorptive surface decreases after the administration of estrogens to patients with primary osteoporosis;[75] this supports the concept of an absolute increase in bone resorption. Others, interpreting similar data, conclude that the defect is decreased osteoblastic activity and that the percentage of resorptive surface cannot be equated with activity of osteoclasts. This is similar to the view held by Albright and colleagues.[2] The fact remains that the disease could result from either an increase in osteoclastic activity with no concomitant increase in osteoblastic ac-

tivity or a failure in the formation of a normal number of osteoblasts. We believe that postmenopausal osteoporosis and senile osteoporosis are heterogeneous conditions. In some patients, the primary abnormality is increased resorption; in others, it is decreased formation; in yet others, both defects may occur. Although the mechanism is not understood, bone resorption and formation are coupled. Thus, estrogen replacement therapy prevents excessive bone resorption by decreasing the activity of osteoclasts, and thus will decrease the amount of bone lost but will not increase the amount of bone formed, since the number of new osteoblasts formed will be decreased.

Epidemiology and etiology

Osteoporosis is a common disease among elderly persons and is a major cause of morbidity and mortality. By roentgenologic examination of the spine, Iskrant and Smith[43] found that 56.7% of all women older than 45 yr of age had significantly decreased bone density. The proportion of patients having decreased bone density (grades 0 and 1) increased from 17.9% at ages 45 through 49 yr to 57.7% at ages 55 through 59 yr to 84.2% at ages 70 through 74 yr. The incidence of fractures as a result of trauma such as falls, was 4.6% in the group with decreased bone density (grades 0 and 1) compared with 2.5% in those without a decrease in bone density (grades 2 and 3). They noted that 70% of all fractures in women older than age 45 yr occurred in those with decreased bone density. Thus, extrapolating from a population sample of 2088 women, they estimated that at least 700,000 of the 1 million fractures that occur yearly in women do so in subjects with decreased bone mass. Other workers, such as Meema and colleagues,[58] Garn and colleagues,[30] and Goldsmith and Johnston,[34] confirmed the high incidence of decreased bone mass in women. Urist[92] estimated that 26% of women older than age 60 yr have sufficient osteoporosis to cause orthopedic problems.

Osteoporosis and its attendant complications are far more common in females than in males. Bruns noted in 1882[8] that the incidence of fractures of the femur was 1:2.5 (males:females)

TABLE 13-1 CAUSES OF GENERALIZED OSTEOPOROSIS

PRIMARY OSTEOPOROSIS
Postmenopausal and senile osteoporosis
Idiopathic osteoporosis of young adults
Acute juvenile osteoporosis
SECONDARY OSTEOPOROSIS
Hormonal
  Hypogonadism
  Cushing's syndrome
  Hyperthyroidism
  Hyperparathyroidism
Nutritional
  Severe malnutrition
  Scurvy
  Malabsorption
Diseases of connective tissue
  Osteogenesis imperfecta
  Ehlers-Danlos syndrome
  Homocystinuria
  Rheumatoid arthritis and related diseases
Diseases of bone marrow
  Multiple myeloma and related diseases
  Diffuse metastatic carcinoma
Paralysis and total immobilization

after the age of 50 yr. Iskrant,[42] using data from the National Health Survey, found that in women older than age 65 yr the rate for fractures of the proximal femur was about eight times that for men. In Caucasians and Blacks, the amount of bone present in fetal skeletons of females is less than that in fetal skeletons of males.[11,92] Blacks have higher bone densities than do Caucasians, and brown- and yellow-skinned people have intermediate bone densities.[34] Osteoporosis is uncommon in Blacks, as suggested by the low frequency of fractures in this population.[5,59] The bone mass of females is smaller than that of males, and women lose bone more rapidly,[34] especially after menopause.[34,57]

Effect of menopause on bone loss

Bone loss is accelerated after menopause.[22,57] This was initially deduced by Albright and colleagues[2] and has been amply documented since then by several workers.[1,13,57] Oophorectomy is followed by accelerated bone loss,[1] and the loss can be prevented by estrogen therapy. Estrogen therapy prevents bone loss in postmenopausal women[52,56,69] and may reduce the frequency of further fractures.[35,40] The role of estrogens in the case of the most common form of primary osteoporosis thus appears well established. It has been suggested that the reduction in bone resorption after estrogen therapy may be mediated by decreasing the sensitivity of bone resorbing cells to circulating endogenous parathyroid hormone.[27,39,46] The main unanswered question is why osteoporosis develops in some menopausal women but not in others. Some[35,40] but not all[78] workers have found that osteoporotic women have lower postmenopausal serum estrogen levels than do control subjects.

Gonadal steroids other than estrogens

Osteoporosis may develop in patients with Klinefelter's syndrome, and those individuals with an adrenal cortical 17-hydroxylase deficiency[54] may develop osteoporosis.

Physical activity

Persons habitually engaged in sustained muscular or weight-bearing physical activity (e.g., athletes) have a bone mass considerably greater than that of sedentary people.[12,18,62] A short-term increase in physical activity, however, has no effect on bone mass.[12] Immobilization causes hypercalciuria and results in osteoporosis if prolonged.[4,14,44]

Space flight will also result in bone loss because of prolonged weightlessness.[93] Nevertheless, it would be incorrect to infer that osteoporotic women are relatively sedentary compared with control subjects or that a lack of physical activity necessarily results in osteoporosis. Regular exercise, however, may modify or prevent involutional bone loss.

Calcium, parathyroid hormone, and vitamin D in primary osteoporosis

Results of studies of several animal models support the view that prolonged calcium deprivation may lead to osteoporosis.[47,79,80] Furthermore, patients with osteoporosis tend to have a lower calcium intake than do age-matched control subjects.[41,63,77] Recker and Heaney[70] have demonstrated a stabilization of bone mass in women administered 2.6 g of calcium carbonate daily at the time of and after menopause. The concept that there is a deficiency in calcium intake in osteoporosis has been challenged by others.[28,31,85]

Alterations in parathyroid hormone and vitamin D metabolism may play a role in the genesis of osteoporosis. In normal persons, the level of serum immunoreactive parathyroid hormone increases with age up to the tenth decade, whereas calcium absorption decreases.[27] The serum immunoreactive parathyroid hormone level also increases in postmenopausal osteoporotic women, but at any given age it is normal or lower than normal; at least it is not increased except in a subset of patients representing about 10 to 15% of the total.[27,72] A lack of estrogens sensitizes bone to the action of parathyroid hormone.[39,65,73]

Transient hypercalcemia might result, producing suppression of parathyroid hormone.

A decrease in circulating parathyroid hormone levels could cause a decrease in renal 25-hydroxyvitamin D 1α-hydroxylase activity and might explain the decreased intestinal calcium absorption noted in some osteoporotic patients.[86] With aging, a primary defect in 25-hydroxyvitamin D 1α-hydroxylase activity may be superimposed, further decreasing calcium absorption.

Serum 25-hydroxyvitamin D levels are normal in patients with osteoporosis.[24,25] Serum 1,25-dihydroxyvitamin D levels are reportedly low when compared with levels in age-matched controls,[24,25] though other workers have not confirmed this.[38] Treatment with estrogens increases the low levels of 1,25-dihydroxyvitamin D_3 toward normal.[26] This could be achieved in one of two ways. Estrogens are known to increase 1,25-dihydroxyvitamin D_3 levels, at least in birds,[48,88] and may do so in patients with osteoporosis either directly or by causing an increase in parathyroid hormone levels. Thus, the sequence of events shown in Figure 13-1 may occur in primary osteoporosis.

It should be emphasized that this is a tentative scheme and that the sequence of events has not been firmly established. Perhaps these events occur concurrently with the basic disease process, and no causal relationship exists. The role of estrogens in the etiology of osteoporosis is clear, and a strong case can be made for treating the disease with various estrogen preparations. Estrogen therapy in postmenopausal women, however, may be associated with an increased incidence of endometrial carcinoma.[95] The use of calcium supplementation in perimenopausal and postmenopausal women also has strong support.[56,69,74] The exact role or necessity of fluoride or the newer vitamin D preparations is unclear at the present time.

Osteomalacia and rickets

Definition

Osteomalacia is a disorder characterized by impaired mineralization of newly formed osteoid tissue. Consequently, the bones are soft and cannot bear mechanical stress adequately. The end results are bending and deformity of bone. Thus, fracture is less common than in osteoporosis in which the bones are more brittle. The bones may be less dense than is normal. Osteomalacia occurs in adults in whom bone growth at the epiphyseal plates has ceased.

Rickets is a disorder of childhood in which the basic defect is similar to that in osteomalacia. In addition, however, there is a defect in mineralization of the matrix of the epiphyseal plate. The bones are soft and deform easily.

Pathogenesis

In osteomalacia and rickets, there is a defect in the mineralization of bone matrix. The most important factor regulating this process is the product of ionic calcium and phosphate in serum, the assumption being that levels in the extracellular fluid surrounding bone cells are similar to those in the blood.[64] Blood is normally supersaturated with calcium and phosphate.[60] Calcification of bone matrix occurs as a result of crystallization. Rachitic blood is undersaturated with calcium and phosphorus.[61] *In vitro* studies[81,82] also demonstrate the importance of calcium and phosphorus in the mineralization of bone matrix.

ESTROGEN ──────▶ ↑SENSITIVITY OF ──────▶ ↑Ca ──▶ ↓PTH ──▶ ↓1. 25(OH)$_2$D$_3$ ──────▶ ↓CALCIUM
DEFICIENCY   BONE TO PTH OR OTHER   ABSORPTION
AT MENOPAUSE   BONE MOBILIZING AGENTS

Rx WITH ESTROGEN ──────▶ ↓Ca ──▶ ↑PTH ──▶ ↑1. 25(OH)$_2$D$_3$ ──▶ ↑Ca ABSORPTION

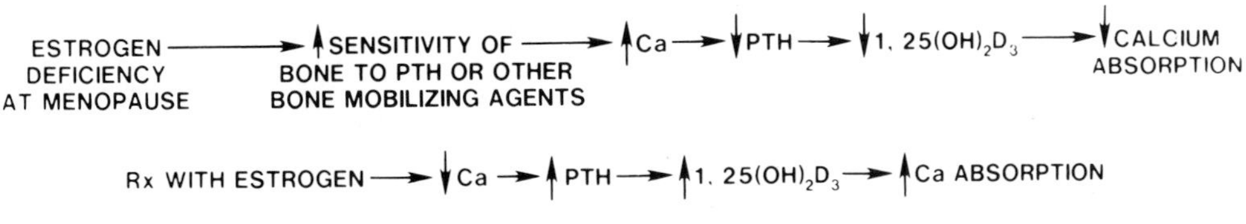

FIGURE 13-1 *Possible sequence of events in primary osteoporosis.*

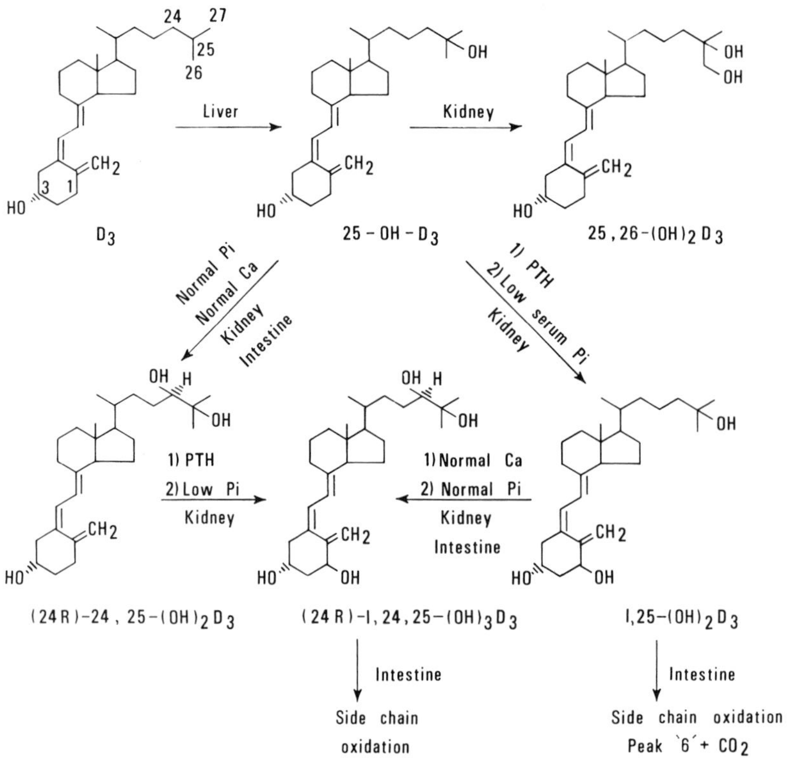

FIGURE 13-2 *Diagram of vitamin D metabolism.*

Vitamin D, through its active metabolite, 1,25-dihydroxyvitamin D, enhances the absorption of calcium and phosphate by the intestine[15,64] and plays an important role in the maintenance of the normal plasma levels of these ions. In osteomalacia, the serum calcium level decreases initially as a result of decreased intestinal absorption. Secondary hyperparathyroidism occurs, and the serum calcium level increases. The serum phosphorus level decreases because of increased renal excretion.

A brief schematic review of vitamin D metabolism is shown in Figure 13-2. Several excellent reviews[15,64] have appeared recently, and the readers are referred to them. At the present time, there is no evidence that vitamin D or its metabolites directly enhance calcification of bone other than by increasing the calcium-phosphorus product in blood.[64] Indeed 1,25-dihydroxyvitamin D_3 inhibits "osteoblast-like" cells and stimulates "osteoclast-like" cells *in vitro*.[94]

Clearly, osteomalacia can be caused by poor intake or absorption of vitamin D, inadequate formation from precursors, or qualitatively or quantitatively (or both) abnormal metabolism of the vitamin. Hypophosphatemia can also produce osteomalacia by decreasing the calcium-phosphorus product. The following is a convenient outline of the pathogenesis of osteomalacia:

1. Inadequate amounts of vitamin D in the diet or failure of formation from precursors in the skin (or both).
2. Malabsorption of vitamin D from the intestine.
3. Defects in the metabolism of vitamin D.
   a. Failure of formation of 25-hydroxyvitamin D, as in hepatic disorders.[19]
   b. Failure of formation of 1,25-dihydroxyvitamin D, as in renal disease.[7,37]
   c. Enhanced metabolism of vitamin D or its metabolites to other inactive compounds, as in long-term anticonvulsant therapy.[20]
   d. Certain forms of inherited vitamin D–resistant rickets (autosomal reces-

sive), type I, responsive to minute amounts of 1,25-dihydroxyvitamin D_3.[6]

  e. Type II vitamin D–resistant rickets,[32] end-organ unresponsiveness.
4. Renal tubular disorders resulting in hypophosphatemia as a consequence of a "phosphate leak," adult and childhood form, hypophosphatemic rickets (X-linked)—unresponsive to physiologic doses of 1,25-dihydroxyvitamin D_3.[51]
5. Hypophosphatemia associated with neoplasms.
6. Hypophosphatasia.
7. Acidosis—possibly as a result of decreased 1,25-dihydroxyvitamin D_3 synthesis or increased 1,25-dihydroxyvitamin D_3 metabolism.[51]
8. Calcium deficiency (rarely).

Histology and bone dynamics

The amount of uncalcified matrix and the number of osteoid seams are increased in osteomalacia and rickets. Bone cell activation is variable. Bone mineralization occurs at extremely slow rates. After tetracycline labeling (two doses administered 10 to 14 d apart), bone biopsy shows a greatly decreased rate of bone mineralization (e.g., 0.1 μm/d instead of approximately 1 μm/d as in normal bone). In rickets, there is inadequate mineralization of the epiphyseal plate, accompanied by disorganization in the arrangement of cartilage cells and widening or cupping of the epiphyseal plate.

Nutritional osteomalacia and rickets are no longer major health problems in this country, as milk is fortified with vitamin D. Nevertheless, osteomalacia and rickets caused by malabsorption, increased metabolism—as in anticonvulsant therapy, and renal disease still occur.

Hyperparathyroid bone disease

Increased secretion of parathyroid hormone results in generalized bone disease. Primary hyperparathyroidism (caused by a parathyroid adenoma or adenomas, carcinoma, or hyperplasia) and secondary hyperparathyroidism (occurring as a result of hypocalcemia resulting from any cause—e.g., osteomalacia, rickets, or chronic renal disease) both result in bone disease. In the former instance, the changes are those resulting from parathyroid hormone action alone, whereas in the latter, other features may be present in addition to those of hyperparathyroidism.

Currently, clinical bone disease caused by hyperparathyroidism is noted less frequently than in the past. The exact reason for this is unclear. Certainly, the earlier diagnosis of hyperparathyroidism as a result of chemical screening for hypercalcemia may account for part of the observed decrease. In these early cases, however, bone biopsy will reveal histologic changes compatible with hyperparathyroidism. The division of hyperparathyroid disease into two subtypes, one manifested primarily as bone disease and the other as renal stone disease, does not appear warranted.[16]

Demineralization of the skeleton, persistent negative calcium balance, subperiosteal resorption, "brown tumors," cysts, fractures, and deformaties develop in patients with hyperparathyroid bone disease. Bone pain, vague musculoskeletal pains, and bone tenderness are common complaints.[3]

The major effect of parathyroid hormone is to cause resorption of bone.[33,87] Osteoclast number and activity are increased. Osteoblast activity is decreased. The number of basic metabolic units activated is increased by parathyroid hormone. Osteoclast and osteoblast pools are increased in size. The sum total of effects of parathyroid hormone will depend on the relative rates of osteoblastic and osteoclastic activity. In general, osteoclastic activity predominates and most hyperparathyroid patients have a persistently negative calcium balance. In many patients, the bone marrow becomes fibrotic.

When studied by the technique of isolated bone cell culture in which two separate bone cell populations exist, parathyroid hormone increases the activity of "osteoclast-like" cells, as evidenced by the increase in acid phosphatase activity and by the increase in hyaluronate synthesis.[53] It decreases the activity of "osteoblast-like" cells in this system. Citrate decarboxylation, prolyl hydroxylase activity, and alkaline phosphatase activity are all decreased. The effects of parathyroid hormone are probably mediated by cyclic-AMP and by changes in the intracellular calcium concentration. Interestingly, 1,25-dihydroxyvitamin D has actions similar to those of parathyroid hormone in this cell culture system.[94] *In vivo*, parathyroid hormone increases renal 25-hydroxyvitamin D 1α-hydroxylase activity and increases circulating levels of 1,25-dihydroxyvitamin D. Thus, the bone resorption in hyperparathyroidism is apparently caused by the action of parathyroid hormone as well as 1,25-dihydroxyvitamin D.

In hyperparathyroidism, bones of the axial skeleton as well as of the appendicular skeleton are involved, hence the name osteitis fibrosa generalisata.[3] The skull, tubular long bones, jaws, and vertebrae are all affected. Cortical bone exhibits thinning and areas of fibrosis and replacement by connective tissue are seen. "Brown tumors" and cysts may be noted. "Brown tumors" are areas of connective tissue containing multinucleate giant cells (probably osteoclasts) into which hemorrhage may have occurred at an earlier time. Degenerated blood pigments impart the brown color to the "tumors." Cysts are cavities lined by fibrous tissue and filled with a proteinaceous fluid. Characteristically, thinning of the periosteum and areas of subperiosteal resorption are evident. The vertebrae exhibit a loss of density, thinning of the trabeculae, and weakening of the end-plates, and the intervertebral disks are expanded. In extreme cases, collapse of the vertebral bodies may occur. Gross spinal deformities such as kyphosis and scoliosis occur in some patients. Thoracic cage abnormalities may be noted. A loss of height occurs. In the skull, demineralization results in a loss of the sharp distinction between the diploe and the inner and outer tables. In the jaw area, "brown tumors" and cysts may occur; the lamina dura of the teeth is lost.

Histologically, there is an increase in the number of osteoclasts. Invasion of the haversian canal walls is noted. Trabeculae are thinned because of an increase in osteoclastic activity.[7] Fibrosis occurs in areas of increased osteoclastic ac-

tivity. The osteoblast number may be increased, but activity is decreased. "Brown tumors" are filled with connective tissue stroma and contain multinucleated giant cells. Cysts are lined with fibrous tissue.

Bone microradiography reveals an increase in the extent of bone-resorbing surfaces. The level of serum calcium is correlated with the extent of the bone-resorbing surfaces.[76]

In secondary hyperparathyroidism, transient hypocalcemia is usually the stimulus to increased parathyroid hormone secretion. The increase in the plasma parathyroid hormone level causes increased mobilization of calcium from bone and a return of serum calcium concentration toward normal. The most frequently encountered form of secondary hyperparathyroidism is that associated with chronic renal failure. Hyperphosphatemia occurs as a result of decreasing renal function. The plasma-ionized calcium level decreases transiently. This is sensed by the parathyroid glands, which increase the secretion of parathyroid hormone. This increase in plasma parathyroid hormone levels causes mobilization of bone calcium and a return of the plasma calcium level toward normal. The increased serum phosphorus level returns to normal as a result of increased renal excretion of phosphorus. To maintain this new steady state, parathyroid hormone levels remain increased. As renal function continues to deteriorate, sequential increases in serum phosphate level are offset by increases in plasma parathyroid hormone levels.[84]

In addition to the abnormalities in parathyroid hormone function, there are changes in the metabolism of vitamin D. 1,25-Dihydroxyvitamin D increases calcium transport in the intestine (see previous section on osteomalacia and rickets). The sole site for the synthesis of this metabolite of vitamin D is the kidney. Deteriorating renal function is associated with decreases in plasma 1,25-dihydroxyvitamin D, which, in turn, result in depressed calcium absorption from the intestine. This increases the tendency to hypocalcemia, and parathyroid hormone levels increase further. The changes in hyperparathyroid bone disease secondary to renal failure are similar in many respects to those of primary hyperparathyroidism; however, the lesions of osteomalacia may also occur. In a small proportion of patients, there may be osteosclerosis of the axial skeleton. The reason for this is unclear.

Secondary hyperparathyroidism occurs in osteomalacia and rickets. Depressed calcium absorption from the kidney as a result of vitamin D deficiency results in hypocalcemia. Parathyroid hormone secretion is stimulated, and the serum calcium concentration returns toward normal. As the kidneys are normal, phosphaturia ensues and the serum phosphorus level decreases. Thus, even when the primary lesion is that of osteomalacia or rickets some changes consistent with hyperparathyroid bone disease may be seen.

Hypoparathyroidism

True hypoparathyroidism is characterized by a low serum calcium concentration, a high serum phosphorus level, and a low level of serum parathyroid hormone. Administration of parathyroid hormone to patients with hypoparathyroidism increases the amount of phosphate and cyclic-AMP excreted in the urine[9] and increases the serum calcium concentration. The serum phosphorus level decreases. Hypoparathyroidism occurs as an isolated idiopathic disorder or in association with multiple endocrine gland deficiencies and pernicious anemia. Thymic aplasia, hypoparathyroidism, and cellular immune deficiency occur as part of the DiGeorge syndrome. Hypoparathyroidism can occur as a complication of thyroidectomy and in rare instances after the administration of radioiodine.

Patients with pseudohypoparathyroidism have the same abnormalities of serum calcium and phosphorus as patients with classic hypoparathyroidism but have increased levels of serum parathyroid hormone. They have end-organ insensitivity to parathyroid hormone.[3] Administration of parathyroid hormone fails to correct the hypocalcemia of this condition and does not increase the amount of phosphorus or cyclic-AMP excreted in the urine.[10] Insensitivity

to parathyroid hormone may be limited to the kidney. Several patients with lesions of hyperparathyroid bone disease have been noted. A further subset of patients with pseudohypoparathyroidism may have normal receptors for parathyroid hormone in the kidney and may generate cyclic-AMP normally in response to an infusion of parathyroid hormone. However, they do not have phosphaturia, and their serum calcium levels remain uncorrected. Patients with pseudohypoparathyroidism have characteristic skeletal abnormalities that include short stature, brachydactyly, and shortening of the fourth and fifth metacarpals. Some patients in these families may have the skeletal defects but not the biochemical abnormalities of the syndrome. Rarely, the converse may be true.

Patients with hypoparathyroidism have low levels of plasma 1,25-dihydroxyvitamin D. Treatment with 1,25-dihydroxyvitamin D is effective in this condition.[49]

Bone mineralization in hypoparathyroidism is normal. Because bone resorption is depressed more than bone formation, the skeleton may be denser than normal. Patients with pseudohypoparathyroidism have brachydactyly as a result of early epiphyseal closure around the elbow. Patients with hypoparathyroidism may have abnormal dentition with hypoplastic, mottled, and irregular teeth.

Treatment is directed at normalizing the serum calcium level. This can be achieved by the administration of vitamin D or its analogues and supplemental calcium.

Paget's disease of bone (osteitis deformans)

Although the cause of Paget's disease is unknown, there is some evidence that it may result from a slow virus infection of bone.[50,66,83] Paget's disease of bone is common (in the United States the incidence is approximately 3%) and usually occurs in persons older than age 40 yr. Monostotic and polyostotic forms of the disease occur. A single focus of involvement may be followed many years later by involvement of another bone. The axial skeleton, skull, pelvis, and long bones of the lower extremities are commonly affected. Involvement of small bones is uncommon. The disease is characterized by a high rate of bone turnover. Osteoclastic activity and osteoblastic activity are increased. There is increased activation of bone cell precursors. The initial phase is generally of increased osteolytic activity—the osteoporotic phase of the disease. This is followed by increased osteoblastic activity. Bone is laid down in an irregular manner, and prominent cement lines are observed between adjacent areas of bone deposition; this creates a mosaic pattern.[45] In the osteoporotic forms of the disease, calcium balance is usually negative. In the osteoblastic phase, calcium balance may become positive as increased amounts of bone are laid down.

Microscopically, there are increased numbers of osteoclasts with prominent nuclei. Resorbed bone is replaced by vascular connective tissue. This is readily apparent in the skull, in which affected areas are visible as purplish patches that are darker than the adjacent unaffected bone. This is because the inner and outer tables are lost, and the dark vascular connective tissue is visible through the thinned bone. Skull roentgenograms reveal radiolucent areas. Later in the disease, there is increased osteoblastic activity during which new bone is laid down in an irregular manner. Finally, osteosclerotic changes may occur. Sarcoma of the affected bone is a frequent complication of the disease.[45] The bloodflow through the involved extremity or bone is increased. Unequivocal demonstration of arteriovenous shunts, however, is not forthcoming.[71] A high-output cardiac state and even congestive heart failure may occur.

Patients with Paget's disease of bone have normal serum calcium and phosphorus levels. During immobilization (as occurs after a fracture), hypercalciuria and hypercalcemia may ensue. Nephrocalcinosis and renal failure are known to result from hypercalcemia occurring during immobilization. Hydroxyproline and hydroxylysine are formed as a result of increased breakdown. As these products are not recycled, they appear in the urine of patients with active disease. An increased level of serum alkaline phosphatase is a marker of increased osteoblastic activity and correlates well with the activity of the disease.

Usually, only symptomatic patients or those with extensive active disease require treatment. About 70% of patients will have a satisfactory response to calcitonin or diphosphonate therapy. Because of its potential toxic effect on the bone marrow, mithramycin, although effective, is rarely indicated.

References

1. Aitken, J. M., Hart, D. M., and Lindsay, R.: Oestrogen replacement therapy for prevention of osteoporosis after oophorectomy, Br. Med. J. 3:515, 1973.
2. Albright, F., Bloomberg, E., and Smith, P. H.: Post-menopausal osteoporosis, Trans. Assoc. Am. Phys. 55:298, 1940.
3. Albright, F., and Reifenstein, E. C.: The parathyroid glands and metabolic bone disease, Selected Studies, Baltimore, Williams & Wilkins Co., 1948.
4. Birge, S. J., and Whedon, G. D.: Bone *In* McNally, M. (ed.): Hypodynamics and Hypogravics, New York, Academic Press, 1968.
5. Bollet, A. J., Engh, G., Parson, W.: Epidemiology of osteoporosis, Arch. Intern. Med. 116:191, 1965.
6. Brooks, M. H., Bell, N. H., Love, L., Stern, P. H., Orfei, E., Queener, S. F., Hamstra, A. J., and DeLuca, H. F.: Vitamin D–dependent rickets type II: resistance of target organs to 1,25-dihydroxyvitamin D, N. Engl. J. Med. 298:996, 1978.
7. Brumbaugh, P. F., Haussler, D. H., Bressler, R., and Haussler, M. R.: Radioreceptor assay for 1,25-dihydroxyvitamin D_3, Science 183:1089, 1974.
8. Bruns, P.: Die Allgemeine lehre von den Knochenbruchen Dtsch. Chir., Vol. 27 Pt. I, Stuttgart, 1882.
9. Chase, L. R., and Aurbach, G. D.: Parathyroid function and the renal excretion of 3'-5'-adenylic acid, Proc. Natl. Acad. Sci. 58:518, 1967.
10. Chase, L. R., Melson, G. L., and Aurbach, G. D.: Pseudohypoparathyroidism: defective exrection of 3',5'-AMP in response to parathyroid hormone, J. Clin. Invest. 48:1832, 1969.
11. Choi, S. C., and Trotter, M.: A statistical study of the multivariate structure and race-sex differ-

ences of American White and Negro fetal skeletons, Am. J. Phys. Anthrop. 3:307, 1970.

12. Dalen, N., and Olsson, K. E.: Bone mineral content and physical activity, Acta Orthop. Scand. 45:170, 1974.

13. Davis, M. E., Strandjord, N. M., and Lanzl, L. H.: Estrogens and the aging process. The detection, prevention, and retardation of osteoporosis, J. Am. Med. Assoc. 196:219, 1966.

14. Deitrick, J. E.: The effect on immobilization on metabolic and physiological functions of normal men, Bull., N.Y. Acad. Med. 24:364, 1948.

15. DeLuca, H. F., and Schnoes, H. K.: Metabolism and mechanism of action of vitamin D, Annual Rev. Biochem. 45:631, 1976.

16. Dent, C. E.: Some problems of hyperparathyroidism, Br. Med. J. 2:1495, 1962.

17. Drezner, M., Neelson, F., and Lebivitz, H. E.: Pseudohypoparathyroidism type II: A possible defect in the reception of the cyclic AMP signal, N. Engl. J. Med. 289:1056, 1973.

18. Eisenberg, E., and Gordan, G. S.: Skeletal dynamics in man measured by nonradioactive strontium, J. Clin. Invest. 40:1809, 1961.

19. Eisman, J. A., Hamstra, A. J., Kream, B. E., and DeLuca, H. F.: A sensitive, precise and convenient method for determination of 1,25-dihydroxyvitamin D in human plasma, Arch. Biochem. Biophys. 176:235, 1976.

20. Fraser, D., Kooh, S. W., Kind, H. P., Holic, M. F., Tanaka, Y., and DeLuca, H. F.: Pathogenesis of hereditary vitamin D–dependent rickets: an inborn error of vitamin D metabolism involving defective conversion of 25-hydroxyvitamin D to 1,25-dihydroxyvitamin D, N. Engl. J. Med. 289:817, 1973.

21. Frost, H. M.: Bone dynamics in metabolic bone disease, J. Bone Joint Surg. 48A:1192, 1966.

22. Frost, H. M.: The bone dynamics in osteoporosis and osteomalacia, Springfield, Charles C Thomas, 1966.

23. Gallagher, J. D., Aaron, J., Horsman, A., Marshall, D. H., Wilkinson, R., and Nordin, B. E. C.: The crush fracture syndrome in postmenopausal women, J. Clin. Endocrinol. Metab. 2:293, 1973.

24. Gallagher, J. C., Riggs, B. L., Eisman, J. A., Arnaud, S. B., and DeLuca, H. F.: Impaired production of 1,25-dihydroxyvitamin D in postmenopausal osteoporosis, Clin. Res. 24:580A, 1976.

25. Gallagher, J. C., Riggs, B. L., Eisman, J. A., Hamstra, A., Arnaud, S. B., and DeLuca, H. F.:

Intestinal calcium absorption and serum vitamin D metabolites in normal subjects and osteoporotic patients. Effect of age and dietary calcium, J. Clin. Invest. 64:729–736, 1979.

26. Gallagher, J. C., Riggs, B. L., Hamstra, A., and DeLuca, H. F.: Effect of estrogen therapy on calcium absorption and vitamin D in post-menopausal osteoporosis, Clin. Res. 26:415A, 1978.

27. Gallagher, J. C., Riggs, B. L., Jerpbak, C. M., and Arnaud, C. D.: Aging and immunoreactive parathyroid hormone in normal and osteoporotic subjects, Clin. Res. 25:623A, 1977.

28. Garn, S. M.: Calcium requirements for bone building and skeletal maintenance, Am. J. Clin. Nutr. 23:1149, 1970.

29. Garn, S. M., Nagy, J. M., and Sandusky, S. T.: Differential sexual demorphism in bone diameters of subjects of European and African ancestry, Am. J. Phys. Anthrop. 37:127, 1972.

30. Garn, S. M., Poznanski, A. K., and Nagy, J. M.: Bone measurement in the differential diagnosis of osteopenia and osteoporosis, Radiology 100:509, 1971.

31. Garn, S. M., Rohmann, C. G., and Wagner, B.: Bone loss as a general phenomenon in man, Fed. Proc. 26:1729, 1967.

32. Glorieux, F. H., Holick, M. F., Scriver, C. R., and DeLuca, H. F.: X-linked hypophosphataemic rickets: Inadequate therapeutic response to 1,25-dihydroxycholecalciferol, Lancet 2:287, 1973.

33. Goldhaber, P.: *In* Gaillard, P., Talmage, R. V., and Bundy, A. (eds.): The Parathyroid Glands, p. 153, University of Chicago Press, 1965.

34. Goldsmith, N. F., and Johnston, J. O.: Mineralization of the bone in an insured population: correlation with reported fractures and other measures of osteoporosis, Int. J. Epidemiol. 2:311, 1973.

35. Gordan, G. S., Picch, J., and Roof, B. S.: Antifracture efficacy of long term estrogens for osteoporosis, Trans. Assoc. Am. Phys. 86:326, 1973.

36. Gordan, G. S., and Vaughan, C.: *In* Clinical Management of the Osteoporoses, Publishing Science Group, Acton, Massachusetts, 1976.

37. Hahn, T. J., Hendin, B. A., Scharp, C. R., and Haddad, J. G.: Effect of chronic anticonvulsant therapy on serum 25-hydroxycalciferol levels in adults, N. Engl. J. Med. 287:900, 1972.

38. Haussler, M. R.: Unpublished observations.

39. Heaney, R. P.: A unified concept of osteoporosis, Am. J. Med. 39:877, 1965.

40. Henneman, P. H., and Wallach, S.: A review of the prolonged use of estrogens and androgens in postmenopausal and senile osteoporosis, Arch. Intern. Med. 100:715, 1957.

41. Hurxthal, L. M., and Vose, G. P.: The relationship of dietary calcium intake to radiographic bone density in normal and osteoporotic persons, Calcif. Tissue Res. 4:245, 1969.

42. Iskrant, A. P.: The etiology of fractured hips in females, Am. J. Publ. Health 58:485, 1968.

43. Iskrant, A. P., and Smith, R. W.: Osteoporosis in women 45 years and over related to subsequent fractures, Publ. Heath Report 84:33, 1969.

44. Issekutz, B., Blizzard, J. J., Birkhead, N. C., and Rodahl, K.: Effect or prolonged bed rest on urinary calcium output, J. Appl. Physiol. 21:1013, 1966.

45. Jaffe, H. L.: Metabolic, degenerative, and inflammatory diseases of bones and joints, Philadelphia, Lea & Febiger, 1972.

46. Jasani, C., Nordin, B. E. C., Smith, D. A., and Swanson, I.: Spinal osteoporosis and the menopause, Proc. R. Soc. Med. 58:441, 1965.

47. Jowsey, J., and Gershon-Cohen, J.: Effect of dietary calcium levels on production and reversal of experimental osteoporosis in cats, Proc. Soc. Exp. Biol. Med. 116:437, 1964.

48. Kenny, A. D.: Vitamin D metabolism: Physiological regulation in egg-laying Japanese quail, Am. J. Physiol. 230:1609, 1976.

49. Kooh, S. W., Fraser, D., DeLuca, H. F., Holick, M. F., Belsey, R. E., Clark, M. B., and Murray, T. M.: Treatment of hypoparathyroidism and pseudohypoparathyroidism with metabolites of vitamin D: Evidence for impaired conversion of 25-hydroxyvitamin D to 1,25-dihydroxyvitamin D, N. Engl. J. Med. 293:840, 1975.

50. Krane, S. M.: Paget's disease of bone, *In* Thorn, G. W., et al (eds.): Harrison's Principles of Internal Medicine, New York, McGraw Hill Book Co., 1977.

51. Lee, S. W., Russel, J., and Avioli, L. V.: 25-Hydroxycholecalciferol to 1,25-dihydroxy-cholecalciferol: conversion impaired by systemic metabolic acidosis, Science 195:994, 1977.

52. Lindsay, R., Aitken, J. M., Anderson, J. B., Hart, D. M., MacDonald, E. B., and Clarke, A. C.: Long-term prevention of postmenopausal osteoporosis by oestrogen, Lancet 1:1038, 1976.

53. Luben, R. A., Wong, G. L., and Cohn, D. V.: Biochemical characterization with parathormone and calcitonin of isolated bone cells: provisional identification of osteoclasts and osteoblasts, Endocrinology 99:526, 1976.

54. Mallin, S. R.: Congenital adrenal hyperplasia secondary to 17 hydroxylase deficiency, Ann. Intern. Med. 70:69, 1969.

55. Marshall, D. H., Crilly, R. G., and Nordin, B. E. C.: Plasma androstenedione and oestrone levels in normal and osteoporotic postmenopausal women, Br. Med. J. 2:1177, 1977.

56. Marshall, D. H., and Nordin, B. E. C.: The prevention and management of postmenopausal osteoporosis, Acta Obstet. Gynecol. Scand. (Suppl.) 65:49, 1977.

57. Meema, H. E., Bunker, M. L., and Meema, S.: Loss of compact bone due to menopause, Am. J. Obstet. Gynecol. 26:333, 1965.

58. Meema, S., Reid, D. B. W., and Meema, H. E.: Age trends of bone mineral mass, muscle width, and subcutaneous fat in normals and osteoporotics, Calcif. Tissue Res. 12:101, 1973.

59. Moldawer, M., Zimmerman, S. J., and Collins, L. C.: Incidence of osteoporosis in elderly whites and elderly negroes, J. Am. Med. Assoc. 194:859, 1965.

60. Neuman, W. F.: On the role of vitamin D in calcification, Am. Med. Assoc. Arch. Pathol. 66:204, 1958.

61. Neuman, W. F., and Neuman, M. W.: The Chemical Dynamics of Bone Mineral, Chicago, University of Chicago Press, 1958.

62. Nilsson, B. E., and Westlin, N. E.: Bone density in athletes, Clin. Orthop. 77:179, 1971.

63. Nordin, B. E. C.: Osteomalacia, osteoporosis and calcium deficiency, Clin. Orthop. 17:235, 1960.

64. Omdahl, J. L., and DeLuca, H. F.: Regulation of vitamin D metabolism and function, Physiol. Rev. 53:327, 1973.

65. Orimo, H., Fujita, T., and Yoshikawa, M.: Increased sensitivity of bone to parathyroid hormone in ovariectomized rats, Endocrinology 90:760, 1972.

66. Paget, J.: On a form of chronic inflammation of bones (osteitis deformans). Medico-Chirurgical Trans. 60:37, 1877.

67. Rasmussen, H.P and Bordier, P.: The cellular basis of metabolic bone disease, N. Engl. J. Med. 289:25, 1973.

68. Rasmussen, H., and Bordier, P.: The Physiological and Cellular Basis of Metabolic Bone Disease, Baltimore, Williams & Wilkins Co., 1974.

69. Recker, R. R., Hassing, G. S., Lau, J. R., and Saville, P. D.: The hyperphosphatemic effect of disodium ethane-1-hydroxy-1, 1-diphosphonate (EHDP): renal handling of phosphorus and the renal response to parathyroid hormone, J. Lab. Clin. Med. 81:258, 1973.

70. Recker, R. R., Saville, P. D., and Heaney, R. P.:

Transcript of Proceedings of Endocrinology and Metabolism Advisory Committee, US FDA Bureau of Drugs, pp. 70–87, Feb. 18, 1977.

71. Rhodes, B. A., Greyson, N. D., Hamilton, C. R., Jr., White, R. I., Jr., Giargiana, F. A., Jr., and Wagner, H. M., Jr.: Absence of anatomic arteriovenous shunts in Paget's disease of bone, N. Engl. J. Med. 287:686, 1972.

72. Riggs, B. L., Arnaud, C. D., Jowsey, J., Goldsmith, R. S., and Kelly, P. J.: Parathyroid function in primary osteoporosis, J. Clin. Invest. 54:181, 1973.

73. Riggs, B. L., Jowsey, J., Goldsmith, R. S., Kelly, P. J., Hoffman, D. L., and Arnaud, C. D.: Short- and long-term effects of estrogen and synthetic anabolic hormone in postmenopausal osteoporosis, J. Clin, Invest. 51:1659, 1972.

74. Riggs, B. L., Jowsey, J., Kelly, P. J., Hoffman, D. L., and Arnaud, C. D.: Effects of oral therapy with calcium and vitamin D in primary osteoporosis, J. Clin. Endocrinol. Metab. 43:1139, 1976.

75. Riggs, B. L., Jowsey, J., Kelly, P. J., Jones, J. D., and Maher, F. T.: Effect of sex hormones on bone in primary osteoporosis, J. Clin. Invest. 48:1065, 1969.

76. Riggs, B. L., Kelly, P. J., Jowsey, J., and Keating, F. R.: Skeletal alterations in hyperparathyroidism, determination of bone formation, resorption and morphologic changes by microradiography, J. Clin. Endocrinol. 25:777, 1965.

77. Riggs, B. L., Kelly, P. J., Kinney, V. R., Scholz, D. A., and Bianco, A. J.: Calcium deficiency and osteoporosis. Observations in one hundred and sixty-six patients and a critical review of the literature, J. Bone Joint Surg. 49A:915, 1967.

78. Riggs, B. L., Ryan, R. J., Wahner, H. W., Jiang, N.-S., and Mattox, V. R.: Serum concentrations of estrogen, testosterone and gonadotropins in osteoporotic and nonosteoporotic postmenopausal women, J. Clin. Endocrinol. Metab. 36:1097, 1973.

79. Saville, P. D., and Krook, L.: Gravimetric and isotopic studies in nutritional hyperparathyroidism in beagles, In Proceedings of the Sixth Symposium on Calcif. Tiss. Res. (Suppl. 2):24, 1968.

80. Shah, B. G., Krishnarau, G. V., and Draper, H. H.: The relationship of calcium and potassium nutrition during adult life and osteoporosis in aged mice, J. Nutr. 92:30, 1967.

81. Shipley, P. G., Kramer, B., and Howland, J.: Calcification of rachitic bones in vitro, Am. J. Dis. Child. 30:37, 1925.

82. Shipley, P. G., Kramer, B., and Howland, J.: Studies upon calcification in vitro, Biochem. J. 20:379, 1926.

83. Singer, F. R.: Paget's Disease of Bone, New York, Plenum Medical Book Co., 1977.

84. Slatopolsky, E., Caglar, S., Pennell, J. P., Taggart, D. D., Canterbury, J. M., Reiss, E., and Bricker, N. S.: On the pathogenesis of hyperparathyroidism in chronic experimental renal insufficiency in the dog, J. Clin. Invest. 50:492, 1971.

85. Smith, R. W., and Frame, B.: Concurrent axial and appendicular osteoporoosis, N. Engl. J. Med. 273:73, 1965.

86. Szymendera, J., Heaney, R. P., and Saville, P. D.: Intestinal calcium absorption: concurrent use of oral and intravenous tracers and calculation by the inverse convolution method, J. Lab. Clin. Med. 79:570, 1972.

87. Talmage, R. V., Kraintz, F. W., Frost, R. C., and Kraintz, L.: Evidence for a dual action of parathyroid extract in maintaining serum calcium and phosphate levels, Endocrinology 52:318, 1953.

88. Tanaka, Y., Castillo, L., and DeLuca, H. F.: Control of renal vitamin D hydroxylases in birds by sex hormones, Proc. Natl. Acad. Sci. 73:2701, 1976.

89. Trotter, M., Broman, G., and Peterson, R. R.: Densities of bones of White and Negro skeletons, J. Bone Joint Surg. 42A:50, 1960.

90. Trotter, M., and Hixon, B. B.: Sequential changes in weight, density, and percentage ash weight of human skeletons from an early fetal period through old age, Anat. Rec. 179:1, 1974.

91. Turnbull, H. M.: Pathogenesis of generalized osteitis fibrosa, Br. J. Surg. 19:254, 1931.

92. Urist, J. R.: Observations bearing on the problem of osteoporosis. In Nicholsen, J., (ed): Bone as a Tissue, New York, McGraw Hill Book Co., 1960.

93. Whedon, G. D., Lutwak, L., Reid, J., Rambaut, P., Whittle, M., Smith, M., and Leach, C.; Mineral and nitrogen metabolic studies on skylab orbital space flights, Trans. Assoc. Am. Phys. 87:95, 1974.

94. Wong, G. L., Luben, R. A., and Cohn, D. V.: 1,25-dihydroxycholecalciferol and parathormone: Effects on isolated osteoclast like and osteoblast like cells, Science 197:663, 1977.

95. Zieland, H. K., and Finkle, W. D.: Increased risk of endometrial carcinoma among users of conjugated estrogens, N. Engl. J. Med. 293:1167, 1975.

Numerals followed by an *f* indicate a figure; *t* following a page number indicates tabular material